Sixth Edition

Medical Terminology

A Living Language

Sixth Edition

Medical Terminology

A Living Language

Bonnie F. Fremgen, PhD

Suzanne S. Frucht, PhD
Associate Professor Emeritus
Northwest Missouri State University
Maryville, MO

PEARSON

Boston Columbus Indianapolis New York San Francisco Hoboken Amsterdam Cape Town
Dubai London Madrid Milan Munich Paris Montreal Toronto Delhi Mexico City Sao Paulo
Sydney Hong Kong Seoul Singapore Taipei Tokyo

Publisher: Julie Levin Alexander
Publisher's Assistant: Sarah Henrich
Executive Editor: John Goucher
Editorial Project Manager: Nicole Ragonese
Editorial Assistant: Amanda Losonsky
Development Editor: Danielle Doller
Director of Marketing: David Gesell
Marketing Manager: Brittany Hammond
Marketing Specialist: Michael Sirinides
Project Management Lead: Cynthia Zonneveld
Project Manager: Patricia Gutierrez
Operations Specialist: MaryAnn Gloriande
Art Director: Andrea Nix
Text Designer: Ilze Lemesis
Cover Designer: Maria Guglielmo Walsh
Cover Art: Palau/Shutterstock
Media Director: Amy Peltier
Lead Media Project Manager: Lorena Cerisano
Full-Service Project Management: Patty Donovan, Laserwords
Composition: Laserwords Pvt. Ltd
Printer/Binder: LSC Communications
Cover Printer: LSC Communications
Text Font: Meridien Com 11/13

Dedication

To my husband for his love and encouragement.

Bonnie Fremgen

To Rick, Kristin, and Chris for their love, support, and friendship. And especially to the newest member of our family, Adrienne.

Suzanne Frucht

To Danielle Doller, whose incredible editing skills (and friendship) have made each edition of this text better.

We would like to extend a special thank you to Garnet Tomich who went above and beyond to help make this edition shine.

Credits and acknowledgments for content borrowed from other sources and reproduced, with permission, in this textbook appear on appropriate page within text.

Library of Congress Cataloging-in-Publication Data

Fremgen, Bonnie F., author.
Medical terminology : a living language / Bonnie F. Fremgen, Suzanne S. Frucht. — Sixth edition.
p. ; cm.
Includes bibliographical references and index.
ISBN 978-0-13-407025-4 — ISBN 0-13-407025-9
I. Frucht, Suzanne S., author. II. Title.
[DNLM: 1. Medicine—Terminology—English. W 15]
R123
610.1'4—dc23
2015001788

5 17

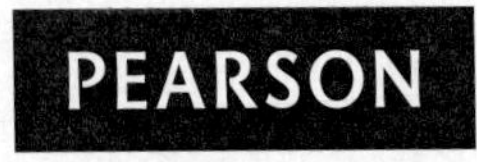

ISBN-10: 0-13-407025-9
ISBN-13: 978-0-13-407025-4

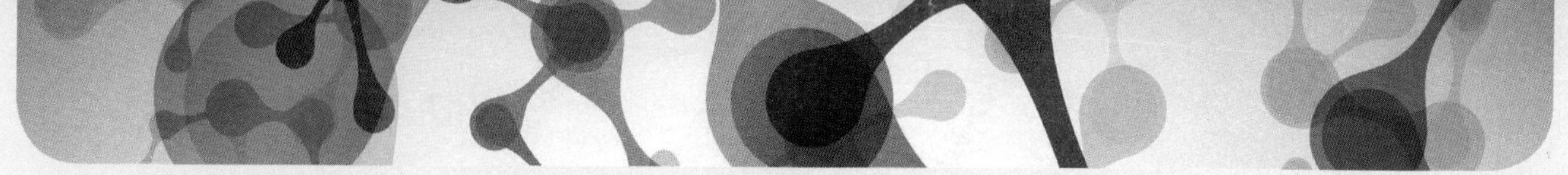

Welcome!

Welcome to the fascinating study of medical language—a vital part of your preparation for a career as a health professional. We are glad that you have joined us. Throughout your career, in a variety of settings, you will use medical terminology to communicate with coworkers and patients. Employing a carefully constructed learning system, ***Medical Terminology: A Living Language*** has helped thousands of readers gain a successful grasp of medical language within a real-world context.

In developing this book we had seven goals in mind:

1. To provide a clear introduction to the basic rules of using word parts to form medical terms.
2. To use phonetic pronunciations that will help you easily pronounce terms by spelling out the word part according to the way it sounds.
3. To help you understand medical terminology within the context of the human body systems. Realizing that this book is designed for a terminology course and not an anatomy and physiology course, we have aimed to stick to only the basics.
4. To help you develop a full range of Latin and Greek word parts used to build medical terms so that you will be able to interpret unfamiliar terms you encounter in the future.
5. To help you visualize medical language with an abundance of real-life photographs and accurate illustrations.
6. To provide you with a wealth of practice applications at the end of each chapter to help you review and master the content as you go along.
7. To create rich multimedia practice opportunities for you by way of MyMedicalTerminologyLab.

Sixth Edition
Medical Terminology
A Living Language
Bonnie F. Fremgen Suzanne S. Frucht

Please turn the page to get a visual glimpse of what makes this book an ideal guide to your exploration of medical terminology.

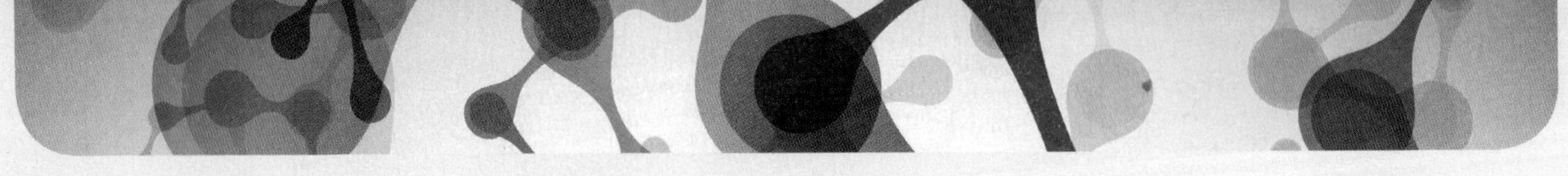

A Guide to What Makes This Book Special

Streamlined Content

Fourteen chapters and only the most essential anatomy and physiology coverage make this book a perfect midsized fit for a one-term course.

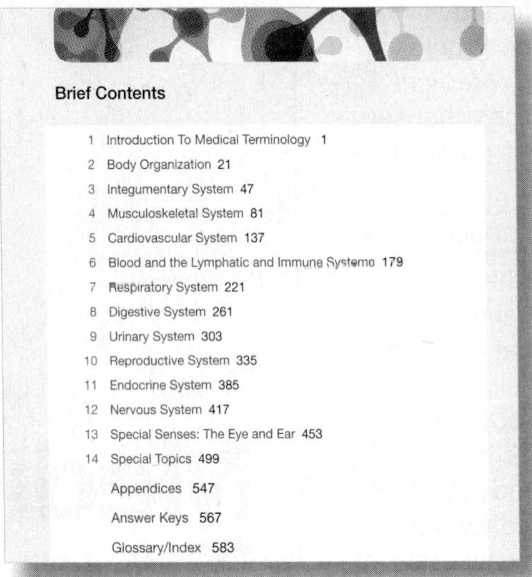

Brief Contents

Chapter-Opening Page Spreads

"At a Glance" and "Illustrated" pages begin each chapter, providing a quick, visual snapshot of what's covered.

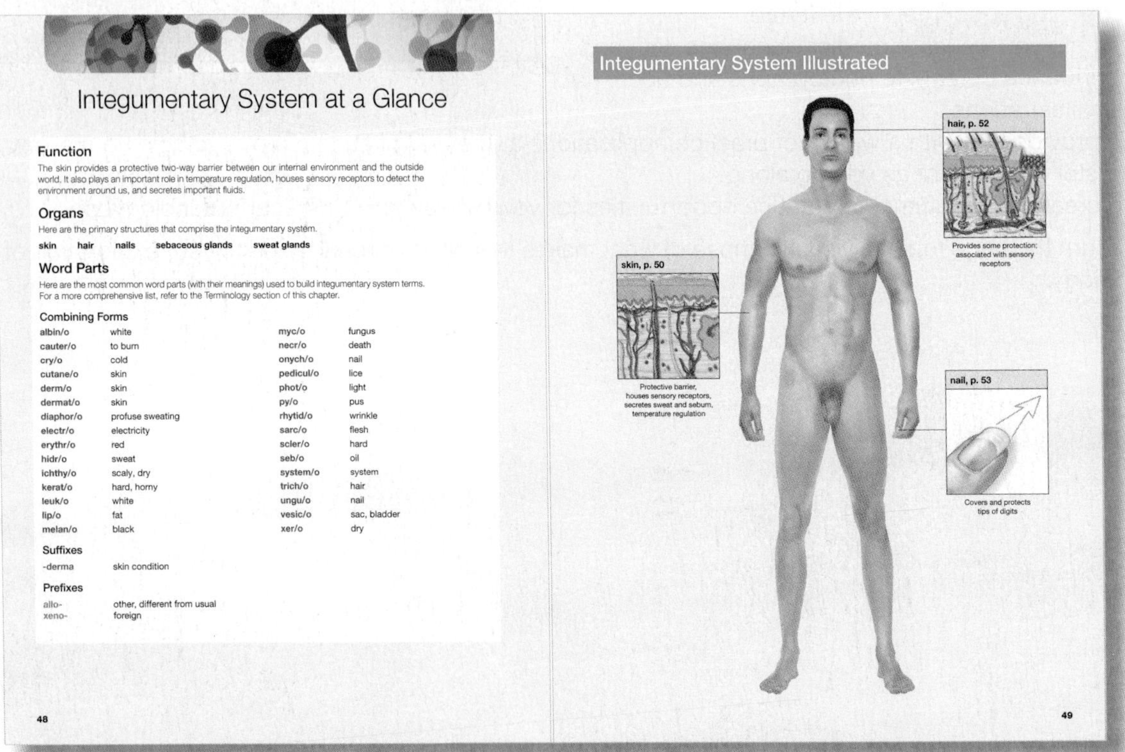

Integumentary System at a Glance

Function

The skin provides a protective two-way barrier between our internal environment and the outside world. It also plays an important role in temperature regulation, houses sensory receptors to detect the environment around us, and secretes important fluids.

Organs

Here are the primary structures that comprise the integumentary system.

skin **hair** **nails** **sebaceous glands** **sweat glands**

Word Parts

Here are the most common word parts (with their meanings) used to build integumentary system terms. For a more comprehensive list, refer to the Terminology section of this chapter.

Combining Forms

albin/o	white	**myc/o**	fungus
cauter/o	to burn	**necr/o**	death
cry/o	cold	**onych/o**	nail
cutane/o	skin	**pedicul/o**	lice
derm/o	skin	**phot/o**	light
dermat/o	skin	**py/o**	pus
diaphor/o	profuse sweating	**rhytid/o**	wrinkle
electr/o	electricity	**sarc/o**	flesh
erythr/o	red	**scler/o**	hard
hidr/o	sweat	**seb/o**	oil
ichthy/o	scaly, dry	**system/o**	system
kerat/o	hard, horny	**trich/o**	hair
leuk/o	white	**ungu/o**	nail
lip/o	fat	**vesic/o**	sac, bladder
melan/o	black	**xer/o**	dry

Suffixes

-derma	skin condition

Prefixes

allo-	other, different from usual
xeno-	foreign

48

Integumentary System Illustrated

49

Key Terms and Pronunciations

Every subsection starts with a list of key terms and pronunciations for those words that will be covered in that section. This sets the stage for comprehension and mastery.

Color-Coded Word Parts—Red combining forms, blue suffixes, and green prefixes allow for quick recognition throughout the book.

NEW! Informative and Interesting Sidebars

The popular Med Term Tip feature offers tidbits of noteworthy information about medical terms that engage learners. New features for the sixth edition are Word Watch and What's In A Name?, which further assist students as they learn medical terminology by helping them not to confuse similar-sounding words and by reinforcing word parts.

mixes with hydrochloric acid and other gastric juices to form a liquid mixture called **chyme**, which then passes through the remaining portion of the digestive system.

Entry into and exit from the stomach is controlled by muscular valves called **sphincters**. These valves open and close to ensure that food can only move forward down the gut tube. The **cardiac sphincter**, named for its proximity to the heart, is located between the esophagus and the fundus; also called the **lower esophageal sphincter** (LES), it keeps food from flowing backward into the esophagus.

The antrum tapers off into the **pyloric sphincter**, which regulates the passage of food into the small intestine. Only a small amount of the chyme is allowed to enter the small intestine with each opening of the sphincter for two important reasons. First, the small intestine is much narrower than the stomach and cannot hold as much as the stomach can. Second, the chyme is highly acidic and must be thoroughly neutralized as it leaves the stomach.

What's In A Name?

Look for these word parts:
cardi/o = heart
hydr/o = water
-ac = pertaining to
-ic = pertaining to

Med Term Tip

It is easier to remember the function of the pyloric sphincter when you note that *pylor/o* means "gatekeeper." This gatekeeper controls the forward movement of food. Sphincters are rings of muscle that can be opened and closed to control entry and exit from hollow organs like the stomach, colon, and bladder.

Small Intestine

duodenum (doo-oh-DEE-num / doo-OD-eh-num)
ileocecal valve (ill-ee-oh-SEE-kal)
ileum (ILL-ee-um)
jejunum (jih-JOO-num)

The small intestine, or small bowel, is the major site of digestion and absorption of nutrients from food. It is located between the pyloric sphincter and the colon (see Figure 8.6 ■). Because the small intestine is concerned with absorption of food products, an abnormality in this organ can cause malnutrition. The small intestine, with an average length of 20 feet, is the longest portion of the alimentary canal and has three sections: the **duodenum**, the **jejunum**, and the **ileum**.

- The duodenum extends from the pyloric sphincter to the jejunum, and is about 10–12 inches long. Digestion is completed in the duodenum after the liquid chyme from the stomach is mixed with digestive juices from the pancreas and gallbladder.
- The jejunum, or middle portion, extends from the duodenum to the ileum and is about eight feet long.

Word Watch

Be careful not to confuse the word root *ile/o* meaning "ileum," a portion of the small intestines, and *ili/o* meaning "ilium," a pelvic bone.

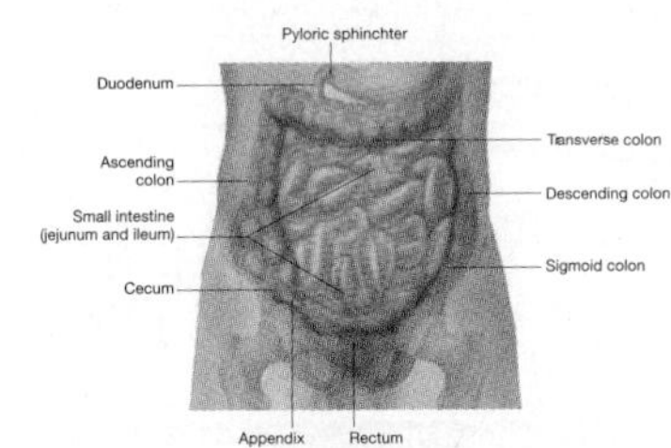

■ **Figure 8.6** The small intestine. Anterior view of the abdominopelvic cavity illustrating how the three sections of small intestine—duodenum, jejunum, ileum—begin at the pyloric sphincter and end at the colon, but are not arranged in a orderly fashion.

Medically Accurate Illustrations

Concepts come to life with vibrant, clear, consistent, and scientifically precise images.

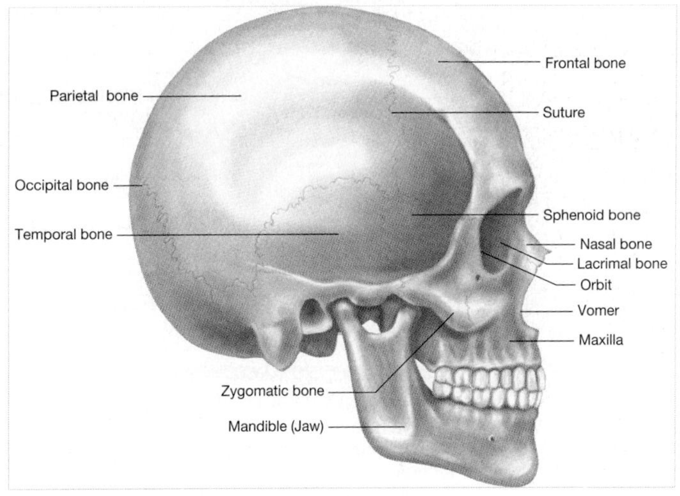

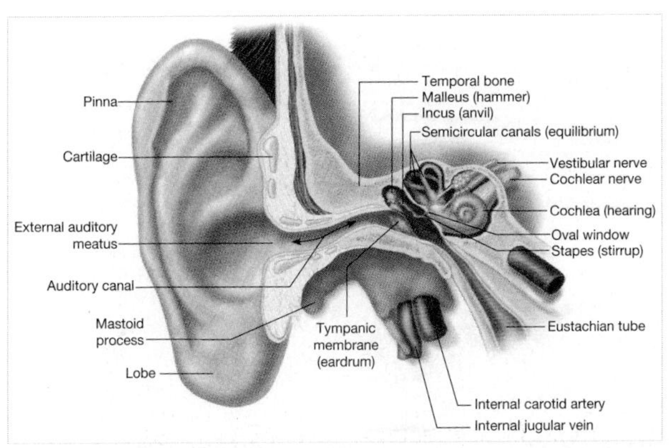

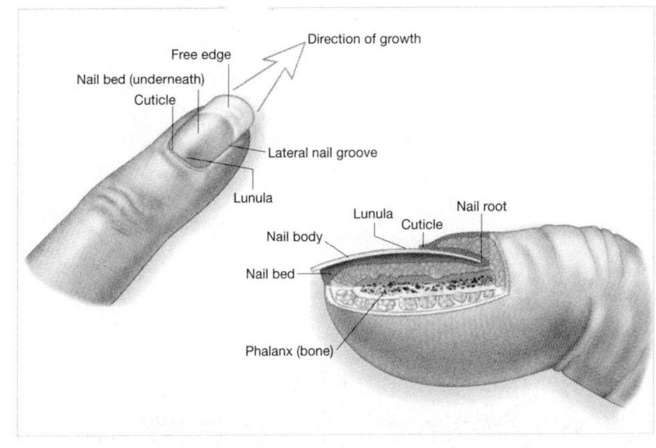

Word Tables

Study lists are categorized and presented in a clear, logical, color-coded format that eases the learning process. The Signs and Symptoms subsection within the Pathology table contains disease-related terms grouped by organ. This allows terms to be categorized into smaller groups, therefore making learning easier. Also the three-column format in the Word Building sections allows for the term (with pronunciation and/or abbreviation), word parts (if appropriate), and definitions to be displayed. The Pharmacology table also includes word parts in a fourth column.

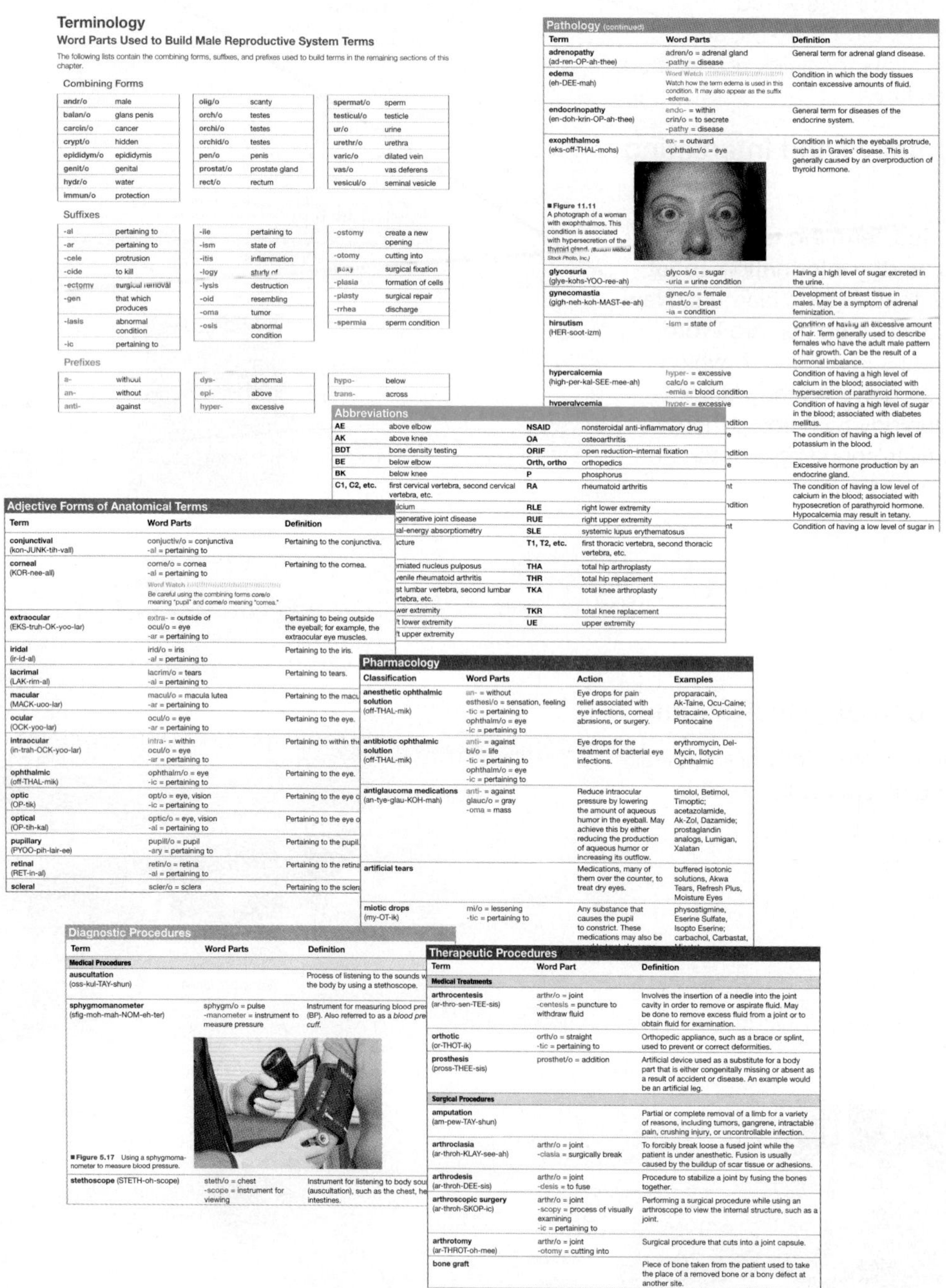

NEW! Practice As You Go

A mix of exercises peppered throughout the chapters to help you take a quick assessment of your understanding of the material discussed.

Practice As You Go

C. Terminology Matching

Match each term to its definition.

1. _______ Wilms' tumor
2. _______ azotemia
3. _______ urinary retention
4. _______ nephroptosis
5. _______ nocturia
6. _______ incontinence
7. _______ hydronephrosis
8. _______ urgency
9. _______ nephrolithiasis
10. _______ polycystic kidney disease

a. kidney stones
b. feeling the need to urinate immediately
c. childhood malignant kidney tumor
d. swelling of the kidney due to urine collecting in the renal pelvis
e. involuntary release of urine
f. frequent urination at night
g. excess nitrogenous waste in bloodstream
h. inability to fully empty bladder
i. a floating kidney
j. multiple cysts in the kidneys

Practice As You Go

A. Complete the Statement

1. The study of the heart is called ________________.
2. The three layers of the heart are ________________, ________________, and ________________.
3. The impulse for the heartbeat (the pacemaker) originates in the ________________.
4. Arteries carry blood ________________ the heart.
5. The four heart valves are ________________, ________________, ________________, and ________________.
6. The ________________ are the receiving chambers of the heart and the ________________ are the pumping chambers.
7. The ________________ circulation carries blood to and from the lungs.
8. The pointed tip of the heart is called the ________________.
9. The ________________ divides the heart into left and right halves.
10. ________________ is the contraction phase of the heartbeat and ________________ is the relaxation phase.

Practice As You Go

B. Give the adjective form for each anatomical structure

1. Blood ________________ or ________________
2. White cell ________________
3. Clotting cell ________________
4. Fibers ________________
5. Red cell ________________

Practice As You Go

E. What Does it Stand For?

1. KUB ________________
2. cath ________________
3. cysto ________________
4. GU ________________
5. ESWL ________________
6. UTI ________________
7. UC ________________
8. RP ________________
9. ARF ________________
10. BUN ________________
11. CRF ________________
12. H_2O ________________

Chapter Review

Practice Exercises—A wide array of workbook exercises at the end of each chapter serve as a fun and challenging study review.

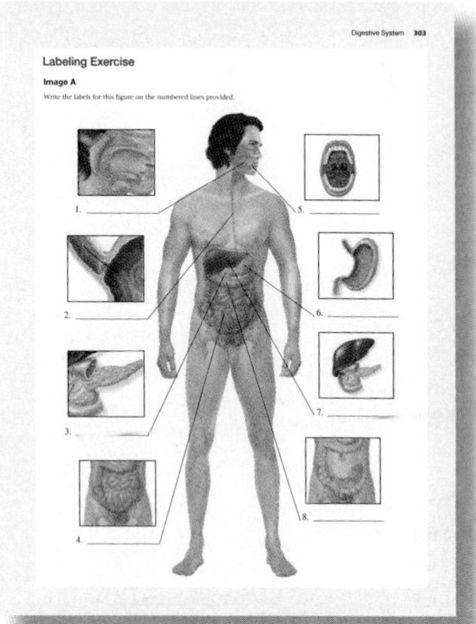
Digestive System 303

Labeling Exercise

Image A

Write the labels for this figure on the numbered lines provided.

1. ______
2. ______
3. ______
4. ______
5. ______
6. ______
7. ______
8. ______

Additionally **Labeling Exercises** provide a visual challenge to reinforce students' grasp of anatomy and physiology concepts.

Real-World Applications—Three critical thinking activities allow students to apply their medical knowledge to true-to-life scenarios:

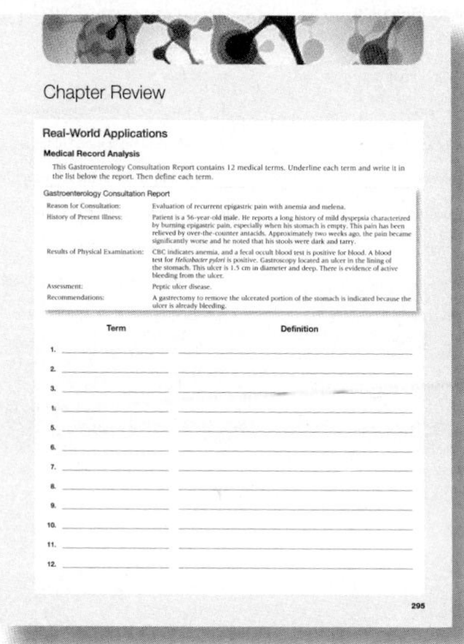
Chapter Review

Real-World Applications

Medical Record Analysis

This Gastroenterology Consultation Report contains 12 medical terms. Underline each term and write it in the list below the report. Then define each term.

Gastroenterology Consultation Report

Reason for Consultation:	Evaluation of recurrent epigastric pain with anemia and melena.
History of Present Illness:	Patient is a 56-year-old male. He reports a long history of mild dyspepsia characterized by burning epigastric pain, especially when his stomach is empty. This pain has been relieved by over-the-counter antacids. Approximately two weeks ago, the pain became significantly worse and he noted that his stools were dark and tarry.
Results of Physical Examination:	CBC indicates anemia, and a fecal occult blood test is positive for blood. A blood test for *Helicobacter pylori* is positive. Gastroscopy located an ulcer in the lining of the stomach. This ulcer is 1.5 cm in diameter and deep. There is evidence of active bleeding from the ulcer.
Assessment:	Peptic ulcer disease.
Recommendations:	A gastrectomy to remove the ulcerated portion of the stomach is indicated because the ulcer is already bleeding.

	Term	Definition
1.		
2.		
3.		
4.		
5.		
6.		
7.		
8.		
9.		
10.		
11.		
12.		

295

1) Medical Record Analysis
Exercises that challenge students to read examples of real medical records and then to apply their medical terminology knowledge in answering related questions.

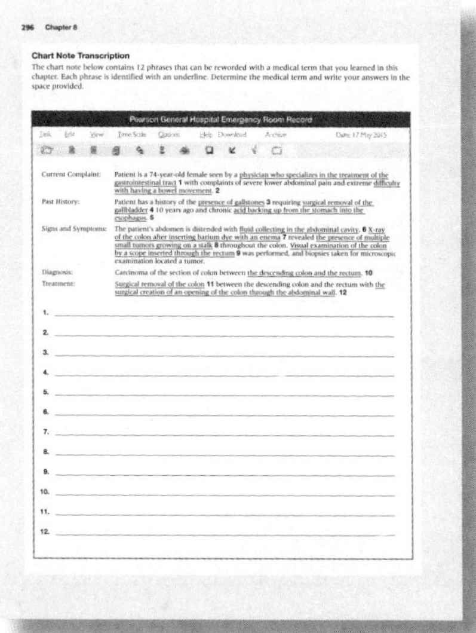
296 Chapter 8

Chart Note Transcription

The chart note below contains 12 phrases that can be reworded with a medical term that you learned in this chapter. Each phrase is identified with an underline. Determine the medical term and write your answers in the space provided.

Pearson General Hospital Emergency Room Record

Task Edit View Time Scale Options Help Download Archive Date: 17 May 2015

Current Complaint:	Patient is a 74-year-old female seen by a physician who specializes in the treatment of the gastrointestinal tract **1** with complaints of severe lower abdominal pain and extreme difficulty with having a bowel movement. **2**
Past History:	Patient has a history of the presence of gallstones **3** requiring surgical removal of the gallbladder **4** 10 years ago and chronic acid backing up from the stomach into the esophagus. **5**
Signs and Symptoms:	The patient's abdomen is distended with fluid collecting in the abdominal cavity. **6** X-ray of the colon after inserting barium dye with an enema **7** revealed the presence of multiple small tumors growing on a stalk **8** throughout the colon. Visual examination of the colon by a scope inserted through the rectum **9** was performed, and biopsies taken for microscopic examination located a tumor.
Diagnosis:	Carcinoma of the section of colon between the descending colon and the rectum. **10**
Treatment:	Surgical removal of the colon **11** between the descending colon and the rectum with the surgical creation of an opening of the colon through the abdominal wall. **12**

1. ______
2. ______
3. ______
4. ______
5. ______
6. ______
7. ______
8. ______
9. ______
10. ______
11. ______
12. ______

2) Chart Note Transcription
Slice-of-real-life exercise that asks students to replace lay terms in a medical chart with the proper medical term.

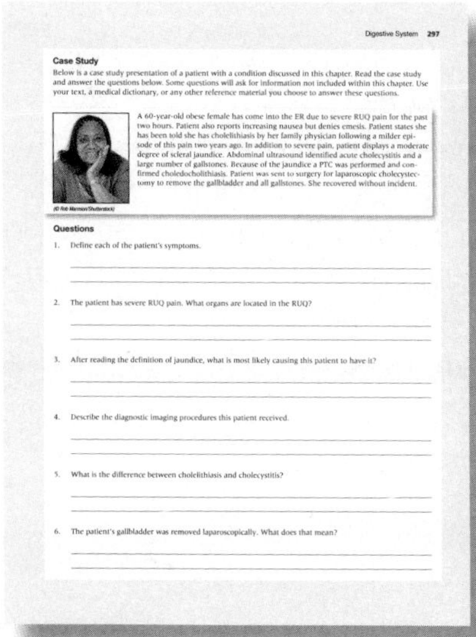
Digestive System 297

Case Study

Below is a case study presentation of a patient with a condition discussed in this chapter. Read the case study and answer the questions below. Some questions will ask for information not included within this chapter. Use your text, a medical dictionary, or any other reference material you choose to answer these questions.

A 60-year-old obese female has come into the ER due to severe RUQ pain for the past two hours. Patient also reports increasing nausea but denies emesis. Patient states she has been told she has cholelithiasis by her family physician following a milder episode of this pain two years ago. In addition to severe pain, patient displays a moderate degree of scleral jaundice. Abdominal ultrasound identified acute cholecystitis and a large number of gallstones. Because of the jaundice a PTC was performed and confirmed choledocholithiasis. Patient was sent to surgery for laparoscopic cholecystectomy to remove the gallbladder and all gallstones. She recovered without incident.

Questions

1. Define each of the patient's symptoms.
2. The patient has severe RUQ pain. What organs are located in the RUQ?
3. After reading the definition of jaundice, what is most likely causing this patient to have it?
4. Describe the diagnostic imaging procedures this patient received.
5. What is the difference between cholelithiasis and cholecystitis?
6. The patient's gallbladder was removed laparoscopically. What does that mean?

3) Case Study
Scenarios that use critical thinking questions to help students develop a firmer understanding of the terminology in context.

The Total Teaching and Learning Package

We are committed to providing students and instructors with exactly the tools they need to be successful in the classroom and beyond. To this end, ***Medical Terminology: A Living Language*** is supported by the most complete and dynamic set of resources available today.

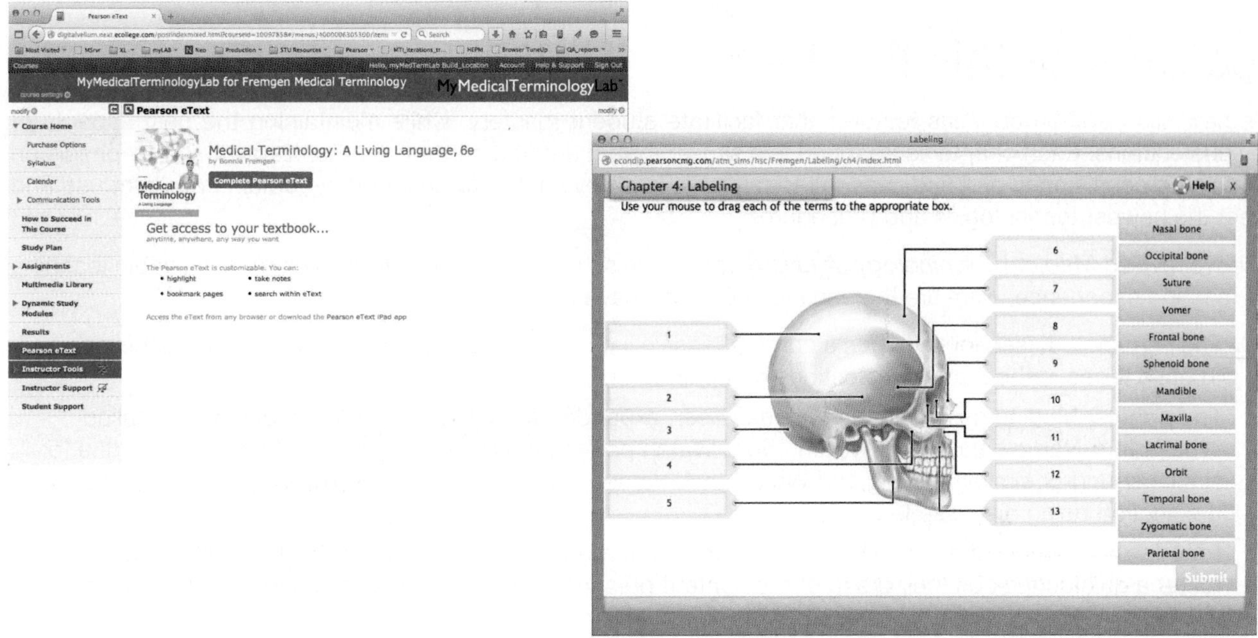

MyMedicalTerminologyLab

The ultimate personalized learning tool is available at **www.mymedicalterminologylab.com**.

This online course correlates with the textbook and is available for purchase separately or for a discount when packaged with the book. MyMedicalTerminologyLab is an immersive study experience that presents students with, quizzes, videos, learning activities and other self-study challenges. The system allows learners to track their own progress through the course and use a personalized study plan to achieve success.

MyMedicalTerminologyLab saves instructors time by providing quality feedback, ongoing individualized assessments for students, and instructor resources all in one place. It offers instructors the flexibility to make technology an integral part of their courses, or a supplementary resource for students.

Visit **www.mymedicalterminologylab.com** to log in to the course or purchase access.

Instructors seeking more information about discount bundle options or for a demonstration, please contact your Pearson sales representative.

Comprehensive Instructional Package

Perhaps the most gratifying part of an educator's work is the "aha" learning moment when the light bulb goes off and a student truly understands a concept—when a connection is made.

Along these lines, Pearson is pleased to help instructors foster more of these educational connections by providing a complete battery of resources to support teaching and learning.

Qualified adopters are eligible to receive a wealth of materials designed to help instructors prepare, present, and assess. For more information, please contact your Pearson sales representative or visit **www.pearsonhighered.com/educator**.

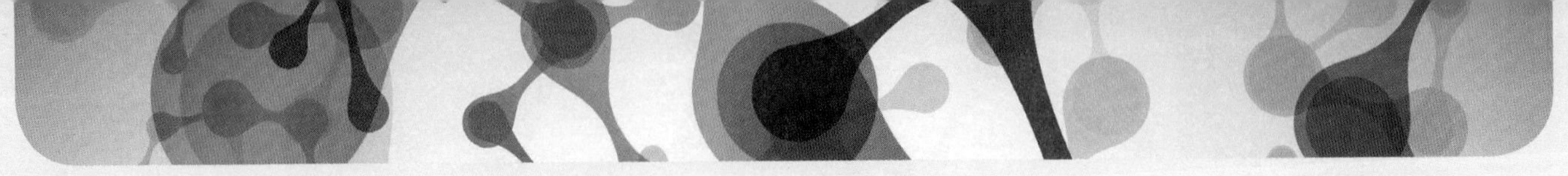

Preface

Since the first edition of ***Medical Terminology: A Living Language*** was published it has been noted for its "clean" and logical format that promotes learning. In this revised edition, we have built upon this strength by enhancing many features to make this text an ideal choice for semester- or quarter-length courses.

Features of this Edition

This new sixth edition contains features that facilitate student mastery, while maintaining the best aspects of previous editions. Each chapter is arranged in a similar format and the content is organized with an emphasis on maintaining consistency and accuracy. All terms have been evaluated to ensure they remain in current use and reflect the newest technologies and procedures.

We have revised ***Medical Terminology: A Living Language*** so that it provides for an even more valuable teaching and learning experience. Here are the enhancements we have made:

- The Terminology section includes a comprehensive list of all combining forms, suffixes, and prefixes used to build terms in the remaining sections of the chapter.
- The popular Med Term Tip margin note has been expanded to include two additional features called **What's In A Name?** and **Word Watch**. Word Watch points out words that may confuse students due to similar sound or similar spelling and What's In A Name? reinforces the breakdown of word parts used in the section being discussed.
- **Practice As You Go** is a "speed bump" feature scattered throughout the chapters that allows the reader to get a quick check on their grasp of the content presented by using a combination of short-answer exercises. Answers are provided at the back of the book.

Organization of the Book

Introductory Chapter

Chapter 1 contains information necessary for an understanding of how medical terms are formed. This includes learning about word roots, combining forms, prefixes, and suffixes, and general rules for building medical terms. Readers will also learn about terminology for medical records and the different healthcare settings. Chapter 2 presents terminology relating to the body organization, including organs and body systems. Here readers will first encounter word-building tables, a feature found in each remaining chapter that lists medical terms and their respective word parts.

Anatomy and Physiology Chapters

Chapters 3–13 are organized by body system. Each chapter begins with the System At A Glance feature, which lists combining forms, prefixes, and/or suffixes with their meanings and is followed by a System Illustrated overview of the organs in the system. The anatomy and physiology section is divided into the various components of the system, and each subsection begins with a list of key medical terms accompanied by a pronunciation guide. Key terms are boldfaced the first time they appear in the narrative. The Terminology section of each chapter begins with a list of all word parts used within the chapter. For ease of learning, the medical terms are divided into five separate sections: adjective forms of anatomical terms, pathology, diagnostic procedures, therapeutic procedures, and pharmacology. The word parts used to build terms are highlighted within each table. An abbreviations section then follows to complete the chapter.

Special Topics Chapter

Chapter 14 contains timely information and appropriate medical terms relevant to the following medical specialties: pharmacology, mental health, diagnostic imaging, rehabilitation services, surgery, and oncology. Knowledge of these topics is necessary for the well-rounded healthcare worker.

Appendices

The appendices contain helpful reference lists of word parts and definitions. This information is intended for quick access. There are three appendices: Word Parts Arranged Alphabetically and Defined, Word Parts Arranged Alphabetically by Definition, and Abbreviations. Finally, all of the key terms appear again in the combination glossary/index at the end of the text.

About the Authors

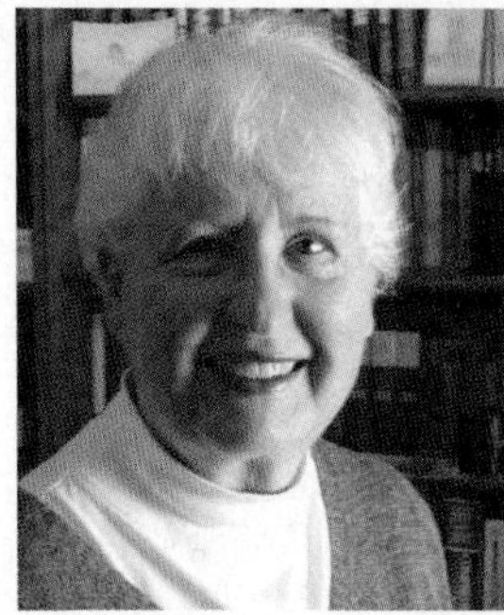

Bonnie F. Fremgen

Bonnie F. Fremgen is a former Associate Dean of the Allied Health Program at Robert Morris College. She has taught medical law and ethics courses as well as clinical and administrative topics. In addition, Dr. Fremgen has served as an advisor for students' career planning. She has broad interests and experiences in the healthcare field, including hospitals, nursing homes, and physicians' offices.

Dr. Fremgen holds a nursing degree as well as a master's in healthcare administration. She received her PhD from the College of Education at the University of Illinois. Dr. Fremgen has performed postdoctoral studies in Medical Law at Loyola University Law School in Chicago. She has authored five textbooks with Pearson.

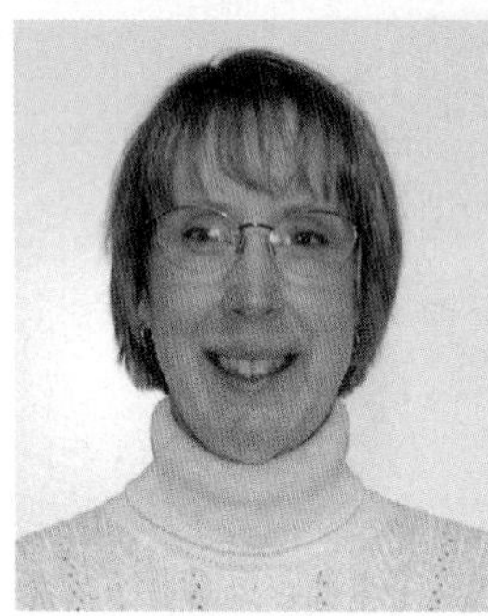

Suzanne S. Frucht

Suzanne S. Frucht is an Associate Professor Emeritus of Anatomy and Physiology at Northwest Missouri State University (NWMSU). She holds baccalaureate degrees in biological sciences and physical therapy from Indiana University, an MS in biological sciences at NWMSU, and a PhD in molecular biology and biochemistry from the University of Missouri–Kansas City.

For 14 years Dr. Frucht worked full time as a physical therapist in various healthcare settings, including acute care hospitals, extended care facilities, and home health. Based on her educational and clinical experience she was invited to teach medical terminology part time in 1988 and became a full-time faculty member three years later as she discovered her love for the challenge of teaching. Dr. Frucht has taught a variety of courses including medical terminology, human anatomy, human physiology, and animal anatomy and physiology. She received the Governor's Award for Excellence in Teaching in 2003. After retiring from teaching in 2008, she continues to be active in student learning through teaching medical terminology as an online course and writing medical terminology texts and anatomy and physiology laboratory manuals.

About the Illustrators

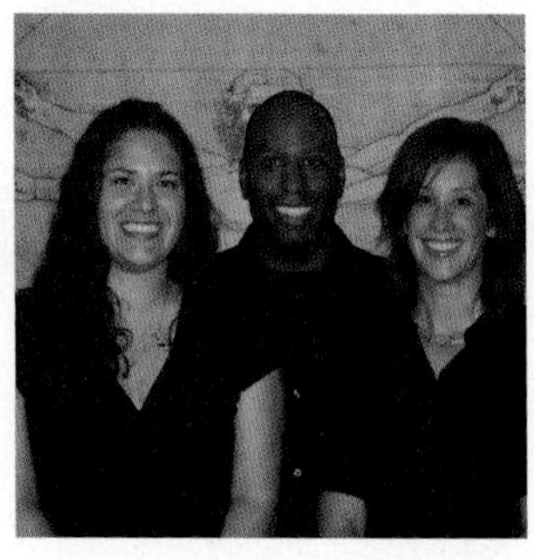

Marcelo Oliver is president and founder of Body Scientific International LLC. He holds an MFA degree in Medical and Biological Illustration from the University of Michigan. For the past 15 years, his passion has been to condense complex anatomical information into visual education tools for students, patients, and medical professionals. For seven years Oliver worked as a medical illustrator and creative director developing anatomical charts used for student and patient education. In the years that followed, he created educational and marketing tools for medical device companies prior to founding Body Scientific International, LLC.

Body Scientific's lead artists in this publication were medical illustrators Liana Bauman and Katie Burgess. Both hold a Master of Science degree in Biomedical Visualization from the University of Illinois at Chicago. Their contribution in the publication was key in the creation and editing of artwork throughout.

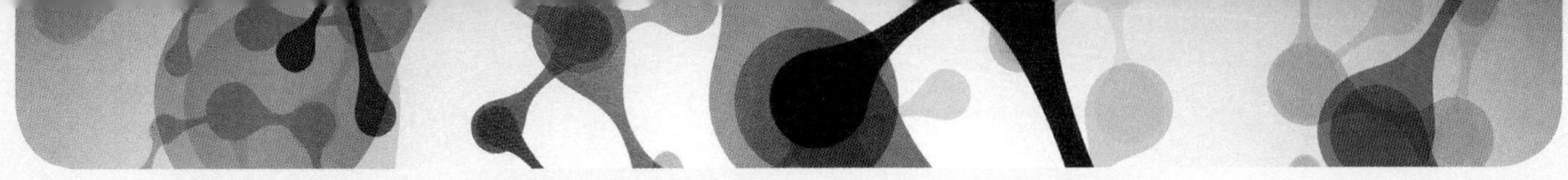

Our Development Team

We would like to express deep gratitude to the over 100 colleagues from schools across the country that have provided us with many hours of their time over the years to help us tailor this book to suit the dynamic needs of instructors and students. These individuals have reviewed manuscript chapters and illustrations for content, accuracy, level, and utility. We sincerely thank them and feel that ***Medical Terminology: A Living Language*** has benefited immeasurably from their efforts, insights, encouragement, and selfless willingness to share their expertise as educators.

Reviewers of the 6th Edition

Nicole Claussen, MS, CST, FAST
Rolla Technical Institute
Rolla, Missouri

Linda A. Costarella, ND
Lake Washington Institute of Technology
Kirkland, Washington

Pamela Dobbins, MS, BS, AAS
Shelton State Community College
Tuscaloosa, Alabama

Carole DuBose, LPN, CST
Choffin School of Surgical Technology
Youngstown, Ohio

Pamela Edwards, MA, NRCMA
Lone Star College System
The Woodlands, Texas

Robert Fanger, MS
Del Mar College
Corpus Christi, Texas

Dolly Horton, CMA (AAMA), EdD
Asheville Buncombe Technical Community College
Asheville, North Carolina

Rebecca Keith, PT, MSHS
Arkansas State University
Jonesboro, Arkansas

Shiela Rojas, MBA
Santa Barbara Business College
Santa Barbara, California

Karen Stenback, MFA, CHHC
Antelope Valley College
Lancaster, California

Maureen Tubbiola, MS, PhD
St. Cloud State University
St. Cloud, Minnesota

Marianne Van Deursen, MS, Ed, CMA (AAMA), MLT
Warren County Community College
Washington, New Jersey

Judith Zappala, MT, ASCP, MBA
Middlesex Community College
Lowell, Massachusetts

Reviewers of Earlier Editions

Yvonne Alles, MBA, RMT
Davenport University
Grand Rapids, Michigan

Rachael C. Alstatter, Program Director
Southern Ohio College
Fairfield, Ohio

Steve Arinder, BS, MPH
Meridian Community College
Meridian, Mississippi

K. William Avery, BSMT, JD, PhD
City College
Gainesville, Florida

Beverly A. Baker, DA, CST
Western Iowa Technical Community College
Sioux City, Iowa

Michael Battaglia, MS
Greenville Technical College
Taylors, South Carolina

Nancy Ridinger Bean, Health Assistant Instructor
Wythe County Vocational School
Wytheville, Virginia

Deborah J. Bedford, CMA, AAS
North Seattle Community College
Seattle, Washington

Barbara J Behrens, PTA, MS
Mercer County Community College
Trenton, New Jersey

Pam Besser, PhD
Jefferson Community and Technical College
Louisville, Kentucky

Norma J. Bird, MEd, BS, CMA
Idaho State University College of Technology
Pocatello, Idaho

Trina Blaschko, RHIT
Chippewa Valley Technical College
Eau Claire, Wisconsin

Richard T. Boan, PhD
Midlands Technical College
Columbia, South Carolina

Susan W. Boggs, RN, BSN, CNOR
Piedmont Technical College
Greenwood, South Carolina

Bradley S. Bowden, PhD
Alfred University
Alfred, New York

Jeannie Bower, BS, NRCAMA
Central Penn College
Summerdale, Pennsylvania

Joan Walker Brittingham
Sussex Tech Adult Division
Georgetown, Delaware

Phyills J. Broughton, Curriculum Coordinator
Pitt Community College
Greenville, North Carolina

Barbara Bussard, Instructor
Southwestern Michigan College
Dowagiac, Michigan

Toni Cade, MBA, RHIA, CCS
University of Louisiana at Lafayette
Lafayette, Louisiana

Gloria H. Coats, RN, MSN
Modesto Junior College
Modesto, California

Lyndal M. Curry, MA, RP
University of South Alabama
Mobile, Alabama

Nancy Dancs, PT
Waukesha County Technical College
Pewaukee, Wisconsin

Theresa H. deBeche, RN, MN, CNS
Louisiana State University at Eunice
Eunice, Louisiana

Bonnie Deister, MS, BSN, CMA-C
Broome Community College
Binghamton, New York

Antoinette Deshaies, RN, BSPA
Glendale Community College
Glendale, Arizona

Carol Eckert, RN, MSN
Southwestern Illinois College
Belleville, Illinois

Jamie Erskine, PhD, RD
University of Northern Colorado
Greeley, Colorado

Mildred K. Fuller, PhD, MT(ASCP), CLS(NCA)
Norfolk State University
Norfolk, Virginia

Deborah Galanski-Maciak
Davenport University
Grand Rapids, Michigan

Debra Getting, Practical Nursing Instructor
Northwest Iowa Community College
Sheldon, Iowa

Ann Queen Giles, MHS, CMA
Western Piedmont Community College
Morganton, North Carolina

Brenda L. Gleason, MSN
Iowa Central Community College
Fort Dodge, Iowa

Steven B. Goldschmidt, DC, CCFC
North Hennepin Community College
Brooklyn Park, Minnesota

Linda S. Gott, RN, MS
Pensacola High School
Pensacola, Florida

Martha Grove, Staff Educator
Mercy Regional Health System
Cincinnati, Ohio

Kathryn Gruber
Globe College
Oakdale, Minnesota

Karen R. Hardney, MSEd
Chicago State University
Chicago, Illinois

Mary Hartman, MS, OTR/L
Genesee Community College
Batavia, New York

Joyce B. Harvey, PhD, RHIA
Norfolk State University
Norfolk, Virginia

Beulah A. Hofmann, RN, BSN, MSN, CMA
Ivy Tech Community College of Indiana
Greencastle, Indiana

Kimberley Hontz, RN
Antonelli Medical and Professional Institute
Pottstown, Pennsylvania

Pamela S. Huber, MS, MT(ASCP)
Erie Community College
Williamsville, New York

Eva I. Irwin
Ivy Tech State College
Indianapolis, Indiana

Susan Jackson, EdS
Valdosta Technical College
Valdosta, Georgia

Mark Jaffe, DPM, MHSA
Nova Southeastern University
Ft. Lauderdale, Florida

Carol Lee Jarrell, MLT, AHI
Brown Mackie College
Merrillville, Indiana

Holly Jodon, MPAS, PA-C
Gannon University
Erie, Pennsylvania

Virginia J. Johnson, CMA
Lakeland Academy
Minneapolis, Minnesota

Marcie C. Jones, BS, CMA
Gwinnett Technical Institute
Lawrenceville, Georgia

Robin Jones, RHIA
Meridian Community College
Meridian, Mississippi

Gertrude A. Kenny, BSN, RN, CMA
Baker College of Muskegon
Muskegon, Michigan

Dianne K. Kuiti, RN
Duluth Business University
Duluth, Minnesota

Andrew La Marca, EMT-P
Mobile Life Support Services
Middletown, New York

Francesca L. Langlow, BS
Delgado Community College
New Orleans, Louisiana

Julie A. Leu, CPC
Creighton University
Omaha, Nebraska

Norma Longoria, BS, COI
South Texas Community College
McAllen, Texas

Jeanne W. Lovelock, RN, MSN
Piedmont Virginia Community College
Charlottesville, Virginia

Jan Martin, RT(R)
Ogeechee Tech College
Statesboro, Georgia

Leslie M. Mazzola, MA
Cuyahoga Community College
Parma, Ohio

Michelle C. McCranie, CPhT
Ogeechee Technical College
Statesboro, Georgia

Lola McGourty, MSN, RN
Bossier Parish Community College
Bossier City, Louisiana

Bridgit R. Moore, EdD, MT(ASCP), CPC
McLennan Community College
Waco, Texas

Christine J. Moore, MEd
Armstrong Atlantic State University
Savannah, Georgia

Connie Morgan
Ivy Tech State College
Kokomo., Indiana

Patricia Moody, RN
Athens Technical College
Athens, Georgia

Catherine Moran, PhD
Breyer State University
Birmingham, Alabama

Katrina B. Myricks
Holmes Community College
Ridgeland, Mississippi

Pam Ncu, CMA
International Business College
Fort Wayne, Indiana

Judy Ortiz MHS, MS, PA-C
Pacific University
Hillsboro, Oregon

Tina M. Peer, BSN, RN
College of Southern Idaho
Twin Falls, ID

Dave Peruski, RN, MSA, MSN
Delta College
University Center, Michigan

Lisa J. Pierce, MSA, RRT
Augusta Technical College
Augusta, Georgia

Sister Marguerite Polcyn, OSF, PhD
Lourdes College
Sylvania, Ohio

Vicki Prater, CMA, RMA, RAHA
Concorde Career Institute
San Bernardino, California

Carolyn Ragsdale CST, BS
Parkland College
Champaign, Illinois

LuAnn Reicks, RNC, BS, MSN
Iowa Central Community College
Fort Dodge, Iowa

Linda Reigel
Glenville State College
Glenville, West Virginia

Ellen Rosen, RN, MN
Glendale Community College
Glendale, California

Georgette Rosenfeld, PhD, RRT, RN
Indian River State College
Fort Pierce, Florida

Brian L. Rutledge, MHSA
Hinds Community College
Jackson, Mississippi

Sue Shibley, MEd, CMT, CCS-P, CPC
North Idaho College
Coeur d'Alene, Idaho

Misty Shuler, RHIA
Asheville Buncombe Technical Community College
Asheville, North Carolina

Patricia A. Slachta, PhD, RN, ACNS-BC, CWOCN
Technical College of the Lowcountry
Beaufort, South Carolina

Donna J. Slovensky, PhD, RHIA, FAHIMA
University of Alabama at Birmingham
Birmingham, Alabama

Connie Smith, RPh
University of Louisiana at Monroe School of Pharmacy
Monroe, Louisiana

Karen Snipe, CPhT, ASBA, MAEd
Trident Technical College
Charleston, South Carolina

Janet Stehling, RHIA
McLennan College
Lorena, Texas

Donna Stern
University of California San Diego
La Jolla, California

Jodi Taylor, AAS, LPN, RMA
Terra State Community College
Fremont, Ohio

Annmary Thomas, MEd, NREMT-P
Community College of Philadelphia
Philadelphia, Pennsylvania

Lenette Thompson, CST, AS
Piedmont Technical College
Greenwood, South Carolina

Scott Throneberry, BS, NREMTP
Calhoun Community College
Decatur, Alabama

Marilyn Turner, RN, CMA
Ogeechee Technical College
Statesboro, Georgia

Joan Ann Verderame, RN, MA
Bergen Community College
Paramus, New Jersey

Twila Wallace, MEd
Central Community College
Columbus, Nebraska

Kathy Wallington
Phillips Junior College
Campbell, California

Linda Walter, RN, MSN
Northwestern Michigan College
Traverse City, Michigan

Jean Watson, PhD
Clark College
Vancouver, Washington

Twila Weiszbrod, MPA
College of the Sequoias
Visalia, California

Sara J. Wellman, RHIT
Indiana University Northwest
Gary, Indiana

Leesa Whicker, BA, CMA
Central Piedmont Community College
Charlotte, NC

Lynn C. Wimett, RN, ANP, EdD
Regis University
Denver, Colorado

Kathy Zaiken, PharmD
Massachusetts College of Pharmacy and Health Sciences
Boston, Massachusetts

Carole A. Zeglin, MSEd, BS, MT, RMA (AMT)
Westmoreland County Community College
Youngwood, Pennsylvania

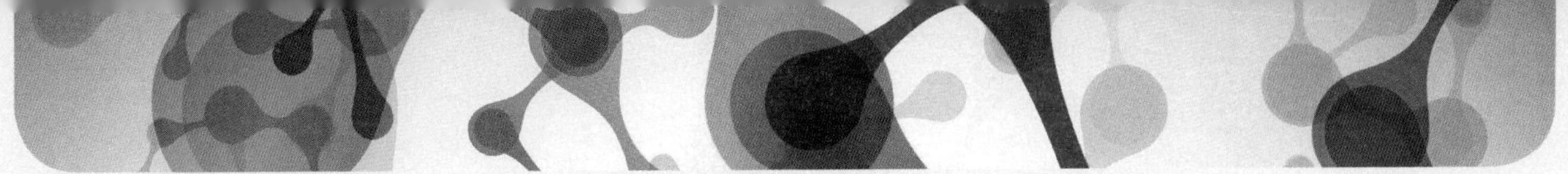

A Commitment to Accuracy

As a student embarking on a career in healthcare you probably already know how critically important it is to be precise in your work. Patients and coworkers will be counting on you to avoid errors on a daily basis. Likewise, we owe it to you—the reader—to ensure accuracy in this book. We have gone to great lengths to verify that the information provided in ***Medical Terminology: A Living Language*** is complete and correct. To this end, here are the steps we have taken:

1. **Editorial Review**—We have assembled a large team of developmental consultants (listed on the preceding pages) to critique every word and every image in this book. Multiple content experts have read each chapter for accuracy.
2. **Medical Illustrations**—A team of medically trained illustrators was hired to prepare each piece of art that graces the pages of this book. These illustrators have a higher level of scientific education than the artists for most textbooks, and they worked directly with the authors and members of our development team to make sure that their work was clear, correct, and consistent with what is described in the text.
3. **Accurate Ancillaries**—Realizing that the teaching and learning ancillaries are often as vital to instruction as the book itself, we took extra steps to ensure accuracy and consistency within these components. We assigned some members of our development team to specifically focus on critiquing every bit of content that comprises the instructional ancillary resources to confirm accuracy.

While our intent and actions have been directed at creating an error-free text, we have established a process for correcting any mistakes that may have slipped past our editors. Pearson takes this issue seriously and therefore welcomes any and all feedback that you can provide along the lines of helping us enhance the accuracy of this text. If you identify any errors that need to be corrected in a subsequent printing, please notify us. Thank you for helping Pearson to reach its goal of providing the most accurate medical terminology textbooks available.

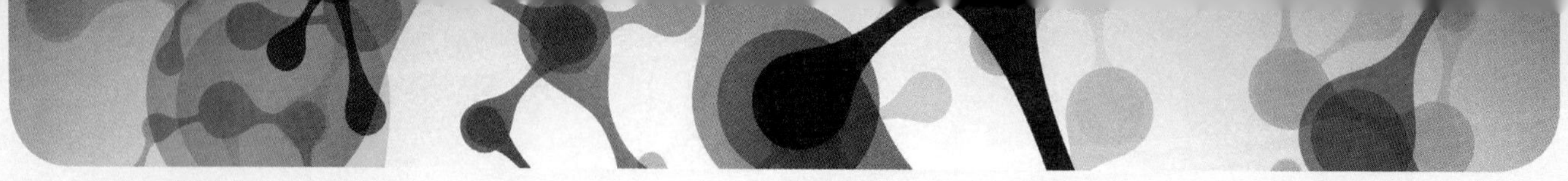

Contents

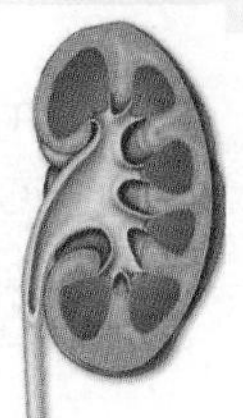

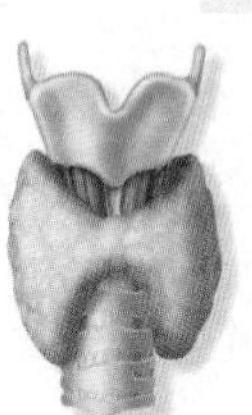

Sixth Edition

Medical Terminology

A Living Language

1

Introduction to Medical Terminology

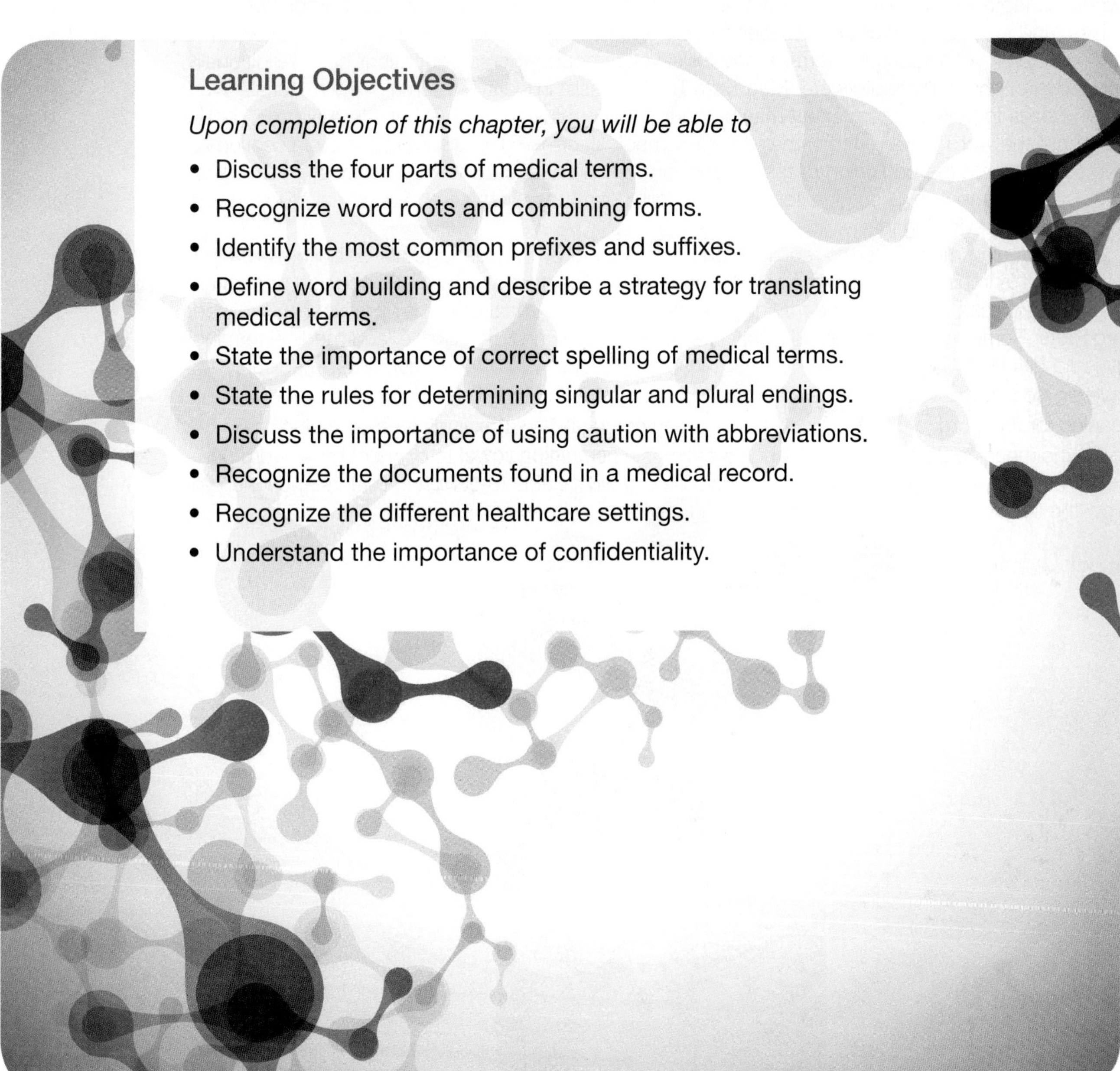

Learning Objectives

Upon completion of this chapter, you will be able to

- Discuss the four parts of medical terms.
- Recognize word roots and combining forms.
- Identify the most common prefixes and suffixes.
- Define word building and describe a strategy for translating medical terms.
- State the importance of correct spelling of medical terms.
- State the rules for determining singular and plural endings.
- Discuss the importance of using caution with abbreviations.
- Recognize the documents found in a medical record.
- Recognize the different healthcare settings.
- Understand the importance of confidentiality.

Medical Terminology at a Glance

Learning medical terminology can initially seem like studying a strange new language. However, once you understand some of the basic rules about how medical terms are formed using word building, it will become much like piecing together a puzzle. The general guidelines for forming words; an understanding of word roots, combining forms, prefixes, and suffixes; pronunciation; and spelling are discussed in this chapter. Chapter 2 introduces you to terms that are used to describe the body as a whole. Chapters 3–13 each focus on a specific body system and present new combining forms, prefixes, and suffixes, as well as exercises to help you gain experience building new medical terms. Finally, Chapter 14 includes the terminology for several important areas of patient care. Additionally, sprinkled throughout all chapters are "Med Term Tips" to assist in clarifying some of the material, "Word Watch" boxes to point out terms that may be particularly confusing, and "What's In A Name?" boxes to highlight the word parts found in the text. New medical terms to be discussed in each section are listed separately at the beginning of the section, and each chapter contains numerous pathological, diagnostic, treatment, and surgical terms. You should use these lists as an additional study tool for previewing and reviewing terms.

Understanding medical terms requires you being able to put words together or build words from their parts. It is impossible to memorize thousands of medical terms; however, once you understand the basics, you can distinguish the meaning of medical terms by analyzing their prefixes, suffixes, and word roots. Remember that there will always be some exceptions to every rule, and medical terminology is no different. We attempt to point out these exceptions where they exist. Most medical terms, however, do follow the general rule that there is a **word root** (indicated by a red color) or fundamental meaning for the word, a **prefix** (indicated by a green color) and a **suffix** (indicated by a blue color) that modify the meaning of the word root, and sometimes a **combining vowel** to connect other word parts. You will be amazed at the seemingly difficult words you will be able to build and understand when you follow the simple steps in word building (see Figure 1.1 ■).

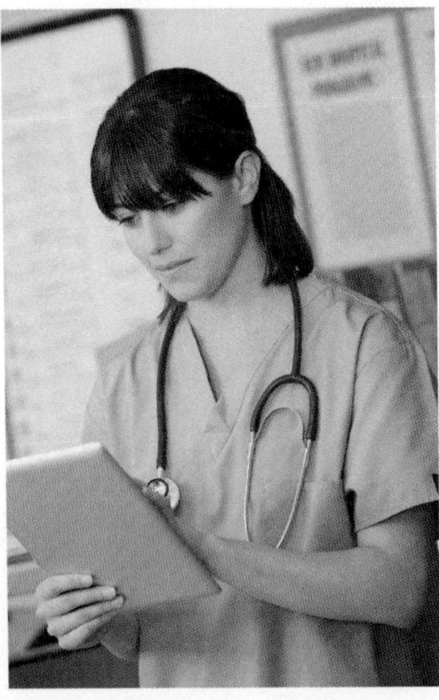

■ **Figure 1.1** Nurse completing a patient report. Healthcare workers use medical terminology in order to accurately and efficiently communicate patient information to each other. *(Monkey Business Images/Shutterstock)*

Building Medical Terms From Word Parts

Four different word parts or elements can be used to construct medical terms:

1. The **word root** is the foundation of the word.	**cardi** ogram = record of the heart
2. A **prefix** is at the beginning of the word.	**peri** cardium = around the heart
3. A **suffix** is at the end of the word.	card **itis** = inflammation of the heart
4. The **combining vowel** is a vowel (usually *o*) that links the word root to another word root or a suffix.	cardi **o** my **o** pathy = disease of the heart muscle

Med Term Tip

Medical terms are built from word parts:

Word Part	Example (Meaning)
Word root	*cardi* (heart)
Prefix	*peri-* (around)
Suffix	*-itis* (inflammation)

When these components are put together, the word *pericarditis* is formed, meaning inflammation around the heart.

The following sections on word roots, combining vowels and forms, prefixes, and suffixes will consider each of these word parts in more detail and present examples of some of those most commonly used.

Practice As You Go

A. Complete the Statement

1. The four components of a medical term are ____________, ____________, ____________, and ____________.
2. The combination of a word root and the combining vowel is called a(n) ____________.
3. The vowel that connects two word roots or a suffix with a word root is usually a(n) ____________.
4. A word part used at the end of a word root to change the meaning of the word is called a(n) ____________.
5. A(n) ____________ is used at the beginning of a word to indicate number, location, or time.

Word Roots

The word root is the foundation of a medical term and provides the general meaning of the word. The word root often indicates the body system or part of the body being discussed, such as *cardi* for heart. At other times the word root may be an action. For example, the word root *cis* means to cut (as in incision).

A term may have more than one word root. For example, **osteoarthritis** (oss-tee-oh-ar-THRY-tis) combines the word root *oste* meaning bone and *arthr* meaning the joint. When the suffix *-itis*, meaning inflammation, is added, we have the entire word, meaning an inflammation involving bone at a joint.

Combining Vowel/Form

To make it possible to pronounce long medical terms with ease and to combine several word parts, a combining vowel is used. This is most often the vowel *o*. Combining vowels are utilized in two places: between a word root and a suffix or between two word roots.

To decide whether or not to use a combining vowel between a word root and a suffix, first look at the suffix. If it begins with a vowel, do not use the combining vowel. If, however, the suffix begins with a consonant, then use a combining vowel. For example: To combine *arthr* with *-scope* will require a combining vowel: **arthroscope** (AR-throh-scope). But to combine *arthr* with *-itis* does not require a combining vowel: **arthritis** (ar-THRY-tis).

The combining vowel is typically kept between two word roots, even if the second word root begins with a vowel. For example, in forming the term **gastroenteritis** (gas-troh-en-ter-EYE-tis), the combining vowel is kept between the two word roots *gastr* and *enter* (gastrenteritis is incorrect). As you can tell from pronouncing these two terms, the combining vowel makes the pronunciation easier.

Med Term Tip

Remember to break down every word into its components (prefix, word root/combining form, and suffix) when learning medical terminology. Do not try to memorize every medical term. Instead, figure out how the word is formed from its components. In a short time you will be able to do this automatically when seeing a new term.

When writing a word root by itself, its **combining form** is typically used. This consists of the word root and its combining vowel written in a word root/vowel form, for example, *cardi/o*. Since it is often simpler to pronounce word roots when they appear in their combining form, we use this format throughout this book.

Common Combining Forms

Some commonly used word roots in their combining form, their meaning, and examples of their use follow. Review the examples to observe when a combining vowel was kept and when it was dropped according to the rules presented above.

COMBINING FORM	MEANING	EXAMPLE (DEFINITION)
bi/o	life	biology (study of life)
carcin/o	cancer	carcinoma (cancerous tumor)
cardi/o	heart	cardiac (pertaining to the heart)
chem/o	chemical	chemotherapy (treatment with chemicals)
cis/o	to cut	incision (process of cutting into)
dermat/o	skin	dermatology (study of the skin)
enter/o	small intestine	enteric (pertaining to the small intestine)
gastr/o	stomach	gastric (pertaining to the stomach)
gynec/o	female	gynecology (study of females)
hemat/o	blood	hematic (pertaining to the blood)
immun/o	immunity	immunology (study of immunity)
laryng/o	larynx	laryngeal (pertaining to the voice box)
nephr/o	kidney	nephromegaly (enlarged kidney)
neur/o	nerve	neural (pertaining to a nerve)
ophthalm/o	eye	ophthalmic (pertaining to the eye)
ot/o	ear	otic (pertaining to the ear)
path/o	disease	pathology (study of disease)
pulmon/o	lung	pulmonary (pertaining to the lungs)
rhin/o	nose	rhinoplasty (surgical repair of the nose)

Practice As You Go

B. Name That Term

Use the suffix **-ology** to write a term for each medical specialty.

1. heart ______
2. stomach ______
3. skin ______
4. eye ______
5. immunity ______
6. kidney ______
7. blood ______
8. female ______
9. nerve ______
10. disease ______

Prefixes

A new medical term is formed when a prefix is added to the front of the term. Prefixes frequently give information about the location of an organ, the number of parts, or the time (frequency). For example, the prefix *bi-* stands for two of something, such as **bilateral** (bye-LAH-ter-al), meaning to have two sides. However, not every term will have a prefix.

Common Prefixes

Some of the more common prefixes, their meanings, and examples of their use are shown below. When written by themselves, prefixes are followed by a hyphen.

PREFIX	MEANING	EXAMPLE (DEFINITION)
a-	without	aphasia (without speech)
an-	without	anoxia (without oxygen)
anti-	against	antibiotic (against life)
auto-	self	autograft (a graft from one's own body)
brady-	slow	bradycardia (slow heartbeat)
de-	without	depigmentation (without pigment)
dys-	painful; difficult; abnormal	dysuria (painful urination); dyspnea (difficulty breathing); dystrophy (abnormal development)

PREFIX	MEANING	EXAMPLE (DEFINITION)
endo-	within; inner	endoscope (instrument to view within); endocardium (inner lining of heart)
epi-	above	epigastric (above the stomach)
eu-	normal	eupnea (normal breathing)
ex-	outward	exostosis (condition of outward, or projecting, bone)
extra-	outside of	extracorporeal (outside of the body)
hetero-	different	heterograft (graft [like a skin graft] from another species)
homo-	same	homograft (graft [like a skin graft] from the same species)
hyper-	excessive	hypertrophy (excessive development)
hypo-	below; insufficient	hypodermic (below the skin); hypoglycemia (insufficient blood sugar)
in-	not; inward	infertility (not fertile); inhalation (to breathe in)
inter-	between	intervertebral (between the vertebrae)
intra-	within	intravenous (within a vein)
macro-	large	macrotia (having large ears)
micro-	small	microtia (having small ears)
neo-	new	neonatology (study of the newborn)
para-	beside; abnormal; two like parts of a pair	paranasal (beside the nose); paresthesia (abnormal sensation); paraplegia (paralysis of two like parts of a pair [the legs])
per-	through	percutaneous (through the skin)
peri-	around	pericardial (around the heart)
post-	after	postpartum (after birth)
pre-	before	preoperative (before a surgical operation)
pro-	before	prolactin (before milk)
pseudo-	false	pseudocyesis (false pregnancy)
re-	again	reinfection (to infect again)
retro-	backward; behind	retrograde (to move backward); retroperitoneal (behind the peritoneum)
sub-	under	subcutaneous (under the skin)
tachy-	fast	tachycardia (fast heartbeat)
trans-	across	transurethral (across the urethra)
ultra-	beyond	ultrasound (beyond sound [high-frequency sound waves])
un-	not	unconscious (not conscious)

Word Watch

Be very careful with prefixes; many have similar spellings but very different meanings. For example:
inter- means "between"; *intra-* means "inside"
per- means "through"; *peri-* means "around"
re- means "again"; *retro-* means "behind"

Number Prefixes

Some common prefixes pertaining to the number of items or measurement, their meanings, and examples of their use are shown below.

PREFIX	MEANING	EXAMPLE (DEFINITION)
bi-	two	bilateral (two sides)
hemi-	half	hemiplegia (paralysis of one side/half of the body)
mono-	one	monoplegia (paralysis of one extremity)
multi-	many	multigravida (woman pregnant more than once)
nulli-	none	nulligravida (woman with no pregnancies)
pan-	all	pansinusitis (inflammation of all the sinuses)
poly-	many	polymyositis (inflammation of many muscles)
quadri-	four	quadriplegia (paralysis of all four limbs)
semi-	partial	semiconscious (partially conscious)
tetra-	four	tetraplegia (paralysis of all four limbs)
tri-	three	triceps (muscle with three heads)

Practice As You Go

C. Prefix Practice

Circle the prefixes in the following terms and then define them in the spaces provided.

1. tachycardia ______________________________
2. pseudocyesis ______________________________
3. hypoglycemia ______________________________
4. intercostal ______________________________
5. eupnea ______________________________
6. postoperative ______________________________
7. monoplegia ______________________________
8. subcutaneous ______________________________

Suffixes

A suffix is attached to the end of a word to add meaning, such as a condition, disease, or procedure. For example, the suffix *-itis*, meaning inflammation, when added to *cardi-* forms the new word **carditis** (car-DYE-tis), meaning inflammation of the heart. Every medical term *must* have a suffix. Most often

Med Term Tip

Remember, if a suffix begins with a vowel, the combining vowel is dropped; for example, *mastitis* rather than *mastoitis*.

the suffix is added to a word root, as in carditis above; however, terms can also be built from a suffix added directly to a prefix, without a word root. For example, the term **dystrophy** (DIS-troh-fee), meaning abnormal development, is built from the prefix *dys-* (meaning abnormal) and the suffix *-trophy* (meaning development).

Common Suffixes

Some common suffixes, their meanings, and examples of their use are shown below. When written by themselves, suffixes are preceded by a hyphen.

SUFFIX	MEANING	EXAMPLE (DEFINITION)
-algia	pain	gastralgia (stomach pain)
-cele	protrusion	cystocele (protrusion of the bladder)
-cyte	cell	erythrocyte (red cell)
-dynia	pain	cardiodynia (heart pain)
-ectasis	dilation	bronchiectasis (dilated bronchi)
-gen	that which produces	pathogen (that which produces disease)
-genic	producing	carcinogenic (cancer producing)
-ia	state, condition	bradycardia (condition of slow heart)
-iasis	abnormal condition	lithiasis (abnormal condition of stones)
-ism	state of	hypothyroidism (state of low thyroid)
-itis	inflammation	dermatitis (inflammation of skin)
-logist	one who studies	cardiologist (one who studies the heart)
-logy	study of	cardiology (study of the heart)
-lytic	destruction	thrombolytic (clot destruction)
-malacia	abnormal softening	chondromalacia (abnormal cartilage softening)
-megaly	enlarged	cardiomegaly (enlarged heart)
-oma	tumor, mass	carcinoma (cancerous tumor)
-opsy	view of	biopsy (view of life)
-osis	abnormal condition	cyanosis (abnormal condition of being blue)
-pathy	disease	myopathy (muscle disease)
-plasm	formation	neoplasm (new formation)
-plegia	paralysis	laryngoplegia (paralysis of larynx)
-ptosis	drooping	blepharoptosis (drooping eyelid)
-rrhage	excessive, abnormal flow	hemorrhage (excessive bleeding)
-rrhagia	abnormal flow condition	cystorrhagia (abnormal flow from the bladder)
-rrhea	discharge	rhinorrhea (discharge from the nose)
-rrhexis	rupture	hysterorrhexis (ruptured uterus)

SUFFIX	MEANING	EXAMPLE (DEFINITION)
-sclerosis	hardening	arteriosclerosis (hardening of an artery)
-stenosis	narrowing	angiostenosis (narrowing of a vessel)
-therapy	treatment	chemotherapy (treatment with chemicals)
-trophy	development	hypertrophy (excessive development)

Adjective Suffixes

The following suffixes are used to convert a word root into an adjective. These suffixes usually are translated as *pertaining to.*

SUFFIX	MEANING	EXAMPLE (DEFINITION)
-ac	pertaining to	cardiac (pertaining to the heart)
-al	pertaining to	duodenal (pertaining to the duodenum)
-an	pertaining to	ovarian (pertaining to the ovary)
-ar	pertaining to	ventricular (pertaining to a ventricle)
-ary	pertaining to	pulmonary (pertaining to the lungs)
-atic	pertaining to	lymphatic (pertaining to lymph)
-eal	pertaining to	esophageal (pertaining to the esophagus)
-iac	pertaining to	chondriac (pertaining to cartilage)
-ic	pertaining to	gastric (pertaining to the stomach)
-ile	pertaining to	penile (pertaining to the penis)
-ine	pertaining to	uterine (pertaining to the uterus)
-ior	pertaining to	superior (pertaining to above)
-nic	pertaining to	embryonic (pertaining to an embryo)
-ory	pertaining to	auditory (pertaining to hearing)
-ose	pertaining to	adipose (pertaining to fat)
-ous	pertaining to	intravenous (pertaining to within a vein)
-tic	pertaining to	acoustic (pertaining to hearing)

Surgical Suffixes

The following suffixes indicate surgical procedures.

SUFFIX	MEANING	EXAMPLE (DEFINITION)
-centesis	puncture to withdraw fluid	arthrocentesis (puncture to withdraw fluid from a joint)
-ectomy	surgical removal	gastrectomy (surgically remove the stomach)
-ostomy	surgically create an opening	colostomy (surgically create an opening for the colon [through the abdominal wall])

Med Term Tip

Surgical suffixes have very specific meanings:
-otomy means "to cut into"
-ostomy means "to surgically create an opening"
-ectomy means "to cut out" or "remove"

SUFFIX	MEANING	EXAMPLE (DEFINITION)
-otomy	cutting into	thoracotomy (cutting into the chest)
-pexy	surgical fixation	nephropexy (surgical fixation of a kidney)
-plasty	surgical repair	dermatoplasty (surgical repair of the skin)
-rrhaphy	to suture	myorrhaphy (suture together muscle)
-tome	instrument to cut	dermatome (instrument to cut skin)

Procedural Suffixes

The following suffixes indicate procedural processes or instruments.

SUFFIX	MEANING	EXAMPLE (DEFINITION)
-gram	record or picture	electrocardiogram (record of heart's electricity)
-graphy	process of recording	electrocardiography (process of recording the heart's electrical activity)
-meter	instrument for measuring	audiometer (instrument to measure hearing)
-metry	process of measuring	audiometry (process of measuring hearing)
-scope	instrument for viewing	gastroscope (instrument to view stomach)
-scopic	pertaining to visually examining	endoscopic (pertaining to visually examining within)
-scopy	process of visually examining	gastroscopy (process of visually examining the stomach)

Practice As You Go

D. Combining Form and Suffix Practice

Join a combining form and a suffix to form words with the following meanings.

1. study of lungs ____________
2. nose discharge ____________
3. abnormal softening of a kidney ____________
4. enlarged heart ____________
5. cutting into the stomach ____________
6. inflammation of the skin ____________
7. surgical removal of the voice box ____________
8. surgical repair of a joint ____________

Word Building

Word building consists of putting together two or more word elements to form a variety of terms. Prefixes and suffixes may be added to a combining form to create a new descriptive term. For example, adding the prefix *hypo-* (meaning below) and the suffix *-ic* (meaning pertaining to) to the combining form *derm/o* (meaning skin) forms **hypodermic** (high-poh-DER-mik), which means pertaining to below the skin.

Interpreting Medical Terms

The following strategy is a reliable method for puzzling out the meaning of an unfamiliar medical term.

STEP	EXAMPLE
1. Divide the term into its word parts.	gastr/o/enter/o/logy
2. Define each word part.	**gastr** = stomach **o** = combining vowel, no meaning **enter** = small intestine **o** = combining vowel, no meaning **-logy** = study of
3. Combine the meaning of the word parts.	stomach, small intestine, study of

Med Term Tip

To gain a quick understanding of a term, it may be helpful to you to read from the end of the word (or the suffix) back to the beginning (the prefix), and then pick up the word root. For example, *pericarditis* reads inflammation (*-itis*) around (*peri-*) the heart (*cardi/o*).

Pronunciation

You may hear different pronunciations for the same terms depending on where a person was born or educated. As long as it is clear which term people are discussing, differing pronunciations are acceptable. Some people are difficult to understand over the telephone or on a transcription tape. If you have any doubt about a term being discussed, ask for the term to be spelled. For example, it is often difficult to hear the difference between the terms **abduction** and **adduction**. However, since the terms refer to opposite directions of movement, it is very important to double-check if there is any question about which term is being used.

Each new term in this book is introduced in boldface type, with the phonetic or "sounds like" pronunciation in parentheses immediately following. The part of the word that should receive the greatest emphasis during pronunciation appears in capital letters, for example, **pericarditis** (per-ih-car-DYE-tis). Each term presented in this book is also pronounced on the accompanying My Medical Terminology Lab website (*www.mymedicalterminologylab.com*). Listen to each word, then pronounce it silently to yourself or out loud.

Spelling

Although you may hear differing pronunciations of the same term, there is only one correct spelling. If you have any doubt about the spelling of a term or of its meaning, always look it up in a medical dictionary. If only one letter of the word is changed, it can make a critical difference for the patient. For example, imagine the problem that could arise if you note for insurance purposes that a portion of a patient's **ileum**, or small intestine, was removed when in reality he had surgery for removal of a piece of his **ilium**, or hip bone.

Med Term Tip

If you have any doubt about the meaning or spelling of a word, look it up in your medical dictionary. Even experienced medical personnel still need to look up a few words.

Some words have the same beginning sounds but are spelled differently. Examples include:

Sounds like *si*

psy	**psychiatry** (sigh-KIGH-ah-tree)
cy	**cytology** (sigh-TALL-oh-gee)

Sounds like *dis*

dys	**dyspepsia** (dis-PEP-see-ah)
dis	**dislocation** (dis-low-KAY-shun)

Singular and Plural Endings

Many medical terms originate from Greek and Latin words. The rules for forming the singular and plural forms of some words follow the rules of these languages rather than English. For example, the heart has a left atrium and a right atrium for a total of two *atria,* not two *atriums.* Other words, such as *virus* and *viruses,* are changed from singular to plural by following English rules. Each medical term needs to be considered individually when changing from the singular to the plural form. The following examples illustrate how to form plurals.

WORDS ENDING IN	SINGULAR	PLURAL
-a	vertebra	vertebrae
-ax	thorax	thoraces
-ex or -ix	appendix	appendices
-is	metastasis	metastases
-ma	sarcoma	sarcomata
-nx	phalanx	phalanges
-on	ganglion	ganglia
-us	nucleus	nuclei
-um	ovum	ova
-y	biopsy	biopsies

Practice As You Go

E. Make It Plural

Change the following singular terms to plural terms.

1. metastasis ______________________
2. ovum ______________________
3. diverticulum ______________________
4. atrium ______________________
5. diagnosis ______________________
6. vertebra ______________________

Abbreviations

Abbreviations are commonly used in the medical profession as a way of saving time. However, some abbreviations can be confusing, such as *SM* for simple mastectomy and *sm* for small. Using incorrect abbreviations can result in problems for a patient, as well as with insurance records and processing. If you have any concern that you will confuse someone by using an abbreviation, spell out the word instead. It is never acceptable to use made-up abbreviations. All types of healthcare facilities will have a list of approved abbreviations, and it is extremely important that you become familiar with this list and follow it closely. Throughout this book abbreviations are included, when possible, immediately following terms. Additionally, a list of common abbreviations for each body system is provided in each chapter. Finally, Appendix III offers a complete alphabetical listing of all the abbreviations used in this text.

The Medical Record

The **medical record** or chart documents the details of a patient's hospital stay. Each healthcare professional that has contact with the patient in any capacity completes the appropriate report of that contact and adds it to the medical chart. This results in a permanent physical record of the patient's day-to-day condition, when and what services he or she received, and the response to treatment. Each institution adopts a specific format for each document and its location within the chart. This is necessary because each healthcare professional must be able to locate quickly and efficiently the information he or she needs in order to provide proper care for the patient. The medical record is also a legal document. Therefore, it is essential that all chart components be completely filled out and signed. Each page must contain the proper patient identification information: the patient's name, age, gender, physician, admission date, and identification number.

While the patient is still in the hospital, a unit clerk is usually responsible for placing documents in the proper place. After discharge, the medical records department ensures that all documents are present, complete, signed, and in the correct order. If a person is readmitted, especially for the same diagnosis, parts of this previous chart can be pulled and added to the current chart for reference (see Figure 1.2 ■). Physicians' offices and other outpatient care providers such as clinics and therapists also maintain a medical record detailing each patient's visit to their facility.

The digital revolution has also impacted healthcare with the increasing use of the **Electronic Medical Record** (EMR). A software program allows you to enter patient information into a computer or tablet, which then organizes and stores the information. You enter information either at a centralized workstation or by using mobile devices at the point of care. Once digitally stored, the information may be analyzed and monitored to detect and prevent potential errors. Since the records are digitally stored, they can be accessed and shared between healthcare providers easily, which reduces unnecessary repetition of tests and inadvertent medication errors. The following list includes the most common elements of a paper chart with a brief description.

History and Physical—Written or dictated by admitting physician; details patient's history, results of physician's examination, initial diagnoses, and physician's plan of treatment

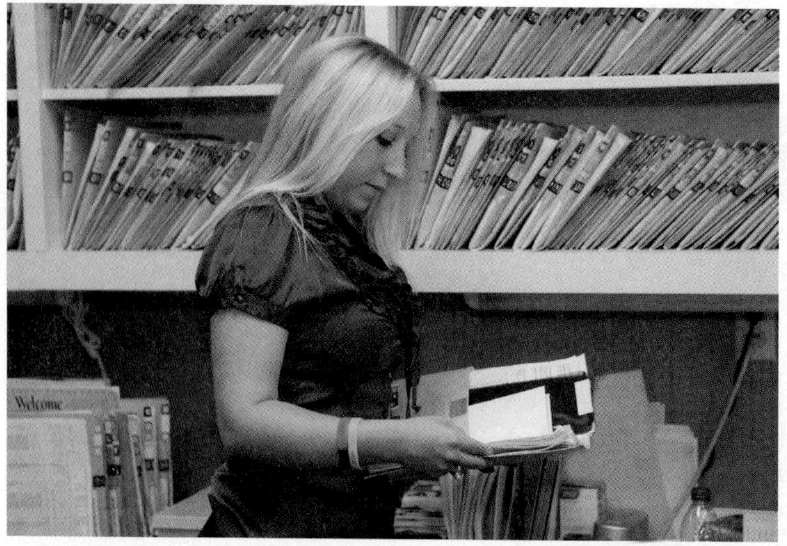

■ **Figure 1.2** Health information professionals maintain accurate, orderly, and permanent patient records. Medical records are securely stored and available for future reference. *(B. Franklin/ Shutterstock)*

Physician's Orders—Complete list of care, medications, tests, and treatments physician orders for patient

Nurse's Notes—Record of patient's care throughout the day; includes vital signs, treatment specifics, patient's response to treatment, and patient's condition

Physician's Progress Notes—Physician's daily record of patient's condition, results of physician's examinations, summary of test results, updated assessment and diagnoses, and further plans for patient's care

Consultation Reports—Reports given by specialists whom physician has asked to evaluate patient

Ancillary Reports—Reports from various treatments and therapies patient has received, such as rehabilitation, social services, or respiratory therapy

Diagnostic Reports—Results of diagnostic tests performed on patient, principally from clinical lab (e.g., blood tests) and medical imaging (e.g., X-rays and ultrasound)

Informed Consent—Document voluntarily signed by patient or a responsible party that clearly describes purpose, methods, procedures, benefits, and risks of a diagnostic or treatment procedure

Operative Report—Report from surgeon detailing an operation; includes pre- and postoperative diagnosis, specific details of surgical procedure itself, and how patient tolerated procedure

Anesthesiologist's Report—Relates details regarding substances (such as medications and fluids) given to patient, patient's response to anesthesia, and vital signs during surgery

Pathologist's Report—Report given by pathologist who studies tissue removed from patient (e.g., bone marrow, blood, or tissue biopsy)

Discharge Summary—Comprehensive outline of patient's entire hospital stay; includes condition at time of admission, admitting diagnosis, test results, treatments and patient's response, final diagnosis, and follow-up plans

Healthcare Settings

The use of medical terminology is widespread. It provides healthcare professionals with a precise and efficient method of communicating very specific patient information to one another, regardless of whether they are in the same type of facility (see Figure 1.3 ■). What follows are descriptions of the different types of settings where medical terminology is used.

Acute Care or General Hospitals—Provide services to diagnose (laboratory, diagnostic imaging) and treat (surgery, medications, therapy) diseases for a short period of time; in addition, they usually provide emergency and obstetrical care

Specialty Care Hospitals—Provide care for very specific types of diseases; for example, a psychiatric hospital

Nursing Homes or Long-Term Care Facilities—Provide long-term care for patients needing extra time to recover from illness or injury before returning home, or for persons who can no longer care for themselves

Ambulatory Care Centers, Surgical Centers, or Outpatient Clinics—Provide services not requiring overnight hospitalization; services range from simple surgeries to diagnostic testing or therapy

Physicians' Offices—Provide diagnostic and treatment services in a private office setting

Health Maintenance Organization (HMO)—Provides wide range of services by a group of primary-care physicians, specialists, and other healthcare professionals in a prepaid system

Home Health Care—Provides nursing, therapy, personal care, or housekeeping services in patient's own home

Rehabilitation Centers—Provide intensive physical and occupational therapy; includes inpatient and outpatient treatment

Hospices—Provide supportive treatment to terminally ill patients and their families

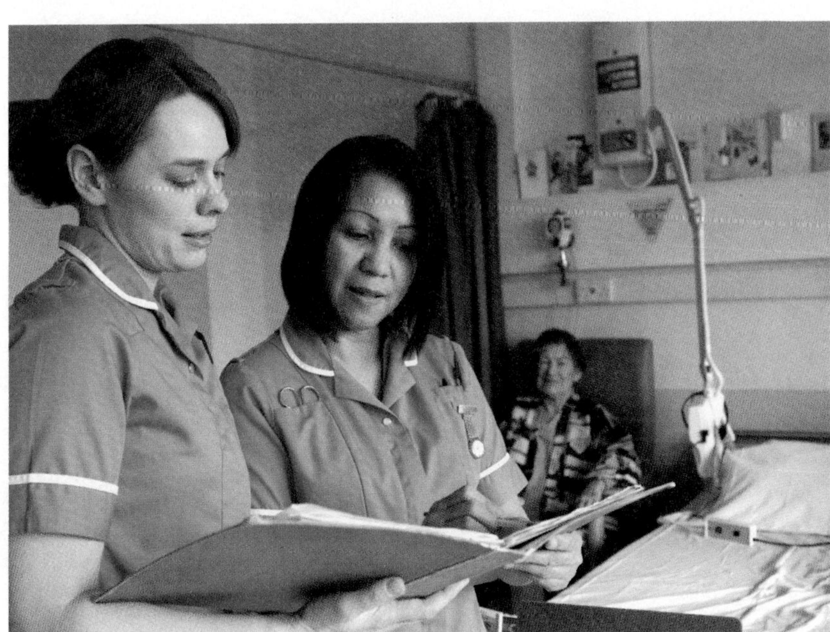

■ **Figure 1.3** A nurse and medical assistant review a patient's chart and plan his or her daily care. *(Life in View/ Science Source)*

Confidentiality

Anyone working with medical terminology and involved in the medical profession must have a firm understanding of confidentiality. Any information or record relating to a patient must be considered privileged. This means that you have a moral and legal responsibility to keep all information about the patient confidential. If you are asked to supply documentation relating to a patient, the proper authorization form must be signed by the patient. Give only the specific information that the patient has authorized. The Health Insurance Portability and Accountability Act of 1996 (HIPAA) set federal standards providing patients with more protection of their medical records and health information, better access to their own records, and greater control over how their health information is used and to whom it is disclosed.

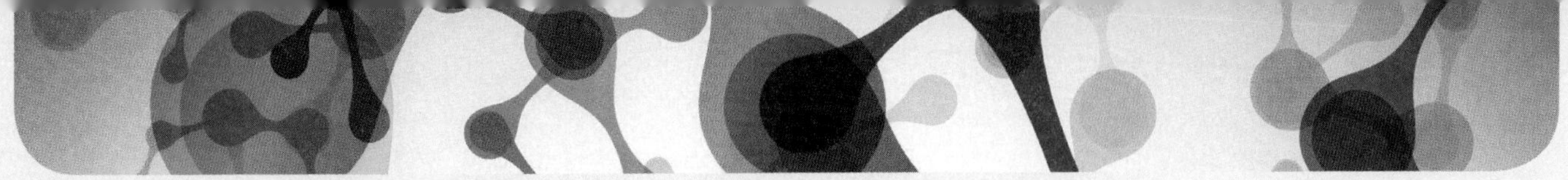

Chapter Review

Practice Exercises

A. Terminology Matching

Match each definition to its term.

1. ________ Provides services for a short period of time	a. rehabilitation center
2. ________ Complete outline of a patient's entire hospital stay	b. nurse's notes
3. ________ Describes purpose, methods, benefits, and risks of procedure	c. ancillary report
4. ________ Contains updated assessment, diagnoses, and further plans for care	d. hospice
5. ________ Provides supportive care to terminally ill patients and families	e. discharge summary
6. ________ Written by the admitting physician	f. physician's progress notes
7. ________ Reports results from study of tissue removed from the patient	g. ambulatory care center
8. ________ Written by the surgeon	h. diagnostic report
9. ________ Provides services not requiring overnight hospital stay	i. long-term care facility
10. ________ Report given by a specialist	j. informed consent
11. ________ Record of a patient's care throughout the day	k. history and physical
12. ________ Clinical lab and medical imaging reports	l. acute care hospital
13. ________ Provides intensive physical and occupational therapy	m. pathologist's report
14. ________ Report of treatment/therapy the patient received	n. consultation report
15. ________ Provides care for patients who need more time to recover	o. operative report

B. Define the Suffix

1. **-plasty** ______________________________
2. **-stenosis** ______________________________
3. **-itis** ______________________________
4. **-al** ______________________________
5. **-algia** ______________________________
6. **-otomy** ______________________________
7. **-megaly** ______________________________

8. **-ectomy** __________

9. **-rrhage** __________

10. **-centesis** __________

11. **-gram** __________

12. **-ac** __________

13. **-malacia** __________

14. **-ism** __________

15. **-rrhaphy** __________

16. **-ostomy** __________

17. **-pexy** __________

18. **-rrhea** __________

19. **-scopy** __________

20. **-oma** __________

C. Name That Prefix

1. inner __________

2. large __________

3. before __________

4. around __________

5. new __________

6. without __________

7. half __________

8. painful, difficult __________

9. excessive __________

10. above __________

11. many __________

12. slow __________

13. self __________

14. across __________

15. two __________

D. Building Medical Terms

Build a medical term by combining the word parts requested in each question.

For example, use the combining form for *spleen* with the suffix meaning *enlargement* to form a word meaning *enlargement of the spleen* (answer: *splenomegaly*).

1. combining form for *heart* ______
   suffix meaning *abnormal softening* ______
   ______ term meaning *softening of the heart*

2. word root form for *stomach* ______
   suffix meaning *to surgically create an opening* ______
   ______ term meaning *creating an opening into the stomach*

3. combining form for *nose* ______
   suffix meaning *surgical repair* ______
   ______ term meaning *surgical repair of the nose*

4. prefix meaning *excessive* ______
   suffix meaning *development* ______
   ______ term meaning *excessive development*

5. combining form meaning *disease* ______
   suffix meaning *the study of* ______
   ______ term meaning *the study of disease*

6. word root meaning *nerve* ______
   suffix for *tumor/mass* ______
   ______ term meaning *nerve tumor*

7. combining form meaning *stomach* ______
   combining form meaning *small intestine* ______
   suffix meaning *study of* ______
   ______ term meaning *study of stomach and small intestine*

8. word root meaning *ear* ______
   suffix meaning *inflammation* ______
   ______ term meaning *ear inflammation*

9. prefix meaning *chemical* ______
   suffix meaning *treatment* ______
   ______ term meaning *chemical treatment*

10. combining form meaning *cancer* ______
    suffix meaning *that which produces* ______
    ______ term meaning *that which produces cancer*

E. Define the Combining Form

1. **bi/o** ______________________________
2. **carcin/o** ______________________________
3. **cardi/o** ______________________________
4. **chem/o** ______________________________
5. **cis/o** ______________________________
6. **dermat/o** ______________________________
7. **enter/o** ______________________________
8. **gastr/o** ______________________________
9. **gynec/o** ______________________________
10. **hemat/o** ______________________________
11. **immun/o** ______________________________
12. **laryng/o** ______________________________
13. **path/o** ______________________________
14. **nephr/o** ______________________________
15. **neur/o** ______________________________
16. **ophthalm/o** ______________________________
17. **ot/o** ______________________________
18. **pulmon/o** ______________________________
19. **rhin/o** ______________________________

2

Body Organization

Learning Objectives

Upon completion of this chapter, you will be able to

- Recognize the combining forms introduced in this chapter.
- Correctly spell and pronounce medical terms and anatomical structures relating to body structure.
- Discuss the organization of the body in terms of cells, tissues, organs, and systems.
- Describe the common features of cells.
- Define the four types of tissues.
- List the major organs found in the 12 organ systems and their related medical specialties.
- Describe the anatomical position.
- Define the body planes.
- Identify regions of the body.
- List the body cavities and their contents.
- Locate and describe the nine anatomical and four clinical divisions of the abdomen.
- Define directional and positional terms.
- Build body organization medical terms from word parts.
- Interpret abbreviations associated with body organization.

Body Organization at a Glance

Arrangement

The body is organized into levels; each is built from the one below it. In other words, the body as a whole is composed of systems, a system is composed of organs, an organ is composed of tissues, and tissues are composed of cells.

Levels

cells **tissues** **organs** **systems** **body**

Word Parts

Presented here are some of the more common combining forms used to build body organizational terms.

Combining Forms

abdomin/o	abdomen
adip/o	fat
anter/o	front
brachi/o	arm
cardi/o	heart
caud/o	tail
cephal/o	head
cervic/o	neck
chondr/o	cartilage
crani/o	skull
crin/o	to secrete
crur/o	leg
cyt/o	cell
dermat/o	skin
dist/o	away from
dors/o	back
enter/o	small intestine
epitheli/o	epithelium
gastr/o	stomach
glute/o	buttock
gynec/o	woman
hemat/o	blood
hist/o	tissue
immun/o	protection
infer/o	below
inguin/o	groin
laryng/o	larynx
later/o	side
lumb/o	loin (low back)
lymph/o	lymph
medi/o	middle
muscul/o	muscle
nephr/o	kidney
neur/o	nerve
ophthalm/o	eye
orth/o	straight, upright
ot/o	ear
pariet/o	cavity wall
ped/o	foot
pelv/o	pelvis
peritone/o	peritoneum
pleur/o	pleura
poster/o	back
proct/o	rectum and anus
proxim/o	near to
pub/o	genital region
pulmon/o	lung
rhin/o	nose
spin/o	spine
super/o	above
thorac/o	chest
ur/o	urine
urin/o	urine
vascul/o	blood vessel
ventr/o	belly
vertebr/o	vertebra
viscer/o	internal organ

Body Organization Illustrated

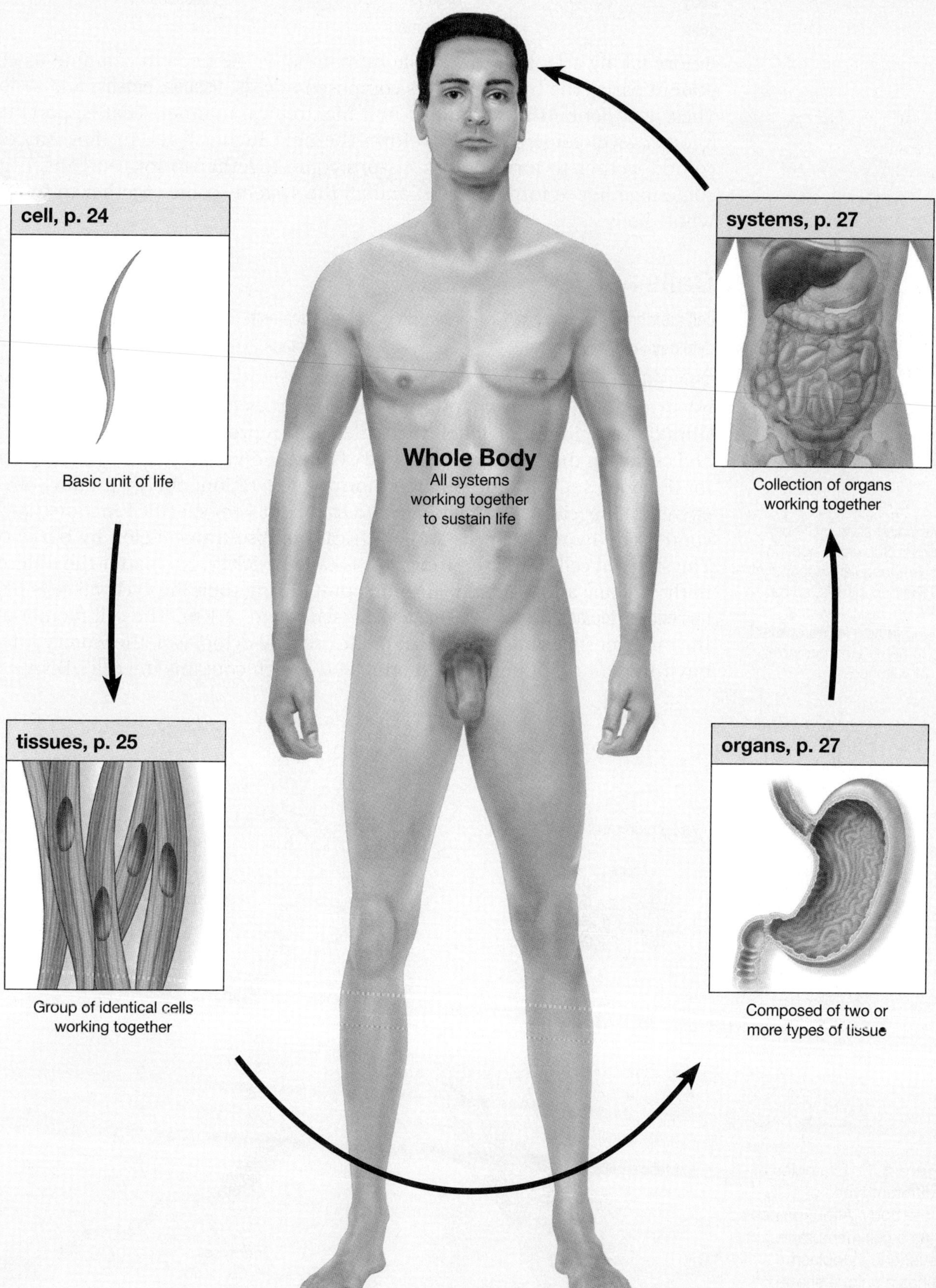

Levels of Body Organization

body **organs** **tissues**
cells **systems**

Before taking a look at the whole human body, we need to examine its component parts. The human **body** is composed of **cells, tissues, organs**, and **systems**. These components are arranged in a hierarchical manner. That is, parts from a lower level come together to form the next higher level. In that way, cells come together to form tissues, tissues come together to form organs, organs come together to form systems, and all the systems come together to form the whole body.

Cells

cell membrane **cytoplasm** (SIGH-toh-plazm)
cytology (sigh-TALL-oh-jee) **nucleus**

What's In A Name?
Look for these word parts:
cyt/o = cell
-logy = study of
-plasm = formation

Med Term Tip
Cells were first seen by Robert Hooke over 300 years ago. To him, the rectangular shapes looked like prison cells, so he named them cells. It was a common practice for early anatomists to name an organ solely on its appearance.

The cell is the fundamental unit of all living things. That is to say, it is the smallest structure of a body that has all the properties of being alive: responding to stimuli, engaging in metabolic activities, and reproducing itself. All the tissues and organs in the body are composed of cells. Individual cells perform functions for the body such as reproduction, hormone secretion, energy production, and excretion. Special cells are also able to carry out very specific functions, such as contraction by muscle cells and electrical impulse transmission by nerve cells. The study of cells and their functions is called **cytology**. No matter the difference in their shape and function, at some point during their life cycle all cells have a **nucleus, cytoplasm**, and a **cell membrane** (see Figure 2.1 ■). The cell membrane is the outermost boundary of a cell. It encloses the cytoplasm, the watery internal environment of the cell, and the nucleus, which contains the cell's DNA.

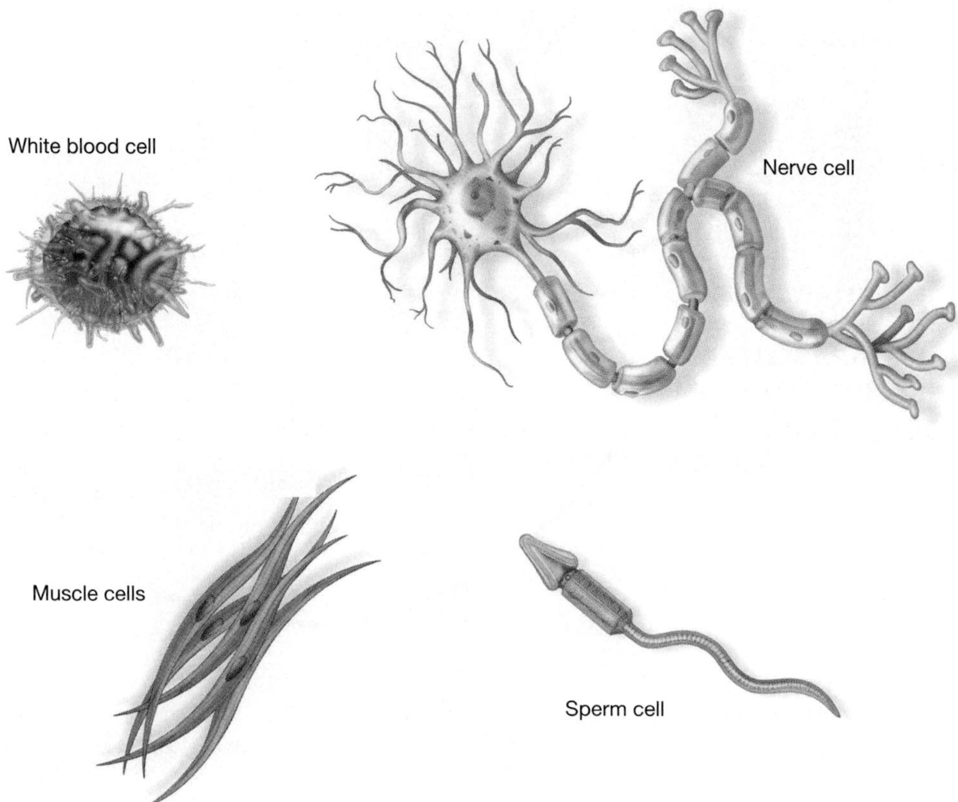

■ **Figure 2.1** Examples of four different types of cells from the body. Although each cell has a cell membrane, nucleus, and cytoplasm, each has a unique shape depending on its location and function.

Tissues

connective tissue
epithelial tissue (ep-ih-THEE-lee-al)
histology (hiss-TALL-oh-jee)
muscular tissue
nervous tissue

Histology is the study of tissue. A tissue is formed when like cells are grouped together and function together to perform a specific activity. The body has four types of tissue: **muscular tissue**, **epithelial tissue**, **connective tissue**, and **nervous tissue** (see Figure 2.2 ■).

What's In A Name?
Look for these word parts:
epitheli/o = epithelium
hist/o = tissue
muscul/o = muscle
-al = pertaining to
-ar = pertaining to
-logy = study of
-ous = pertaining to

Muscular Tissue

cardiac muscle
smooth muscle
muscle fibers
skeletal muscle

Muscular tissue produces movement in the body through contraction, or shortening in length, and is composed of individual muscle cells called **muscle fibers**. Muscle tissue forms one of three basic types of muscles: **skeletal muscle**, **smooth muscle**, or **cardiac muscle**. Skeletal muscle is attached to bone. Smooth muscle is found in internal organs such as the intestine, uterus, and blood vessels. Cardiac muscle is found only in the heart.

What's In A Name?
Look for these word parts:
cardi/o = heart
-ac = pertaining to
-al = pertaining to

Epithelial Tissue

epithelium (ep-ih-THEE-lee-um)

Epithelial tissue, or **epithelium**, is found throughout the body and is composed of close-packed cells that form the covering for and lining of body structures. For example, both the top layer of skin and the lining of the stomach are epithelial tissue (see Figure 2.2). In addition to forming a protective barrier, epithelial tissue may be specialized to absorb substances (such as nutrients from the intestine), secrete substances (such as sweat glands), or excrete wastes (such as the kidney tubules).

Med Term Tip
The term *epithelium* comes from the prefix *epi-* meaning "on top of" and the combining form *theli/o* meaning "nipple" (referring to any projection from the surface).

Connective Tissue

adipose (ADD-ih-pohs)
bone
cartilage (CAR-tih-lij)
tendons

Connective tissue is the supporting and protecting tissue in body structures. Because connective tissue performs many different functions depending on its location, it appears in many different forms so that each is able to perform the task required at that location. For example, **bone** provides structural support for the whole body. **Cartilage** is the shock absorber in joints. **Tendons** tightly connect skeletal muscles to bones. **Adipose** provides protective padding around body structures (see Figure 2.2).

What's In A Name?
Look for these word parts:
adip/o = fat
-ose = pertaining to

Nervous Tissue

brain
nerves
neurons
spinal cord

Nervous tissue is composed of cells called **neurons** (see Figure 2.2). This tissue forms the **brain**, **spinal cord**, and a network of **nerves** throughout the entire body, allowing for the conduction of electrical impulses to send information between the brain and the rest of the body.

What's In A Name?
Look for these word parts:
neur/o = nerve
spin/o = spine
-al = pertaining to

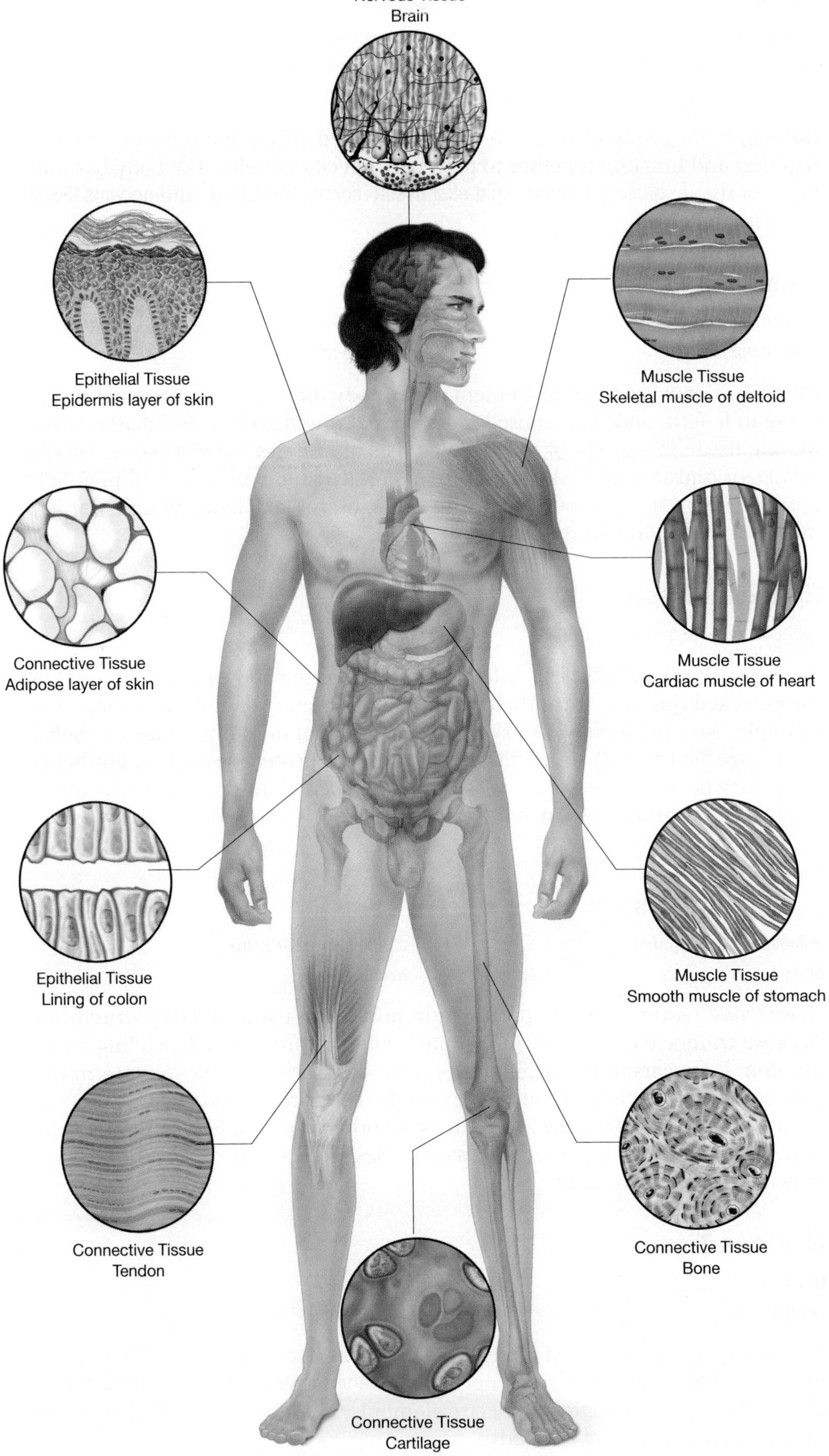

■ **Figure 2.2** The appearance of different types of tissues—muscle, epithelial, nervous, connective—and their location within the body.

Practice as You Go

A. Complete the Statement

1. The levels of organization of the body in order from smallest to largest are: ____________________, ____________________, ____________________, ____________________, ____________________.
2. No matter its shape, all cells have a ____________________, ____________________, and ____________________.
3. ____________________ tissue lines internal organs and serves as a covering for the skin.
4. ____________________ muscle is located in the heart, ____________________ muscle is attached to bones, and ____________________ muscle is found in internal organs.
5. Cartilage and tendons are examples of ____________________ tissue.
6. Nervous tissue is composed of ____________________.

Organs and Systems

Organs are composed of several different types of tissue that work as a unit to perform special functions. For example, the stomach contains smooth muscle tissue, nervous tissue, and epithelial tissue that allow it to contract to mix food with digestive juices.

A system is composed of several organs working in a coordinated manner to perform a complex function or functions. To continue with our example, the stomach plus the other digestive system organs—the oral cavity, esophagus, liver, pancreas, small intestine, and colon—work together to ingest, digest, and absorb our food.

Table 2.1 ■ presents the organ systems that are discussed in this book along with the major organs found in each system, the system functions, and the medical specialties that treat conditions of that system.

Table 2.1 Organ Systems of the Human Body

System and Medical Specialty	Word Parts	Structures	Functions
Integumentary System (in-teg-you-MEN-tah-ree) **dermatology** (der-mah-TALL-oh-jee)	-ary = pertaining to dermat/o = skin -logy = study of	• Skin • Hair • Nails • Sweat glands • Sebaceous glands	Forms protective two-way barrier and aids in temperature regulation.

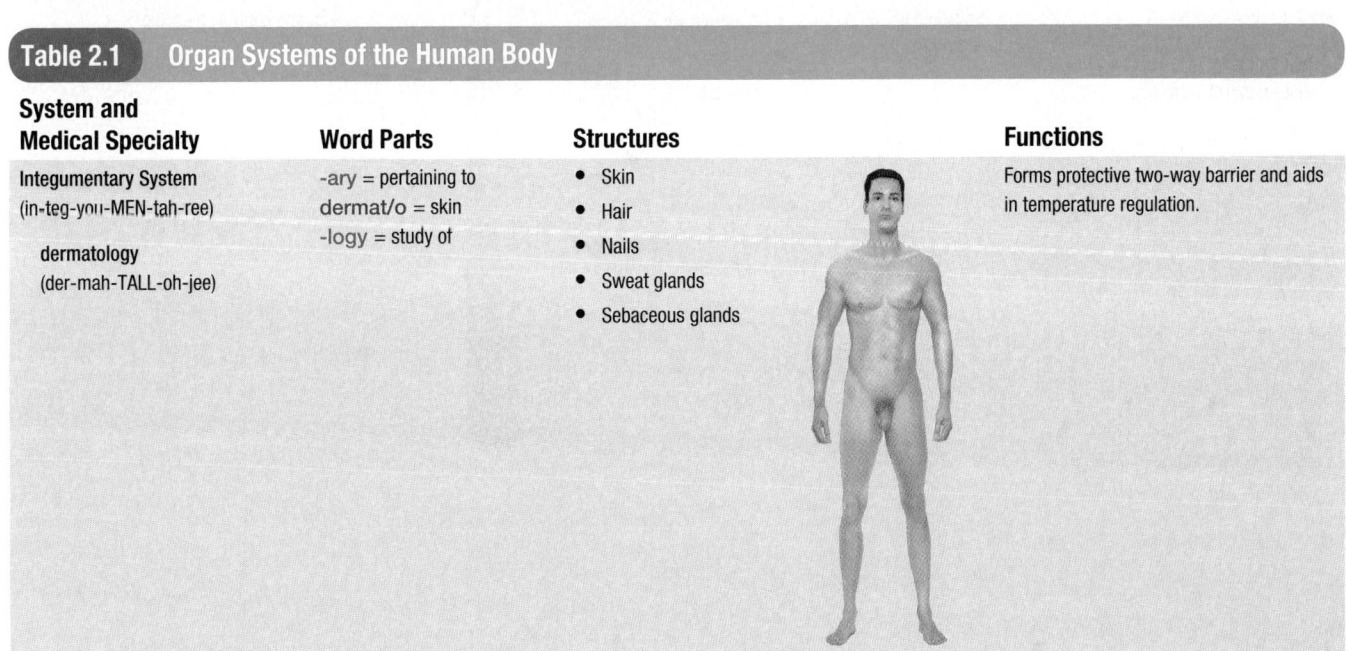

Table 2.1 Organ Systems of the Human Body (continued)

System and Medical Specialty	Word Parts	Structures		Functions
Musculoskeletal System (MS) (mus-qu-low-SKEL-et-all) **orthopedics** (or-thoh-PEE-diks) **orthopedic surgery** (or-thoh-PEE-dik)	muscul/o = muscle -al = pertaining to orth/o = straight ped/o = foot -ic = pertaining to	• Bones • Joints • Muscles	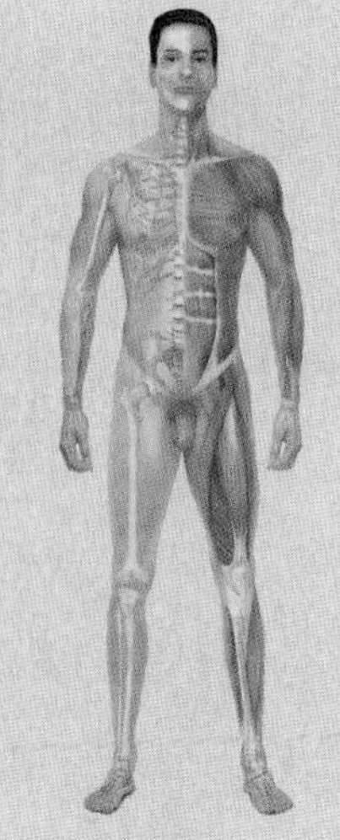	Skeleton supports and protects the body, forms blood cells, and stores minerals. Muscles produce movement.
Cardiovascular System (CV) (car-dee-oh-VAS-kew-lar) **cardiology** (car-dee-ALL-oh-jee)	cardi/o = heart vascul/o = blood vessel -ar = pertaining to -logy = study of	• Heart • Arteries • Veins	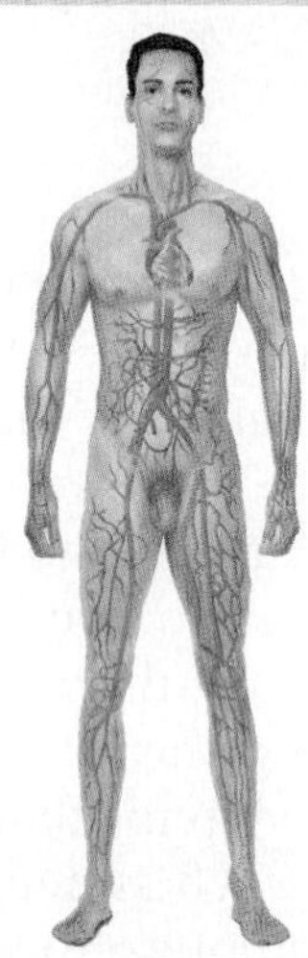	Pumps blood throughout the entire body to transport nutrients, oxygen, and wastes.
Blood (Hematic System) (he-MAT-tik) **hematology** (hee-mah-TALL-oh-jee)	hemat/o = blood -ic = pertaining to -logy = study of	• Plasma • Erythrocytes • Leukocytes • Platelets	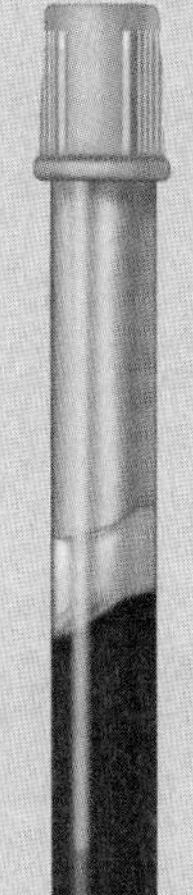	Transports oxygen, protects against pathogens, and controls bleeding.

Table 2.1 Organ Systems of the Human Body (continued)

System and Medical Specialty	Word Parts	Structures		Functions
Lymphatic System (lim-FAT-ik) **immunology** (im-yoo-NALL-oh-jee)	lymph/o = lymph -atic = pertaining to immun/o = protection -logy = study of	• Lymph nodes • Lymphatic vessels • Spleen • Thymus gland • Tonsils	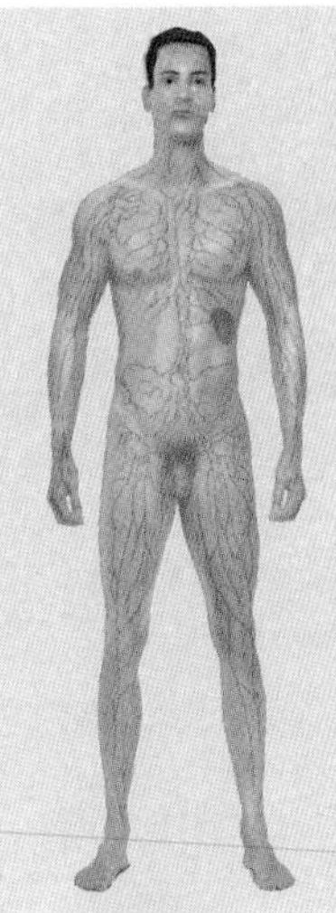	Protects the body from disease and invasion from pathogens.
Respiratory System **otorhinolaryngology** (ENT) (oh-toh-rye-noh-lair-ing-GALL-oh-jee) **pulmonology** (pull-mon-ALL-oh-jee) **thoracic surgery** (tho-RASS-ik)	-ory = pertaining to ot/o = ear rhin/o = nose laryng/o = larynx pulmon/o = lung thorac/o = chest -ic = pertaining to -logy = study of	• Nasal cavity • Pharynx • Larynx • Trachea • Bronchial tubes • Lungs	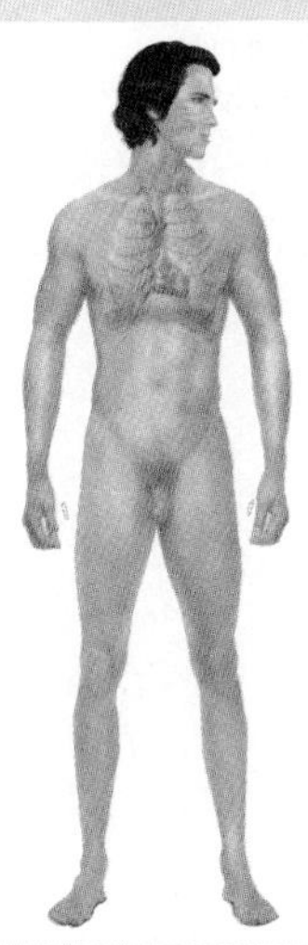	Obtains oxygen and removes carbon dioxide from the body.
Digestive or Gastrointestinal System (GI) **gastroenterology** (gas-troh-en-ter-ALL-oh-jee) **proctology** (prok-TOL-oh-jee)	gastr/o = stomach enter/o = small intestine proct/o = rectum and anus -al = pertaining to -logy = study of	• Oral cavity • Pharynx • Esophagus • Stomach • Small intestine • Colon • Liver • Gallbladder • Pancreas • Salivary glands	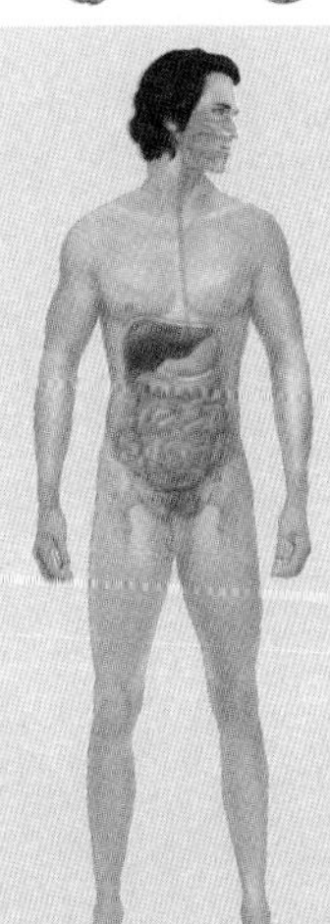	Ingests, digests, and absorbs nutrients for the body.

Table 2.1 Organ Systems of the Human Body (continued)

System and Medical Specialty	Word Parts	Structures		Functions
Urinary System (YOO-rih-nair-ee) **nephrology** (neh-FROL-oh-jee) **urology** (yoo-RALL-oh-jee)	urin/o = urine -ary = pertaining to nephr/o = kidney ur/o = urine -logy = study of	• Kidneys • Ureters • Urinary bladder • Urethra	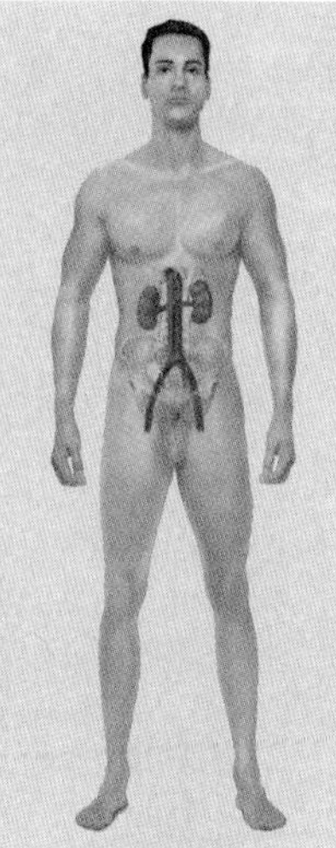	Filters waste products out of the blood and removes them from the body.
Female Reproductive System **gynecology** (GYN) (gigh-neh-KOL-oh-jee) **obstetrics** (OB) (ob-STET-riks)	gynec/o = female -logy = study of	• Ovary • Fallopian tubes • Uterus • Vagina • Vulva • Breasts	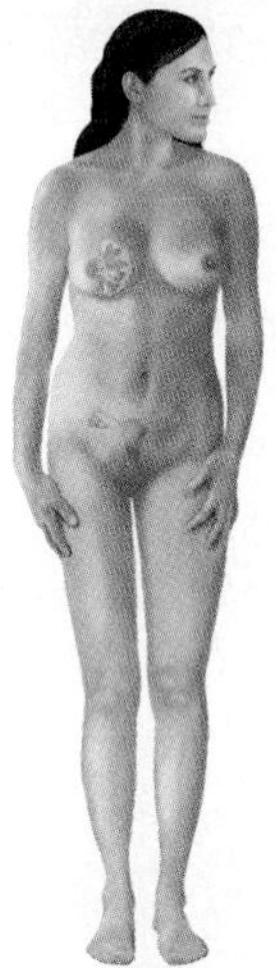	Produces eggs for reproduction and provides place for growing baby.
Male Reproductive System **urology** (yoo-RALL-oh-jee)	ur/o = urine -logy = study of	• Testes • Epididymis • Vas deferens • Penis • Seminal vesicles • Prostate gland • Bulbourethral gland	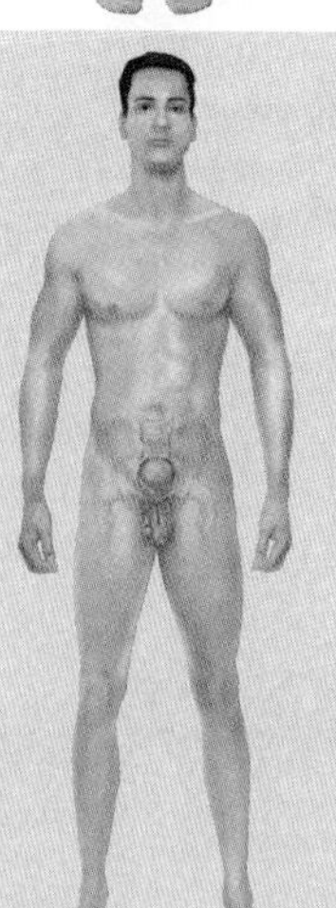	Produces sperm for reproduction.

Table 2.1 Organ Systems of the Human Body (continued)

System and Medical Specialty	Word Parts	Structures		Functions
Endocrine System (EN-doh-krin) **endocrinology** (en-doh-krin-ALL-oh-jee)	endo- = within crin/o = to secrete -ine = pertaining to -logy = study of	• Pituitary gland • Pineal gland • Thyroid gland • Parathyroid glands • Thymus gland • Adrenal glands • Pancreas • Ovaries • Testes	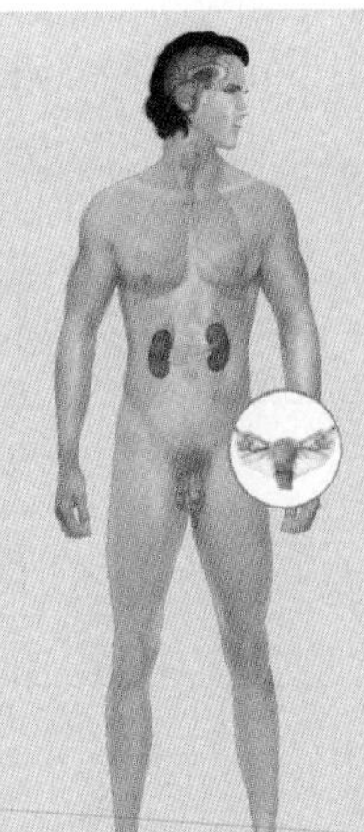	Regulates metabolic activities of the body.
Nervous System **neurology** (noo-RALL-oh-jee) **neurosurgery** (noo-roh-SIR-jer-ee)	-ous = pertaining to neur/o = nerve -logy = study of	• Brain • Spinal cord • Nerves	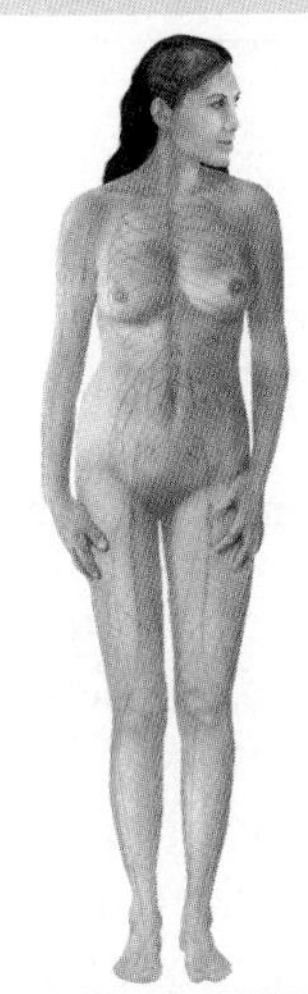	Receives sensory information and coordinates the body's response.
Special Senses **ophthalmology** (off-thal-MALL-oh-jee)	ophthalm/o = eye -logy = study of	• Eye	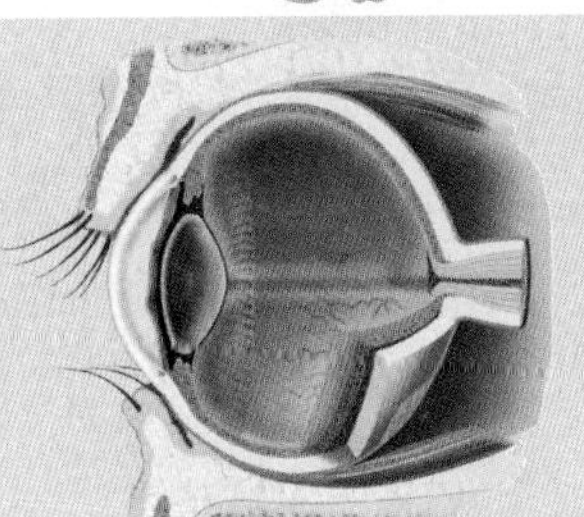	Vision
otorhinolaryngology (ENT) (oh-toh-rye-noh-lair-ing-GALL-oh-jee)	ot/o = ear rhin/o = nose laryng/o = larynx -logy = study of	• Ear	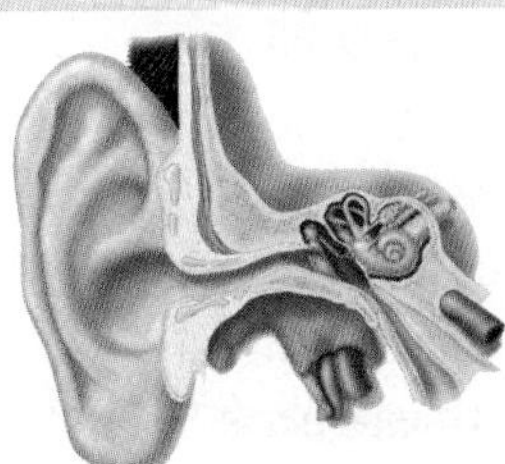	Hearing and balance

Practice as You Go

B. Organ System and Function Challenge

For each organ listed below, identify the name of the system it belongs to and then match it to its function.

	Organ	System	Function
1. ________	skin	________________	a. supports the body
2. ________	heart	________________	b. provides place for growing baby
3. ________	stomach	________________	c. filters waste products from blood
4. ________	uterus	________________	d. provides two-way barrier
5. ________	bones	________________	e. produces movement
6. ________	lungs	________________	f. produces sperm
7. ________	kidney	________________	g. ingests, digests, and absorbs nutrients
8. ________	testes	________________	h. coordinates body's response
9. ________	brain	________________	i. pumps blood through blood vessels
10. ________	muscles	________________	j. obtains oxygen

Body

anatomical position

What's In A Name?
Look for this word part:
-al = pertaining to

As seen from the previous sections, the body is the sum of all the systems, organs, tissues, and cells found within it. It is important to learn the anatomical terminology that applies to the body as a whole in order to correctly identify specific locations and directions when dealing with patients. The **anatomical position** is used when describing the positions and relationships of structures in the human body. A body in the anatomical position is standing erect with the arms at the sides of the body, the palms of the hands facing forward, and the eyes looking straight ahead. In addition, the legs are parallel with the feet, and the toes are pointing forward (see Figure 2.3 ■). For descriptive purposes the assumption is always that the person is in the anatomical position even if the body or parts of the body are in any other position.

Body Planes

coronal plane (kor-RONE-al)
coronal section
cross-section
frontal plane
frontal section
horizontal plane
longitudinal section
median plane
sagittal plane (SAJ-ih-tal)
sagittal section
transverse plane
transverse section

The terminology for body planes is used to assist medical personnel in describing the body and its parts. To understand body planes, imagine cuts slicing through the body at various angles. This imaginary slicing allows us to use more specific language when describing parts of the body. These body planes, illustrated in Figure 2.4 ■, include the following:

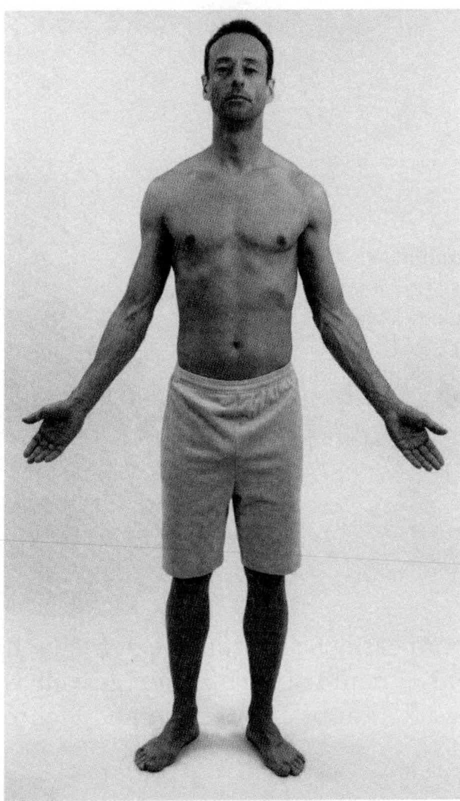

■ **Figure 2.3** The anatomical position: standing erect, gazing straight ahead, arms down at sides, palms facing forward, fingers extended, legs together, and toes pointing forward. *(Patrick Watson, Pearson Education)*

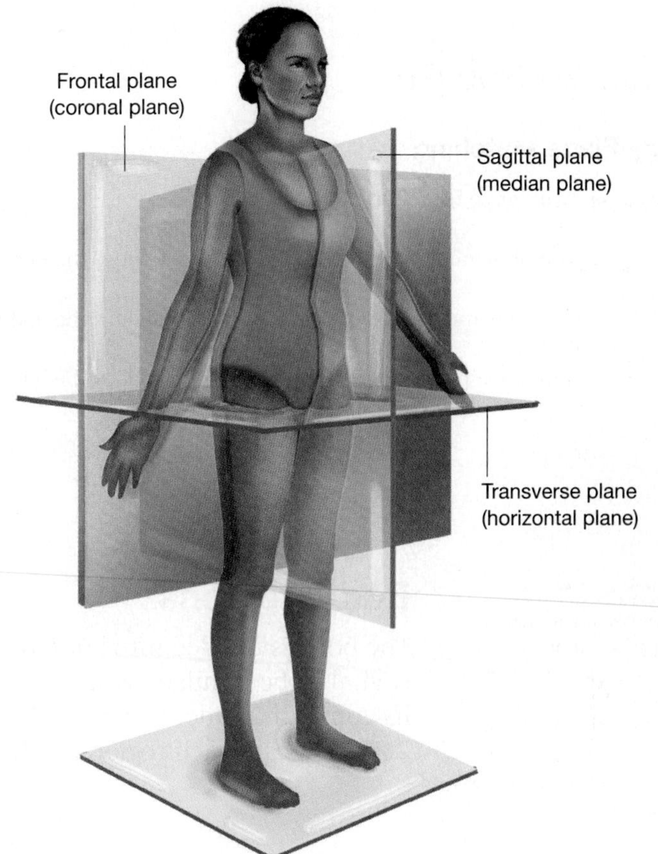

■ **Figure 2.4** The planes of the body. The sagittal plane is vertical from front to back, the frontal plane is vertical from left to right, and the transverse plane is horizontal.

1. **Sagittal plane:** This vertical plane runs lengthwise from front to back and divides the body or any of its parts into right and left portions. The right and left sides do not have to be equal. If the sagittal plane passes through the middle of the body, thus dividing it into equal right and left halves, it is called a **midsagittal** or **median plane**. A cut along the sagittal plane yields a **sagittal section** view of the inside of the body.
2. **Frontal plane:** The frontal, or **coronal plane**, divides the body into front and back portions; a vertical lengthwise plane is running from side to side. A cut along the frontal plane yields a **frontal** or **coronal section** view of the inside of the body.
3. **Transverse plane:** The transverse, or **horizontal plane**, is a crosswise plane that runs parallel to the ground. This imaginary cut would divide the body or its parts into upper and lower portions. A cut along the transverse plane yields a **transverse section** view of the inside of the body.

The terms **cross-section** and **longitudinal section** are frequently used to describe internal views of structures. A lengthwise slice along the long axis of a structure produces a longitudinal section. A slice perpendicular to the long axis of the structure produces a cross-section view.

What's In A Name?

Look for these word parts:
medi/o = middle
trans- = across
-al = pertaining to
-an = pertaining to

Practice As You Go

C. Body Plane Matching

Match each body plane to its definition.

1. ________ frontal plane
2. ________ sagittal plane
3. ________ transverse plane

a. divides the body into right and left
b. divides the body into upper and lower
c. divides the body into anterior and posterior

Med Term Tip

As you learn medical terminology, it is important that you remember not to use common phrases and terms any longer. Many people commonly use the term *stomach* (an organ) when they actually mean *abdomen* (a body region).

Body Regions

The body is divided into large regions that can easily be identified externally. It is vital to be familiar with both the anatomical name of each region as well as its common name. See Table 2.2 ■ for a description of each region and Figure 2.5 ■ to locate each region on the body.

Table 2.2 Terms Describing Body Regions

Region	Word Parts	Description
abdominal region (ab-DOM-ih-nal)	abdomin/o = abdomen -al = pertaining to	Abdomen; on anterior side of trunk
brachial region (BRAY-kee-all)	brachi/o = arm -al = pertaining to	Upper extremities (UE) or arms
cephalic region (seh-FAL-ik)	cephal/o = head -ic = pertaining to	Head
cervical region (SER-vih-kal)	cervic/o = neck -al = pertaining to	Neck; connects head to trunk
crural region (KREW-ral)	crur/o = leg -al = pertaining to	Lower extremities (LE) or legs
dorsum (DOOR-sum)	dors/o = back of body	Back; on posterior side of trunk
gluteal region (GLOO-tee-all)	glute/o = buttock -al = pertaining to	Buttocks; on posterior side of trunk
pelvic region (PELL-vik)	pelv/o = pelvis -ic = pertaining to	Pelvis; on anterior side of trunk
pubic region (PEW-bik)	pub/o = genital -ic = pertaining to	Region containing external genitals; on anterior side of trunk
thoracic region (tho-RASS-ik)	thorac/o = chest -ic = pertaining to	Chest; on anterior side of trunk; also called thorax
trunk		Contains all body regions other than head, neck, and extremities; also called torso
vertebral region (VER-tee-bral)	vertebr/o = vertebra -al = pertaining to	Overlies spinal column or vertebrae; on posterior side of trunk

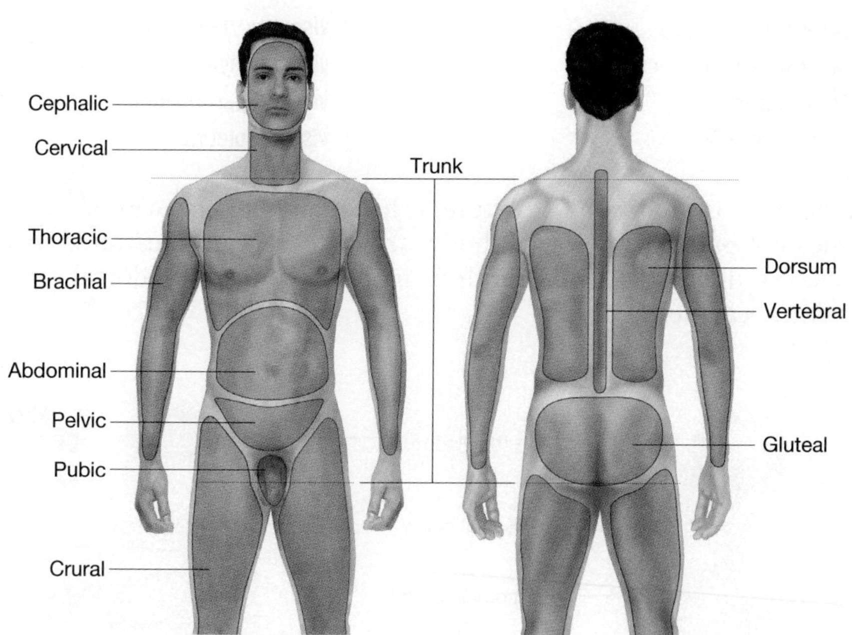

■ **Figure 2.5** Anterior and posterior views of the body illustrating the location of various body regions.

Practice As You Go

D. Body Region Practice

For each term below, write the corresponding body region.

1. head ______________________
2. genitals ______________________
3. leg ______________________
4. buttocks ______________________
5. neck ______________________
6. arm ______________________
7. back ______________________
8. chest ______________________

Body Cavities

abdominal cavity
abdominopelvic cavity (ab-dom-ih-noh-PELL-vik)
cranial cavity (KRAY-nee-al)
diaphragm (DYE-ah-fram)
mediastinum (mee-dee-ass-TYE-num)
parietal layer (pah-RYE-eh-tal)
parietal peritoneum
parietal pleura
pelvic cavity
pericardial cavity (pair-ih-CAR-dee-al)
peritoneum (pair-ih-toh-NEE-um)

pleura (PLOO-rah)
pleural cavity (PLOO-ral)
spinal cavity
thoracic cavity
viscera (VISS-er-ah)
visceral layer (VISS-er-al)
visceral peritoneum
visceral pleura

The body is not a solid structure; it has many open spaces or cavities. The cavities are part of the normal body structure and are illustrated in Figure 2.6 ■. We can divide the body into four major cavities—two dorsal cavities and two ventral cavities.

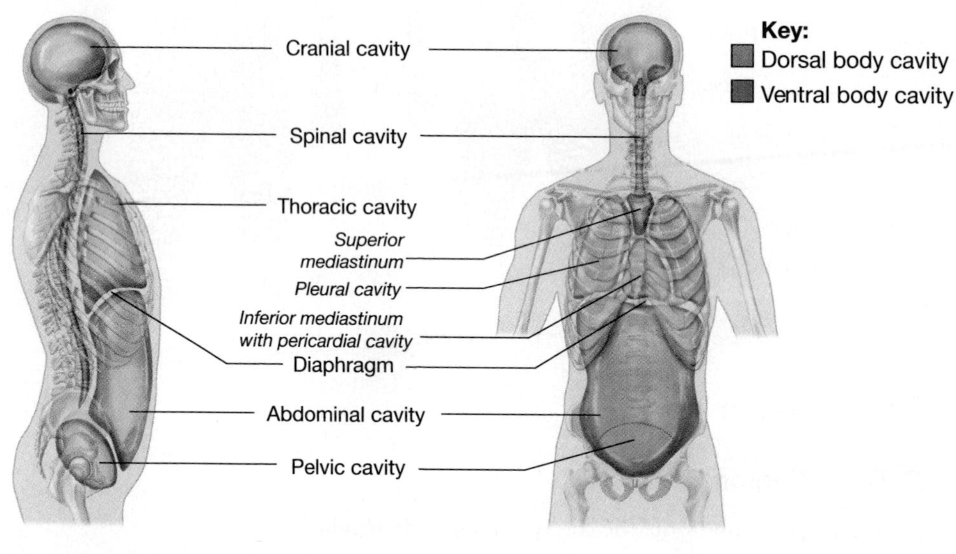

■ **Figure 2.6** The dorsal (red) and ventral (purple) body cavities.

What's In A Name?

Look for these word parts:
abdomin/o = abdomen
crani/o = skull
pelv/o = pelvis
pariet/o = cavity wall
pleur/o = pleura
spin/o = spine
thorac/o = chest
viscer/o = internal organ
peri- = around
-al = pertaining to
-ic = pertaining to

Med Term Tip

The kidneys are the only major abdominopelvic organ located outside the sac formed by the peritoneum. Because they are found behind this sac, their position is referred to as *retroperitoneal* (retro- = behind; peritone/o = peritoneum; -al = pertaining to).

The dorsal cavities include the **cranial cavity**, containing the brain, and the **spinal cavity**, containing the spinal cord.

The ventral cavities include the **thoracic cavity** and the **abdominopelvic cavity**. The thoracic cavity contains the two lungs and a central region between them called the **mediastinum**. The heart, aorta, esophagus, trachea, and thymus gland are some of the structures located in the mediastinum. There is an actual physical wall between the thoracic cavity and the abdominopelvic cavity called the **diaphragm**. The diaphragm is a muscle used for breathing. The abdominopelvic cavity is generally subdivided into a superior **abdominal cavity** and an inferior **pelvic cavity**. The organs of the digestive, excretory, and reproductive systems are located in these cavities. The organs within the ventral cavities are referred to as a group as the internal organs or **viscera**. Table 2.3 ■ describes the body cavities and their major organs.

All of the ventral cavities are lined by, and the viscera are encased in, a two-layer membrane called the **pleura** in the thoracic cavity and the **peritoneum** in the abdominopelvic cavity. The outer layer that lines the cavities is called the **parietal layer** (i.e., **parietal pleura** and **parietal peritoneum**), and the inner layer that encases the viscera is called the **visceral layer** (i.e., **visceral pleura** and **visceral peritoneum**).

Within the thoracic cavity, the pleura is subdivided, forming the **pleural cavity**, containing the lungs, and the **pericardial cavity**, containing the heart. The larger abdominopelvic cavity is usually subdivided into regions in order to precisely refer to different areas. Two different methods of subdividing this cavity are used: the anatomical divisions and the clinical divisions. Choose a method partly

Table 2.3 Body Cavities and Their Major Organs

Cavity	Major Organs
Dorsal cavities	
Cranial cavity	Brain
Spinal cavity	Spinal cord
Ventral cavities	
Thoracic cavity	Pleural cavity: lungs Pericardial cavity: heart Mediastinum: heart, esophagus, trachea , thymus gland, aorta
Abdominopelvic cavities	
Abdominal cavity	Stomach, spleen, liver, gallbladder, pancreas, and portions of the small intestine and colon
Pelvic cavity	Urinary bladder, ureters, urethra, and portions of the small intestine and colon Female: uterus, ovaries, fallopian tubes, vagina Male: prostate gland, seminal vesicles, portion of vas deferens

on personal preference and partly on which system best describes the patient's condition. See Table 2.4 ■ for a description of these methods for dividing the abdominopelvic cavity.

Table 2.4 Methods of Subdividing the Abdominopelvic Cavity

Anatomical Divisions of the Abdomen

- Right hypochondriac (high-poh-KON-dree-ak): Right lateral region of upper row beneath the lower ribs
- Epigastric (ep-ih-GAS-trik): Middle area of upper row above the stomach
- Left hypochondriac: Left lateral region of the upper row beneath the lower ribs
- Right lumbar: Right lateral region of the middle row at the waist
- Umbilical (um-BILL-ih-kal): Central area over the navel
- Left lumbar: Left lateral region of the middle row at the waist
- Right inguinal (ING-gwih-nal): Right lateral region of the lower row at the groin
- Hypogastric (high-poh-GAS-trik): Middle region of the lower row beneath the navel
- Left inguinal: Left lateral region of the lower row at the groin

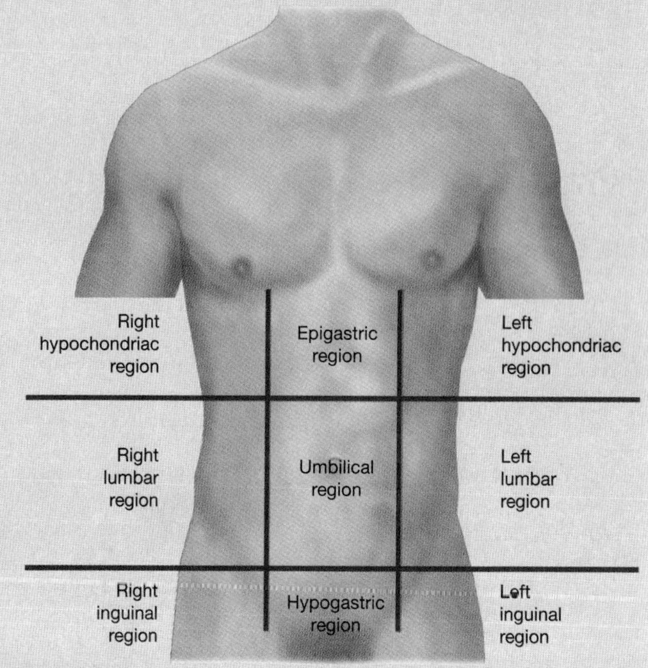

What's In A Name?

Look for these word parts:
chondr/o = cartilage
gastr/o = stomach
inguin/o = groin
lumb/o = loin (low back)
epi- = above
hypo- = below
-al = pertaining to
-ar = pertaining to
-iac = pertaining to
-ic = pertaining to

Med Term Tip

To visualize the nine anatomical divisions, imagine a tic-tac-toe diagram over this region.

Med Term Tip

The term *hypochondriac*, literally meaning "below the cartilage" (of the ribs), has come to refer to a person who believes he or she is sick when there is no obvious cause for illness. These patients commonly complain of aches and pains in the hypochondriac region.

Table 2.4 Methods of Subdividing the Abdominopelvic Cavity (continued)

Clinical Divisions of the Abdomen

- Right upper quadrant (RUQ): Contains majority of liver, gallbladder, small portion of pancreas, right kidney, small intestines, and colon
- Right lower quadrant (RLQ): Contains small intestine and colon, right ovary and fallopian tube, appendix, and right ureter
- Left upper quadrant (LUQ): Contains small portion of liver, spleen, stomach, majority of pancreas, left kidney, small intestines, and colon
- Left lower quadrant (LLQ): Contains small intestine and colon, left ovary and fallopian tube, and left ureter
- Midline organs: uterus, bladder, prostate gland

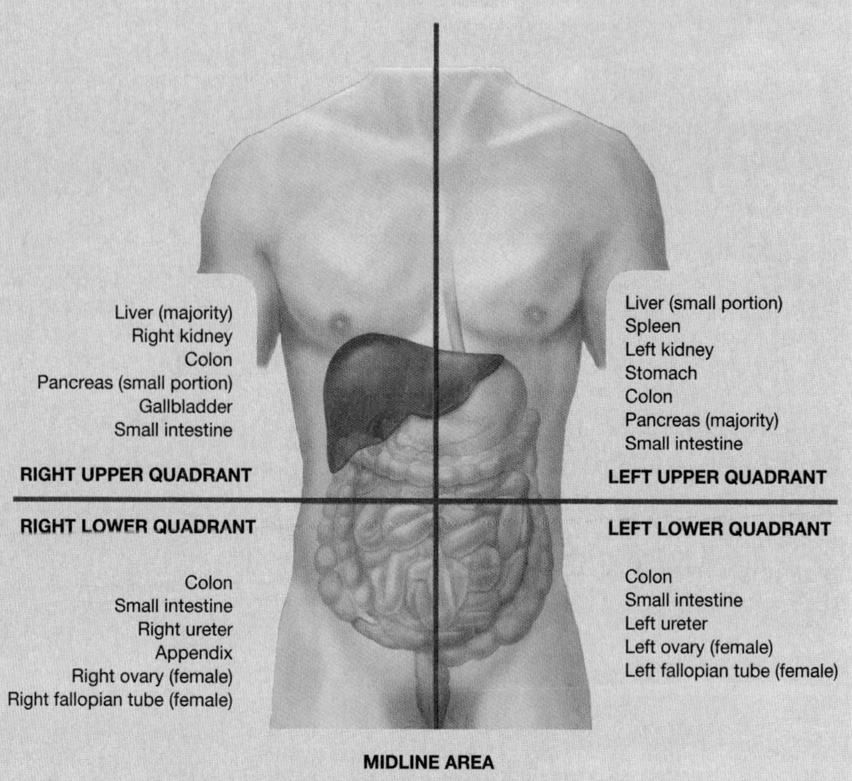

Practice As You Go

E. Complete the Statement

1. In the ________________ position the body is standing erect with arms at sides and palms facing forward.
2. The ________________ quadrant of the abdomen contains the appendix.
3. The dorsal cavities are the ________________ cavity and the ________________ cavity.
4. There are ________________ anatomical divisions in the abdominal cavity.
5. The ________________ region of the abdominal cavity is located in the right lower lateral region near the groin.
6. Within the thoracic cavity the lungs are found in the ________________ cavity and the heart is found in the ________________ cavity.

Directional and Positional Terms

Directional and positional terms describe one process's, organ's, or system's relationship to another. Table 2.5 ■ presents commonly used terms for describing the position of the body or its parts. They are listed in pairs that have opposite meanings; for example, superior versus inferior, anterior versus posterior, medial versus lateral, proximal versus distal, superficial versus deep, and supine versus prone. Directional terms are illustrated in Figure 2.7 ■.

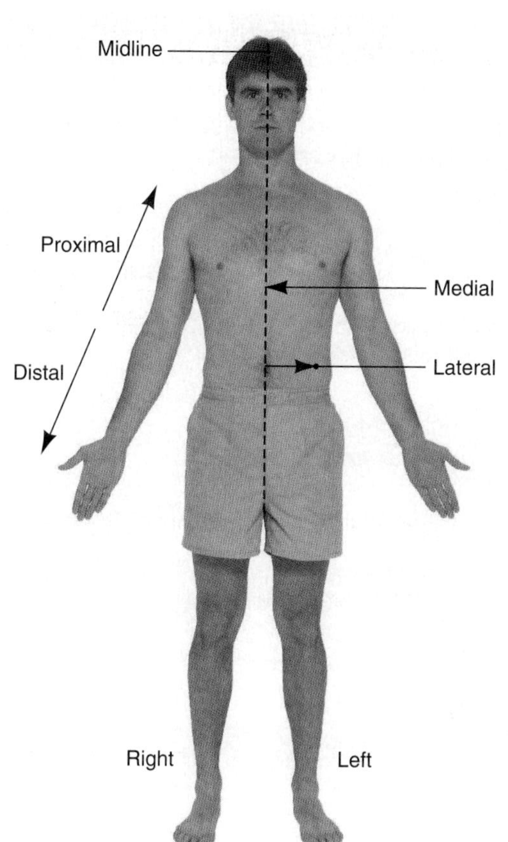

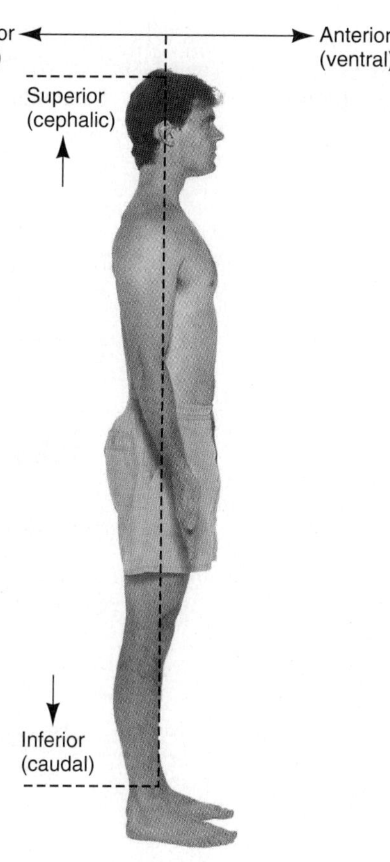

■ **Figure 2.7** Anterior and lateral views of the body illustrating directional terms. *(Michal Heron, Pearson Education)*

Table 2.5 Terms for Describing Body Position

Term	Word parts	Description
superior (soo-PEE-ree-or) or **cephalic** (seh-FAL-ik)	super/o = above -ior = pertaining to cephal/o = head -ic = pertaining to	More toward the head, or above another structure. Example: The adrenal glands are superior to the kidneys.
inferior (in-FEE-ree-or) or **caudal** (KAWD-al)	infer/o = below -ior = pertaining to caud/o = tail -al = pertaining to	More toward the feet or tail, or below another structure. Example: The intestine is inferior to the heart.
anterior (an-TEE-ree-or) or **ventral** (VEN-tral)	anter/o = front -ior = pertaining to ventr/o = belly -al = pertaining to	More toward the front or belly side of the body. Example: The navel is located on the anterior surface of the body.
posterior (poss-TEE-ree-or) or **dorsal** (DOR-sal)	poster/o = back -ior = pertaining to dors/o = back -al = pertaining to	More toward the back or spinal cord side of the body. Example: The posterior wall of the right kidney was excised.
medial (MEE-dee-al)	medi/o = middle -al = pertaining to	Refers to the middle or near the middle of the body or the structure. Example: The heart is medially located in the chest cavity.
lateral (LAT-er-al)	later/o = side -al = pertaining to	Refers to the side. Example: The ovaries are located lateral to the uterus.
proximal (PROK-sim-al)	proxim/o = near to -al = pertaining to	Located nearer to the point of attachment to the body. Example: In the anatomical position, the elbow is proximal to the hand.
distal (DISS-tal)	dist/o = away from -al = pertaining to	Located farther away from the point of attachment to the body. Example: The hand is distal to the elbow.
apex (AY-peks)		Tip or summit of an organ. Example: We hear the heartbeat by listening over the apex of the heart.

Table 2.5 Terms for Describing Body Position (continued)

Term	Word parts	Description
base		Bottom or lower part of an organ. Example: On the X-ray, a fracture was noted at the base of the skull.
superficial		More toward the surface of the body. Example: The cut was superficial.
deep		Further away from the surface of the body. Example: An incision into an abdominal organ is a deep incision.
supine (soo-PINE)		The body is lying horizontally and facing upward. Example: The patient is in the supine position for abdominal surgery. ■ **Figure 2.8A** The supine position. *(Richard Logan, Pearson Education)*
prone (PROHN)		The body is lying horizontally and facing downward. Example: The patient is placed in the prone position for spinal surgery. ■ **Figure 2.8B** The prone position. *(Richard Logan, Pearson Education)*

Abbreviations

AP	anteroposterior	**LUQ**	left upper quadrant
CV	cardiovascular	**MS**	musculoskeletal
ENT	ear, nose, and throat	**OB**	obstetrics
GI	gastrointestinal	**PA**	posteroanterior
GYN	gynecology	**RLQ**	right lower quadrant
lat	lateral	**RUQ**	right upper quadrant
LE	lower extremity	**UE**	upper extremity
LLQ	left lower quadrant		

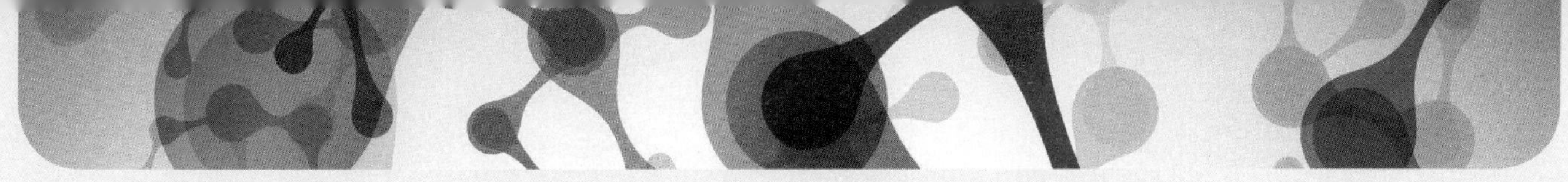

Chapter Review

Practice Exercises

A. Prefix Practice

Circle the prefixes in the following terms and define in the space provided.

1. epigastric ____
2. pericardium ____
3. hypochondriac ____
4. retroperitoneal ____

B. Terminology Matching

Match each term to its definition.

1. ________ distal	a. away from the surface
2. ________ prone	b. toward the surface
3. ________ lateral	c. located closer to point of attachment to the body
4. ________ inferior	d. caudal
5. ________ deep	e. tip or summit of an organ
6. ________ apex	f. lying face down
7. ________ base	g. cephalic
8. ________ posterior	h. ventral
9. ________ superficial	i. dorsal
10. ________ supine	j. lying face up
11. ________ anterior	k. to the side
12. ________ medial	l. middle
13. ________ proximal	m. bottom or lower part of an organ
14. ________ superior	n. located further away from point of attachment to the body

C. What's the Abbreviation?

1. musculoskeletal ______________________
2. lateral ______________________
3. right upper quadrant ______________________
4. cardiovascular ______________________
5. gastrointestinal ______________________
6. anteroposterior ______________________
7. obstetrics ______________________
8. left lower quadrant ______________________

D. Build a Medical Term

Build terms for each expression using the correct combining forms and suffixes.

1. pertaining to spinal cord side ______________________
2. pertaining to the chest ______________________
3. pertaining to above ______________________
4. pertaining to the tail ______________________
5. pertaining to internal organs ______________________
6. pertaining to the side ______________________
7. pertaining to away from ______________________
8. pertaining to nerves ______________________
9. study of the lungs ______________________
10. pertaining to the muscles ______________________
11. pertaining to the belly side ______________________
12. pertaining to the front ______________________
13. pertaining to the head ______________________
14. pertaining to the middle ______________________

E. Define the Combining Form

1. **viscer/o** ______________________
2. **poster/o** ______________________
3. **abdomin/o** ______________________
4. **thorac/o** ______________________
5. **medi/o** ______________________

6. **ventr/o** ____________________

7. **anter/o** ____________________

8. **hist/o** ____________________

9. **epitheli/o** ____________________

10. **crani/o** ____________________

11. **cyt/o** ____________________

12. **proxim/o** ____________________

13. **cephal/o** ____________________

F. Terminology Matching

Match each organ to its body cavity.

1. ________ gallbladder
2. ________ appendix
3. ________ urinary bladder
4. ________ small intestines
5. ________ right kidney
6. ________ left ovary
7. ________ stomach
8. ________ colon
9. ________ right ureter
10. ________ pancreas (majority)

a. right upper quadrant
b. left upper quadrant
c. right lower quadrant
d. left lower quadrant
e. all quadrants
f. midline structure

G. Fill in the Blank

cardiology	otorhinolaryngology	urology	gynecology
ophthalmology	gastroenterology	dermatology	orthopedics

1. John is a musician who plays an electric bass guitar and is experiencing difficulty in hearing soft voices. He would consult a physician in ______________________.
2. Ruth is a stock trader with the Chicago Board of Trade. She has had a pounding and racing heartbeat. She would consult a physician specializing in ______________________.
3. Mary Ann is experiencing excessive bleeding from the uterus. She would consult a ______________________ doctor.
4. José has fractured his wrist in a fall. A physician in ______________________ would see him for an examination.
5. A physician who performs eye exams specializes in the field of ______________________.
6. When her daughter had repeated bladder infections, Mrs. Cortez sought the opinion of a specialist in ______________________.
7. Martha could not get rid of a persistent skin rash with over-the-counter creams. She decided to make an appointment with a specialist in ______________________.
8. After reviewing his X-ray, the specialist in ______________________ informed Mr. Sparks that he had a stomach ulcer.

Labeling Exercise

Image A

Write the labels for this figure on the numbered lines provided.

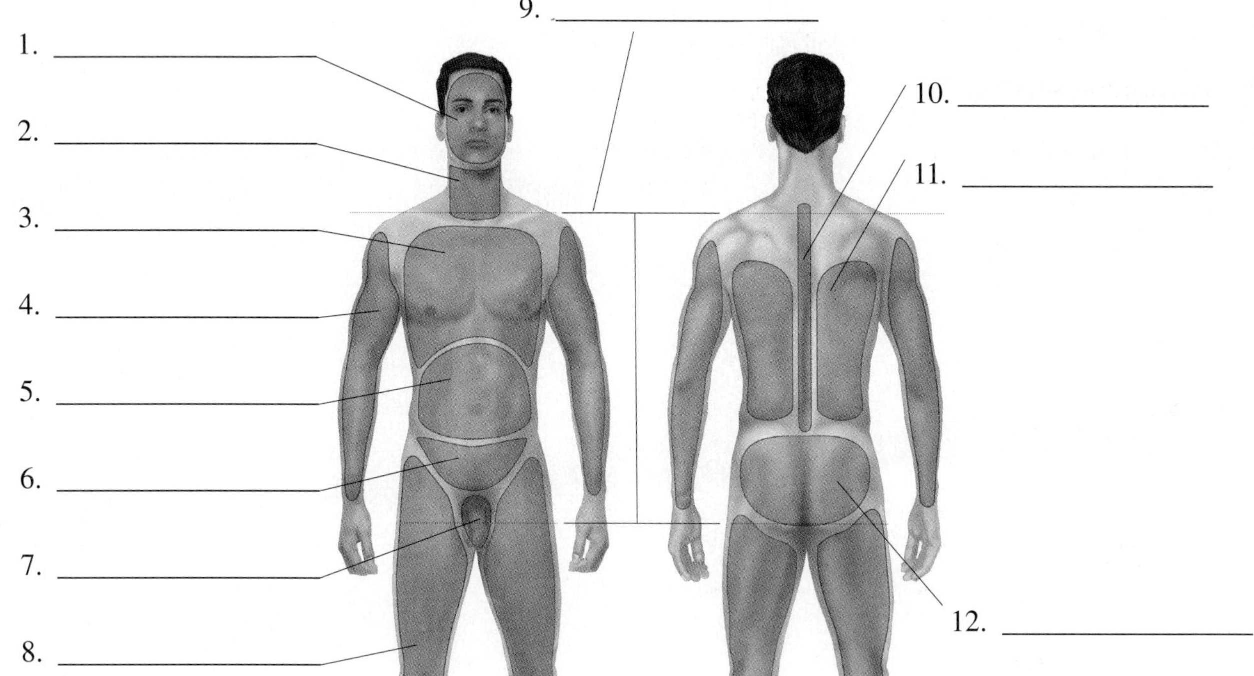

Image B

Write the labels for this figure on the numbered lines provided.

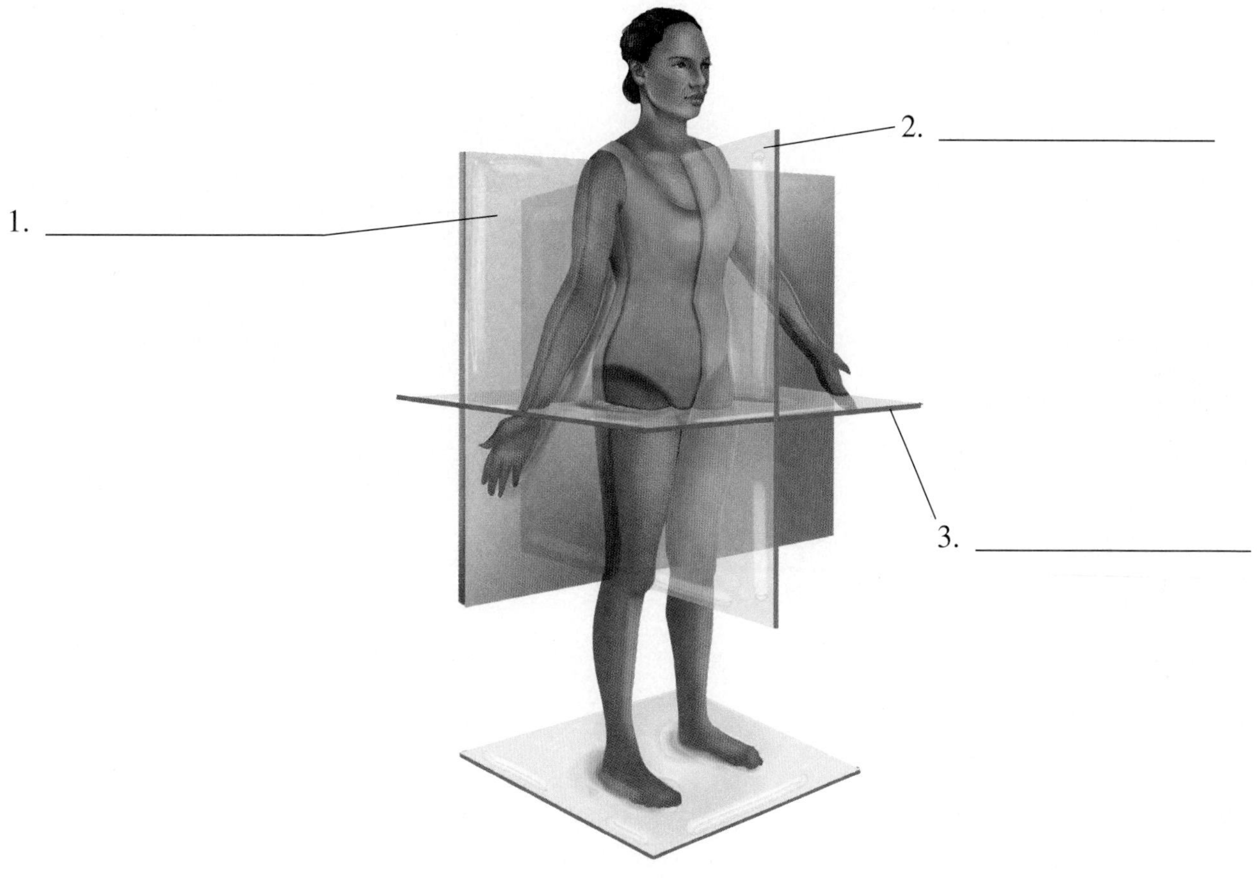

3

Integumentary System

Learning Objectives

Upon completion of this chapter, you will be able to

- Identify and define the combining forms, prefixes, and suffixes introduced in this chapter.
- Correctly spell and pronounce medical terms and major anatomical structures relating to the integumentary system.
- List and describe the four purposes of the skin.
- Describe the layers of the skin and the subcutaneous layer and their functions.
- List and describe the accessory organs of the skin.
- Identify and define integumentary system anatomical terms.
- Identify and define selected integumentary system pathology terms.
- Identify and define selected integumentary system diagnostic procedures.
- Identify and define selected integumentary system therapeutic procedures.
- Identify and define selected medications relating to the integumentary system.
- Define selected abbreviations associated with the integumentary system.

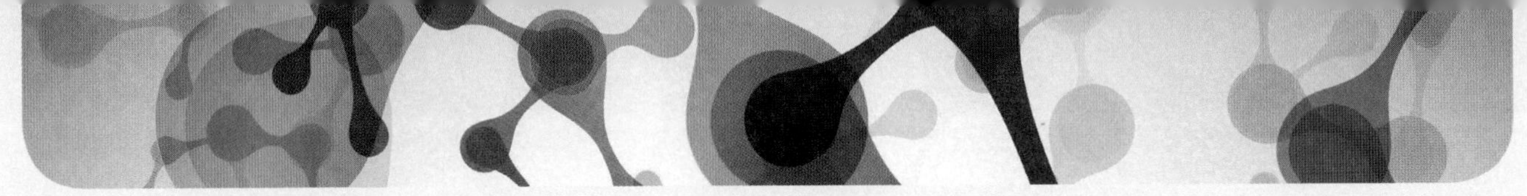

Integumentary System at a Glance

Function

The skin provides a protective two-way barrier between our internal environment and the outside world. It also plays an important role in temperature regulation, houses sensory receptors to detect the environment around us, and secretes important fluids.

Organs

Here are the primary structures that comprise the integumentary system.

skin **hair** **nails** **sebaceous glands** **sweat glands**

Word Parts

Here are the most common word parts (with their meanings) used to build integumentary system terms. For a more comprehensive list, refer to the Terminology section of this chapter.

Combining Forms

albin/o	white
cauter/o	to burn
cry/o	cold
cutane/o	skin
derm/o	skin
dermat/o	skin
diaphor/o	profuse sweating
electr/o	electricity
erythr/o	red
hidr/o	sweat
ichthy/o	scaly, dry
kerat/o	hard, horny
leuk/o	white
lip/o	fat
melan/o	black
myc/o	fungus
necr/o	death
onych/o	nail
pedicul/o	lice
phot/o	light
py/o	pus
rhytid/o	wrinkle
sarc/o	flesh
scler/o	hard
seb/o	oil
system/o	system
trich/o	hair
ungu/o	nail
vesic/o	sac, bladder
xer/o	dry

Suffixes

-derma	skin condition

Prefixes

allo-	other, different from usual
xeno-	foreign

Integumentary System Illustrated

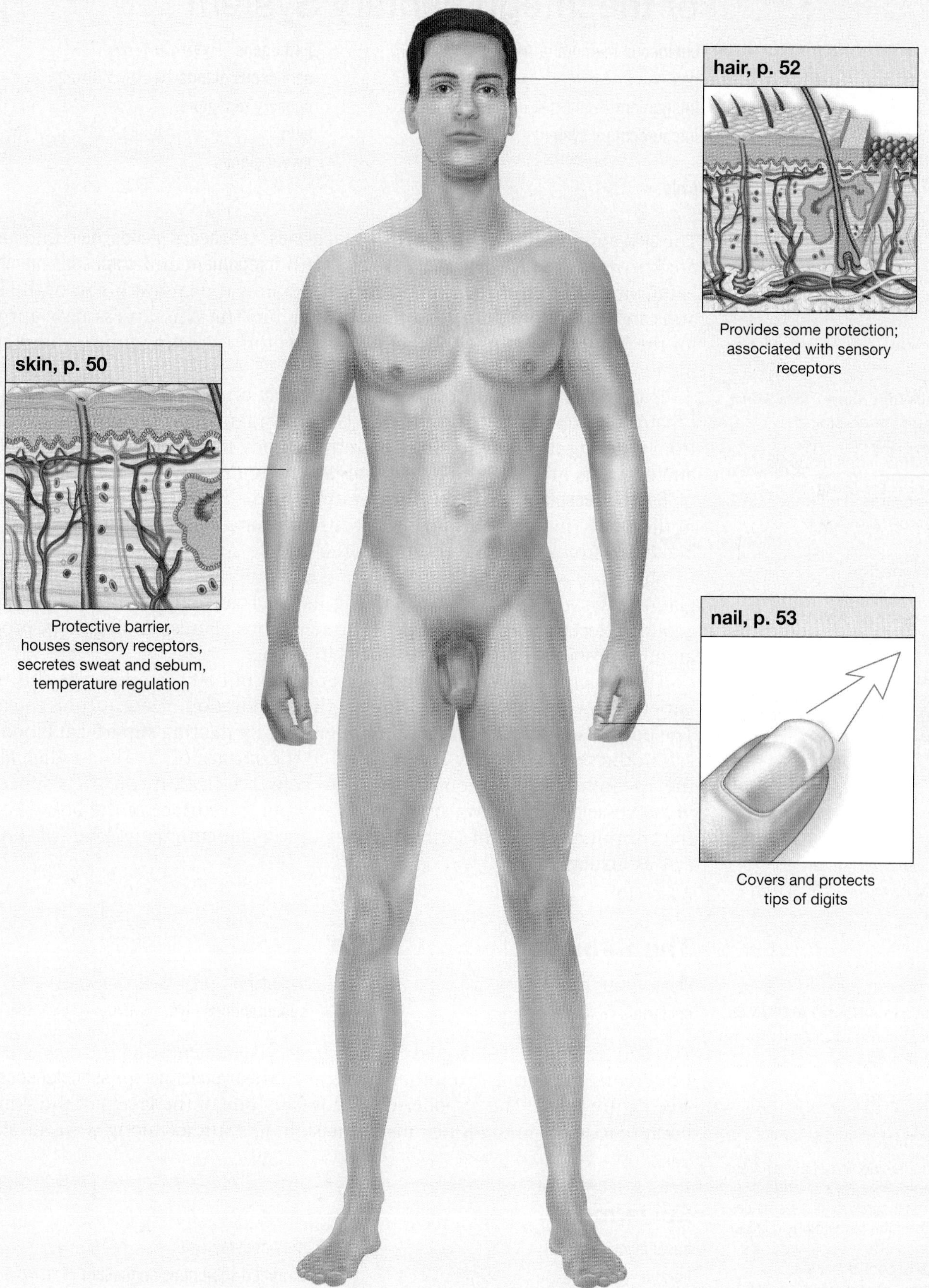

Anatomy and Physiology of the Integumentary System

cutaneous membrane (kew-TAY-nee-us)
hair
integument (in-TEG-you-mint)
integumentary system (in-teg-you-MEN-tah-ree)
nails
pathogens (PATH-oh-jenz)
sebaceous glands (see-BAY-shus)
sensory receptors
skin
sweat glands

The **skin** and its accessory organs—**sweat glands**, **sebaceous glands**, **hair**, and **nails**—are known as the **integumentary system**, with **integument** and **cutaneous membrane** being alternate terms for skin. In fact, the skin is the largest organ of the body and can weigh more than 20 pounds in an adult. The skin serves many purposes for the body: protecting, housing nerve receptors, secreting fluids, and regulating temperature.

What's In A Name?
Look for these word parts:
path/o = disease
-gen = that which produces
-ary = pertaining to
-ory = pertaining to
-ous = pertaining to

Med Term Tip
Flushing of the skin, a normal response to an increase in environmental temperature or to a fever, is caused by an increased blood flow to the skin of the face and neck. However, in some people, it is also a response to embarrassment, called blushing, and is not easily controlled.

The primary function of the skin is protection. It forms a two-way barrier capable of keeping **pathogens** (disease-causing organisms) and harmful chemicals from entering the body. It also stops critical body fluids from escaping the body and prevents injury to the internal organs lying underneath the skin.

Sensory receptors that detect temperature, pain, touch, and pressure are located in the skin. The messages for these sensations are conveyed to the spinal cord and brain from the nerve endings in the middle layer of the skin.

Fluids are produced in two types of skin glands: sweat and sebaceous. Sweat glands assist the body in maintaining its internal temperature by creating a cooling effect as sweat evaporates. The sebaceous glands, or oil glands, produce an oily substance that lubricates the skin surface.

The structure of skin aids in the regulation of body temperature through a variety of means. As noted previously, the evaporation of sweat cools the body. The body also lowers its internal temperature by dilating superficial blood vessels in the skin. This brings more blood to the surface of the skin, which allows the release of heat. If the body needs to conserve heat, it constricts superficial blood vessels, keeping warm blood away from the surface of the body. Finally, the continuous layer of fat that makes up the subcutaneous layer of the skin acts as insulation.

The Skin

dermis (DER-mis)
epidermis (ep-ih-DER-mis)
hypodermis (high-poh-DER-mis)
subcutaneous layer (sub-kyoo-TAY-nee-us)

What's In A Name?
Look for these word parts:
derm/o = skin
epi- = above
hypo- = below

Med Term Tip
An understanding of the different layers of the skin is important for healthcare workers because much of the terminology relating to types of injections and medical conditions, such as burns, is described using these designations.

The skin is composed of two layers, the superficial **epidermis** and the deeper **dermis**. Underlying the dermis is another layer called the **hypodermis**, or **subcutaneous layer** (see Figure 3.1 ■). The hypodermis is not truly one of the layers of the skin, but because it assists in the functions of the skin, it is studied along with the skin.

Epidermis

basal layer (BAY-sal)
keratin (KAIR-ah-tin)
melanin (MEL-ah-nin)
melanocytes (mel-AN-oh-sights)
stratified squamous epithelium (STRAT-ih-fyde/SKWAY-mus / ep-ih-THEE-lee-um)

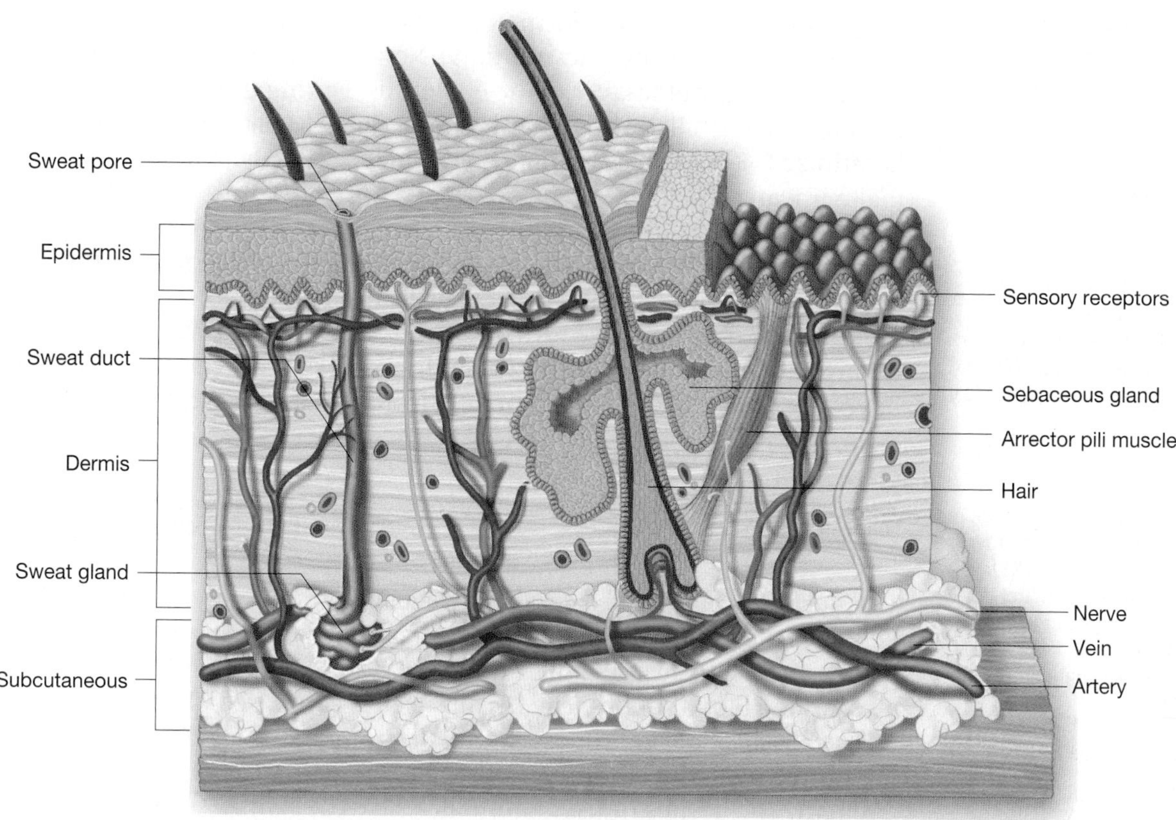

■ **Figure 3.1** Skin structure, including the layers of the skin, the subcutaneous layer, and the accessory organs: sweat gland, sebaceous gland, and hair.

The epidermis is composed of **stratified squamous epithelium** (see Figure 3.2 ■). This type of epithelial tissue consists of flat scale-like cells arranged in overlapping layers or strata. The epidermis does not have a blood supply or any connective tissue, so it is dependent for nourishment on the deeper layers of skin.

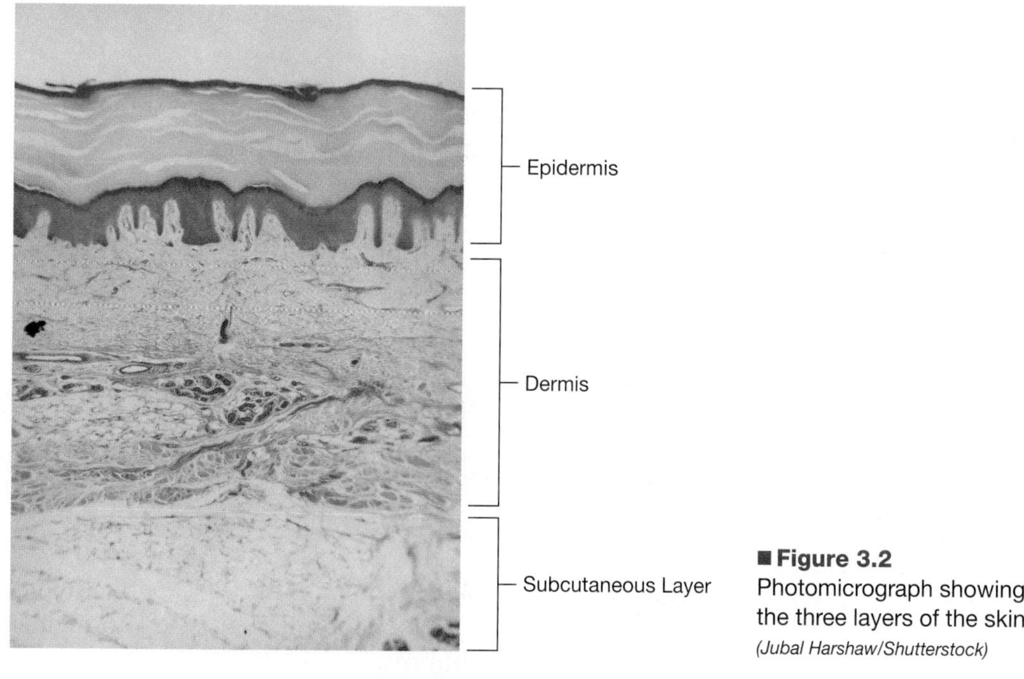

■ **Figure 3.2** Photomicrograph showing the three layers of the skin.
(Jubal Harshaw/Shutterstock)

What's In A Name?
Look for these word parts:
bas/o = base
melan/o = black
-al = pertaining to
-cyte = cell
-ous = pertaining to

Med Term Tip
We lose 30,000–50,000 old, dead skin cells per minute and replace them with new, younger cells. In fact, because of this process, the epidermis is completely replaced every 25 days.

Med Term Tip
A suntan can be thought of as a protective response to the rays of the sun. However, when the melanin in the skin is not able to absorb all the rays of the sun, the skin burns and DNA may be permanently and dangerously damaged.

Med Term Tip
Ridges formed in the dermis of our fingertips are what give each of us unique fingerprints. These do not change during a person's lifetime and so are a reliable means of identification. In fact, fingerprints are still visible on Egyptian mummies.

The deepest layer within the epidermis is called the **basal layer**. Cells in this layer continually grow and multiply. New cells that are forming push the old cells toward the outer layer of the epidermis. During this process the cells shrink, die, and become filled with a hard protein called **keratin**. These dead, overlapping, keratinized cells allow the skin to act as an effective barrier to infection and also make it waterproof.

The basal layer also contains special cells called **melanocytes**, which produce the black pigment **melanin**. Not only is this pigment responsible for the color of the skin, but it also protects against damage from the ultraviolet (UV) rays of the sun. This damage may be in the form of leather-like skin and wrinkles, which are not hazardous, or it may be one of several forms of skin cancer. Dark-skinned people have more melanin and are generally less likely to get wrinkles or skin cancer.

Dermis

collagen fibers (KOL-ah-jen)
corium (KOH-ree-um)

The dermis, also referred to as the **corium**, is the middle layer of skin, located between the epidermis and the subcutaneous layer (see Figure 3.2). Its name means "true skin." Unlike the thinner epidermis, the dermis is living tissue with a very good blood supply. The dermis itself is composed of connective tissue and **collagen fibers**. Collagen fibers are made from a strong, fibrous protein present in connective tissue, forming a flexible "glue" that gives connective tissue its strength. The dermis houses hair follicles, sweat glands, sebaceous glands, blood vessels, lymph vessels, sensory receptors, nerve fibers, and muscle fibers.

Subcutaneous Layer

lipocytes (LIP-oh-sights)

What's In A Name?
Look for these word parts:
lip/o = fat
-cyte = cell

The subcutaneous layer (or hypodermis) is a continuous layer of fat that separates the dermis from deeper tissues (see Figure 3.2). It is composed of fat cells called **lipocytes**. Its functions include protecting deeper tissues of the body from trauma, acting as insulation from heat and cold, and serving as a source of energy in a starvation situation.

Accessory Organs

The accessory organs of the skin are the anatomical structures located within the dermis, including the hair, nails, sebaceous glands, and sweat glands.

Hair

arrector pili (ah-REK-tor / pee-lie)
hair follicle (FALL-ikl)
hair root
hair shaft

Med Term Tip
Our hair turns gray as part of the normal aging process when we no longer produce melanin.

The fibers that make up hair are composed of the protein keratin, the same hard protein material that fills the cells of the epidermis. The process of hair formation is much like the process of growth in the epidermal layer of the skin. The deeper cells in the **hair root** force older keratinized cells to move upward, forming the **hair shaft**. The hair shaft grows toward the skin surface within the **hair follicle**. Melanin gives hair its color. Sebaceous glands release oil directly into the hair follicle. Each hair has a small slip of smooth muscle attached to it called the **arrector pili** muscle (see Figure 3.3 ■). When this muscle contracts the hair shaft stands up, resulting in "goose bumps."

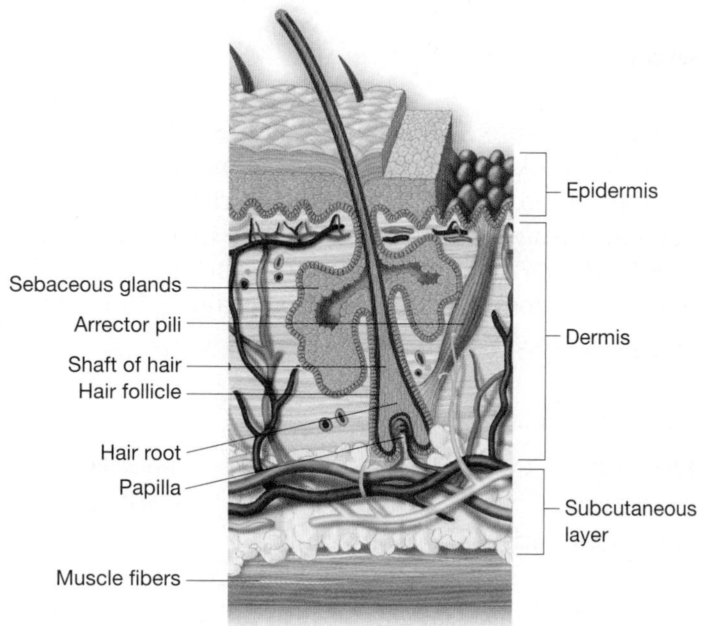

■ **Figure 3.3** Structure of a hair and its associated sebaceous gland.

Nails

cuticle (KEW-tikl)
free edge
lunula (LOO-nyoo-lah)
nail bed
nail body
nail root

Nails are a flat plate of keratin called the **nail body** that covers the ends of fingers and toes. The nail body is connected to the tissue underneath by the **nail bed**. Nails grow longer from the **nail root**, which is found at the base of the nail and is covered and protected by the soft tissue **cuticle**. The **free edge** is the exposed edge that is trimmed when nails become too long. The light-colored half-moon area at the base of the nail is the **lunula** (see Figure 3.4 ■).

Med Term Tip

Because of its rich blood supply and light color, the nail bed is an excellent place to check patients for low oxygen levels in their blood. Deoxygenated blood is a very dark purple-red and gives skin a bluish tinge called *cyanosis*.

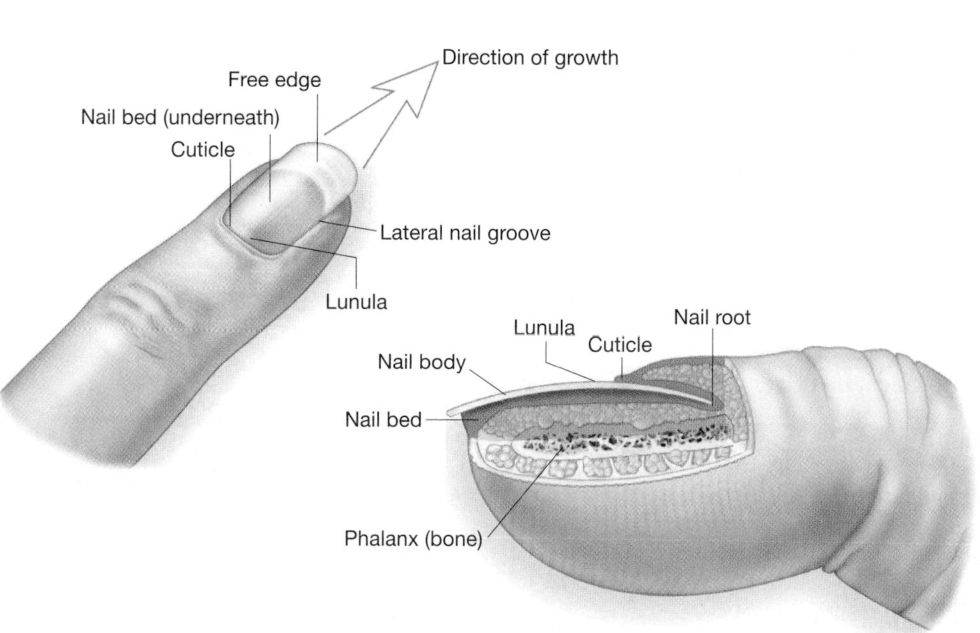

■ **Figure 3.4** External and internal structures of nails.

Sebaceous Glands

sebum

Sebaceous glands, found in the dermis, secrete the oil **sebum**, which lubricates the hair and skin, thereby helping to prevent drying and cracking. These glands secrete sebum directly into hair follicles, rather than a duct (see Figure 3.1). Secretion from the sebaceous glands increases during adolescence, playing a role in the development of acne. Sebum secretion begins to diminish as age increases. A loss of sebum in old age, along with sun exposure, can account for wrinkles and dry skin.

Sweat Glands

apocrine glands (APP-oh-krin)
perspiration
sudoriferous glands (sue-doh-RIF-er-us)
sweat duct
sweat pore

What's In A Name?
Look for these word parts:
crin/o = to secrete
-ous = pertaining to

Word Watch
Be careful when using *hydr/o* meaning "water" and *hidr/o* meaning "sweat."

About 2 million sweat glands, also called **sudoriferous glands**, are found throughout the body. These highly coiled glands are located in the dermis. Sweat travels to the surface of the skin in a **sweat duct**. The surface opening of a sweat duct is called a **sweat pore** (see Figure 3.1).

Sweat glands function to cool the body as sweat evaporates. Sweat or **perspiration** contains a small amount of waste product but is normally colorless and odorless. However, there are sweat glands called **apocrine glands** in the pubic and underarm areas that secrete a thicker sweat, which can produce an odor when it comes into contact with bacteria on the skin. This is what we recognize as body odor.

Practice As You Go

A. Complete the Statement

1. The two layers of skin are the superficial ____________________ and deeper ____________________.
2. The ____________________ separates the dermis from underlying tissue.
3. The ____________________ layer is the only living layer of the epidermis.
4. The hypodermis is composed primarily of ____________________.
5. Sensory receptors are located in the ____________________ layer of skin.
6. Nails and hair are composed of a hard protein called ____________________.
7. ____________________ is the pigment that gives skin its color.
8. Another name for the dermis is ____________________.
9. The nail body is connected to underlying tissue by the ____________________.
10. ____________________ glands release their product directly into hair follicles while ____________________ glands release their product into a duct.

Terminology

Word Parts Used to Build Integumentary System Terms

The following lists contain the combining forms, suffixes, and prefixes used to build terms in the remaining sections of this chapter.

Combining Forms

albin/o	white
angi/o (see Chapter 5)	vessel
bas/o	base
bi/o	life
carcin/o	cancer
cauter/o	to burn
chem/o	chemical
cis/o	to cut
cortic/o (see Chapter 4)	outer layer
cry/o	cold
cutane/o	skin
cyt/o	cell
derm/o	skin
dermat/o	skin

diaphor/o	profuse sweating
electr/o	electricity
erythr/o	red
esthesi/o (see Chapter 12)	feeling
hem/o (see Chapter 6)	blood
hidr/o	sweat
ichthy/o	scaly, dry
kerat/o	hard, horny
leuk/o	white
lip/o	fat
melan/o	black
myc/o	fungus
necr/o	death

onych/o	nail
pedicul/o	lice
phot/o	light
py/o	pus
rhytid/o	wrinkle
sarc/o	flesh
scler/o	hard
seb/o	oil
septic/o (see Chapter 6)	infection
system/o	system
trich/o	hair
ungu/o	nail
vesic/o	sac
xer/o	dry

Suffixes

-al	pertaining to
-derma	skin condition
-ectomy	surgical removal
-emia (see Chapter 6)	blood condition
-ia	state, condition
-iasis	abnormal condition
-ic	pertaining to

-ism	state of
-itis	inflammation
-logy	study of
-malacia	abnormal softening
-oma	mass, tumor
-opsy	view of
-osis	abnormal condition

-ous	pertaining to
-phagia (see Chapter 8)	eat, swallow
-plasty	surgical repair
-rrhea	discharge
-tic	pertaining to
-tome	instrument to cut
-ule	small

Prefixes

allo-	other
an-	without
anti-	against
auto-	self

de-	without
epi-	above
hyper-	excessive
hypo-	below

intra-	within
para-	beside
sub-	under
xeno-	foreign

Adjective Forms of Anatomical Terms

Term	Word Parts	Definition
cutaneous (kyoo-TAY-nee-us)	cutane/o = skin -ous = pertaining to	Pertaining to the skin.
dermal (DER-mal)	derm/o = skin -al = pertaining to	Pertaining to the skin.
epidermal (ep-ih-DER-mal)	epi- = above derm/o = skin -al = pertaining to	Pertaining to upon the skin.
hypodermic (high-poh-DER-mik)	hypo- = below derm/o = skin -ic = pertaining to	Pertaining to under the skin.
intradermal (ID) (in-trah-DER-mal)	intra- = within derm/o = skin -al = pertaining to	Pertaining to within the skin.
subcutaneous (Subc, Subq) (sub-kyoo-TAY-nee-us)	sub- = under cutane/o = skin -ous = pertaining to	Pertaining to under the skin.
ungual (UNG-gwal)	ungu/o = nail -al = pertaining to	Pertaining to the nails.

Practice As You Go

B. Give the adjective form for each anatomical structure.

1. A nail ____________________
2. The skin ____________________ or ____________________
3. Above the skin ____________________
4. Below the skin ____________________ or ____________________
5. Within the skin ____________________

Pathology

Term	Word Parts	Definition
Medical Specialties		
dermatology (Derm, derm) (der-mah-TALL-oh-jee)	dermat/o = skin -logy = study of	Branch of medicine involving diagnosis and treatment of conditions and diseases of the integumentary system. Physician is a *dermatologist*.
plastic surgery		Surgical specialty involved in repair, reconstruction, or improvement of body structures such as the skin that are damaged, missing, or misshapen. Physician is a *plastic surgeon.*
Signs and Symptoms		
abrasion (ah-BRAY-zhun)		A scraping-away of the skin surface by friction.
anhidrosis (an-hi-DROH-sis)	an- = without hidr/o = sweat -osis = abnormal condition	Abnormal condition of no sweat.
comedo (KOM-ee-doh)		Collection of hardened sebum in hair follicle. Also called a *blackhead.*
contusion		Injury caused by a blow to the body; causes swelling, pain, and bruising. The skin is not broken.
cyst (SIST) ■ **Figure 3.5** Cyst.		Fluid-filled sac under the skin.
depigmentation (dee-pig-men-TAY-shun)	de- = without	Loss of normal skin color or pigment.
diaphoresis (dye-ah-for-REE-sis)	diaphor/o = profuse sweating	Profuse sweating.
ecchymosis (ek-ih-MOH-sis) ■ **Figure 3.6** Male lying supine with large ecchymosis on lateral rib cage and shoulder. *(Michal Heron, Pearson Education)*	-osis = abnormal condition	Skin discoloration caused by blood collecting under the skin following blunt trauma to the skin. A bruise.

Pathology (continued)

Term	Word Parts	Definition
erythema (er-ih-THEE-mah)	erythr/o = red hem/o = blood	Redness or flushing of the skin.
erythroderma (eh-rith-roh-DER-mah)	erythr/o = red -derma = skin condition	The condition of having reddened or flushed skin.
eschar (ES-kar)		A thick layer of dead tissue and tissue fluid that develops over a deep burn area.
fissure (FISH-er) ■ **Figure 3.7** Fissure.	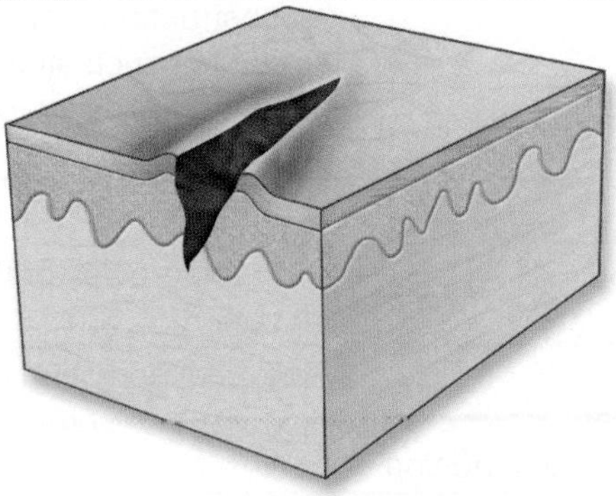	Crack-like lesion or groove on the skin.
hirsutism (HER-soot-izm)	-ism = state of	Excessive hair growth over the body.
hyperemia (high-per-EE-mee-ah)	hyper- = excessive -emia = blood condition	Redness of the skin due to increased blood flow.
hyperhidrosis (high-per-hi-DROH-sis)	hyper- = excessive hidr/o = sweat -osis = abnormal condition	Abnormal condition of excessive sweat.
hyperpigmentation (high-per-pig-men-TAY-shun)	hyper- = excessive	Abnormal amount of pigmentation in the skin.
ichthyoderma (ick-thee-oh-DER-mah)	ichthy/o = scaly, dry -derma = skin condition	The condition of having scaly and dry skin.
lesion (LEE-shun)		A general term for a wound, injury, or abnormality.
leukoderma (loo-koh-DER-mah)	leuk/o = white -derma = skin condition	Having skin that appears white because the normal skin pigment is absent. May be all of the skin or just in some areas.
lipoma (lip-OH-mah)	lip/o = fat -oma = mass	Fatty mass.
macule (MACK-yool) ■ **Figure 3.8** Macule.	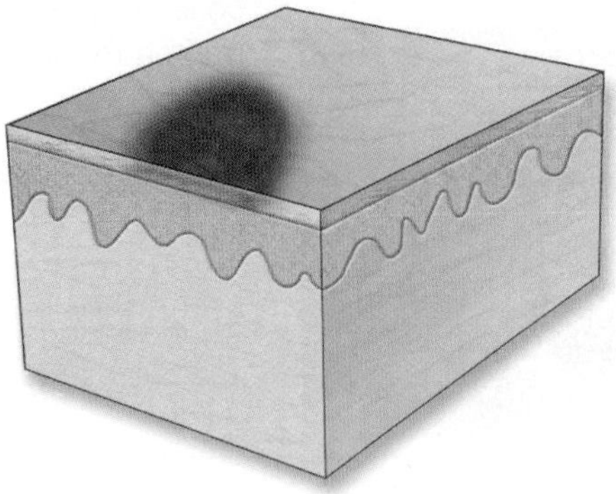 -ule = small	Flat, discolored area that is flush with the skin surface. An example would be a freckle or a birthmark.

Pathology (continued)

Term	Word Parts	Definition
necrosis (neh-KROH-sis)	necr/o = death -osis = abnormal condition	Abnormal condition of death.
nevus (NEV-us)		Pigmented skin blemish, birthmark, or mole. Usually benign but may become cancerous.
nodule (NOD-yool)	-ule = small	Firm, solid mass of cells in the skin larger than 0.5 cm in diameter.
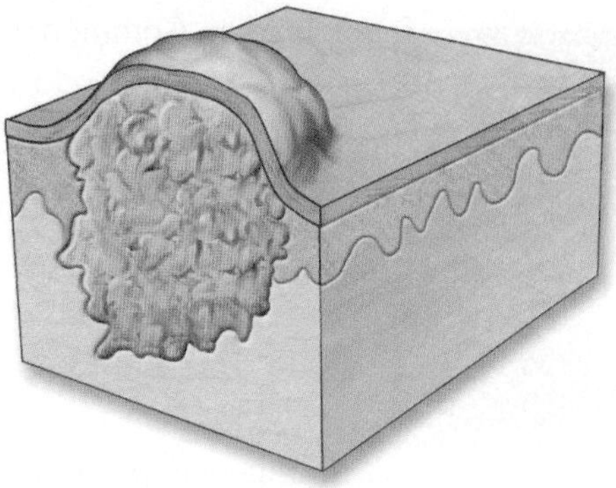 ■ **Figure 3.9** Nodule.		
onychomalacia (on-ih-koh-mah-LAY-she-ah)	onych/o = nail -malacia = abnormal softening	Softening of the nails.
pallor (PAL-or)		Abnormal paleness of the skin.
papule (PAP-yool)	-ule = small	Small, solid, circular raised spot on the surface of the skin less than 0.5 cm in diameter.
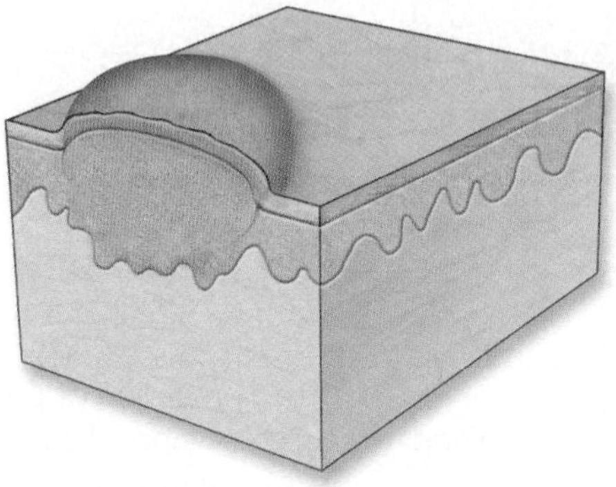 ■ **Figure 3.10** Papule.		
petechiae (peh-TEE-kee-eye)		Pinpoint purple or red spots from minute hemorrhages under the skin.
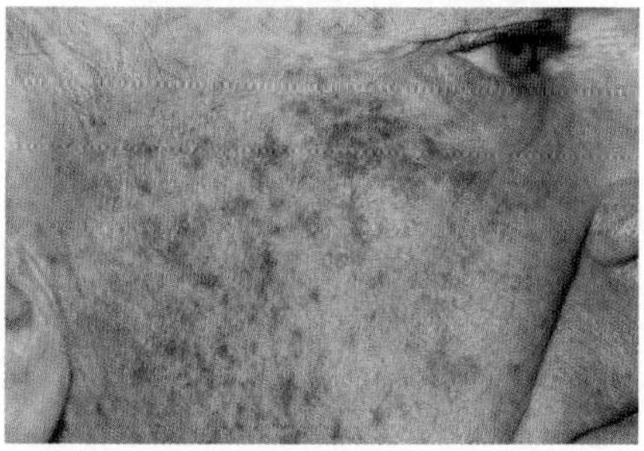 ■ **Figure 3.11** Petechiae, pinpoint skin hemorrhages. *(Dr. P. Marazzi/Science Source)*		

Pathology (continued)

Term	Word Parts	Definition
photosensitivity (foh-toh-sen-sih-TIH-vih-tee)	phot/o = light	Condition in which the skin reacts abnormally when exposed to light, such as the ultraviolet (UV) rays of the sun.
pruritus (proo-RIGH-tus)		Severe itching.
purpura (PER-pew-rah)	*Purpura* is the Latin term for purple	Hemorrhages into the skin due to fragile blood vessels that appear dark brown/ purplish. Commonly seen in older adults.
■ **Figure 3.12** Purpura, hemorrhaging into the skin due to fragile blood vessels. *(Scimat/Science Source)*		
purulent (PYUR-yoo-lent)		Containing pus or an infection that is producing pus. Pus consists of dead bacteria, white blood cells, and tissue debris.
pustule (PUS-tyool)	-ule = small	Raised spot on the skin containing pus.
■ **Figure 3.13** Pustule.		
pyoderma (pye-oh-DER-mah)	py/o = pus -derma = skin condition	The presence of pus on or in the layers of skin. A sign of a bacterial infection.
scleroderma (sklair-ah-DER-mah)	scler/o = hard -derma = skin condition	A condition in which the skin has lost its elasticity and become hardened.
seborrhea (seb-or-EE-ah)	seb/o = oil -rrhea = discharge	Oily discharge.
suppurative (SUP-pure-a-tiv)		Containing or producing pus.

Pathology (continued)

Term	Word Parts	Definition
ulcer (ULL-ser) 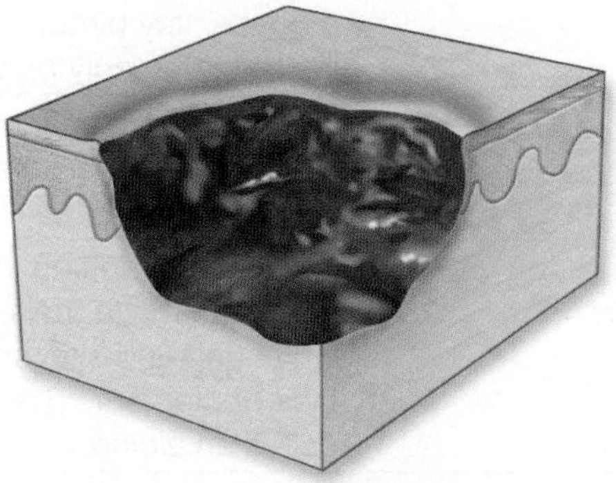 ■ **Figure 3.14** Ulcer.		Open sore or lesion in skin or mucous membrane.
urticaria (er-tih-KAY-ree-ah)	-ia = state, condition	Also called *hives*; a skin eruption of pale reddish wheals with severe itching. Usually associated with food allergy, stress, or drug reactions.
vesicle (VESS-ikl) 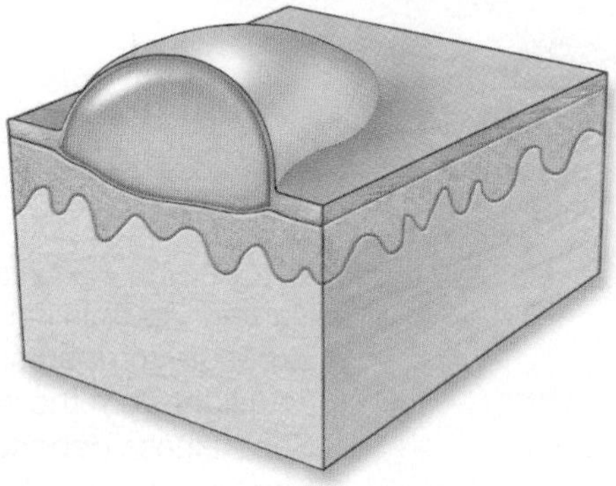 ■ **Figure 3.15** Vesicle.	vesic/o = sac	A blister; small, fluid-filled raised spot on the skin.
wheal (WEEL) 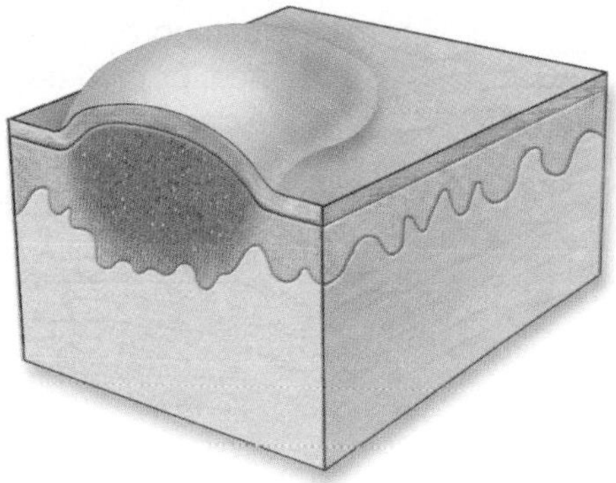 ■ **Figure 3.16** Wheal.		Small, round, swollen area on the skin; typically seen in allergic skin reactions such as *hives* and usually accompanied by urticaria.
xeroderma (zee-roh-DER-mah)	xer/o = dry -derma = skin condition	Condition in which the skin is abnormally dry.
Skin		
abscess (AB-sess)		A collection of pus in the skin.
acne (ACK-nee)		Inflammatory disease of the sebaceous glands and hair follicles resulting in papules and pustules.

Pathology (continued)

Term	Word Parts	Definition
acne rosacea (ACK-nee roh-ZAY-she-ah)		Chronic form of acne seen in adults involving redness, tiny pimples, and broken blood vessels, primarily on the nose and cheeks.
acne vulgaris (ACK-nee vul-GAY-ris)		Common form of acne seen in teenagers. Characterized by comedos, papules, and pustules.
albinism (al-BIH-nizm)	albin/o = white -ism = state of	A genetic condition in which the body is unable to make melanin. Characterized by white hair and skin and red pupils due to the lack of pigment. The person with albinism is called an *albino*.
basal cell carcinoma (BCC) (BAY-sal / sell / kar-sin-NOH-ma) ■ **Figure 3.17** Basal cell carcinoma. A frequent type of skin cancer that rarely metastasizes. *(Centers for Disease Control)*	bas/o = base -al = pertaining to carcin/o = cancer -oma = tumor	Cancerous tumor of the basal cell layer of the epidermis. A frequent type of skin cancer that rarely metastasizes or spreads. These cancers can arise on sun-exposed skin.
burn		Damage to the skin that can result from exposure to open fire, electricity, ultraviolet (UV) light from the sun, or caustic chemicals. Seriousness depends on the amount of body surface involved and the depth of the burn as determined by the amount of damage to each layer. Skin and burns are categorized as first degree, second degree, or third degree. See Figure 3.18 ■ for a description of the damage associated with each degree of burn. Extent of a burn is estimated using the Rule of Nines (see Figure 3.19 ■).

Pathology (continued)

Term	Word Parts	Definition

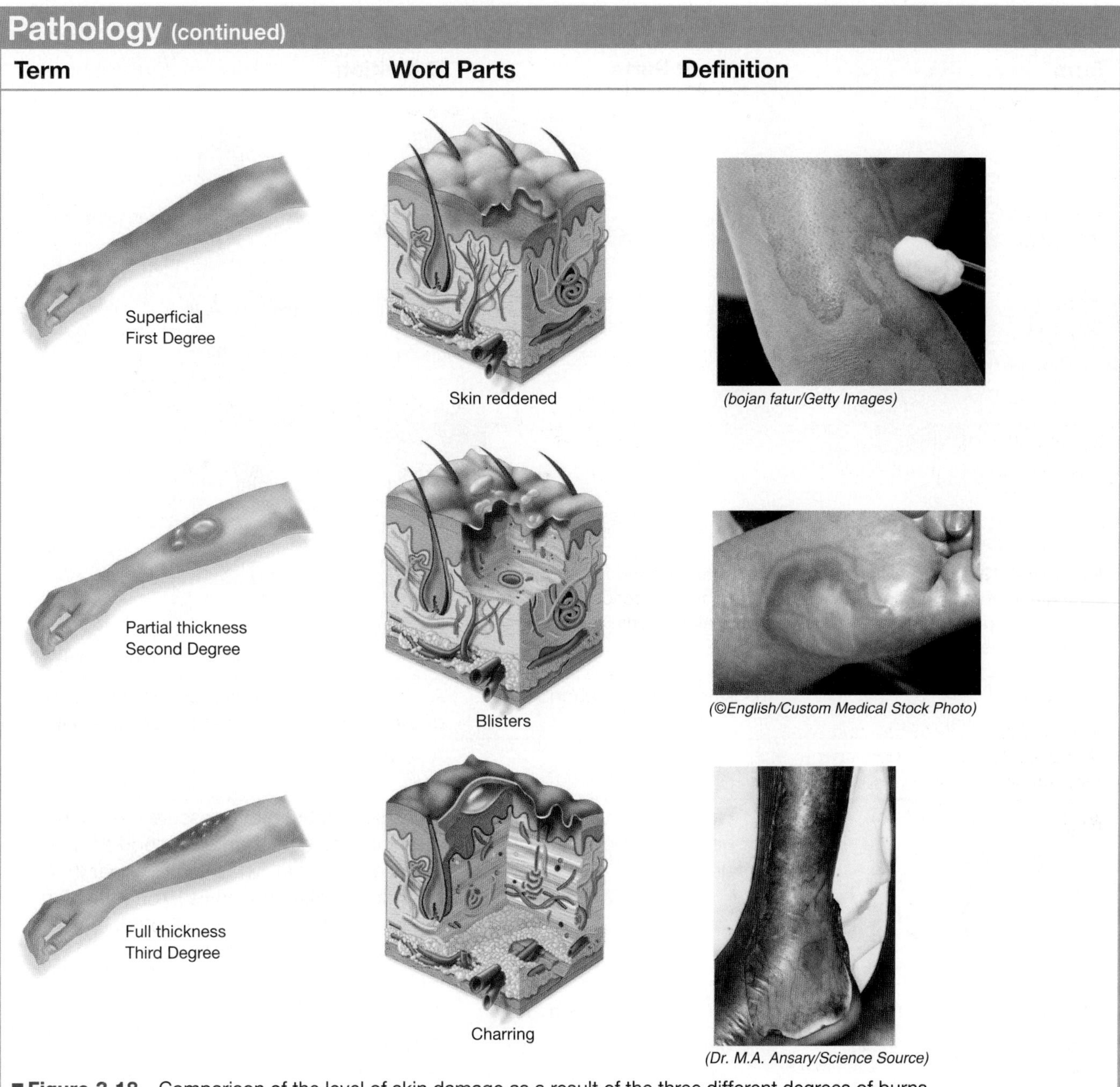

■ **Figure 3.18** Comparison of the level of skin damage as a result of the three different degrees of burns.

Pathology (continued)

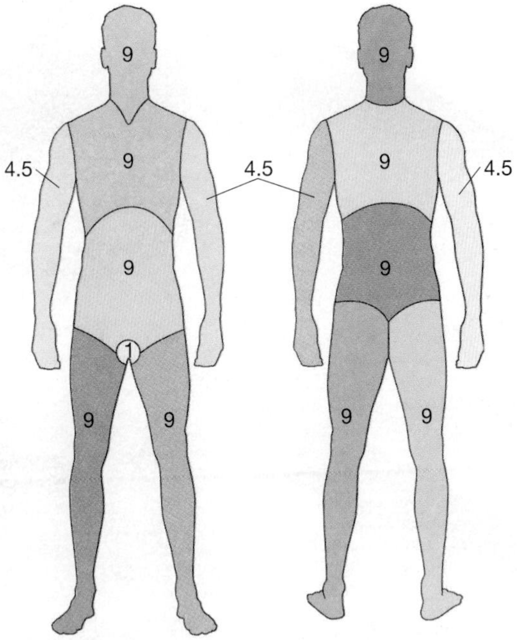

■ **Figure 3.19** Rule of Nines. A method for determining percentage of body burned. Each differently colored section represents a percentage of the body surface. All sections added together will equal 100%.

Term	Word Parts	Definition
cellulitis (sell-you-LYE-tis)	-itis = inflammation	A diffuse, acute infection and inflammation of the connective tissue found in the skin.
cicatrix (SICK-ah-trix)		A scar.
decubitus ulcer (decub) (dee-KYOO-bih-tus)	Comes from the Latin word *decumbo*, meaning "lying down"	Open sore caused by pressure over bony prominences cutting off the blood flow to the overlying skin. These can appear in bedridden patients who lie in one position too long and can be difficult to heal. Also called *bedsore* or *pressure sore.*
dermatitis (der-mah-TYE-tis)	dermat/o = skin -itis = inflammation	Inflammation of the skin.
dermatosis (der-mah-TOH-sis)	dermat/o = skin -osis = abnormal condition	A general term indicating the presence of an abnormal skin condition.
dry gangrene (GANG-green)		Late stages of gangrene characterized by the affected area becoming dried, blackened, and shriveled; referred to as *mummified.*
eczema (EK-zeh-mah)		Superficial dermatitis of unknown cause accompanied by redness, vesicles, itching, and crusting.
gangrene (GANG-green)		Tissue necrosis usually due to deficient blood supply.
ichthyosis (ick-thee-OH-sis)	ichthy/o = scaly, dry -osis = abnormal condition	Condition in which the skin becomes dry, scaly, and keratinized.

Pathology (continued)

Term	Word Parts	Definition
impetigo (im-peh-TYE-goh)		A highly infectious bacterial infection of the skin with pustules that rupture and become crusted over.
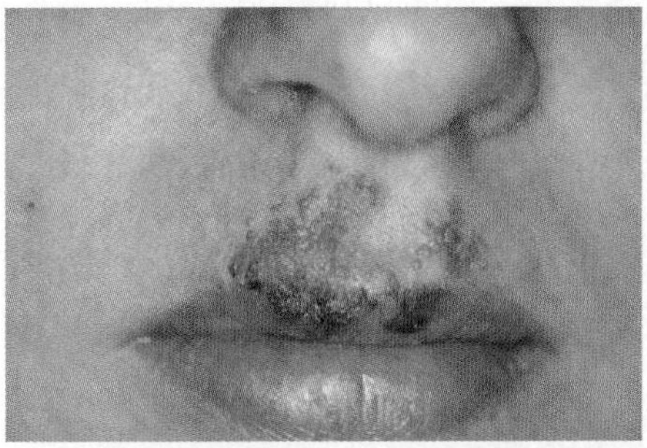 ■ **Figure 3.20** Impetigo, a highly contagious bacterial infection. *(Biophoto Associates)*		
Kaposi's sarcoma (KAP-oh-seez / sar-KOH-mah)	sarc/o = flesh -oma = tumor	Form of skin cancer frequently seen in acquired immunodeficiency syndrome (AIDS) patients. Consists of brownish-purple papules that spread from the skin and metastasize to internal organs.
keloid (KEE-loyd)		Formation of a raised and thickened hypertrophic scar after an injury or surgery.
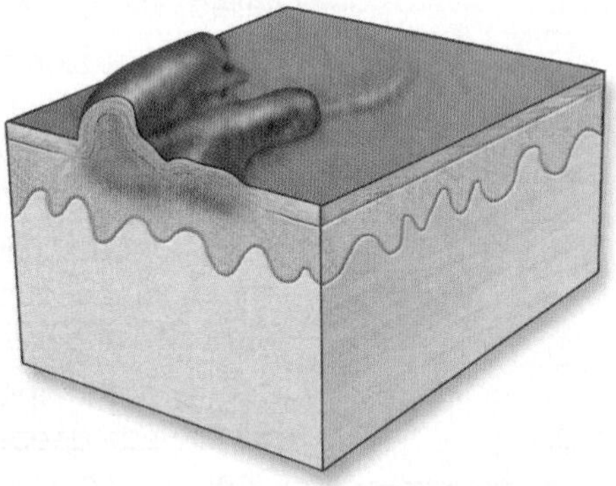 ■ **Figure 3.21** Keloid.		
keratosis (kair-ah-TOH-sis)	kerat/o = hard, horny -osis = abnormal condition	Term for any skin condition involving an overgrowth and thickening of the epidermis layer.
laceration		A torn or jagged wound; incorrectly used to describe a cut.
malignant melanoma (MM) (mah-LIG-nant / mel-a-NOH-ma)	melan/o = black -oma = tumor	Dangerous form of skin cancer caused by an uncontrolled growth of melanocytes. May quickly metastasize or spread to internal organs.
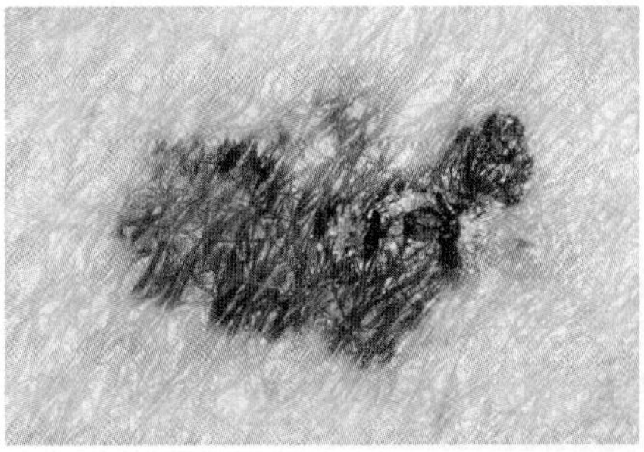 ■ **Figure 3.22** Malignant melanoma. This photograph demonstrates the highly characteristic color of this tumor. *(National Cancer Institute)*		

Pathology (continued)

Term	Word Parts	Definition
pediculosis (peh-dik-you-LOH-sis)	pedicul/o = lice -osis = abnormal condition	Infestation with lice. The eggs laid by the lice are called nits and cling tightly to hair.
psoriasis (soh-RYE-ah-sis)	-iasis = abnormal condition	Chronic inflammatory condition consisting of papules forming "silvery scale" patches with circular borders.

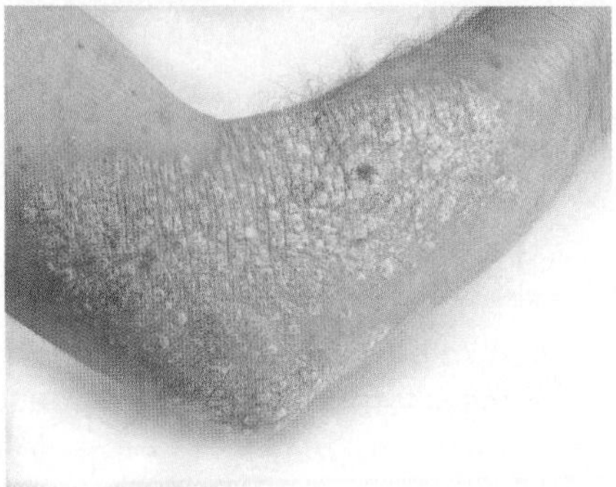

■ **Figure 3.23** Psoriasis. This photograph demonstrates the characteristic white skin patches of this condition. *(phasinphoto/ Shutterstock)*

Term	Word Parts	Definition
rubella (roo-BELL-ah)		Contagious viral skin infection. Commonly called *German measles.*
scabies (SKAY-bees)		Contagious skin disease caused by an egg-laying mite that burrows through the skin and causes redness and intense itching; often seen in children.
sebaceous cyst (see-BAY-shus / SIST)	seb/o = oil	Sac under the skin filled with sebum or oil from a sebaceous gland. This can grow to a large size and may need to be excised.
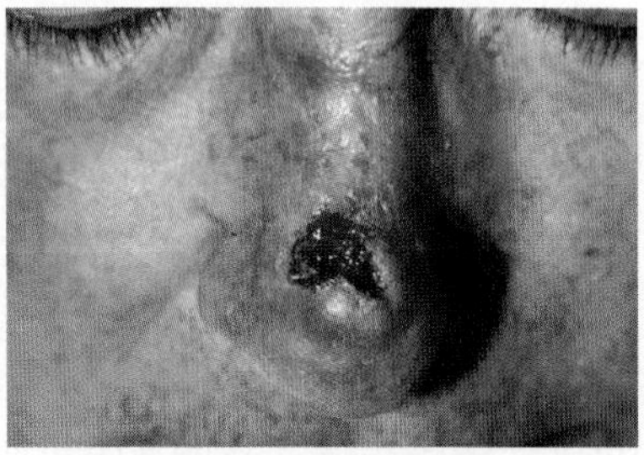 **squamous cell carcinoma** (SCC) (SKWAY-mus/sell/kar-sih-NOH-mah)	carcin/o = cancer -oma = tumor	Cancer of the epidermis layer of skin that may invade deeper tissue and metastasize. Often begins as a sore that does not heal.

■ **Figure 3.24** Squamous cell carcinoma. *(National Cancer Institute)*

Term	Word Parts	Definition
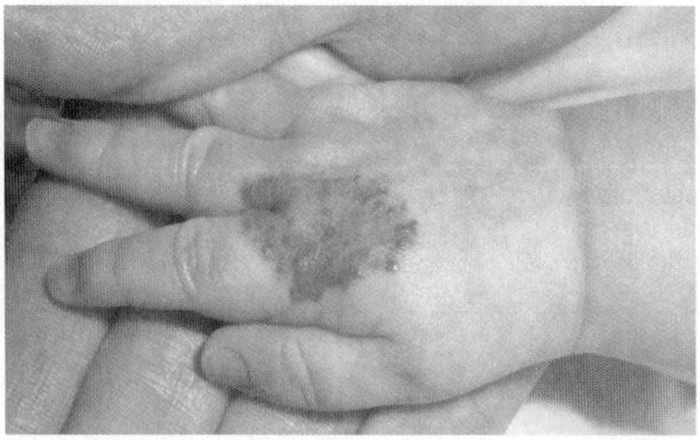 **strawberry hemangioma** (hee-man-jee-OH-ma)	hem/o = blood angi/o = vessel -oma = mass	Congenital collection of dilated blood vessels causing a red birthmark that fades a few months after birth.

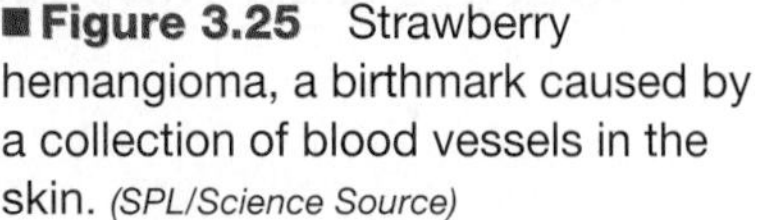

■ **Figure 3.25** Strawberry hemangioma, a birthmark caused by a collection of blood vessels in the skin. *(SPL/Science Source)*

Pathology (continued)

Term	Word Parts	Definition
systemic lupus erythematosus (SLE) (sis-TEM-ik / LOO-pus / air-ih-them-ah-TOH-sis)	system/o = system -ic = pertaining to erythr/o = red	Chronic disease of the connective tissue that injures the skin, joints, kidneys, nervous system, and mucous membranes. This is an autoimmune condition meaning that the body's own immune system attacks normal tissue of the body. May produce a characteristic red, scaly butterfly rash across the cheeks and nose.
tinea (TIN-ee-ah)		Fungal skin disease resulting in itching, scaling lesions.
tinea capitis (TIN-ee-ah / CAP-it-is)	*Capitis* is the Latin term for the head	Fungal infection of the scalp. Commonly called *ringworm.*
tinea pedis (TIN-ee-ah / PED-is)	*Pedis* is the Latin term for the foot	Fungal infection of the foot. Commonly called *athlete's foot.*
varicella (vair-ih-SELL-ah) ■ **Figure 3.26** Varicella or chickenpox, a viral skin infection. In this photograph, the rash is beginning to form scabs. *(Beneda Miroslav/Shutterstock)*		Contagious viral skin infection. Commonly called *chickenpox.*
verruca (ver-ROO-kah)		Commonly called *warts*; a benign growth caused by a virus. Has a rough surface that is removed by chemicals and/or laser therapy.
vitiligo (vit-ill-EYE-go)		Disappearance of pigment from the skin in patches, causing a milk-white appearance. Also called *leukoderma.*
wet gangrene (GANG-green)		An area of gangrene that becomes secondarily infected by pus-producing bacteria.
Hair		
alopecia (al-oh-PEE-she-ah)		Absence or loss of hair, especially of the head. Commonly called *baldness.*
carbuncle (CAR-bung-kl)		Furuncle involving several hair follicles.
furuncle (FOO-rung-kl)		Bacterial infection of a hair follicle. Characterized by redness, pain, and swelling. Also called a *boil.*
trichomycosis (trik-oh-my-KOH-sis)	trich/o = hair myc/o = fungus -osis = abnormal condition	Abnormal condition of hair fungus.

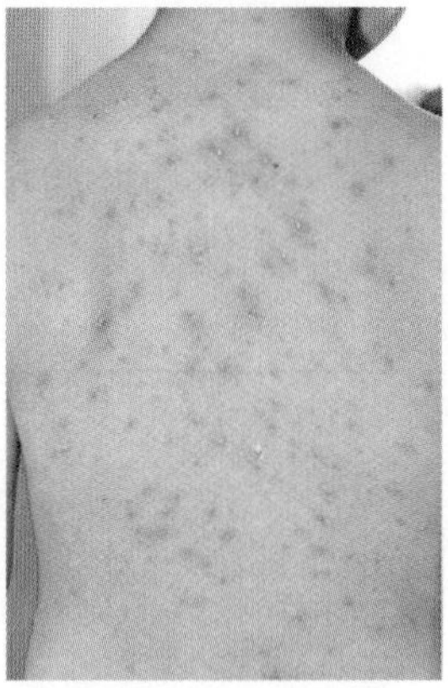

Pathology (continued)

Term	Word Parts	Definition
Nails		
onychia (oh-NICK-ee-ah)	onych/o = nail -ia = state, condition	Infected nail bed.
onychomycosis (on-ih-koh-my-KOH-sis)	onych/o = nail myc/o = fungus -osis = abnormal condition	Abnormal condition of nail fungus.
onychophagia (on-ih-koh-FAY-jee-ah)	onych/o = nail -phagia = eat, swallow	Nail eating (nail biting).
paronychia (pair-oh-NICK-ee-ah)	para- = beside onych/o = nail -ia = state, condition	Infection of the skin fold around a nail.

■ **Figure 3.27** Paronychia.
(Scott Camazine/Getty Images)

Practice As You Go

C. Match each pathology term with its definition.

1. ________ eczema	a. decubitus ulcer
2. ________ nevus	b. lack of skin pigment
3. ________ lipoma	c. acne commonly seen in adults
4. ________ urticaria	d. hardened skin
5. ________ bedsore	e. redness, vesicles, itching, crusts
6. ________ acne rosacea	f. birthmark
7. ________ acne vulgaris	g. excessive hair growth
8. ________ hirsutism	h. caused by deficient blood supply
9. ________ alopecia	i. fatty tumor
10. ________ gangrene	j. hives
11. ________ scleroderma	k. baldness
12. ________ albinism	l. acne of adolescence

Diagnostic Procedures

Term	Word Parts	Definition
Clinical Laboratory Tests		
culture and sensitivity (C&S)		Laboratory test that grows a colony of bacteria removed from an infected area in order to identify the specific infecting bacteria and then determine its sensitivity to a variety of antibiotics.
Biopsy Procedures		
biopsy (BX, bx) (BYE-op-see) Word Watch Be careful when using *bi-* meaning "two" and *bi/o* meaning "life."	bi/o = life -opsy = view of	Piece of tissue removed by syringe and needle, knife, punch, or brush to examine under a microscope. Used to aid in diagnosis.
exfoliative cytology (ex-FOH-lee-ah-tiv/ sigh-TALL-oh-jee)	cyt/o = cell -logy = study of	Scraping cells from tissue and then examining them under a microscope.
frozen section (FS)		Thin piece of tissue cut from a frozen specimen for rapid examination under a microscope.
fungal scrapings	-al = pertaining to	Scrapings, taken with a curette or scraper, of tissue from lesions are placed on a growth medium and examined under a microscope to identify fungal growth.

Therapeutic Procedures

Term	Word Parts	Definition
Skin Grafting		
allograft (AL-oh-graft)	allo- = other	Skin graft from one person to another; donor is usually a cadaver. Also called *homograft* (homo = same).
autograft (AW-toh-graft)	auto- = self	Skin graft from a person's own body.

■ **Figure 3.28** A freshly applied autograft. Note that the donor skin has been perforated so that it can be stretched to cover a larger burned area. *(Bob Ingelhart/Getty Images)*

Term	Word Parts	Definition
dermatome (DER-mah-tohm)	derm/o = skin -tome = instrument to cut	Instrument for cutting the skin or thin transplants of skin.
dermatoplasty (DER-mah-toh-plas-tee)	dermat/o = skin -plasty = surgical repair	Skin grafting; transplantation of skin.
skin graft (SG)		Transfer of skin from a normal area to cover another site. Used to treat burn victims and after some surgical procedures. Also called *dermatoplasty.*

Therapeutic Procedures (continued)

xenograft (ZEN-oh-graft)	xeno- = foreign	Skin graft from an animal of another species (usually a pig) to a human. Also called *heterograft* (hetero- = other).
Surgical Procedures		
cauterization (kaw-ter-ih-ZAY-shun)	cauter/o = to burn	Destruction of tissue by using caustic chemicals, electric currents, or by heating or freezing.
cryosurgery (cry-oh-SER-jer-ee)	cry/o = cold	Use of extreme cold to freeze and destroy tissue.
curettage (koo-REH-tahzh)		Removal of superficial skin lesions with a curette (surgical instrument shaped like a spoon) or scraper.
debridement (de-BREED-mint)		Removal of foreign material and dead or damaged tissue from a wound.
electrocautery (ee-leck-troh-KAW-teh-ree)	electr/o = electricity	To destroy tissue with an electric current.
incision and drainage (I&D)	cis/o = to cut	Making an incision to create an opening for the drainage of material such as pus.
onychectomy (on-ee-KECK-toh-mee)	onych/o = nail -ectomy = surgical removal	Removal of a nail.
Plastic Surgery Procedures		
chemabrasion (kee-moh-BRAY-zhun)	chem/o = chemical	Abrasion using chemicals. Also called a *chemical peel.*
dermabrasion (DERM-ah-bray-shun)	derm/o = skin	Abrasion or rubbing using wire brushes or sandpaper. Performed to remove acne scars, tattoos, and scar tissue.
laser therapy		Removal of skin lesions and birthmarks using a laser beam that emits intense heat and power at a close range. The laser converts frequencies of light into one small, powerful beam.
liposuction (LIP-oh-suck-shun)	lip/o = fat	Removal of fat beneath the skin by means of suction.
rhytidectomy (rit-ih-DECK-toh-mee)	rhytid/o = wrinkle -ectomy = surgical removal	Surgical removal of excess skin to eliminate wrinkles. Commonly referred to as a *face lift.*

Practice As You Go

D. Match each procedure term with its definition.

1. ________ debridement a. surgical removal of wrinkled skin
2. ________ cauterization b. instrument to cut thin slices of skin
3. ________ chemabrasion c. removing a piece of tissue for examination
4. ________ dermatoplasty d. use of extreme cold to destroy tissue
5. ________ biopsy e. skin grafting
6. ________ rhytidectomy f. removal of lesions with scraper
7. ________ curettage g. removal of skin with brushes
8. ________ dermabrasion h. removal of damaged skin
9. ________ dermatome i. destruction of tissue with electric current
10. ________ cryosurgery j. chemical peel

Pharmacology

Classification	Word Parts	Action	Examples
anesthetic (an-es-THET-tic)	an- = without esthesi/o = feeling -tic = pertaining to	Deadens pain when applied to the skin.	lidocaine, Xylocaine; procaine, Novocain
antibiotic (an-tye-bye-AW-tic)	anti- = against bi/o = life -tic = pertaining to	Kills bacteria causing skin infections.	bacitracin/neomycin/polymixinB, Neosporin ointment
antifungal (an-tye-FUNG-all)	anti- = against -al = pertaining to	Kills fungi infecting the skin.	miconazole, Monistat; clotrimazole, Lotrimin
antiparasitic (an-tye-pair-ah-SIT-tic)	anti- = against -ic = pertaining to	Kills mites or lice.	lindane, Kwell; permethrin, Nix
antipruritic (an-tye-proo-RIGH-tik)	anti- = against -ic = pertaining to	Reduces severe itching.	diphenhydramine, Benadryl; camphor/pramoxine/zinc, Caladryl
antiseptic (an-tye-SEP-tic)	anti- = against septic/o = infection -tic = pertaining to	Kills bacteria in skin cuts and wounds or at a surgical site.	isopropyl alcohol; hydrogen peroxide
corticosteroid cream	cortic/o = outer layer	A cream containing a hormone produced by the adrenal cortex that has very strong anti-inflammatory properties.	hydrocortisone, Cortaid; triamcinolone, Kenalog

Abbreviations

BCC	basal cell carcinoma	**MM**	malignant melanoma
BX, bx	biopsy	**SCC**	squamous cell carcinoma
C&S	culture and sensitivity	**SG**	skin graft
decub	decubitus ulcer	**SLE**	systemic lupus erythematosus
Derm, derm	dermatology	**STSG**	split-thickness skin graft
FS	frozen section	**Subc, Subq**	subcutaneous
I&D	incision and drainage	**UV**	ultraviolet
ID	intradermal		

Word Watch

Be careful when using the abbreviation *ID* meaning "intradermal" and *I&D* meaning "incision and drainage."

Practice As You Go

E. Give the abbreviation for each term.

1. frozen section ______
2. incision and drainage ______
3. intradermal ______
4. subcutaneous ______
5. ultraviolet ______
6. biopsy ______
7. culture and sensitivity ______
8. basal cell carcinoma ______
9. decubitus ulcer ______
10. dermatology ______

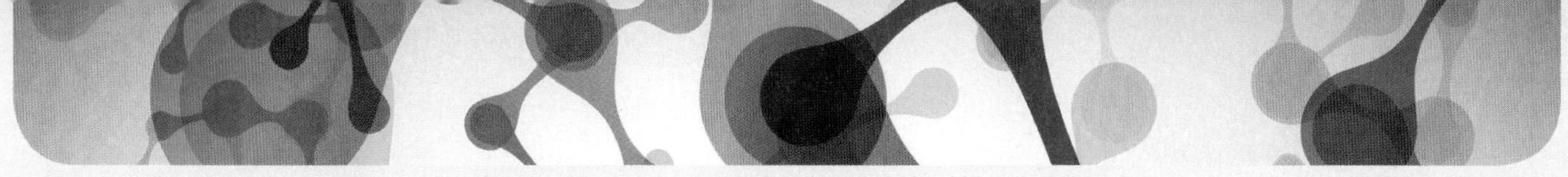

Chapter Review

Real-World Applications

Medical Record Analysis

This Dermatology Consultation Report contains 11 medical terms. Underline each term and write it in the list below the report. Then define each term.

Dermatology Consultation Report

Reason for Consultation:	Possible recurrence of basal cell carcinoma, left cheek.
History of Present Illness:	Patient is a 74-year-old male first seen by his regular physician five years ago for persistent facial lesions. Biopsies revealed basal cell carcinoma in two lesions, one on the nasal tip and the other on the left cheek. These were successfully excised. The patient noted that the left cheek lesion returned approximately one year ago. Patient reports pruritus and states the lesion is growing larger.
Results of Physical Exam:	Examination revealed a 10 × 14 mm lesion on left cheek 20 mm anterior to the ear. The lesion displays marked erythema and poorly defined borders. The area immediately around the lesion shows depigmentation with vesicles.
Assessment:	Recurrence of basal cell carcinoma.
Recommendations:	Due to the lesion's size, shape, and reoccurrence, deep excision of the carcinoma through the epidermis and dermis layers followed by dermatoplasty is recommended.

	Term	Definition
1.	______________	______________________________
2.	______________	______________________________
3.	______________	______________________________
4.	______________	______________________________
5.	______________	______________________________
6.	______________	______________________________
7.	______________	______________________________
8.	______________	______________________________
9.	______________	______________________________
10.	______________	______________________________
11.	______________	______________________________

Chart Note Transcription

The chart note below contains 10 phrases that can be reworded with a medical term that you learned in this chapter. Each phrase is identified with an underline. Determine the medical term and write your answers in the spaces provided.

Pearson General Hospital Consultation Report

Task Edit View Time Scale Options Help Download Archive Date: 17 May 2015

Current Complaint:	A 64-year-old female with an open sore **1** on her right leg is seen by the specialist in treating diseases of the skin. **2**
Past History:	Patient states she first noticed an area of pain, severe itching, **3** and redness of the skin **4** just below her right knee about 6 weeks ago. One week later raised spots containing pus **5** appeared. Patient states the raised spots containing pus ruptured and the open sore appeared.
Signs and Symptoms:	Patient has a deep open sore 5 × 3 cm: It is 4 cm distal to the knee on the lateral aspect of the right leg. It appears to extend into the middle skin layer, **6** and the edges show signs of tissue death. **7** The open sore has a small amount of drainage but there is no odor. A sample of the drainage that was grown in the lab to identify the microorganism and determine the best antibiotic **8** of the drainage revealed *Staphylococcus* bacteria in the open sore.
Diagnosis:	Inflammation of connective tissue in the skin. **9**
Treatment:	Removal of damaged tissue **10** of the open sore followed by application of an antibiotic cream. Patient was instructed to return to the skin disease specialist's office in two weeks, or sooner if the open sore does not heal or if it begins draining pus.

1. ______________________

2. ______________________

3. ______________________

4. ______________________

5. ______________________

6. ______________________

7. ______________________

8. ______________________

9. ______________________

10. ______________________

Case Study

Below is a case study presentation of a patient with a condition discussed in this chapter. Read the case study and answer the questions below. Some questions will ask for information not included within this chapter. Use your text, a medical dictionary, or any other reference material you choose to answer these questions.

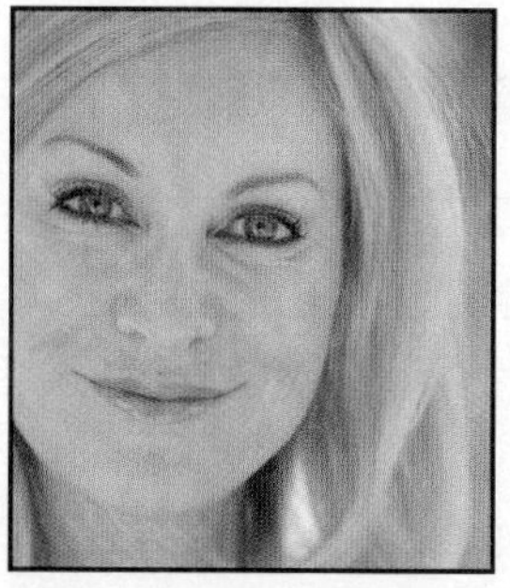
(Monkey Business Images/Shutterstock)

A 40-year-old female is seen in the dermatologist's office, upon the recommendation of her internist, for a workup for suspected SLE. Her presenting symptoms include erythema rash across her cheeks and nose, photosensitivity resulting in raised rash in sun-exposed areas, patches of alopecia, and pain and stiffness in her joints. The dermatologist examines the patient and orders exfoliative cytology and fungal scrapings to rule out other sources of the rash. Her internist had already placed the patient on oral anti-inflammatory medication for joint pain. The dermatologist orders corticosteroid cream for the rash. The patient is advised to use a sunscreen and make a follow-up appointment for results of the biopsy.

Questions

1. What pathological condition does the internist think this patient might have? Look this condition up in a reference source, and include a short description of it. SLE is an autoimmune disease. Use a reference source to look up the name of another autoimmune disease.

____

____

2. List and define each of the patient's presenting symptoms in your own words.

____

____

3. What diagnostic tests did the dermatologist perform? Describe it in your own words. Why were they important in helping the dermatologist make a diagnosis?

____

____

4. Each physician initiated a treatment. Describe them in your own words.

____

____

5. What do you think the term "workup" means?

____

____

Practice Exercises

A. Define the Word Parts

	Definition	Example from Chapter
1. **cry/o**		
2. **cutane/o**		
3. **diaphor/o**		
4. **py/o**		
5. **cauter/o**		
6. **ungu/o**		
7. **lip/o**		
8. **hidr/o**		
9. **rhytid/o**		
10. **seb/o**		
11. **trich/o**		
12. **necr/o**		
13. **-derma**		
14. **allo-**		
15. **xeno-**		

B. Describe the Type of Burn

1. first degree ______________________________
2. second degree ______________________________
3. third degree ______________________________

C. Define the Term

1. macule ______________________________
2. papule ______________________________
3. cyst ______________________________
4. fissure ______________________________

5. pustule ______

6. wheal ______

7. vesicle ______

8. ulcer ______

9. nodule ______

10. laceration ______

D. Word Building Practice

The combining form **dermat/o** refers to the skin. Use it to write a term that means:

1. inflammation of the skin ______
2. any abnormal skin condition ______
3. an instrument for cutting the skin ______
4. specialist in skin ______
5. surgical repair of the skin ______
6. study of the skin ______

The combining form **melan/o** means black. Use it to write a term that means:

7. black tumor ______
8. black cell ______

The suffix **-derma** means skin. Use it to write a term that means:

9. scaly skin ______
10. white skin ______
11. red skin ______

The combining form **onych/o** refers to the nail. Use it to write a term that means:

12. abnormal softening of the nails ______
13. infection around the nail ______
14. nail eating (biting) ______
15. removal of the nail ______

E. What Does it Stand For?

1. C&S ______
2. BCC ______
3. derm ______

4. SG ______________________________

5. decub ______________________________

6. MM ______________________________

F. Fill in the Blank

impetigo	tinea	keloid	exfoliative cytology	xeroderma
petechiae	frozen section	paronychia	scabies	Kaposi's sarcoma

1. The winter climates can cause dry skin. The medical term for this is ______________________________.
2. Kim has experienced small pinpoint purplish spots caused by bleeding under the skin. This is called ______________.
3. Janet has a fungal skin disease. This is called ______________________________.
4. A contagious skin disease caused by a mite is ______________________________.
5. An infection around the entire nail is called ______________________________.
6. A form of skin cancer affecting AIDS patients is called ______________________________.
7. Latrivia has a bacterial skin infection that results in pustules crusting and rupturing. It is called ______________.
8. James's burn scar became a hypertrophic ______________________________.
9. For a(n) ______________________________ test, cells scraped off the skin are examined under a microscope.
10. During surgery a ______________________________ was ordered for a rapid exam of tissue cut from a tumor.

G. Pharmacology Challenge

Fill in the classification for each drug description, then match the brand name.

	Drug Description	Classification	Brand Name
1.	________ kills fungi	______________	a. Kwell
2.	________ reduces severe itching	______________	b. Cortaid
3.	________ kills mites and lice	______________	c. Benadryl
4.	________ powerful anti-inflammatory	______________	d. Neosporin
5.	________ deadens pain	______________	e. Monistat
6.	________ kills bacteria	______________	f. Xylocaine

Labeling Exercise

Image A

Write the labels for this figure on the numbered lines provided.

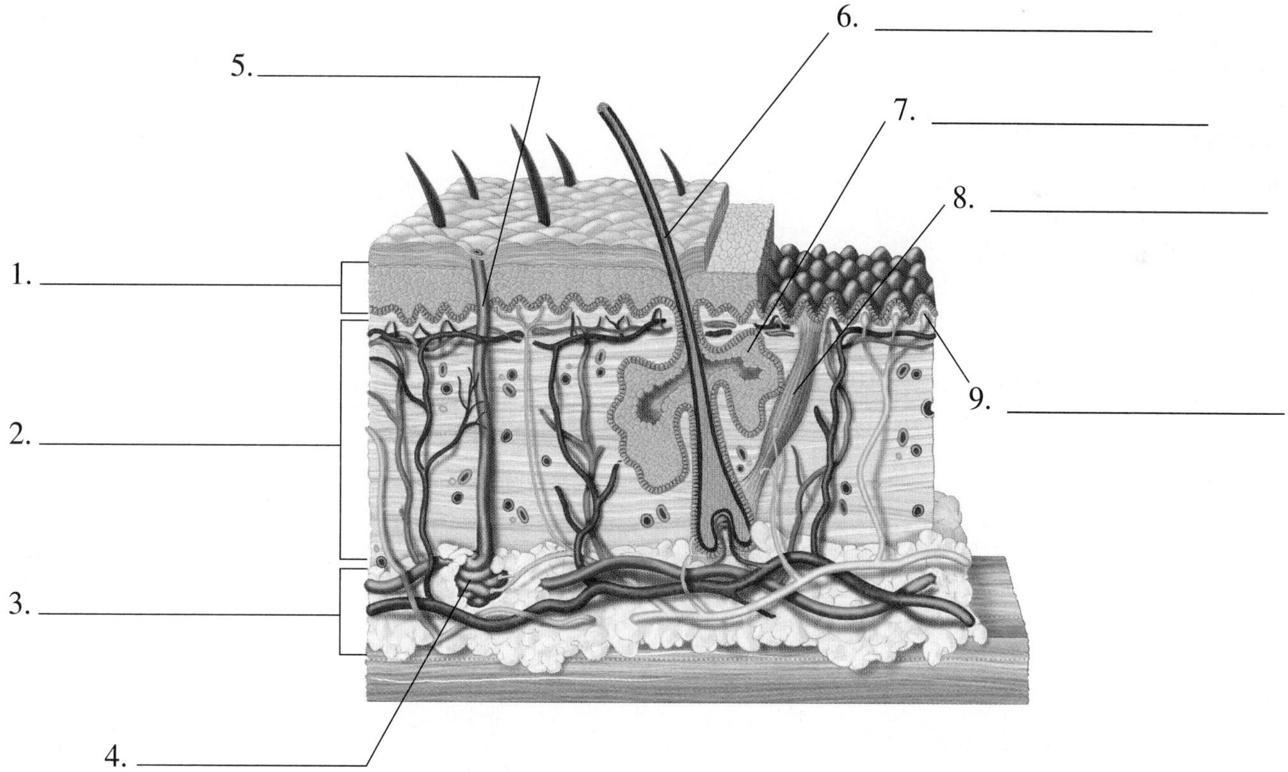

Image B

Write the labels for this figure on the numbered lines provided.

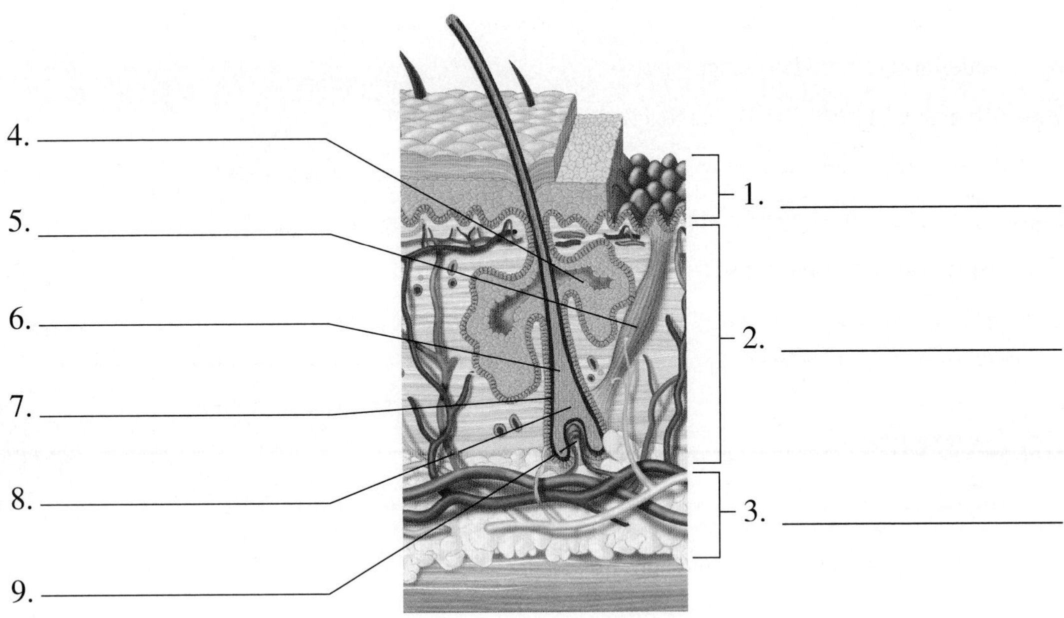

Image C

Write the labels for this figure on the numbered lines provided.

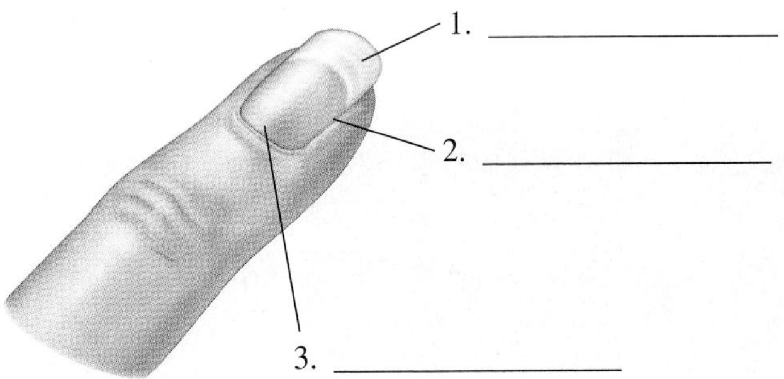

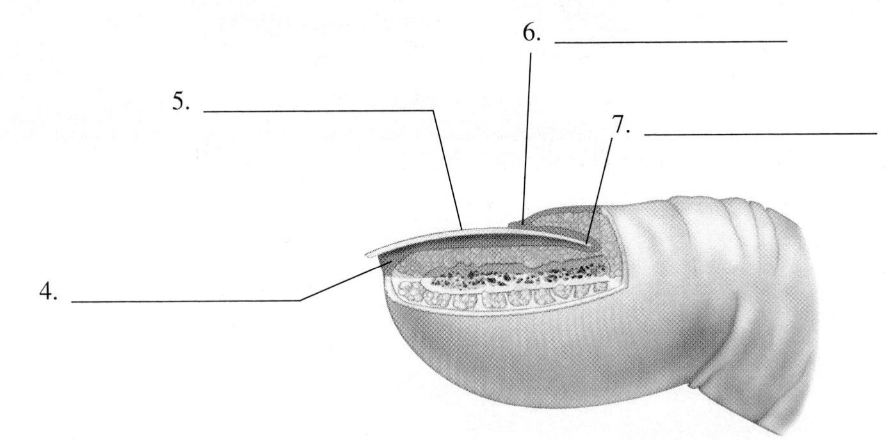

4

Musculoskeletal System

Learning Objectives

Upon completion of this chapter, you will be able to

- Identify and define the combining forms, suffixes, and prefixes introduced in this chapter.
- Correctly spell and pronounce medical terms and major anatomical structures relating to the musculoskeletal system.
- Locate and describe the major organs of the musculoskeletal system and their functions.
- Correctly place bones in either the axial or the appendicular skeleton.
- List and describe the components of a long bone.
- Identify bony projections and depressions.
- Identify the parts of a synovial joint.
- Describe the characteristics of the three types of muscle tissue.
- Use movement terminology correctly.
- Identify and define musculoskeletal system anatomical terms.
- Identify and define selected musculoskeletal system pathology terms.
- Identify and define selected musculoskeletal system diagnostic procedures.
- Identify and define selected musculoskeletal system therapeutic procedures.
- Identify and define selected medications relating to the musculoskeletal system.
- Define selected abbreviations associated with the musculoskeletal system.

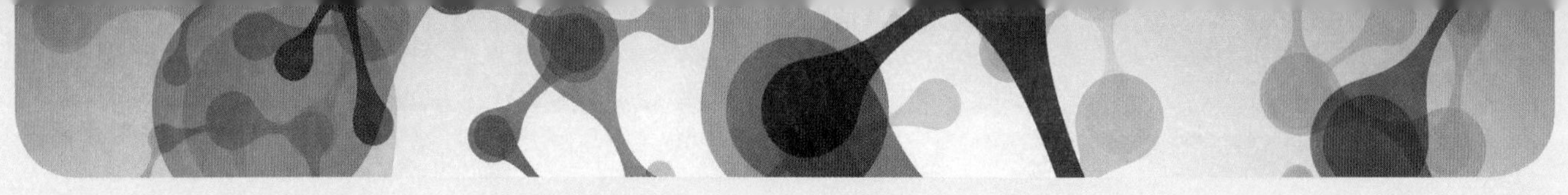

Section I: Skeletal System at a Glance

Function

The skeletal system consists of 206 bones that make up the internal framework of the body, called the skeleton. The skeleton supports the body, protects internal organs, serves as a point of attachment for skeletal muscles for body movement, produces blood cells, and stores minerals.

Organs

Here are the primary structures that comprise the skeletal system:

bones **joints**

Word Parts

Here are the most common word parts (with their meanings) used to build skeletal system terms. For a more comprehensive list, refer to the Terminology section of this chapter.

Combining Forms

ankyl/o	stiff joint
arthr/o	joint
articul/o	joint
burs/o	sac
carp/o	carpus
cervic/o	neck
chondr/o	cartilage
clavicul/o	clavicle
coccyg/o	coccyx
cortic/o	outer layer
cost/o	rib
crani/o	skull
femor/o	femur
fibul/o	fibula
humer/o	humerus
ili/o	ilium
ischi/o	ischium
kyph/o	hump
lamin/o	lamina (part of vertebra)
lord/o	bent backward
lumb/o	loin (low back between ribs and pelvis)
mandibul/o	mandible
maxill/o	maxilla
medull/o	inner region
metacarp/o	metacarpus
metatars/o	metatarsus
myel/o	bone marrow, spinal cord
orth/o	straight
oste/o	bone
patell/o	patella
pector/o	chest
ped/o	child; foot
pelv/o	pelvis
phalang/o	phalanges
pod/o	foot
prosthet/o	addition
pub/o	pubis
radi/o	radius; ray (X-ray)
sacr/o	sacrum
scapul/o	scapula
scoli/o	crooked
spin/o	spine
spondyl/o	vertebrae
stern/o	sternum
synovi/o	synovial membrane
synov/o	synovial membrane
tars/o	tarsus
thorac/o	chest
tibi/o	tibia
uln/o	ulna
vertebr/o	vertebra

(continued on page 84)

Skeletal System Illustrated

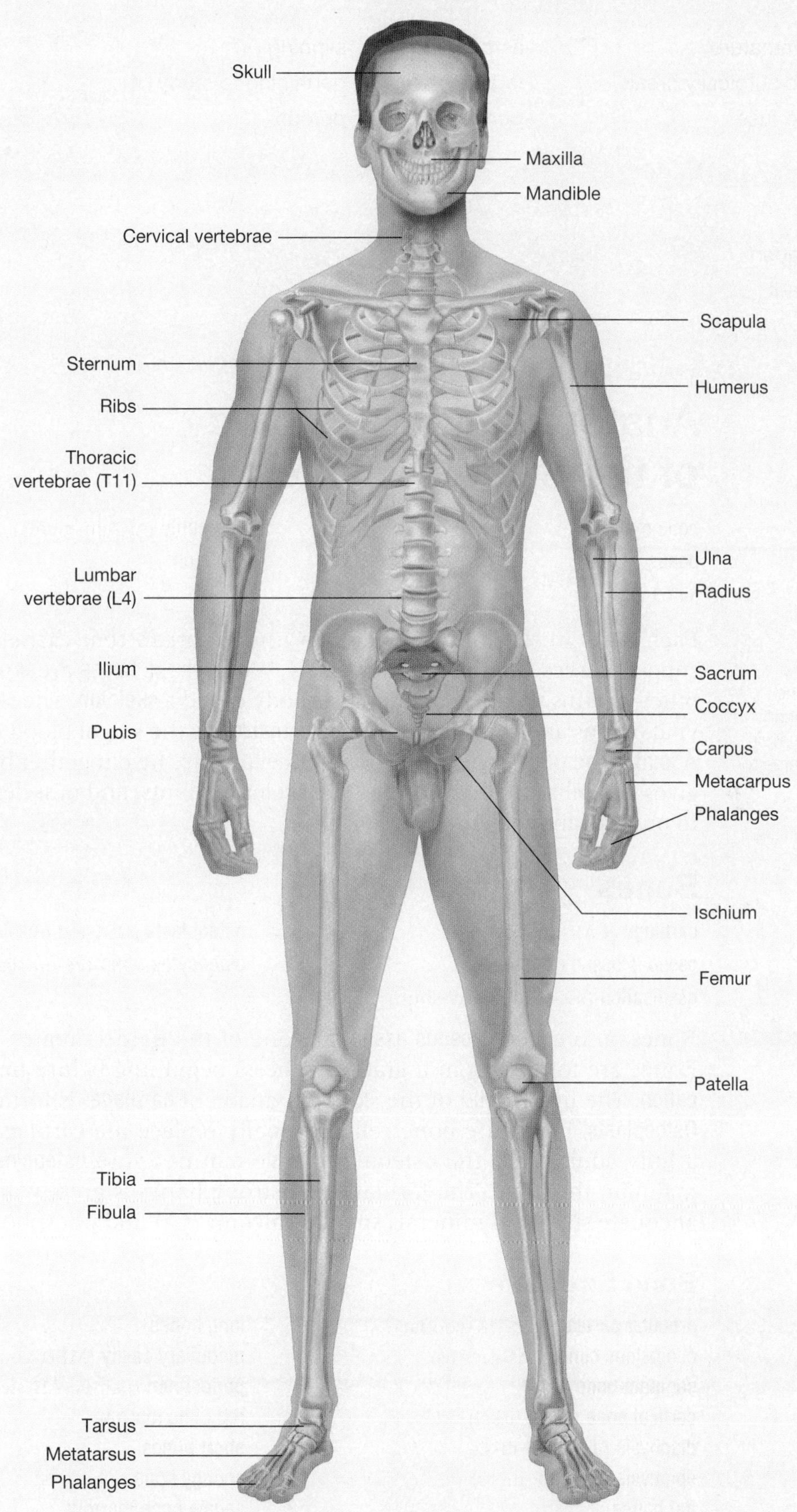

Suffixes

-blast	immature	**-listhesis**	slipping
-clasia	to surgically break	**-logic**	pertaining to study of
-desis	to fuse	**-porosis**	porous

Prefixes

dis-	apart
non-	not

Anatomy and Physiology of the Skeletal System

bone marrow
bones
joints
ligaments (LIG-ah-ments)
skeleton

Med Term Tip

The term *skeleton*, from the Greek word *skeltos* meaning "dried up," was originally used in reference to a dried-up mummified body, but over time came to be used for bones.

Each bone in the human body is a unique organ that carries its own blood supply, nerves, and lymphatic vessels. When these **bones** are connected to each other it forms the framework of the body called a **skeleton.** The skeleton protects vital organs and stores minerals. **Bone marrow** is the site of blood cell production. A **joint** is the place where two bones meet and are held together by **ligaments.** This gives flexibility to the skeleton. The skeleton, joints, and muscles work together to produce movement.

Bones

cartilage (CAR-tih-lij)
osseous tissue (OSS-ee-us)
ossification (oss-sih-fih-KAY-shun)
osteoblasts (OSS-tee-oh-blasts)
osteocytes (OSS-tee-oh-sights)

What's In A Name?

Look for these word parts:
oste/o = bone
-blast = immature
-cyte = cell
-ous = pertaining to

Bones, also called **osseous tissue**, are one of the hardest materials in the body. Bones are formed from a gradual process beginning before birth called **ossification.** The first model of the skeleton, made of **cartilage**, is formed in the fetus. **Osteoblasts**, immature bone cells, gradually replace the cartilage with bone. In a fully adult bone, the osteoblasts have matured into **osteocytes** that work to maintain the bone. The formation of strong bones is greatly dependent on an adequate supply of minerals such as calcium (Ca) and phosphorus (P).

Bone Structure

articular cartilage (ar-TIK-yoo-lar)
cancellous bone (CAN-sell-us)
compact bone
cortical bone (KOR-ti-kal)
diaphysis (dye-AFF-ih-sis)
epiphysis (eh-PIFF-ih-sis)
flat bones
irregular bones
long bones
medullary cavity (MED-you-lair-ee)
periosteum (pair-ee-AH-stee-um)
red bone marrow
short bones
spongy bone
yellow bone marrow

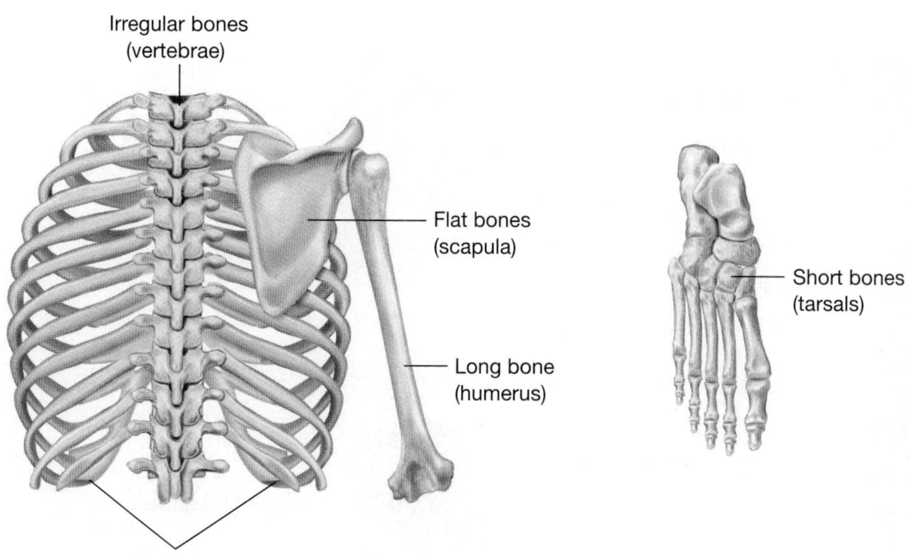

■ **Figure 4.1** Classification of bones by shape.

Several different types of bones are found throughout the body and fall into four categories based on their shape: **long bones**, **short bones**, **flat bones**, and **irregular bones** (see Figure 4.1 ■). Long bones are longer than they are wide; examples are the femur and humerus. Short bones are roughly as long as they are wide; examples are the carpals and tarsals. Irregular bones received their name because the shapes of the bones are very irregular; for example, the vertebrae are irregular bones. Flat bones are usually plate-shaped bones such as the sternum, scapulae, and pelvis.

The majority of bones in the human body are long bones. These bones have similar structure with a central shaft or **diaphysis** that widens at each end, which is called an **epiphysis**. Each epiphysis is covered by a layer of cartilage called **articular cartilage** to prevent bone from rubbing directly on bone. The remaining surface of each bone is covered with a thin connective tissue membrane called the **periosteum**, which contains numerous blood vessels, nerves, and lymphatic vessels. The dense and hard exterior surface bone is called **cortical** or **compact bone. Cancellous** or **spongy bone** is found inside the bone. As its name indicates, spongy bone has spaces in it, giving it a spongelike appearance. These spaces contain **red bone marrow**, which manufactures most of the blood cells and is found in some parts of all bones.

The center of the diaphysis contains an open canal called the **medullary cavity**. Early in life this cavity also contains red bone marrow, but as we age the red bone marrow of the medullary cavity gradually converts to **yellow bone marrow**, which consists primarily of fat cells. Figure 4.2 ■ contains an illustration of the structure of long bones.

What's In A Name?

Look for these word parts:
articul/o = joint
cortic/o = outer layer
medull/o = inner region
oste/o = bone
peri- = around
-al = pertaining to
-ar = pertaining to
-ary = pertaining to

Med Term Tip

Do not confuse a long bone with a large bone. A long bone is not necessarily a large bone. The bones of your fingers are short in length, but since they are longer than they are wide, they are classified as long bones.

Med Term Tip

The term *diaphysis* comes from the Greek term meaning "to grow between."

Bone Projections and Depressions

condyle (KON-dile)
epicondyle (ep-ih-KON-dile)
fissure (FISH-er)
foramen (for-AY-men)
fossa (FOSS-ah)
head
neck
process
sinus (SIGH-nus)
trochanter (tro-KAN-ter)
tubercle (TOO-ber-kl)
tuberosity (too-ber-OSS-ih-tee)

Bones have many projections and depressions; some are rounded and smooth in order to articulate with another bone in a joint. Others are rough to provide muscles with attachment points. The general term for any bony

Med Term Tip

The elbow, commonly referred to as the *funny bone*, is actually a projection of the ulna called the olecranon process.

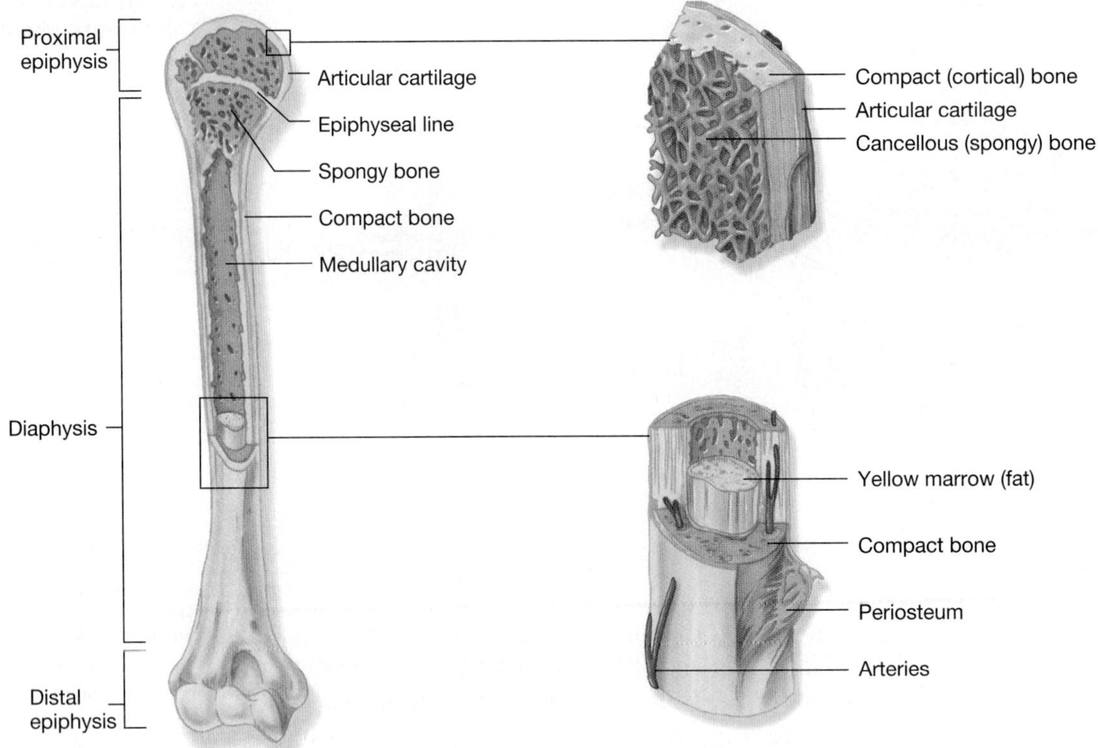

■ **Figure 4.2** Components of a long bone. The entire long bone is on the left side accompanied by a blow-up of the proximal epiphysis and a section of the diaphysis.

projection is a **process**. Then there are specific terms to describe the different shapes and locations of various processes. These terms are commonly used on operative reports and in physicians' records for clear identification of areas on the individual bones. Some of the common bony processes include the following:

1. The **head** is a large, smooth, ball-shaped end on a long bone. It may be separated from the body or shaft of the bone by a narrow area called the **neck**.
2. A **condyle** refers to a smooth, rounded portion at the end of a bone.
3. The **epicondyle** is a projection located above or on a condyle.
4. The **trochanter** refers to a large rough process for the attachment of a muscle.
5. A **tubercle** is a small, rough process that provides the attachment for tendons and muscles.
6. The **tuberosity** is a large, rough process that provides the attachment of tendons and muscles.

What's In A Name?
Look for these word parts:
epi- = above

See Figure 4.3 ■ for an illustration of the processes found on the femur.

Additionally, bones have hollow regions or depressions, the most common of which are the:

7. **Sinus**: a hollow cavity within a bone.
8. **Foramen**: a smooth, round opening for nerves and blood vessels.
9. **Fossa**: consists of a shallow cavity or depression on the surface of a bone.
10. **Fissure**: a slit-type opening.

Skeleton

appendicular skeleton (app-en-DIK-yoo-lar) **axial skeleton** (AK-see-al)

What's In A Name?
Look for these word parts:
-al = pertaining to
-ar = pertaining to

The human skeleton has two divisions: the **axial skeleton** and the **appendicular skeleton**. Figures 4.4 and 4.8 illustrate these two skeletons.

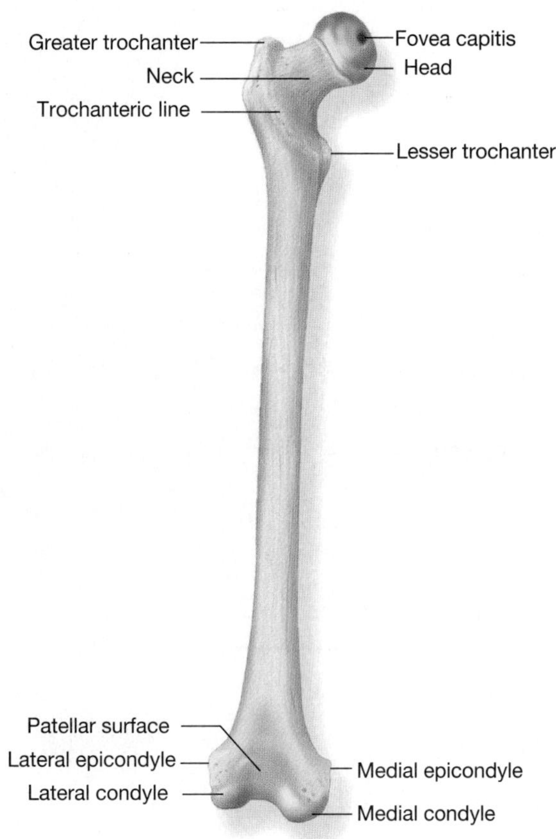

■ **Figure 4.3** Bony processes found on the femur.

Axial Skeleton

cervical vertebrae
coccyx (COCK-six)
cranium (KRAY-nee-um)
ethmoid bone (ETH-moyd)
facial bones
frontal bone
hyoid bone (HIGH-oyd)
intervertebral disk (in-ter-VER-teh-bral)
lacrimal bone (LACK-rim-al)
lumbar vertebrae
mandible (MAN-dih-bl)
maxilla (mack-SIH-lah)
nasal bone
occipital bone (ock-SIP-eh-tal)
palatine bone (PAL-ah-tine)
parietal bone (pah-RYE-eh-tal)
rib cage
sacrum (SAY-crum)
sphenoid bone (SFEE-noyd)
sternum (STER-num)
temporal bone (TEM-por-al)
thoracic vertebrae
vertebral column (VER-teh-bral)
vomer bone (VOH-mer)
zygomatic bone (zeye-go-MAT-ik)

Med Term Tip

Newborn infants have about 300 bones at birth that will fuse into 206 bones as an adult.

The axial skeleton includes the bones of the head, neck, spine, chest, and trunk of the body (see Figure 4.4 ■). These bones form the central axis for the whole body and protect many of the internal organs such as the brain, lungs, and heart.

The head or skull is divided into two parts consisting of the **cranium** and **facial bones**. These bones surround and protect the brain, eyes, ears, nasal cavity, and oral cavity from injury. The muscles for chewing and moving the head are attached to the cranial bones. The cranium encases the brain and consists of the **frontal**, **parietal**, **temporal**, **ethmoid**, **sphenoid**, and **occipital bones**. The facial bones surround the mouth, nose, and eyes, and include the **mandible**, **maxilla**,

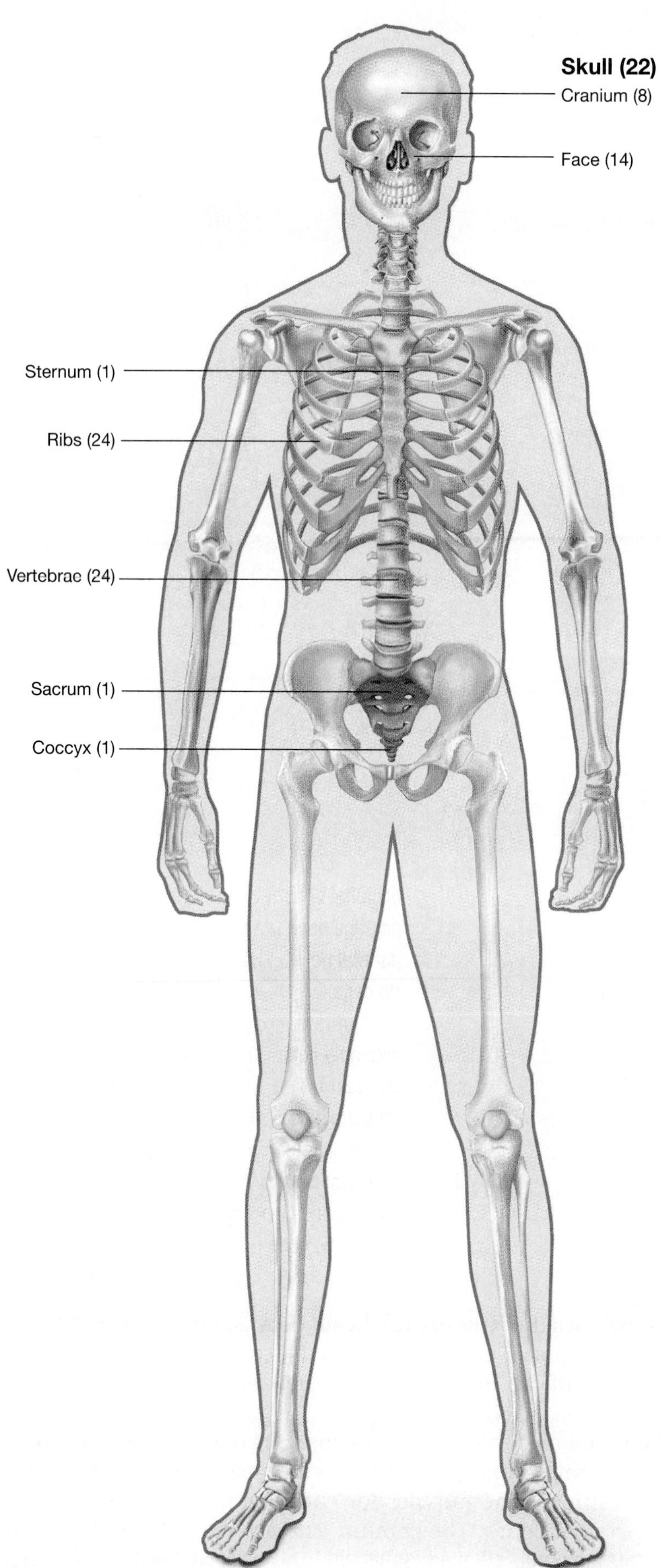

■ **Figure 4.4** Bones of the axial skeleton.

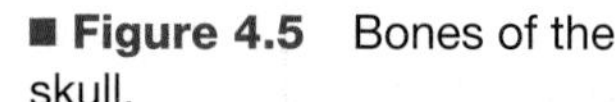

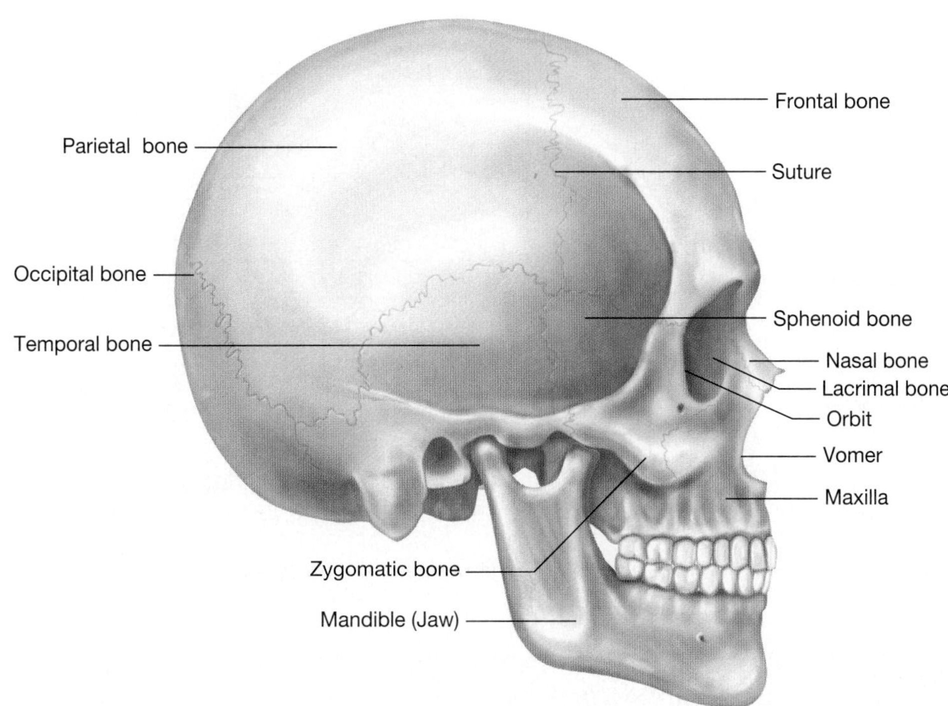

■ **Figure 4.5** Bones of the skull.

zygomatic, **vomer**, **palatine**, **nasal**, and **lacrimal bones**. The cranial and facial bones are illustrated in Figure 4.5 ■ and described in Table 4.1 ■.

The **hyoid bone** is a single U-shaped bone suspended in the neck between the mandible and larynx. It is a point of attachment for swallowing and speech muscles.

The trunk of the body consists of the **vertebral column**, **sternum**, and **rib cage**. The vertebral or spinal column is divided into five sections: **cervical vertebrae**, **thoracic vertebrae**, **lumbar vertebrae**, **sacrum**, and **coccyx** (see Figure 4.6 ■ and Table 4.2 ■). Located between each pair of vertebrae, from the cervical through the lumbar regions, is an **intervertebral disk**. Each disk is composed of fibrocartilage to provide a cushion between the vertebrae. The rib cage has 12 pairs of ribs attached at the back to the vertebral column. Ten of the pairs are also attached to the sternum in the front (see Figure 4.7 ■). The lowest two pairs are called *floating ribs* and

Med Term Tip

The term *coccyx* comes from the Greek word for the cuckoo because the shape of these small bones extending off the sacrum resembles this bird's bill.

Table 4.1 Bones of the Skull

Name	Number	Description
Cranial Bones		
Frontal bone	1	Forehead
Parietal bone	2	Upper sides of cranium and roof of skull
Occipital bone	1	Back and base of skull
Temporal bone	2	Sides and base of cranium
Sphenoid bone	1	Bat-shaped bone that forms part of the base of the skull, floor, and sides of eye orbit
Ethmoid bone	1	Forms part of eye orbit, nose, and floor of cranium
Facial Bones		
Lacrimal bone	2	Inner corner of each eye
Nasal bone	2	Form part of nasal septum and support bridge of nose
Maxilla	1	Upper jaw
Mandible	1	Lower jawbone; only movable bone of the skull
Zygomatic bone	2	Cheekbones
Vomer bone	1	Base of nasal septum
Palatine bone	1	Hard palate (PAH lat) roof of oral cavity and floor of nasal cavity

What's In A Name?

Look for these word parts:
-al = pertaining to
-ar = pertaining to
-oid = resembling
-tic = pertaining to

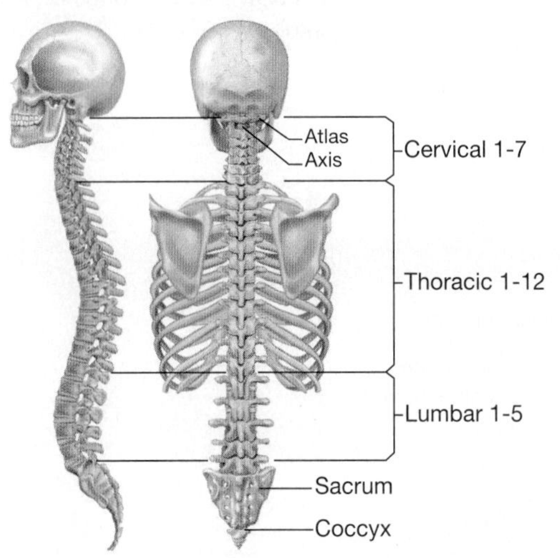

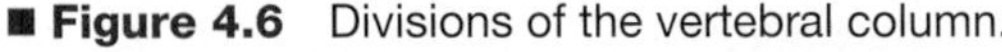

■ **Figure 4.6** Divisions of the vertebral column.

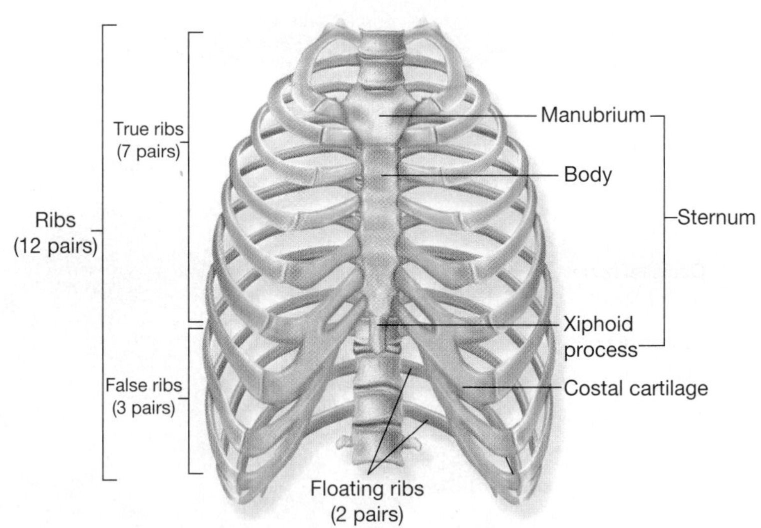

■ **Figure 4.7** The structure of the rib cage.

Table 4.2 Bones of the Vertebral/Spinal Column

Name	Number	Description
Cervical vertebra	7	Vertebrae in the neck region
Thoracic vertebra	12	Vertebrae in the chest region with ribs attached
Lumbar vertebra	5	Vertebrae in the small of the back, about waist level
Sacrum	1	Five vertebrae that become fused into one triangular-shaped flat bone at the base of the vertebral column
Coccyx	1	Three to five very small vertebrae attached to the sacrum, often become fused

are attached only to the vertebral column. The rib cage serves to provide support for organs, such as the heart and lungs.

Appendicular Skeleton

carpus (CAR-pus)
clavicle (CLAV-ih-kl)
femur (FEE-mer)
fibula (FIB-yoo-lah)
humerus (HYOO-mer-us)
ilium (ILL-ee-um)
innominate bone (ih-NOM-ih-nayt)
ischium (ISS-kee-um)
lower extremities
metacarpus (met-ah-CAR-pus)
metatarsus (met-ah-TAHR-sus)
os coxae (OSS / KOK-sigh)
patella (pah-TELL-ah)
pectoral girdle (PEK-toh-ral)
pelvic girdle (PEL-vik)
phalanges (fah-LAN-jeez)
pubis (PYOO-bis)
radius (RAY-dee-us)
scapula (SKAP-yoo-lah)
tarsus (TAHR-sus)
tibia (TIB-ee-ah)
ulna (UHL-nah)
upper extremities

What's In A Name?

Look for these word parts:
pector/o = chest
pelv/o = pelvis
-al = pertaining to
-ic = pertaining to

Med Term Tip

The term *girdle*, meaning something that encircles or confines, refers to the entire bony structure of the shoulder and the pelvis. If just one bone from these areas is being discussed, like the ilium of the pelvis, it would be named as such. If, however, the entire pelvis is being discussed, it would be called the pelvic girdle.

The appendicular skeleton consists of the **pectoral girdle**, **upper extremities**, **pelvic girdle**, and **lower extremities** (see Figure 4.8 ■). These are the bones for our appendages or limbs and along with the muscles attached to them, they are responsible for body movement.

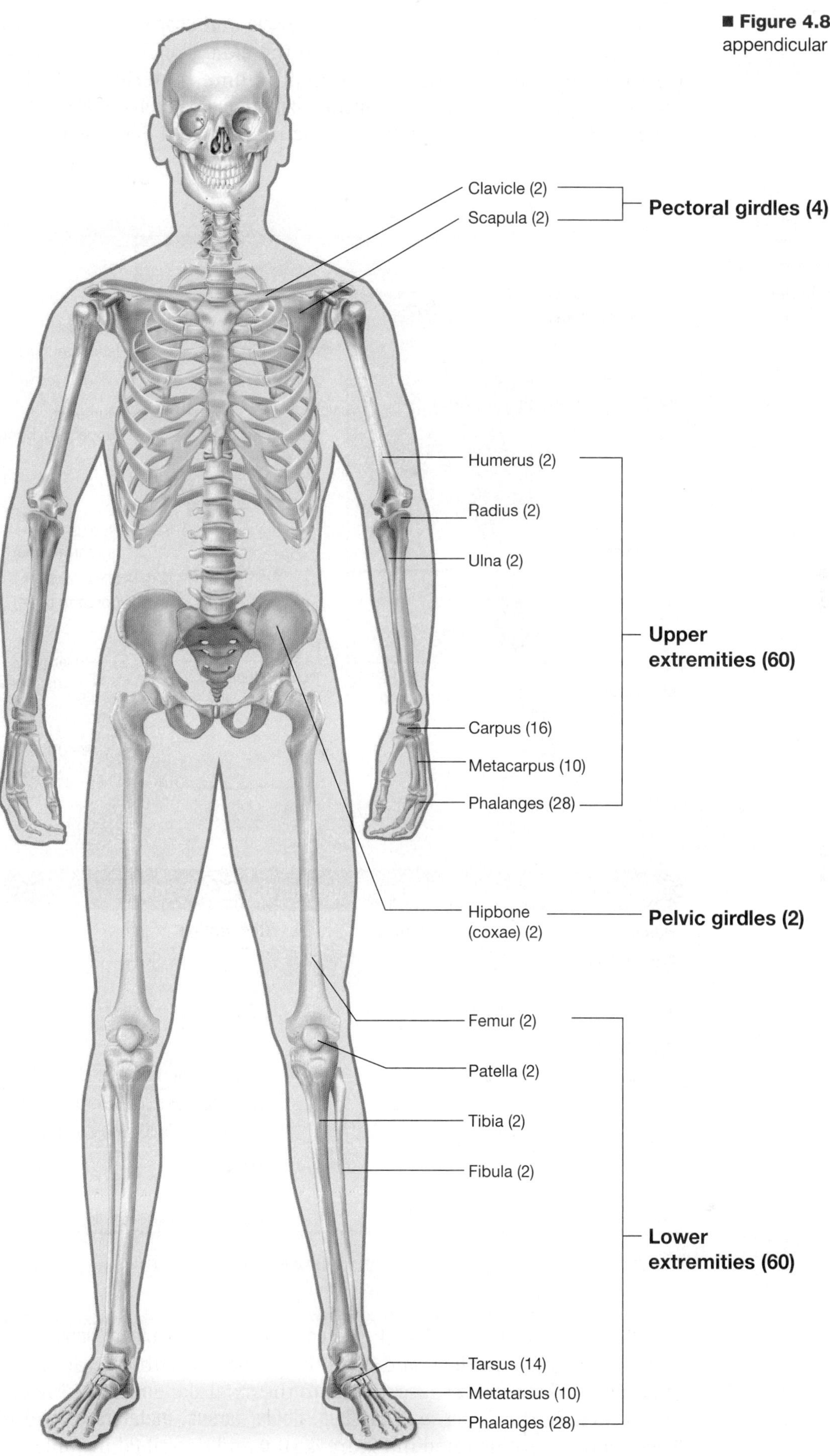

■ **Figure 4.8** Bones of the appendicular skeleton.

The pectoral girdle consists of the **clavicle** and **scapula** bones. It functions to attach the upper extremity, or arm, to the axial skeleton by articulating with the sternum anteriorly and the vertebral column posteriorly. The bones of the upper extremity include the **humerus**, **ulna**, **radius**, **carpus**, **metacarpus**, and **phalanges**. These bones are illustrated in Figure 4.9 ■ and described in Table 4.3 ■.

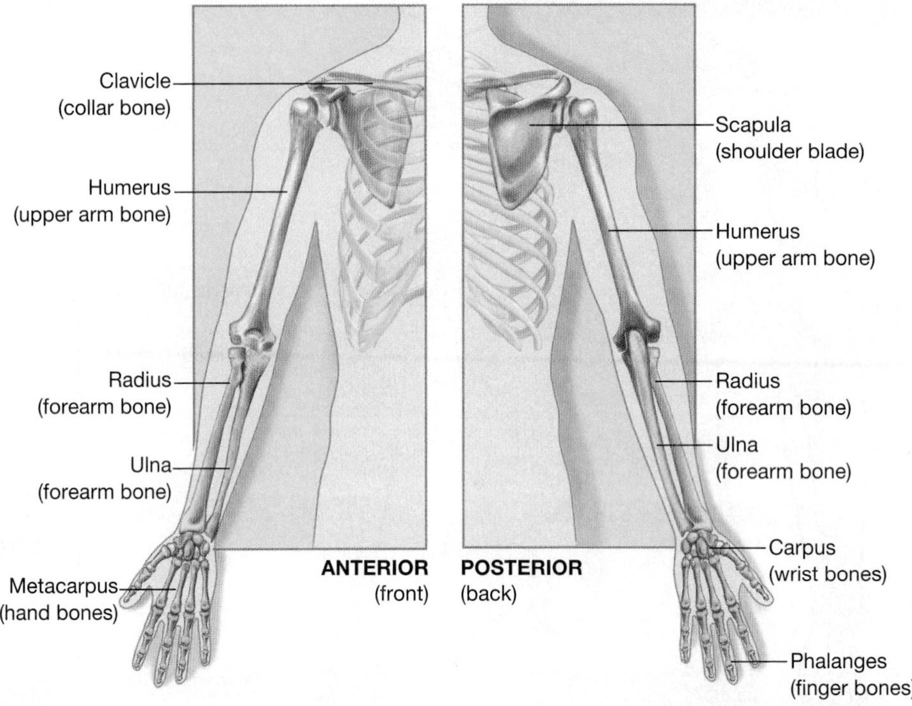

■ **Figure 4.9** Anatomical and common names for the pectoral girdle and upper extremity.

Table 4.3 Bones of the Pectoral Girdle and Upper Extremity

Name	Number	Description
Pectoral Girdle		
Clavicle	2	Collar bone
Scapula	2	Shoulder blade
Upper Extremity		
Humerus	2	Upper arm bone
Radius	2	Forearm bone on thumb side of lower arm
Ulna	2	Forearm bone on little finger side of lower arm
Carpus	16	Bones of wrist
Metacarpus	10	Bones in palm of hand
Phalanges	28	Finger bones; three in each finger and two in each thumb

The pelvic girdle is called the **os coxae** or the **innominate bone** or hipbone. It contains the **ilium**, **ischium**, and **pubis**. It articulates with the sacrum posteriorly to attach the lower extremity, or leg, to the axial skeleton. The lower extremity bones include the **femur**, **patella**, **tibia**, **fibula**, **tarsus**, **metatarsus**, and phalanges. These bones are illustrated in Figure 4.10 ■ and described in Table 4.4 ■

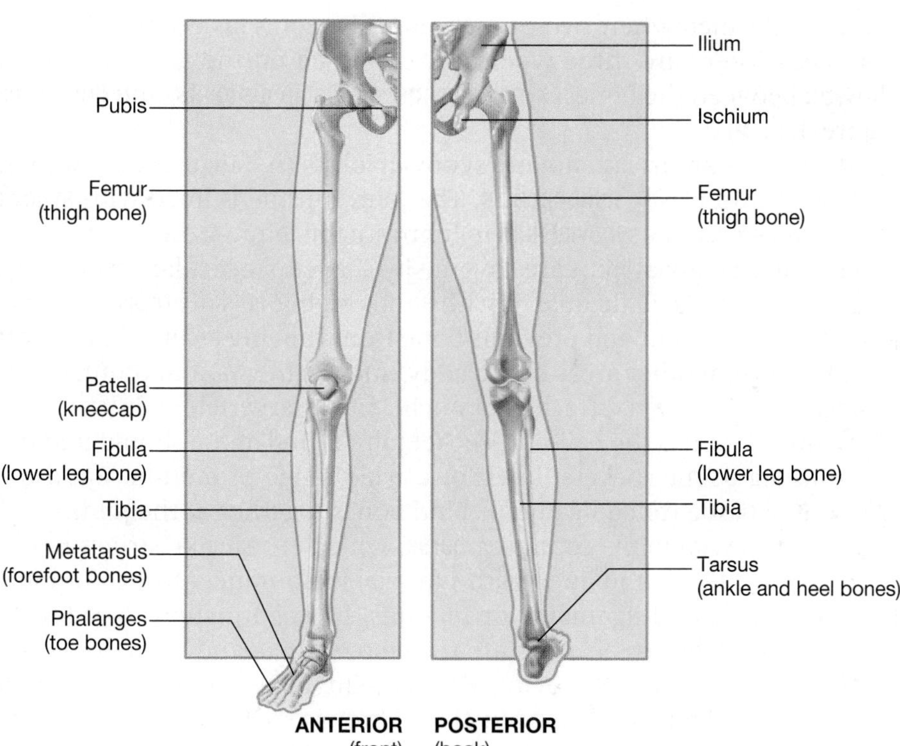

■ **Figure 4.10** Anatomical and common names for the pelvic girdle and lower extremity.

Table 4.4 Bones of the Pelvic Girdle and Lower Extremity

Name	Number	Description
Pelvic Girdle/Os Coxae		
Ilium	2	Part of the hipbone
Ischium	2	Part of the hipbone
Pubis	2	Part of the hipbone
Lower Extremity		
Femur	2	Upper leg bone; thigh bone
Patella	2	Kneecap
Tibia	2	Shin bone; thicker lower leg bone
Fibula	2	Thinner, long bone in lateral side of lower leg
Tarsus	14	Ankle and heel bones
Metatarsus	10	Forefoot bones
Phalanges	28	Toe bones; three in each toe and two in each great toe

Joints

articulation (ar-tik-yoo-LAY-shun)
bursa (BER-sah)
cartilaginous joints (car-tih-LAJ-ih-nus)
fibrous joints (FYE-bruss)
joint capsule
synovial fluid
synovial joint (sin-OH-vee-al)
synovial membrane

Joints are formed when two or more bones meet. This is also referred to as an **articulation**. There are three types of joints based on the amount of movement allowed between the bones: **synovial joints**, **cartilaginous joints**, and **fibrous joints** (see Figure 4.11 ■).

Most joints are freely moving synovial joints (see Figure 4.12 ■), which are enclosed by an elastic **joint capsule**. The joint capsule is lined with **synovial membrane**, which secretes **synovial fluid** to lubricate the joint. As noted earlier, the ends of bones in a synovial joint are covered by a layer of articular cartilage. Cartilage is very tough, but still flexible. It withstands high levels of stress to act as a shock absorber for the joint and prevents bone from rubbing against bone. Cartilage is found in several other areas of the body, such as the nasal septum, external ear, eustachian tube, larynx, trachea, bronchi, and intervertebral disks. One example of a synovial joint is the ball-and-socket joint found at the shoulder and hip. The ball rotating in the socket allows for a wide range of motion. Bands of strong connective tissue called ligaments bind bones together at the joint.

What's In A Name?

Look for these word parts:
articul/o = joint
fibr/o = fibers
synovi/o = synovial membrane
-al = pertaining to
-ous = pertaining to

Some synovial joints contain a **bursa**, which is a saclike structure composed of connective tissue and lined with synovial membrane. Most commonly found between bones and ligaments or tendons, bursas function to reduce friction. Some common bursa locations are the elbow, knee, and shoulder joints.

Med Term Tip

Bursitis is an inflammation of the bursa located between bony prominences such as at the shoulder. Housemaid's knee, a term thought to have originated from the damage to the knees that occurred when maids knelt to scrub floors, is a form of bursitis and carries the medical name *prepatellar bursitis.*

Not all joints are freely moving. Fibrous joints allow almost no movement since the ends of the bones are joined by thick fibrous tissue, which may even fuse into solid bone. The sutures of the skull are an example of a fibrous joint. Cartilaginous joints allow for slight movement but hold bones firmly in place by a solid piece of cartilage. An example of this type of joint is the pubic symphysis, the point at which the left and right pubic bones meet in the front of the lower abdomen.

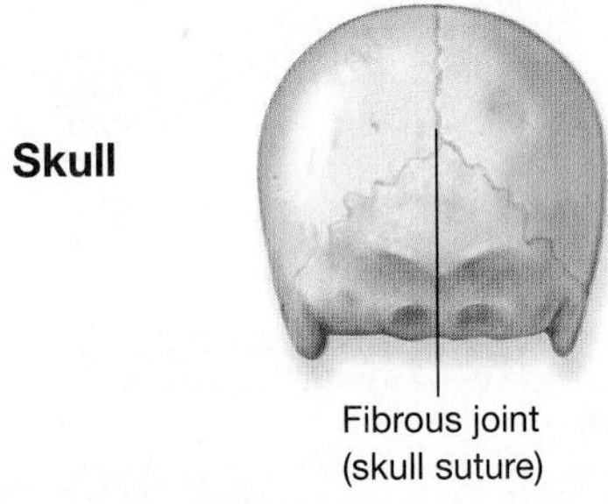

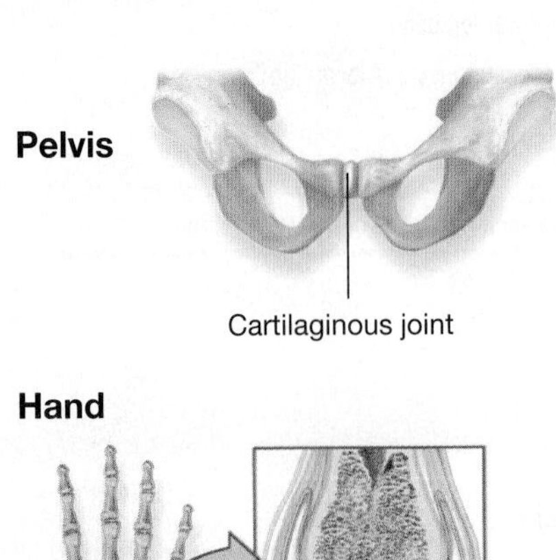

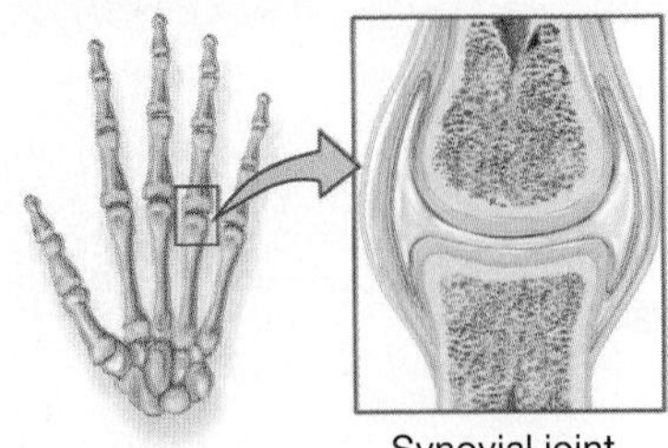

■ **Figure 4.11** Examples of three types of joints found in the body.

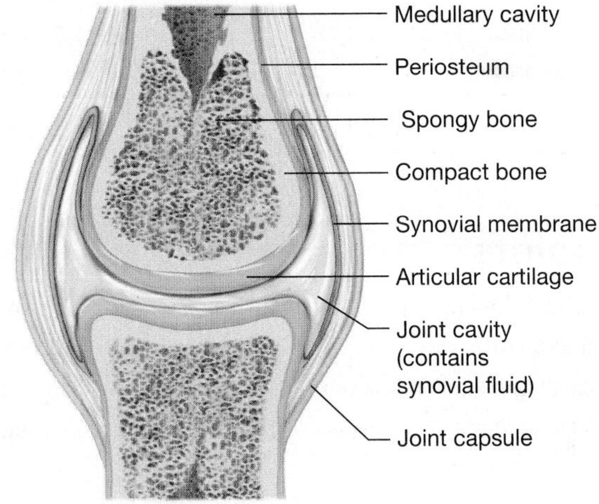

■ **Figure 4.12** Structure of a generalized synovial joint.

Practice As You Go

A. Complete the Statement

1. The two divisions of the human skeleton are the ________________ and ________________.
2. The five functions of the skeletal system are to ________________, ________________, ________________, ________________, and ________________.
3. ________________ bones are roughly as long as they are wide.
4. The membrane covering bones is called the ________________.
5. Another name for spongy bone is ________________ bone.
6. ________________ joints are the most common joints in the body.
7. A ________________ is a smooth, round opening in bones.
8. The ________________ is the shaft of a long bone.

Terminology

Word Parts Used to Build Skeletal System Terms

The following lists contain the combining forms, suffixes, and prefixes used to build terms in the remaining sections of this chapter.

Combining Forms

ankyl/o	stiff joint
arthr/o	joint
burs/o	bursa
carp/o	carpus
cervic/o	neck
chondr/o	cartilage
clavicul/o	clavicle
coccyg/o	coccyx
cortic/o	outer layer
cost/o	rib
crani/o	skull
cutane/o	skin
erythr/o	red

femor/o	femur
fibul/o	fibula
humer/o	humerus
ili/o	ilium
ischi/o	ischium
kyph/o	hump
lamin/o	lamina
lord/o	bent backward
lumb/o	loin
mandibul/o	mandible
maxill/o	maxilla
medull/o	inner region
metacarp/o	metacarpus

metatars/o	metatarsus
myel/o	bone marrow, spinal cord
orth/o	straight
oste/o	bone
patell/o	patella
path/o	disease
ped/o	child; foot
phalang/o	phalanges
pod/o	foot
prosthet/o	addition
pub/o	pubis
radi/o	radius, ray (X-ray)

Combining Forms (continued)

sacr/o	sacrum
sarc/o	flesh
scapul/o	scapula
scoli/o	crooked
spin/o	spine

spondyl/o	vertebra
stern/o	sternum
synov/o	synovial membrane
system/o	system

tars/o	tarsus
thorac/o	chest
tibi/o	tibia
uln/o	ulna
vertebr/o	vertebra

Suffixes

-ac	pertaining to
-al	pertaining to
-algia	pain
-ar	pertaining to
-ary	pertaining to
-centesis	puncture to withdraw fluid
-clasia	surgically break
-desis	to fuse
-eal	pertaining to
-ectomy	surgical removal
-genic	producing
-gram	record
-graphy	process of recording

-iatry	medical treatment
-ic	pertaining to
-itis	inflammation
-listhesis	slipping
-logy	study of
-malacia	abnormal softening
-metry	process of measuring
-oma	tumor
-ory	pertaining to
-osis	abnormal condition
-otomy	cutting into
-ous	pertaining to

-pathy	disease
-plasty	surgical repair
-porosis	porous
-scope	instrument for viewing
-scopic	pertaining to visually examining
-scopy	process of visually examining
-stenosis	narrowing
-tic	pertaining to
-tome	instrument to cut

Prefixes

anti-	against
bi-	two
dis-	apart

ex-	outward
inter-	between
intra-	within

non-	not
per-	through
sub-	under

Adjective Forms of Anatomical Terms

Term	Word Parts	Definition
carpal (CAR-pal)	carp/o = carpus -al = pertaining to	Pertaining to the carpus.
cervical (CER-vih-kal)	cervic/o = neck -al = pertaining to	Pertaining to the neck.
clavicular (cla-VIK-yoo-lar)	clavicul/o = clavicle -ar = pertaining to	Pertaining to the clavicle.
coccygeal (cock-SIH-gee-al)	coccyg/o = coccyx -eal = pertaining to	Pertaining to the coccyx.
costal (KOS-tal)	cost/o = rib -al = pertaining to	Pertaining to the rib.

Adjective Forms of Anatomical Terms (continued)

Term	Word Parts	Definition
cranial (KRAY-nee-all)	crani/o = skull -al = pertaining to	Pertaining to the skull.
femoral (FEM-or-all)	femor/o = femur -al = pertaining to	Pertaining to the femur.
fibular (FIB-yoo-lar)	fibul/o = fibula -ar = pertaining to	Pertaining to the fibula.
humeral (HYOO-mer-all)	humer/o = humerus -al = pertaining to	Pertaining to the humerus.
iliac (ILL-ee-ack)	ili/o = ilium -ac = pertaining to	Pertaining to the ilium.
intervertebral (in-ter-VER-teh-bral)	inter- = between vertebr/o = vertebra -al = pertaining to	Pertaining to between vertebrae.
intracranial (in-trah-KRAY-nee-al)	intra- = within crani/o = skull -al = pertaining to	Pertaining to within the skull.
ischial (ISS-kee-al)	ischi/o = ischium -al = pertaining to	Pertaining to the ischium.
lumbar (LUM-bar)	lumb/o = low back -ar = pertaining to	Pertaining to the low back.
mandibular (man-DIB-yoo-lar)	mandibul/o = mandible -ar = pertaining to	Pertaining to the mandible.
maxillary (mack-sih-LAIR-ree)	maxill/o = maxilla -ary = pertaining to	Pertaining to the maxilla.
metacarpal (met-ah-CAR-pal)	metacarp/o = metacarpus -al = pertaining to	Pertaining to the metacarpus.
metatarsal (met-ah-TAHR-sal)	metatars/o = metatarsus -al = pertaining to	Pertaining to the metatarsus.
patellar (pa-TELL-ar)	patell/o = patella -ar = pertaining to	Pertaining to the patella.
phalangeal (fay-lan-JEE-all)	phalang/o = phalanges -eal = pertaining to	Pertaining to the phalanges.
pubic (PYOO-bik)	pub/o = pubis -ic = pertaining to	Pertaining to the pubis.
radial (RAY-dee-all)	radi/o = radius -al = pertaining to	Pertaining to the radius.
sacral (SAY-kral)	sacr/o = sacrum -al = pertaining to	Pertaining to the sacrum.
scapular (SKAP-yoo-lar)	scapul/o = scapula -ar = pertaining to	Pertaining to the scapula.
sternal (STER-nal)	stern/o = sternum -al = pertaining to	Pertaining to the sternum.
tarsal (TAHR-sal)	tars/o = tarsus -al = pertaining to	Pertaining to the tarsus.

Adjective Forms of Anatomical Terms (continued)

Term	Word Parts	Definition
thoracic (tho-RASS-ik)	thorac/o = thorax -ic = pertaining to	Pertaining to the thorax.
tibial (TIB-ee-all)	tibi/o = tibia -al = pertaining to	Pertaining to the tibia.
ulnar (UHL-nar)	uln/o = ulna -ar = pertaining to	Pertaining to the ulna.
vertebral (VER-teh-bral)	vertebr/o = vertebra -al = pertaining to	Pertaining to a vertebra.

Practice As You Go

B. Adjective Form Practice

Give the adjective form for the following bones.

1. femur ________________
2. sternum ________________
3. clavicle ________________
4. coccyx ________________
5. maxilla ________________
6. tibia ________________
7. patella ________________
8. phalanges ________________
9. humerus ________________
10. pubis ________________

Pathology

Term	Word Parts	Definition
Medical Specialties		
chiropractic (ki-roh-PRAK-tik)	-tic = pertaining to	Healthcare profession concerned with diagnosis and treatment of malalignment conditions of the spine and musculoskeletal system with the intention of affecting the nervous system and improving health. Healthcare professional is a *chiropractor.*

Pathology (continued)

Term	Word Parts	Definition
orthopedics (Orth, ortho) (or-thoh-PEE-diks)	**orth/o** = straight **ped/o** = child, foot -ic = pertaining to	Branch of medicine specializing in the diagnosis and treatment of conditions of the musculoskeletal system; also called *orthopedic surgery.* Physician is an *orthopedist* or *orthopedic surgeon.* Name derived from straightening (*orth/o*) deformities in children (*ped/o*).
orthotics (or-THOT-iks)	**orth/o** = straight -tic = pertaining to	Healthcare profession specializing in making orthopedic appliances such as braces and splints. Person skilled in making and adjusting these appliances is an *orthotist.*
podiatry (po-DYE-ah-tree)	**pod/o** = foot -iatry = medical treatment	Healthcare profession specializing in diagnosis and treatment of disorders of the feet and lower legs. Healthcare professional is a *podiatrist.*
prosthetics (pross-THET-iks)	**prosthet/o** = addition -ic = pertaining to	Healthcare profession specializing in making artificial body parts. Person skilled in making and adjusting prostheses is a *prosthetist.*
Signs and Symptoms		
arthralgia (ar-THRAL-jee-ah)	**arthr/o** = joint -algia = pain	Joint pain.
bursitis (ber-SIGH-tis)	**burs/o** = bursa -itis = inflammation	Inflammation of a bursa.
callus (KAL-us)		The mass of bone tissue that forms at a fracture site during its healing.
chondromalacia (kon-droh-mah-LAY-she-ah)	**chondr/o** = cartilage -malacia = abnormal softening	Softening of the cartilage.
crepitation (krep-ih-TAY-shun)		The noise produced by bones or cartilage rubbing together in conditions such as arthritis. Also called *crepitus.*
ostealgia (oss-tee-AL-jee-ah)	**oste/o** = bone -algia = pain	Bone pain.
osteomyelitis (oss-tee-oh-mi-ell-EYE-tis)	**oste/o** = bone **myel/o** = bone marrow -itis = inflammation	Inflammation of bone and bone marrow.
synovitis (sih-no-VIGH-tis)	**synov/o** = synovial membrane -itis = inflammation	Inflammation of synovial membrane.

Pathology (continued)

Term	Word Parts	Definition
Fractures		
closed fracture		Fracture in which there is no open skin wound. Also called a *simple fracture.*

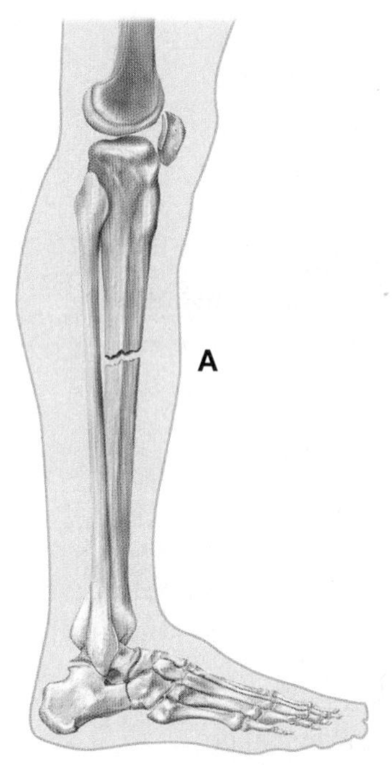

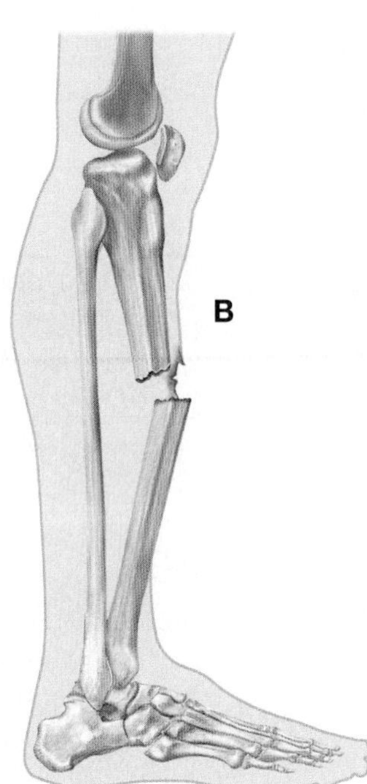

■ **Figure 4.13** A) Closed (or simple) fracture and B) open (or compound) fracture.

Term	Word Parts	Definition
Colles' fracture (COL-eez)		A common type of wrist fracture.

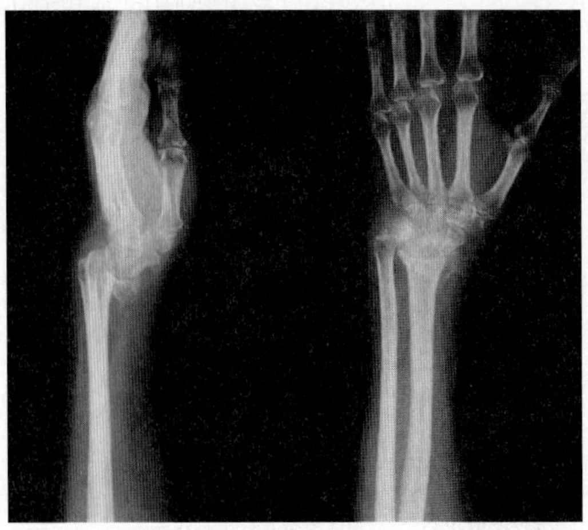

■ **Figure 4.14** Colles' fracture. *(Akawath/Shutterstock)*

Term	Word Parts	Definition
comminuted fracture (kom-ih-NYOOT-ed)		Fracture in which the bone is shattered, splintered, or crushed into many small pieces or fragments.
compound fracture		Fracture in which the bone has broken through the skin. Also called an *open fracture* (see Figure 4.13B ■).

Pathology (continued)

Term	Word Parts	Definition
compression fracture		Fracture involving loss of height of a vertebral body. It may be the result of trauma, but in older people, especially women, it may be caused by conditions like osteoporosis.
fracture (FX, Fx)		A broken bone.
greenstick fracture		Fracture in which there is an incomplete break; one side of bone is broken and the other side is bent. This type of fracture is commonly found in children due to their softer and more pliable bone structure.
impacted fracture		Fracture in which bone fragments are pushed into each other.
oblique fracture (oh-BLEEK)		Fracture at an angle to the bone.

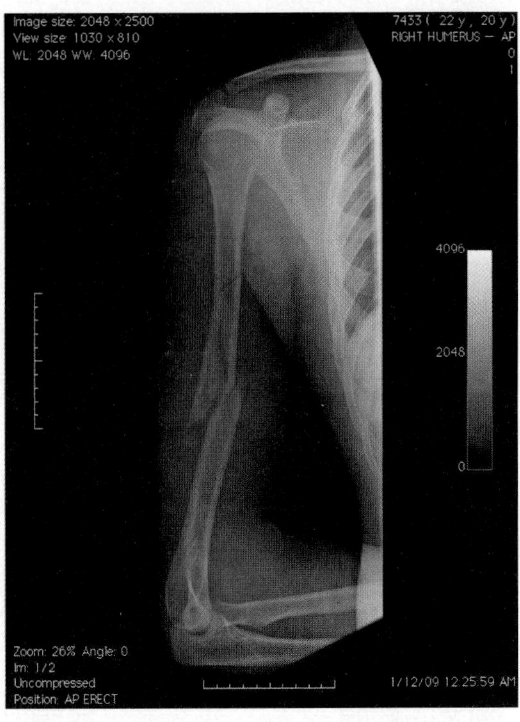

■ **Figure 4.15** X-ray showing oblique fracture of the humerus. *(Du Cane Medical Imaging Ltd./Science Source)*

Term	Word Parts	Definition
pathologic fracture (path-ah-LOJ-ik)	path/o = disease -logic = pertaining to study of	Fracture caused by diseased or weakened bone.
spiral fracture	-al = pertaining to	Fracture in which the fracture line spirals around the shaft of the bone. Can be caused by a twisting injury and is often slower to heal than other types of fractures.
stress fracture		A slight fracture caused by repetitive low-impact forces, like running, rather than a single forceful impact.

Pathology (continued)

Term	Word Parts	Definition
transverse fracture ■ **Figure 4.16** X-ray showing transverse fracture of radius. *(James Stevenson/Science Source)*		Complete fracture that is straight across the bone at right angles to the long axis of the bone.
Bones		
chondroma (kon-DROH-mah)	chondr/o = cartilage -oma = tumor	A tumor, usually benign, that forms in cartilage.
Ewing's sarcoma (YOO-wings / sar-KOH-mah)	sarc/o = flesh -oma = tumor	Malignant growth found in the shaft of long bones that spreads through the periosteum. Removal is the treatment of choice because this tumor will metastasize or spread to other organs.
exostosis (eck-sos-TOH-sis)	ex- = outward oste/o = bone -osis = abnormal condition	A bony, outward projection from the surface of a bone; also called a *bone spur*.
myeloma (my-ah-LOH-mah)	myel/o = bone marrow -oma = tumor	A tumor that forms in bone marrow tissue.
osteochondroma (oss-tee-oh-kon-DROH-mah)	oste/o = bone chondr/o = cartilage -oma = tumor	A tumor, usually benign, that consists of both bone and cartilage tissue.
osteogenic sarcoma (oss-tee-oh-JEN-ik / sark-OH-mah)	oste/o = bone -genic = producing sarc/o = flesh -oma = tumor	The most common type of bone cancer. Usually begins in osteocytes found at the ends of long bones.
osteomalacia (oss-tee-oh-mah-LAY-she-ah)	oste/o = bone -malacia = abnormal softening	Softening of the bones caused by a deficiency of calcium. It is thought to be caused by insufficient sunlight and vitamin D in children.
osteopathy (oss-tee-OPP-ah-thee)	oste/o = bone -pathy = disease	A general term for bone disease.

Pathology (continued)

Term	Word Parts	Definition
osteoporosis (oss-tee-oh-por-ROH-sis)	oste/o = bone -porosis = porous	Decrease in bone mass producing a thinning and weakening of the bone with resulting fractures. The bone becomes more porous, especially in the spine and pelvis.
Paget's disease (PAH-jets)		A fairly common metabolic disease of the bone from unknown causes. It usually attacks middle-aged and older adults and is characterized by bone destruction and deformity. Named for Sir James Paget, a British surgeon.
rickets (RIK-ets)		Deficiency in calcium and vitamin D found in early childhood that results in bone deformities, especially bowed legs.
Spinal Column		
ankylosing spondylitis (ang-kih-LOH-sing / spon-dih-LYE-tis)	ankyl/o = stiff joint spondyl/o = vertebra -itis = inflammation	Inflammatory spinal condition resembling rheumatoid arthritis and results in gradual stiffening and fusion of the vertebrae. More common in men than in women.
herniated nucleus pulposus (HNP) (HER-nee-ated / NOO-klee-us / pull-POH-sus) ■ **Figure 4.17** Magnetic resonance imaging (MRI) image demonstrating a back herniated disc. *(Michelle Milano/ Shutterstock)*		Herniation or protrusion of an intervertebral disk; also called *herniated disk* or *ruptured disk.* May require surgery.
kyphosis (ki-FOH-sis)	kyph/o = hump -osis = abnormal condition	Abnormal increase in the outward curvature of the thoracic spine. Also known as *hunchback* or *humpback.* See Figure 4.18 ■ for an illustration of abnormal spine curvatures.

Pathology (continued)

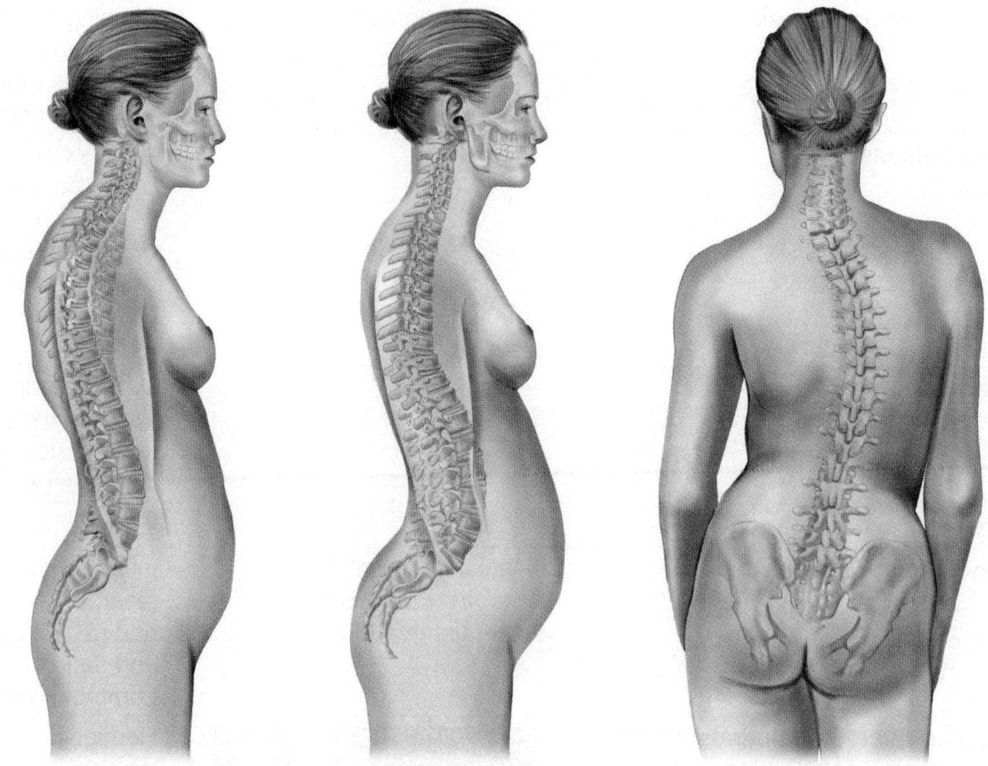

■ **Figure 4.18** Abnormal spinal curvatures: kyphosis, lordosis, and scoliosis.

Kyphosis (excessive posterior thoracic curvature - hunchback)

Lordosis (excessive anterior lumbar curvature - swayback)

Scoliosis (lateral curvature)

Term	Word Parts	Definition
lordosis (lor-DOH-sis)	lord/o = bent backward -osis = abnormal condition	Abnormal increase in the forward curvature of the lumbar spine. Also known as *swayback*. See again Figure 4.18 for an illustration of abnormal spine curvatures.
scoliosis (skoh-lee-OH-sis)	scoli/o = crooked -osis = abnormal condition	Abnormal lateral curvature of the spine. See again Figure 4.18 for an illustration of abnormal spine curvatures.
spina bifida (SPY-nah / BIF-ih-dah)	spin/o = spine bi- = two	Congenital anomaly occurring when a vertebra fails to fully form around the spinal cord.
spinal stenosis (ste-NOH-sis)	spin/o = spine -al = pertaining to	Narrowing of the spinal canal causing pressure on the cord and nerves.
	Word Watch Watch how the term *stenosis* is used in this condition. It most often appears as the suffix ***-stenosis***. However, in this case, it is used as a freestanding word.	
spondylolisthesis (spon-dih-loh-liss-THEE-sis)	spondyl/o = vertebra -listhesis = slipping	The forward sliding of a lumbar vertebra over the vertebra below it.
spondylosis (spon-dih-LOH-sis)	spondyl/o = vertebra -osis = abnormal condition	Specifically refers to ankylosing of the spine, but commonly used in reference to any degenerative condition of the vertebral column.

Pathology (continued)

Term	Word Parts	Definition
whiplash		Cervical muscle and ligament sprain or strain as a result of a sudden movement forward and backward of the head and neck. Can occur as a result of a rear-end auto collision.
Joints		
bunion (BUN-yun)		Inflammation of the bursa of the first metatarsophalangeal joint (base of the big toe).
dislocation	dis- = apart	Occurs when the bones in a joint are displaced from their normal alignment and the ends of the bones are no longer in contact.
osteoarthritis (OA) (oss-tee-oh-ar-THRY-tis)	oste/o = bone arthr/o = joint -itis = inflammation	Arthritis resulting in degeneration of the bones and joints, especially those bearing weight. Results in bone rubbing against bone. Also called degenerative joint disease (DJD).
rheumatoid arthritis (RA) (ROO-mah-toyd / ar-THRY-tis)	arthr/o = joint -itis = inflammation	Chronic form of arthritis with inflammation of the joints, swelling, stiffness, pain, and changes in the cartilage that can result in crippling deformities; considered to be an autoimmune disease.

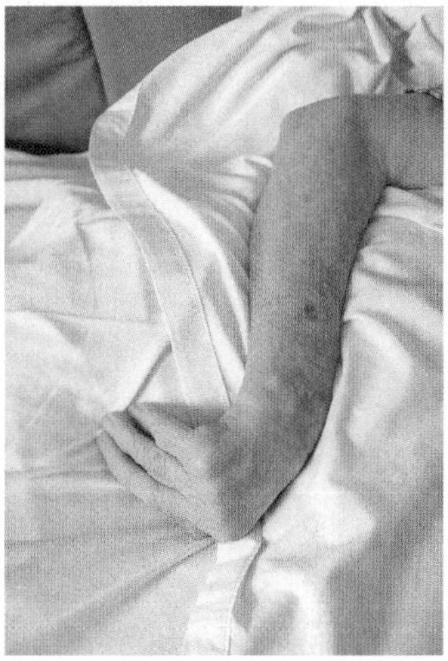

■ **Figure 4.19** Patient with typical rheumatoid arthritis contractures. *(Michal Heron, Pearson Education)*

Pathology (continued)

Term	Word Parts	Definition
sprain		Damage to the ligaments surrounding a joint due to overstretching, but no dislocation of the joint or fracture of the bone.
subluxation (sub-LUCKS-a-shun)	sub- = under	An incomplete dislocation, the joint alignment is disrupted, but the ends of the bones remain in contact.
systemic lupus erythematosus (SLE) (sis-TEM-ik / LOOP-us / air-ih-them-ah-TOH-sis)	system/o = system -ic = pertaining to erythr/o = red	Chronic inflammatory autoimmune disease of connective tissue affecting many systems that may include joint pain and arthritis. May be mistaken for rheumatoid arthritis.
talipes (TAL-ih-peez)		Congenital deformity causing misalignment of the ankle joint and foot. Also referred to as a *clubfoot*.

Practice As You Go

C. Fracture Type Matching

Match each fracture type to its definition.

1. ________ comminuted	a. fracture line is at an angle
2. ________ greenstick	b. fracture line curves around the bone
3. ________ compound	c. bone is splintered or crushed
4. ________ simple	d. bone is pressed into itself
5. ________ impacted	e. fracture line is straight across bone
6. ________ transverse	f. skin has been broken
7. ________ oblique	g. no open wound
8. ________ spiral	h. bone only partially broken

Diagnostic Procedures

Term	Word Part	Definition
Diagnostic Imaging		
arthrogram (AR-throh-gram)	**arthr/o** = joint **-gram** = record	X-ray record of a joint, usually taken after the joint has been injected by a contrast medium.
arthrography (ar-THROG-rah-fee)	**arthr/o** = joint **-graphy** = process of recording	Process of X-raying a joint, usually after injection of a contrast medium into the joint space.
bone scan		Nuclear medicine procedure in which the patient is given a radioactive dye and then scanning equipment is used to visualize bones. It is especially useful in identifying stress fractures, observing progress of treatment for osteomyelitis, and locating cancer metastases to the bone.
dual-energy absorptiometry (DXA) (ab-sorp-she-AHM-eh-tree)	**-metry** = process of measuring	Measurement of bone density using low-dose X-ray for the purpose of detecting osteoporosis.
myelography (my-eh-LOG-rah-fee)	**myel/o** = spinal cord **-graphy** = process of recording	Study of the spinal column after injecting opaque contrast material; particularly useful in identifying herniated nucleus pulposus pinching a spinal nerve. **Med Term Tip** The combining form *myel/o* means "marrow" and is used for both the spinal cord and bone marrow. To the ancient Greek philosophers and physicians, the spinal cord appeared to be much like the marrow found in the medullary cavity of a long bone.
radiography	**radi/o** = ray **-graphy** = process of recording	Diagnostic imaging procedure using X-rays to study the internal structure of the body; especially useful for visualizing bones and joints.
Endoscopic Procedures		
arthroscope (AR-throh-skope)	**arthr/o** = joint **-scope** = instrument for viewing	Instrument used to view inside a joint.
arthroscopy (ar-THROS-koh-pee)	**arthr/o** = joint **-scopy** = process of visually examining	Examination of the interior of a joint by entering the joint with an *arthroscope.* The arthroscope contains a small television camera that allows the physician to view the interior of the joint on a monitor during the procedure. Some joint conditions can be repaired during arthroscopy.

Therapeutic Procedures

Term	Word Part	Definition
Medical Treatments		
arthrocentesis (ar-throh-sen-TEE-sis)	arthr/o = joint -centesis = puncture to withdraw fluid	Involves the insertion of a needle into the joint cavity in order to remove or aspirate fluid. May be done to remove excess fluid from a joint or to obtain fluid for examination.
orthotic (or-THOT-ik)	orth/o = straight -tic = pertaining to	Orthopedic appliance, such as a brace or splint, used to prevent or correct deformities.
prosthesis (pross-THEE-sis)	prosthet/o = addition	Artificial device used as a substitute for a body part that is either congenitally missing or absent as a result of accident or disease. An example would be an artificial leg.
Surgical Procedures		
amputation (am-pew-TAY-shun)		Partial or complete removal of a limb for a variety of reasons, including tumors, gangrene, intractable pain, crushing injury, or uncontrollable infection.
arthroclasia (ar-throh-KLAY-see-ah)	arthr/o = joint -clasia = surgically break	To forcibly break loose a fused joint while the patient is under anesthetic. Fusion is usually caused by the buildup of scar tissue or adhesions.
arthrodesis (ar-throh-DEE-sis)	arthr/o = joint -desis = to fuse	Procedure to stabilize a joint by fusing the bones together.
arthroscopic surgery (ar-throh-SKOP-ic)	arthr/o = joint -scopic = pertaining to visually examining	Performing a surgical procedure while using an arthroscope to view the internal structure, such as a joint.
arthrotomy (ar-THROT-oh-mee)	arthr/o = joint -otomy = cutting into	Surgical procedure that cuts into a joint capsule.
bone graft		Piece of bone taken from the patient used to take the place of a removed bone or a bony defect at another site.
bunionectomy (bun-yun-ECK-toh-mee)	-ectomy = surgical removal	Removal of the bursa at the joint of the great toe.
bursectomy (ber-SEK-toh-mee)	burs/o = bursa -ectomy = surgical removal	Surgical removal of a bursa.
chondrectomy (kon-DREK-toh-mee)	chondr/o = cartilage -ectomy = surgical removal	Surgical removal of cartilage.
chondroplasty (KON-droh-plas-tee)	chondr/o = cartilage -plasty = surgical repair	Surgical repair of cartilage.
craniotomy (kray-nee-OTT-oh-mee)	crani/o = skull -otomy = cutting into	Surgical procedure that cuts into the skull.
laminectomy (lam-ih-NEK-toh-mee)	lamin/o = lamina -ectomy = surgical removal	Removal of the vertebral posterior arch to correct severe back problems and pain caused by compression of a spinal nerve.
osteoclasia (oss-tee-oh-KLAY-see-ah)	oste/o = bone -clasia = surgically break	Surgical procedure involving the intentional breaking of a bone to correct a deformity.
osteotome (OSS-tee-oh-tohm)	oste/o = bone -tome = instrument to cut	Instrument used to cut bone.

Therapeutic Procedures (continued)

Term	Word Part	Definition
osteotomy (oss-tee-OTT-ah-mee)	oste/o = bone -otomy = cutting into	Surgical procedure that cuts into a bone.
percutaneous diskectomy (per-kyoo-TAY-nee-us / disk-EK-toh-mee)	per- = through cutane/o = skin -ous = pertaining to -ectomy = surgical removal	A thin catheter tube is inserted into the intervertebral disk through the skin and the herniated or ruptured disk material is sucked out or a laser is used to vaporize it.
spinal fusion	spin/o = spine -al = pertaining to	Surgical immobilization of adjacent vertebrae. This may be done for several reasons, including correction for a herniated disk.
synovectomy (sih-no-VEK-toh-mee)	synov/o = synovial membrane -ectomy = surgical removal	Surgical removal of the synovial membrane.
total hip arthroplasty (THA) (ar-throh-PLAS-tee)	arthr/o = joint -plasty = surgical repair	Surgical reconstruction of a hip by implanting a prosthetic or artificial hip joint. Also called *total hip replacement (THR).*

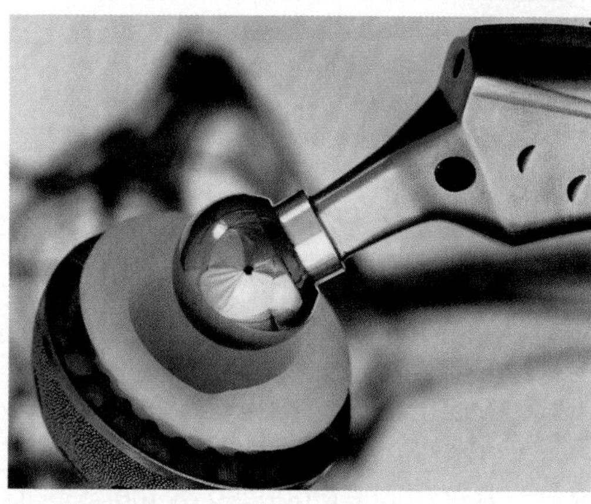

■ **Figure 4.20**
Prosthetic hip joint. *(Lawrence Livermore National Library/Science Photo Library/Science Source)*

Term	Word Part	Definition
total knee arthroplasty (TKA) (ar-throh-PLAS-tee)	arthr/o = joint -plasty = surgical repair	Surgical reconstruction of a knee joint by implanting a prosthetic knee joint. Also called *total knee replacement (TKR).*
Fracture Care		
cast		Application of a solid material to immobilize an extremity or portion of the body as a result of a fracture, dislocation, or severe injury. It may be made of plaster of Paris or fiberglass.
fixation		Procedure to stabilize a fractured bone while it heals. *External fixation* includes casts, splints, and pins inserted through the skin. *Internal fixation* includes pins, plates, rods, screws, and wires that are applied during an *open reduction.*

Therapeutic Procedures (continued)

Term	Word Part	Definition
reduction		Correcting a fracture by realigning the bone fragments. *Closed reduction* is doing this manipulation without entering the body. *Open reduction* is the process of making a surgical incision at the site of the fracture to do the reduction. This is necessary when bony fragments need to be removed or *internal fixation* such as plates or pins are required.
traction		Applying a pulling force on a fractured or dislocated limb or the vertebral column in order to restore normal alignment.

Pharmacology

Classification	Word Parts	Action	Examples
bone reabsorption inhibitors		Conditions that result in weak and fragile bones, such as osteoporosis and Paget's disease, are improved by medications that reduce the reabsorption of bones.	alendronate, Fosamax; ibandronate, Boniva
calcium supplements and vitamin D therapy		Maintaining high blood levels of calcium in association with vitamin D helps maintain bone density; used to treat osteomalacia, osteoporosis, and rickets.	calcium carbonate, Oystercal, Tums; calcium citrate, Cal-Citrate, Citracal
corticosteroids	cortic/o = outer layer	A hormone produced by the adrenal cortex that has very strong anti-inflammatory properties. It is particularly useful in treating rheumatoid arthritis.	prednisone; methylprednisolone, Medrol; dexamethasone, Decadron
nonsteroidal anti-inflammatory drugs (NSAIDs)	non- = not -al = pertaining to anti- = against -ory = pertaining to	A large group of drugs (other than corticosteroids) that provide mild pain relief and anti-inflammatory benefits for conditions such as arthritis.	ibuprofen, Advil, Motrin; naproxen, Aleve, Naprosyn; salicylates, Aspirin

Abbreviations

AE	above elbow	**NSAID**	nonsteroidal anti-inflammatory drug
AK	above knee	**OA**	osteoarthritis
BDT	bone density testing	**ORIF**	open reduction–internal fixation
BE	below elbow	**Orth, ortho**	orthopedics
BK	below knee	**P**	phosphorus
C1, C2, etc.	first cervical vertebra, second cervical vertebra, etc.	**RA**	rheumatoid arthritis
Ca	calcium	**RLE**	right lower extremity
DJD	degenerative joint disease	**RUE**	right upper extremity
DXA	dual-energy absorptiometry	**SLE**	systemic lupus erythematosus
FX, Fx	fracture	**T1, T2, etc.**	first thoracic vertebra, second thoracic vertebra, etc.
HNP	herniated nucleus pulposus	**THA**	total hip arthroplasty
JRA	juvenile rheumatoid arthritis	**THR**	total hip replacement
L1, L2, etc.	first lumbar vertebra, second lumbar vertebra, etc.	**TKA**	total knee arthroplasty
LE	lower extremity	**TKR**	total knee replacement
LLE	left lower extremity	**UE**	upper extremity
LUE	left upper extremity		

Practice As You Go

D. What's the Abbreviation?

1. total knee replacement ______________________
2. herniated nucleus pulposus ______________________
3. upper extremity ______________________
4. fifth lumbar vertebra ______________________
5. above the knee ______________________
6. fracture ______________________
7. nonsteroidal anti-inflammatory drug ______________________

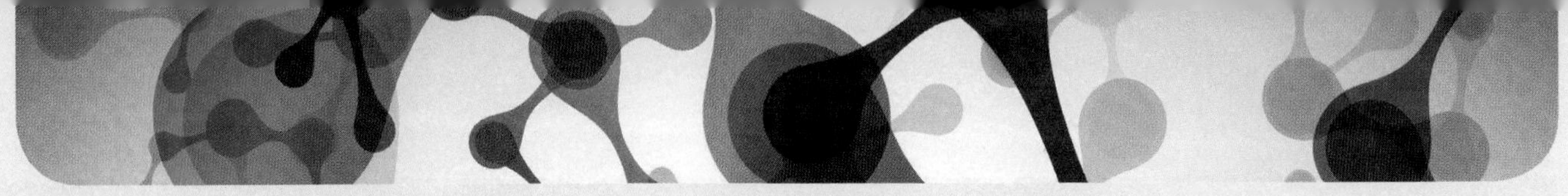

Section II: Muscular System at a Glance

Function

Muscles are bundles, sheets, or rings of tissue that produce movement by contracting and pulling on the structures to which they are attached.

Organs

Here is the primary structure that comprises the muscular system:

muscles

Word Parts

Here are the most common word parts (with their meanings) used to build muscular system terms. For a more comprehensive list, refer to the Terminology section of this chapter.

Combining Forms

duct/o	to bring
extens/o	to stretch out
fasci/o	fibrous band
fibr/o	fibers
flex/o	to bend
kinesi/o	movement
muscul/o	muscle
my/o	muscle
myos/o	muscle
plant/o	sole of foot
rotat/o	to revolve
ten/o	tendon
tend/o	tendon
tendin/o	tendon
vers/o	to turn

Suffixes

-asthenia	weakness
-ion	action
-kinesia	movement
-tonia	tone
-trophic	pertaining to development

Prefixes

ab-	away from
ad-	toward
circum-	around
e-	outward

Muscular System Illustrated

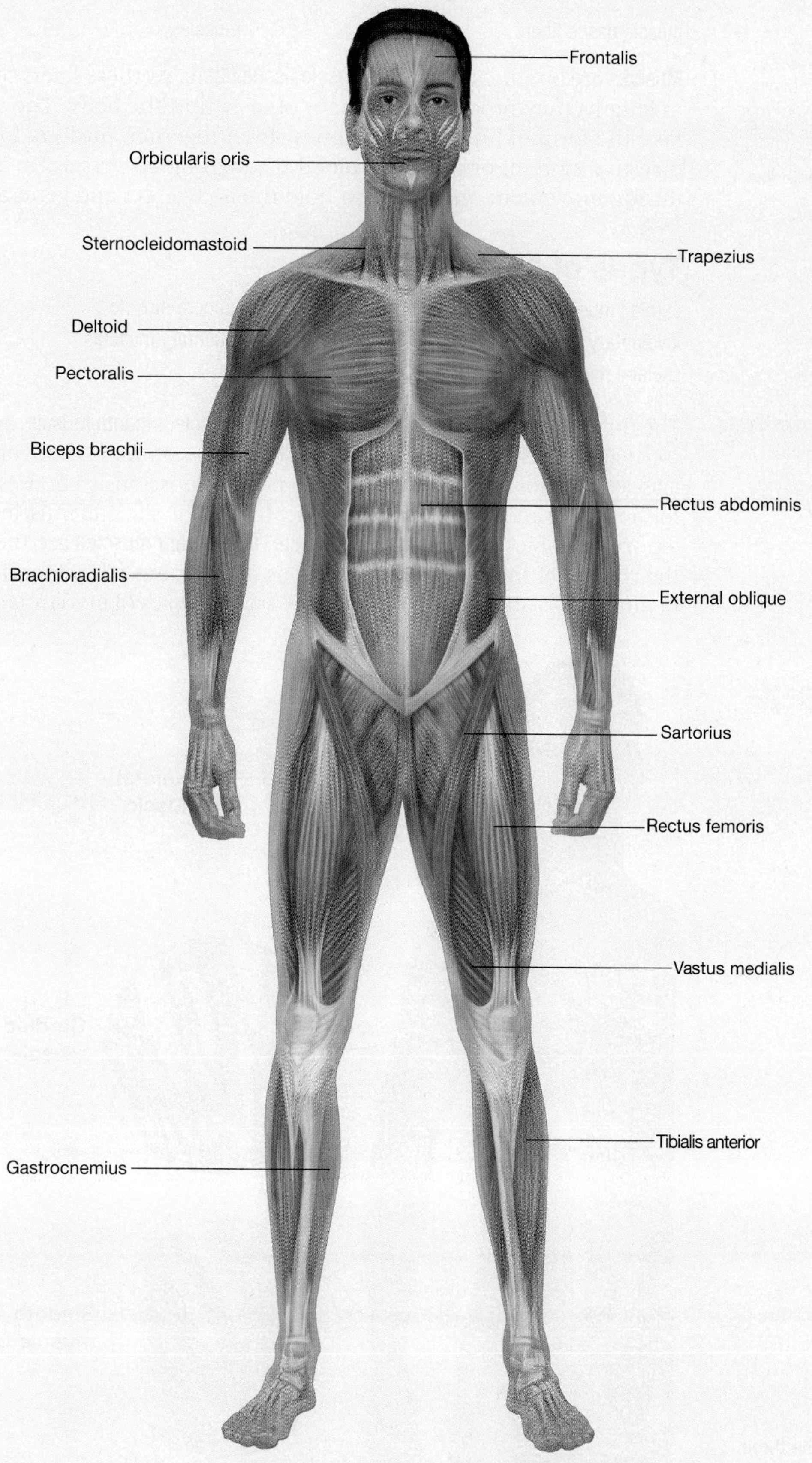

Anatomy and Physiology of the Muscular System

muscle tissue fibers
muscles

Med Term Tip

The term *muscle* is the diminutive form of the Latin word *mus* or "little mouse." This is thought to describe how the skin ripples when a muscle contracts, like a little mouse running.

Muscles are bundles of parallel **muscle tissue fibers**. As these fibers contract (shorten in length) they produce movement of or within the body. The movement may take the form of bringing two bones closer together, pushing food through the digestive system, or pumping blood through blood vessels. In addition to producing movement, muscles also hold the body erect and generate heat.

Types of Muscles

cardiac muscle
involuntary muscles
skeletal muscle
smooth muscle
voluntary muscles

What's In A Name?

Look for these word parts:
cardi/o = heart
-ac = pertaining to
in- = not

The three types of muscle tissue are **skeletal muscle**, **smooth muscle**, and **cardiac muscle** (see Figure 4.21 ■). Muscle tissue may be either voluntary or involuntary. **Voluntary muscles** are those muscles for which a person consciously chooses to contract and for how long and how hard to contract them. The skeletal muscles of the arm and leg are examples of this type of muscle. **Involuntary muscles** are the muscles under the control of the subconscious regions of the brain. The smooth muscles found in internal organs and cardiac muscles are examples of involuntary muscle tissue.

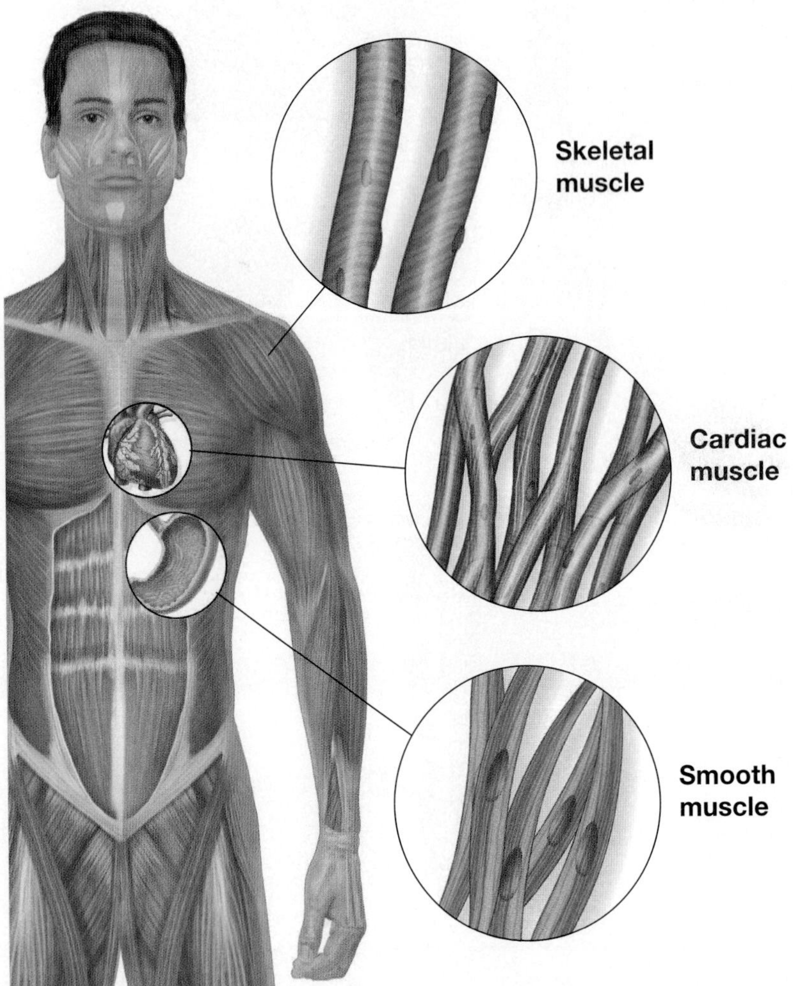

■ **Figure 4.21** The three types of muscles: skeletal, smooth, and cardiac.

Skeletal Muscle

fascia (FASH-ee-ah)
motor neurons
myoneural junction (MY-oh-NOO-rall)
striated muscles (stry-a-ted)
tendon (TEN-dun)

A skeletal muscle is directly or indirectly attached to a bone and produces voluntary movement of the skeleton. It is also referred to as a **striated muscle** because of its striped appearance under the microscope (see Figure 4.22 ■). Each muscle is wrapped in layers of fibrous connective tissue called **fascia**. The fascia tapers at each end of a skeletal muscle to form a very strong **tendon**. The tendon then inserts into the periosteum covering a bone to anchor the muscle to the bone. Skeletal muscles are stimulated by **motor neurons** of the nervous system. The point at which the motor nerve contacts a muscle fiber is called the **myoneural junction**.

Med Term Tip

The human body has more than 400 skeletal muscles, which account for almost 50% of the body's weight.

Smooth Muscle

visceral muscle (vis-seh-ral)

Smooth muscle tissue is found in association with internal organs. For this reason, it is also referred to as **visceral muscle**. The name smooth muscle refers to the muscle's microscopic appearance; it lacks the striations of skeletal muscle (see again Figure 4.22). Smooth muscle is found in the walls of the hollow organs, such as the stomach, tube-shaped organs, such as the respiratory airways, and blood vessels. It is responsible for the involuntary muscle action associated with movement of the internal organs, such as churning food, constricting a blood vessel, and uterine contractions.

What's In A Name?

Look for these word parts:
cardi/o = heart
my/o = muscle
neur/o = nerve
viscer/o = internal organ
-al = pertaining to

Cardiac Muscle

myocardium (my-oh-CAR-dee-um)

Cardiac muscle, or **myocardium**, makes up the wall of the heart (see again Figure 4.22). With each involuntary contraction the heart squeezes to pump blood out of its chambers and through the blood vessels. This muscle is more thoroughly described in Chapter 5, Cardiovascular System.

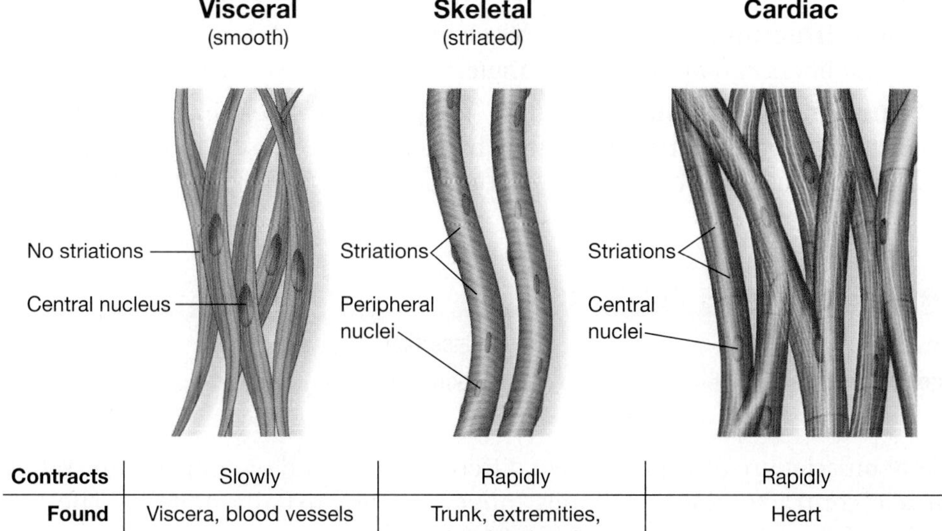

	Visceral	Skeletal	Cardiac
Contracts	Slowly	Rapidly	Rapidly
Found	Viscera, blood vessels	Trunk, extremities, head and neck	Heart
Control	Involuntary	Voluntary	Involuntary

■ **Figure 4.22** Characteristics of the three types of muscles.

Practice As You Go

E. Complete the Statement

1. Another name for visceral muscle is ____________________ muscle.
2. Nerves contact skeletal muscle fibers at the ____________________ junction.
3. The three types of muscle are ____________________, ____________________, and ____________________.

Naming Skeletal Muscles

biceps (BYE-seps)
extensor carpi
external oblique
flexor carpi
gluteus maximus (GLOO-tee-us / MACKS-ih-mus)
rectus abdominis (REK-tus / ab-DOM-ih-nis)
sternocleidomastoid (STER-noh-KLY-doh MASS-toid)

The name of a muscle often reflects its location, origin and insertion, size, action, fiber direction, or number of attachment points, as illustrated by the following examples:

- **Location:** the term ***rectus abdominis*** means straight (rectus) abdominal muscle.
- **Origin and insertion:** the **sternocleidomastoid** is named for its two origins (**stern/o** for sternum and **cleid/o** for clavicle) and single insertion (mastoid process).
- **Size:** when gluteus, meaning rump area, is combined with maximus, meaning large, we have the term **gluteus maximus**.
- **Action:** the **flexor carpi** and **extensor carpi** muscles are named as such because they produce flexion and extension at the wrist.
- **Fiber direction:** the **external oblique** muscle is an abdominal muscle whose fibers run at an oblique angle.
- **Number of attachment points:** the prefix **bi-**, meaning two, can form the medical term **biceps**, which refers to the muscle in the upper arm that has two heads or connecting points.

What's In A Name?
Look for these word parts:
cleid/o = clavicle
extens/o = to stretch out
flex/o = to bend
stern/o = sternum
-al = pertaining to
bi- = two
ex- = outward

Skeletal Muscle Actions

action
antagonistic pairs
insertion
origin

Skeletal muscles are attached to two different bones and overlap a joint. When a muscle contracts, the two bones move, but not usually equally. The less movable of the two bones is considered to be the starting point of the muscle and is called the **origin**. The more movable bone is considered to be where the muscle ends and is called the **insertion** (see Figure 4.23 ■). The type of movement a muscle produces is called its **action**. Muscles are often arranged around joints in **antagonistic pairs**, meaning that they produce opposite actions. For example, one muscle will bend a joint while its antagonist is responsible for straightening the joint. Some common terminology for muscle actions are described in Table 4.5 ■.

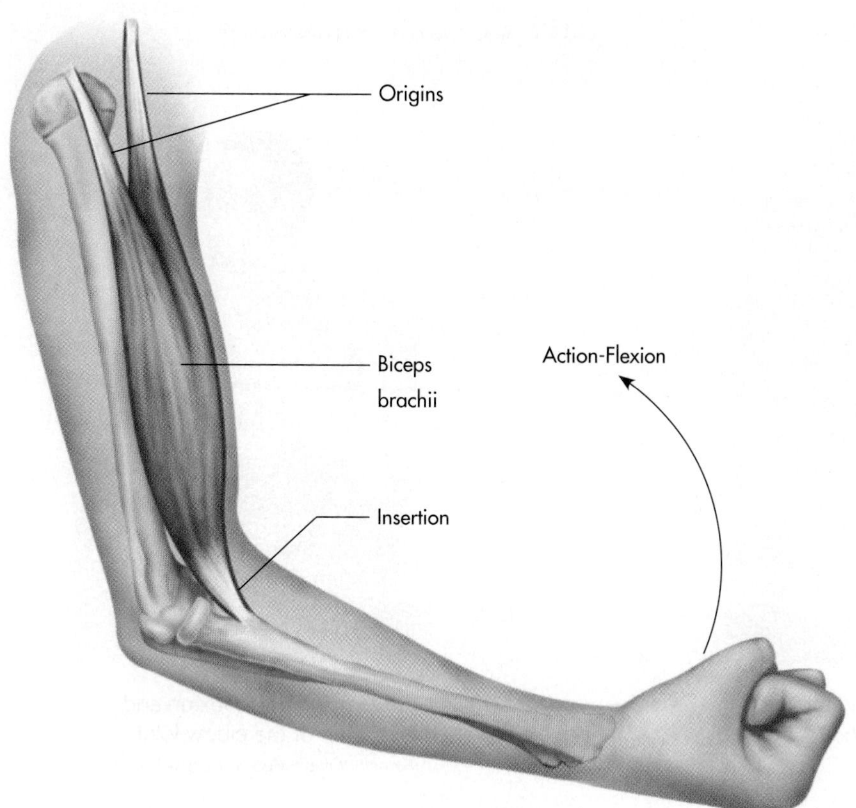

■ **Figure 4.23** Origin and insertion of a muscle

Table 4.5 Muscle Actions Grouped by Antagonistic Pairs

Action	Word Parts	Description
abduction (ab-DUCK-shun)	ab- = away from duct/o = to bring -ion = action	Movement away from midline of the body (see Figure 4.24 ■)
adduction (ah-DUCK-shun)	ad- = toward duct/o = to bring -ion = action	Movement toward midline of the body (see again Figure 4.24)
flexion (FLEK-shun)	flex/o = to bend -ion = action	Act of bending or being bent (see Figure 4.25 ■)
extension (eks-TEN-shun)	extens/o = to stretch out -ion = action	Movement that brings limb into or toward a straight condition (see again Figure 4.25)
dorsiflexion (dor-see-FLEK-shun)	dors/o = back of body flex/o = to bend -ion = action	Backward bending, as of hand or foot (see Figure 4.26A ■)
plantar flexion (PLAN-tar / FLEK-shun)	plant/o = sole of foot -ar = pertaining to flex/o = to bend -ion = action	Bending sole of foot; pointing toes downward (see Figure 4.26B ■)

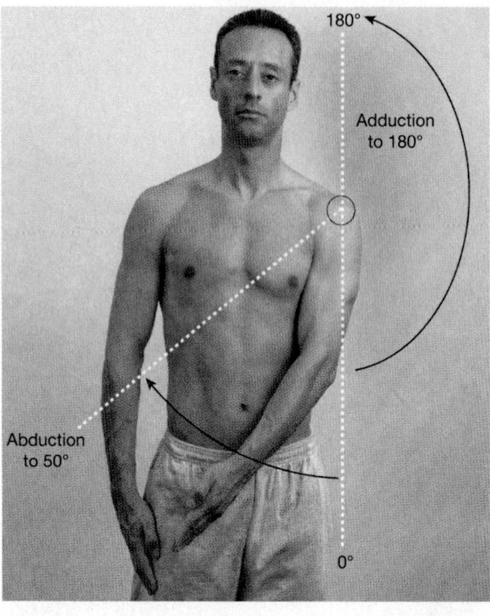

■ **Figure 4.24** Abduction and adduction of the shoulder joint. *(Patrick Watson, Pearson Education)*

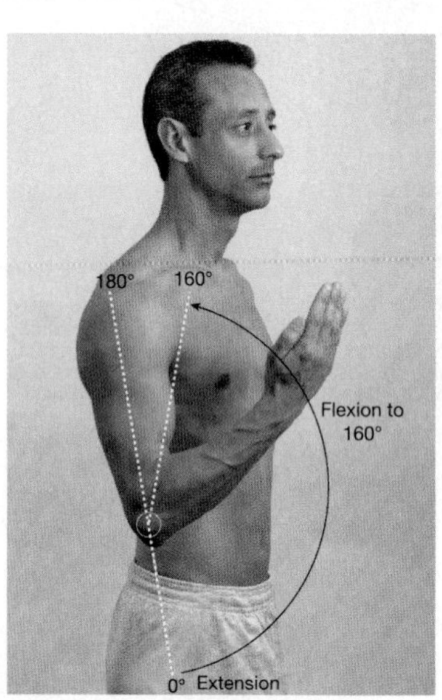

■ **Figure 4.25** Flexion and extension of the elbow joint. *(Patrick Watson, Pearson Education)*

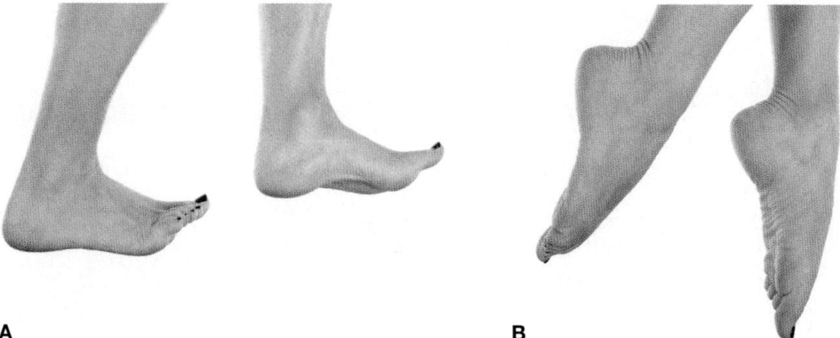

■ **Figure 4.26** Dorsiflexion (A) and plantar flexion (B) of the ankle joint. *(Poulsons Photography/ Shutterstock)*

Table 4.5 Muscle Actions Grouped by Antagonistic Pairs (continued)

Action	Word Parts	Description
eversion (ee-VER-zhun)	e- = outward vers/o = to turn -ion = action	Turning outward (see Figure 4.27 ■)
inversion (in-VER-zhun)	in- = inward vers/o = to turn -ion = action	Turning inward (see again Figure 4.27)
pronation (proh-NAY-shun)		To turn downward or backward as with the hand or foot (see Figure 4.28 ■)
supination (soo-pin-NAY-shun)		Turning the palm or foot upward (see again Figure 4.28)
elevation		To raise a body part, as in shrugging the shoulders
depression		A downward movement, as in dropping the shoulders
The circular actions described below are an exception to the antagonistic pair arrangement.		
circumduction (sir-kum-DUCK-shun)	circum- = around duct/o = to bring -ion = action	Movement in a circular direction from a central point as if drawing a large, imaginary circle in the air
opposition	Med Term Tip Primates are the only animals with opposable thumbs.	Moving thumb away from palm; the ability to move the thumb into contact with the other fingers
rotation	rotat/o = to revolve -ion = action	Moving around a central axis

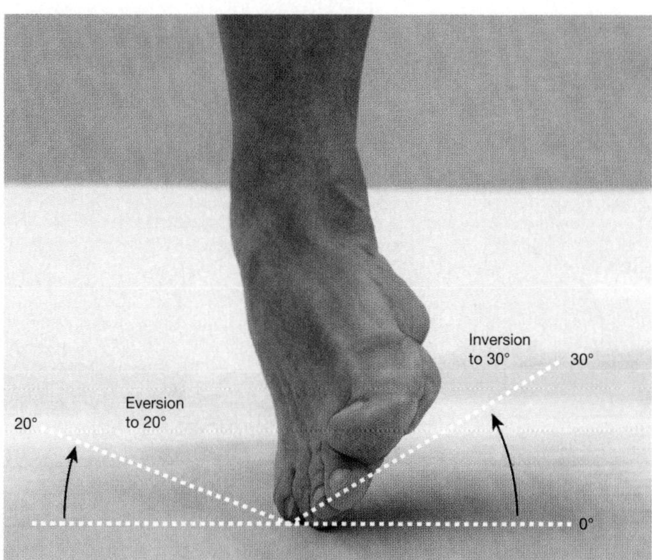

■ **Figure 4.27** Eversion and inversion of the foot. *(Patrick Watson, Pearson Education)*

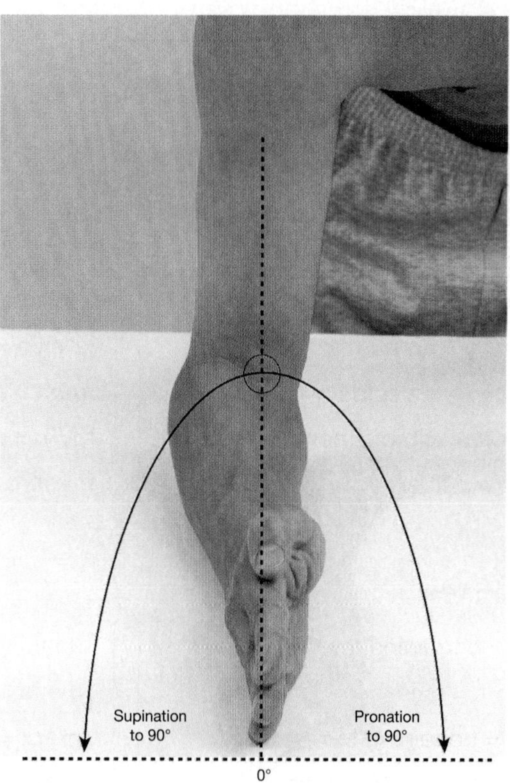

■ **Figure 4.28** Pronation and supination of the forearm. *(Patrick Watson, Pearson Education)*

Practice As You Go

F. Terminology Matching

Match each term to its definition.

1. ________ abduction	a.	backward bending of the foot
2. ________ rotation	b.	bending the foot to point toes toward the ground
3. ________ plantar flexion	c.	straightening motion
4. ________ extension	d.	motion around a central axis
5. ________ dorsiflexion	e.	motion away from the body
6. ________ flexion	f.	moving the thumb away from the palm
7. ________ adduction	g.	motion toward the body
8. ________ opposition	h.	bending motion

Terminology

Word Parts Used to Build Muscular System Terms

The following lists contain the combining forms, suffixes, and prefixes used to build terms in the remaining sections of this chapter.

Combining Forms

bi/o = life	**kinesi/o** = movement	**ten/o** = tendon
carp/o = carpus	**later/o** = side	**tend/o** = tendon
electr/o = electricity	**muscul/o** = muscle	**tendin/o** = tendon
fasci/o = fibrous band	**my/o** = muscle	
fibr/o = fibers	**myos/o** = muscle	

Suffixes

-al = pertaining to	**-desis** = to fuse	**-itis** = inflammation
-algia = pain	**-dynia** = pain	**-kinesia** = movement
-ar = pertaining to	**-gram** = record	**-logy** = study of
-asthenia = weakness	**-graphy** = process of recording	**-opsy** = view of

Suffixes (continued)

-otomy = cutting into
-ous = pertaining to
-pathy = disease
-plasty = surgical repair

-rrhaphy = suture
-rrhexis = rupture
-tonia = tone

-trophic = pertaining to development
-trophy = development

Prefixes

a- = without
brady- = slow
dys- = abnormal; difficult

epi- = above
hyper- = excessive
hypo- = insufficient

poly- = many
pseudo- = false

Adjective Forms of Anatomical Terms

Term	Word Parts	Definition
fascial (FAS-ee-all)	fasci/o = fibrous band -al = pertaining to	Pertaining to fascia.
muscular (MUSS-kew-lar)	muscul/o = muscle -ar = pertaining to	Pertaining to muscles.
musculoskeletal (MUSS-kew-loh-SKEL-eh-tal)	muscul/o = muscle -al = pertaining to	Pertaining to the muscles and skeleton.
tendinous (TEN-din-us)	tendin/o = tendon -ous = pertaining to	Pertaining to tendons.

Pathology

Term	Word Parts	Definition
Medical Specialties		
kinesiology (kih-NEE-see-oh-loh-jee)	kinesi/o = movement -logy = study of	The science that studies movement, how it is produced, and the muscles involved.
Signs and Symptoms		
adhesion		Scar tissue forming in the fascia surrounding a muscle, making it difficult to stretch the muscle.
atonia	a- = without -tonia = tone	The lack of muscle tone.
atrophy (AT-rah-fee)	a- = without -trophy = development	Poor muscle development as a result of muscle disease, nervous system disease, or lack of use; commonly referred to as *muscle wasting.*
bradykinesia (brad-ee-kih-NEE-see-ah)	brady- = slow -kinesia = movement	Having slow movements.

Pathology (continued)

Term	Word Parts	Definition
contracture (kon-TRACK-chur)		Abnormal shortening of muscle fibers, tendons, or fascia, making it difficult to stretch the muscle.
dyskinesia (dis-kih-NEE-see-ah)	dys- = difficult, abnormal -kinesia = movement	Having difficult or abnormal movement.
dystonia	dys- = abnormal -tonia = tone	Having abnormal muscle tone.
hyperkinesia (high-per-kih-NEE-see-ah)	hyper- = excessive -kinesia = movement	Having an excessive amount of movement.
hypertonia	hyper- = excessive -tonia = tone	Having excessive muscle tone.
hypertrophy (high-PER-troh-fee)	hyper- = excessive -trophy = development	Increase in muscle bulk as a result of use, as with lifting weights.
hypokinesia (HI-poh-kih-NEE-see-ah)	hypo- = insufficient -kinesia = movement	Having an insufficient amount of movement.
hypotonia	hypo- = insufficient -tonia = tone	Having insufficient muscle tone.
intermittent claudication (klaw-dih-KAY-shun)		Attacks of severe pain and lameness caused by ischemia of the muscles, typically the calf muscles; brought on by walking even very short distances.
myalgia (my-AL-jee-ah)	my/o = muscle -algia = pain	Muscle pain.
myasthenia (my-ass-THEE-nee-ah)	my/o = muscle -asthenia = weakness	Muscle weakness.
myotonia	my/o = muscle -tonia = tone	Muscle tone.
spasm		Sudden, involuntary, strong muscle contraction.
tenodynia (ten-oh-DIN-ee-ah)	ten/o = tendon -dynia = pain	Tendon pain.
Muscles		
fasciitis (fas-ee-EYE-tis)	fasci/o = fibrous band -itis = inflammation	Inflammation of fascia.
fibromyalgia (figh-broh-my-AL-jee-ah)	fibr/o = fibers my/o = muscle -algia = pain	Condition with widespread aching and pain in the muscles and soft tissue.
lateral epicondylitis (ep-ih-kon-dih-LYE-tis)	later/o = side -al = pertaining to epi- = above -itis = inflammation	Inflammation of the muscle attachment to the lateral epicondyle of the elbow. Often caused by strongly gripping. Commonly called *tennis elbow.*
muscular dystrophy (MD) (MUSS-kew-ler / DIS-troh-fee)	muscul/o = muscle -ar = pertaining to dys- = abnormal -trophy = development	Inherited disease causing a progressive muscle degeneration, weakness, and atrophy.
myopathy (my-OPP-ah-thee)	my/o = muscle -pathy = disease	A general term for muscle disease.

Pathology (continued)

Term	Word Parts	Definition
myorrhexis (my-oh-REK-sis)	**my/o** = muscle **-rrhexis** = rupture	Tearing a muscle.
polymyositis (pol-ee-my-oh-SIGH-tis)	**poly-** = many **myos/o** = muscle **-itis** = inflammation	The simultaneous inflammation of two or more muscles.
pseudohypertrophic muscular dystrophy (soo-doh-HIGH-per-troh-fic)	**pseudo-** = false **hyper-** = excessive **-trophic** = pertaining to development **muscul/o** = muscle **-ar** = pertaining to **dys-** = abnormal **-trophy** = development	A type of inherited muscular dystrophy in which the muscle tissue is gradually replaced by fatty tissue, giving the appearance of a healthy and strong muscle. Also called *Duchenne's muscular dystrophy.*
torticollis (tore-tih-KOLL-iss)		Severe neck spasms pulling the head to one side. Commonly called *wryneck* or a *crick in the neck.*
Tendons, Muscles, and/or Ligaments		
carpal tunnel syndrome (CTS)	**carp/o** = carpus **-al** = pertaining to	Repetitive motion disorder with pain caused by compression of the finger flexor tendons and median nerve as they pass through the carpal tunnel of the wrist.
ganglion cyst (GANG-lee-on)		Cyst that forms on tendon sheath, usually on hand, wrist, or ankle.
repetitive motion disorder		Group of chronic disorders involving the tendon, muscle, joint, and nerve damage, resulting from the tissue being subjected to pressure, vibration, or repetitive movements for prolonged periods.
rotator cuff injury		The rotator cuff consists of the joint capsule of the shoulder joint reinforced by the tendons from several shoulder muscles. The high degree of flexibility at the shoulder joint puts the rotator cuff at risk for strain and tearing.
strain		Damage to the muscle, tendons, or ligaments due to overuse or overstretching.
tendinitis (ten-dih-NIGH-tis)	**tendin/o** = tendon **-itis** = inflammation	Inflammation of a tendon.

Diagnostic Procedures

Term	Word Parts	Definition
Clinical Laboratory Test		
creatine phosphokinase (CPK) (KREE-ah-teen / foss-foe-KYE-nase)		Muscle enzyme found in skeletal muscle and cardiac muscle. Blood levels become elevated in disorders such as heart attack, muscular dystrophy, and other skeletal muscle pathologies.

Diagnostic Procedures (continued)

Term	Word Parts	Definition
Additional Diagnostic Procedures		
deep tendon reflexes (DTR)		Muscle contraction in response to a stretch caused by striking the muscle tendon with a reflex hammer. Test used to determine if muscles are responding properly.
electromyogram (EMG) (ee-lek-troh-MY-oh-gram)	electr/o = electricity my/o = muscle -gram = record	The hardcopy record produced by electromyography.
electromyography (EMG) (ee-lek-troh-my-OG-rah-fee)	electr/o = electricity my/o = muscle -graphy = process of recording	Study and record of the strength and quality of muscle contractions as a result of electrical stimulation.
muscle biopsy (BYE-op-see)	bi/o = life -opsy = view of	Removal of muscle tissue for pathological examination.

Therapeutic Procedures

Term	Word Parts	Definition
Surgical Procedures		
carpal tunnel release	carp/o = carpus -al = pertaining to	Surgical cutting of the ligament in the wrist to relieve nerve pressure caused by carpal tunnel syndrome, which can result from repetitive motion such as typing.
fasciotomy (fas-ee-OT-oh-mee)	fasci/o = fibrous band -otomy = cutting into	A surgical procedure that cuts into fascia.
myoplasty (MY-oh-plas-tee)	my/o = muscle -plasty = surgical repair	A surgical procedure to repair a muscle.
myorrhaphy (MY-or-ah-fee)	my/o = muscle -rrhaphy = suture	To suture a muscle.
tendoplasty (TEN-doh-plas-tee)	tend/o = tendon -plasty = surgical repair	A surgical procedure to repair a tendon.
tendotomy (tend-OT-oh-mee)	tend/o = tendon -otomy = cutting into	A surgical procedure that cuts into a tendon.
tenodesis (ten-oh-DEE-sis)	ten/o = tendon -desis = fuse	Surgical procedure to stabilize a joint by anchoring down the tendons of the muscles that move the joint.
tenoplasty (TEN-oh-plas-tee)	ten/o = tendon -plasty = surgical repair	A surgical procedure to repair a tendon.
tenorrhaphy (tah-NOR-ah-fee)	ten/o = tendon -rrhaphy = suture	To suture a tendon.

Pharmacology

Classification	Word Parts	Action	Examples
skeletal muscle relaxants	-al = pertaining to	Medication to relax skeletal muscles in order to reduce muscle spasms. Also called *antispasmodics.*	cyclobenzaprine, Flexeril; carisoprodol, Soma

Abbreviations

CTS	carpal tunnel syndrome	**EMG**	electromyogram
CPK	creatine phosphokinase	**IM**	intramuscular
DTR	deep tendon reflex	**MD**	muscular dystrophy

Practice As You Go

G. What's the Abbreviation?

1. intramuscular ______________________________
2. deep tendon reflex ______________________________
3. muscular dystrophy ______________________________
4. electromyogram ______________________________
5. carpal tunnel syndrome ______________________________

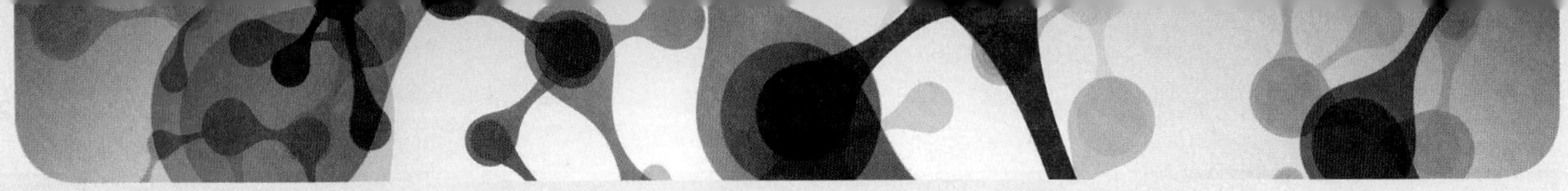

Chapter Review

Real-World Applications

Medical Record Analysis

This Discharge Summary contains 10 medical terms. Underline each term and write it in the list below the report. Then define each term. You will find Chapter 14 of your textbook helpful with the rehabilitation terms.

Discharge Summary

Admitting Diagnosis:	Osteoarthritis bilateral knees.
Final Diagnosis:	Osteoarthritis bilateral knees with right TKA
History of Present Illness:	Patient is a 68-year-old male. He reports he has experienced occasional knee pain and swelling since he injured his knees playing football in high school. These symptoms became worse while he was in his 50s and working on a concrete surface. The right knee has always been more painful than the left. He saw his orthopedic surgeon six months ago because of constant knee pain and swelling severe enough to interfere with sleep and all activities. He required a cane to walk. CT scan indicated severe bilateral osteoarthritis. He is admitted to the hospital at this time for TKR right knee.
Summary of Hospital Course:	Patient tolerated the surgical procedure well. He began intensive physical therapy for lower extremity ROM and strengthening exercises and gait training with a walker. He received occupational therapy instruction in ADLs, especially dressing and personal care. He was able to transfer himself out of bed by the third post-op day and was able to ambulate 150 ft with a walker and dress himself on the fifth post-op day.
Discharge Plans:	Patient was discharged home with his wife one week post-op. He will continue rehabilitation as an outpatient. Return to office for post-op checkup in one week.

	Term	Definition
1.		
2.		
3.		
4.		
5.		
6.		
7.		
8.		
9.		
10.		

Chart Note Transcription

The chart note below contains 11 phrases that can be reworded with a medical term that you learned in this chapter. Each phrase is identified with an underline. Determine the medical term and write your answers in the space provided.

Pearson General Hospital Emergency Room Record

Task Edit View Time Scale Options Help Download Archive Date: 17 May 2015

Current Complaint:	An 82-year-old female was transported to the Emergency Room via ambulance with severe left hip pain following a fall on the ice.
Past History:	Patient suffered a broken wrist bone **1** 2 years earlier that required immobilization by solid material. **2** Following this broken bone, **3** her physician who specializes in treatment of bone conditions **4** diagnosed her with moderate porous bones **5** on the basis of a computer-assisted X-ray. **6**
Signs and Symptoms:	Patient reported severe left hip pain, rating it as 8 on a scale of 1 to 10. She held her hip in a bent position **7** and could not tolerate movement toward a straight position. **8** X-rays of the left hip and leg were taken.
Diagnosis:	Shattered broken bone **9** in the neck of the left thigh bone. **10**
Treatment:	Implantation of an artificial hip joint **11** on the left.

1. ______________________

2. ______________________

3. ______________________

4. ______________________

5. ______________________

6. ______________________

7. ______________________

8. ______________________

9. ______________________

10. ______________________

11. ______________________

Case Study

Below is a case study presentation of a patient with a condition covered by this chapter. Read the case study and answer the questions below. Some questions will ask for information not included within this chapter. Use your text, a medical dictionary, or any other reference material you choose to answer these questions.

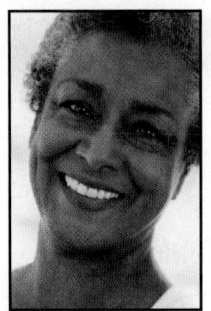

(Monkey Business Images/Shutterstock)

Mary Pearl, age 60, has come into the physician's office complaining of swelling, stiffness, and arthralgia, especially in her elbows, wrists, and hands. A bone scan revealed acute inflammation in multiple joints with damaged articular cartilage and an erythrocyte sedimentation rate blood test indicated a significant level of acute inflammation in the body. A diagnosis of acute episode of rheumatoid arthritis was made. The physician ordered nonsteroidal anti-inflammatory medication and physical therapy. The therapist initiated a treatment program of hydrotherapy and AROM exercises.

Questions

1. What pathological condition does this patient have? Look this condition up in a reference source and include a short description of it.

____

____

2. What type of long-term damage may occur in a patient with rheumatoid arthritis?

____

____

3. Describe the other major type of arthritis mentioned in your textbook.

____

____

4. What two diagnostic procedures did the physician order? Describe them in your own words. What were the results? (One of these procedures is described in Chapter 6 of your text.)

____

____

5. What treatments were ordered? Explain what the physical therapy procedures involve (refer to Chapter 14).

____

____

6. This patient is experiencing an acute episode. Explain what this phrase means and contrast it with chronic.

____

____

Practice Exercises

A. Word Building Practice

The combining form **oste/o** refers to bone. Use it to write a term that means:

1. bone cell ____________________
2. immature bone cell ____________________
3. porous bone ____________________
4. disease of the bone ____________________
5. cutting into a bone ____________________
6. instrument to cut bone ____________________
7. inflammation of the bone and bone marrow ____________________
8. abnormal softening of bone ____________________
9. bone and cartilage tumor ____________________

The combining form **my/o** refers to muscle. Use it to write a term that means:

10. muscle disease ____________________
11. surgical repair of muscle ____________________
12. suture of muscle ____________________
13. record of muscle electricity ____________________
14. muscle weakness ____________________

The combining form **ten/o** refers to tendons. Use it to write a term that means:

15. tendon pain ____________________
16. tendon suture ____________________

The combining form **arthr/o** refers to the joints. Use it to write a term that means:

17. to fuse a joint ____________________
18. surgical repair of a joint ____________________
19. cutting into a joint ____________________
20. inflammation of a joint ____________________
21. puncture to withdraw fluid from a joint ____________________
22. pain in the joints ____________________

The combining form **chondr/o** refers to cartilage. Use it to write a term that means:

23. surgical removal of cartilage ____________________
24. cartilage tumor ____________________
25. abnormal softening of cartilage ____________________

B. Name That Suffix

	Suffix	Example from Chapter
1. to fuse	______	______
2. weakness	______	______
3. slipping	______	______
4. to surgically break	______	______
5. movement	______	______
6. porous	______	______

C. Spinal Column Practice

Name the five regions of the spinal column and indicate the number of bones in each area.

	Name	Number of Bones
1.	______	______
2.	______	______
3.	______	______
4.	______	______
5.	______	______

D. Prefix and Suffix Practice

Circle the prefix and/or suffix. Place a *P* for prefix or an *S* for suffix over these word parts, then define the term.

1. arthroscopy______
2. intervertebral______
3. chondromalacia______
4. diskectomy______
5. intracranial______
6. spondylosis______

E. Define the Combining Form

	Definition	Example from Chapter
1. **lamin/o**	______	______
2. **ankyl/o**	______	______
3. **chondr/o**	______	______

	Definition	Example from Chapter
4. **spondyl/o**	____________	____________
5. **my/o**	____________	____________
6. **orth/o**	____________	____________
7. **kyph/o**	____________	____________
8. **tend/o**	____________	____________
9. **myel/o**	____________	____________
10. **articul/o**	____________	____________

F. Fill in the Blank

carpal tunnel syndrome	rickets	lateral epicondylitis	systemic lupus erythematosus
scoliosis	osteogenic sarcoma	pseudohypertrophic muscular dystrophy	
herniated nucleus pulposus	osteoporosis		
	spondylolisthesis		

1. Mrs. Lewis, age 84, broke her hip. Her physician will be running tests for what potential ailment? ____________
2. Jamie, age six months, is being given orange juice and vitamin supplements to avoid what condition? ____________
3. George has severe elbow pain after playing tennis four days in a row. He may have ____________.
4. Marshall's doctor told him that he had a ruptured disk. The medical term for this is ____________.
5. Mr. Jefferson's physician has discovered a tumor at the end of his femur. He has been admitted to the hospital for a biopsy to rule out what type of bone cancer? ____________
6. The school nurse has asked Janelle to bend over so that she may examine her back to see if she is developing a lateral curve. What is the nurse looking for? ____________
7. Gerald has experienced a gradual loss of muscle strength over the past five years even though his muscles look large and healthy. The doctors believe he has an inherited muscle disease. What is that disease? ____________
8. Roberta has suddenly developed arthritis in her hands and knees. Rheumatoid arthritis had been ruled out, but what other autoimmune disease might Roberta have? ____________
9. Mark's X-ray demonstrated forward sliding of a lumbar vertebra; the radiologist diagnosed ____________.
10. The orthopedist determined that Marcia's repetitive wrist movements at work caused her to develop ____________

G. Name That Anatomical Name

1. kneecap ____________
2. ankle bones ____________
3. collar bone ____________
4. thigh bone ____________

5. toe bones ______
6. wrist bones ______
7. shin bone ______
8. shoulder blade ______
9. finger bones ______

H. What Does it Stand For?

1. DJD______
2. EMG______
3. C1______
4. T6______
5. IM______
6. DTR______
7. JRA______
8. LLE______
9. ortho______
10. CTS______

I. Define the Term

1. chondroplasty______
2. bradykinesia______
3. osteoporosis______
4. lordosis______
5. atrophy______
6. myeloma______
7. prosthesis______
8. craniotomy______
9. arthrocentesis______
10. bursitis______

J. Pharmacology Challenge

Fill in the classification for each drug description, then match the brand name.

	Drug Description	Classification	Brand Name
1.	_______ Treats mild pain and is an anti-inflammatory	_______________	a. Flexeril
2.	_______ Hormone with anti-inflammatory properties	_______________	b. Aleve
3.	_______ Reduces muscle spasms	_______________	c. Fosamax
4.	_______ Treats conditions of weakened bones	_______________	d. Oystercal
5.	_______ Maintains blood calcium levels	_______________	e. Medrol

Labeling Exercise

Image A

Write the labels for this figure on the numbered lines provided.

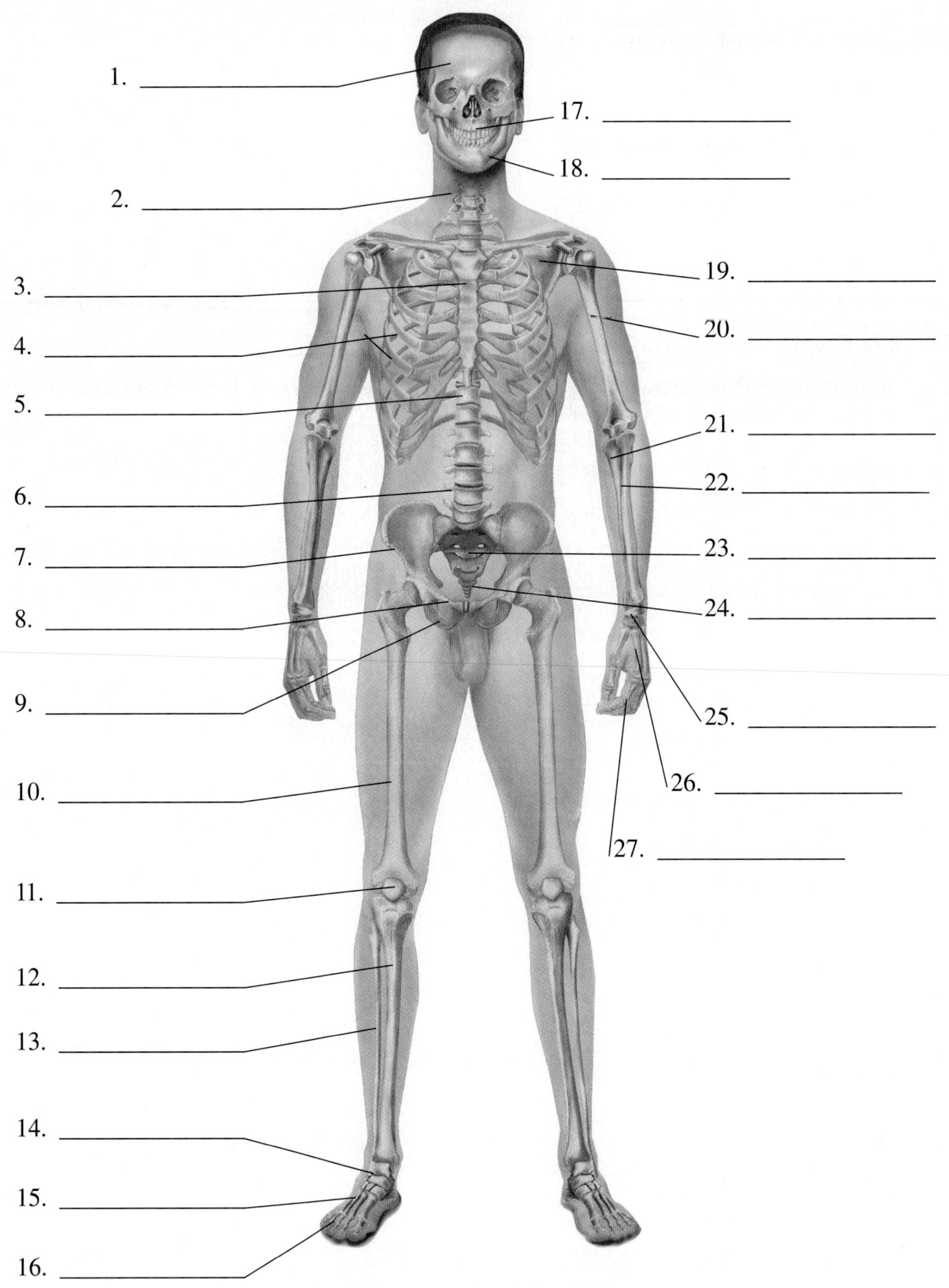

Image B

Write the labels for this figure on the numbered lines provided.

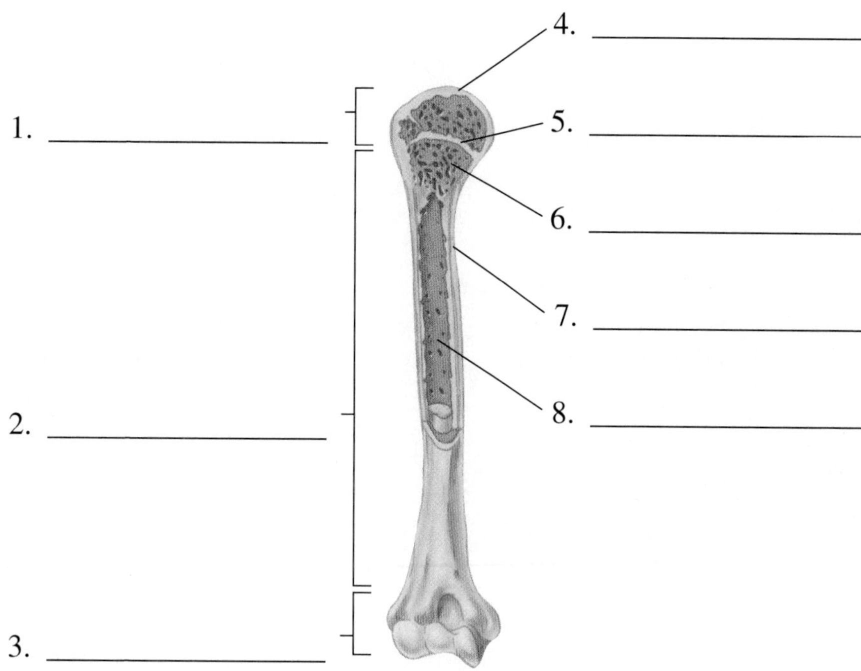

Image C

Write the labels for this figure on the numbered lines provided.

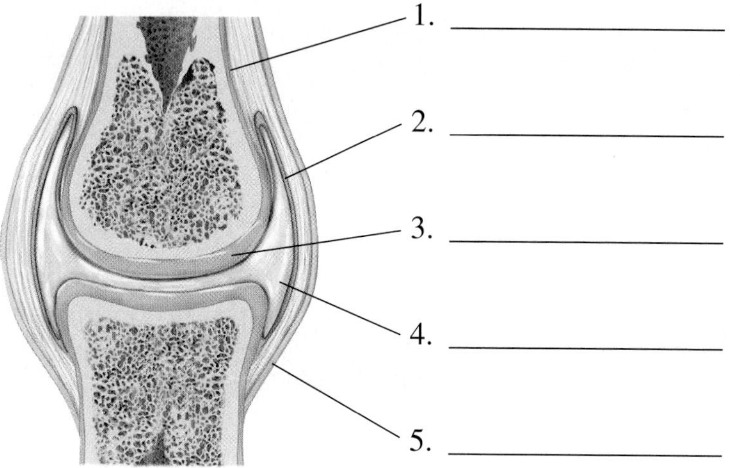

5

Cardiovascular System

Learning Objectives

Upon completion of this chapter, you will be able to

- Identify and define the combining forms, suffixes, and prefixes introduced in this chapter.
- Correctly spell and pronounce medical terms and major anatomical structures relating to the cardiovascular system.
- Describe the major organs of the cardiovascular system and their functions.
- Describe the anatomy of the heart.
- Describe the flow of blood through the heart.
- Explain how the electrical conduction system controls the heartbeat.
- List and describe the characteristics of the three types of blood vessels.
- Define pulse and blood pressure.
- Identify and define cardiovascular system anatomical terms.
- Identify and define selected cardiovascular system pathology terms.
- Identify and define selected cardiovascular system diagnostic procedures.
- Identify and define selected cardiovascular system therapeutic procedures.
- Identify and define selected medications relating to the cardiovascular system.
- Define selected abbreviations associated with the cardiovascular system.

Cardiovascular System at a Glance

Function

The cardiovascular system consists of the pump and vessels that distribute blood to all areas of the body. This system allows for the delivery of needed substances to the cells of the body as well as for the removal of wastes.

Organs

Here are the primary structures that comprise the cardiovascular system:

blood vessels

- **arteries**
- **capillaries**
- **veins**

heart

Word Parts

Here are the most common word parts (with their meanings) used to build cardiovascular system terms. For a more comprehensive list, refer to the Terminology section of this chapter.

Combining Forms

angi/o	vessel
aort/o	aorta
arteri/o	artery
ather/o	fatty substance
atri/o	atrium
cardi/o	heart
coron/o	heart
corpor/o	body
embol/o	plug
isch/o	to hold back
myocardi/o	heart muscle
phleb/o	vein
sept/o	wall
son/o	sound
sphygm/o	pulse
steth/o	chest
thromb/o	clot
valv/o	valve
valvul/o	valve
varic/o	dilated vein
vascul/o	blood vessel
vas/o	vessel
ven/o	vein
ventricul/o	ventricle

Suffixes

-cardia	heart condition
-manometer	instrument to measure pressure
-ole	small
-spasm	involuntary muscle contraction
-tension	pressure
-tonic	pertaining to tone
-ule	small

Prefixes

di-	two

Cardiovascular System Illustrated

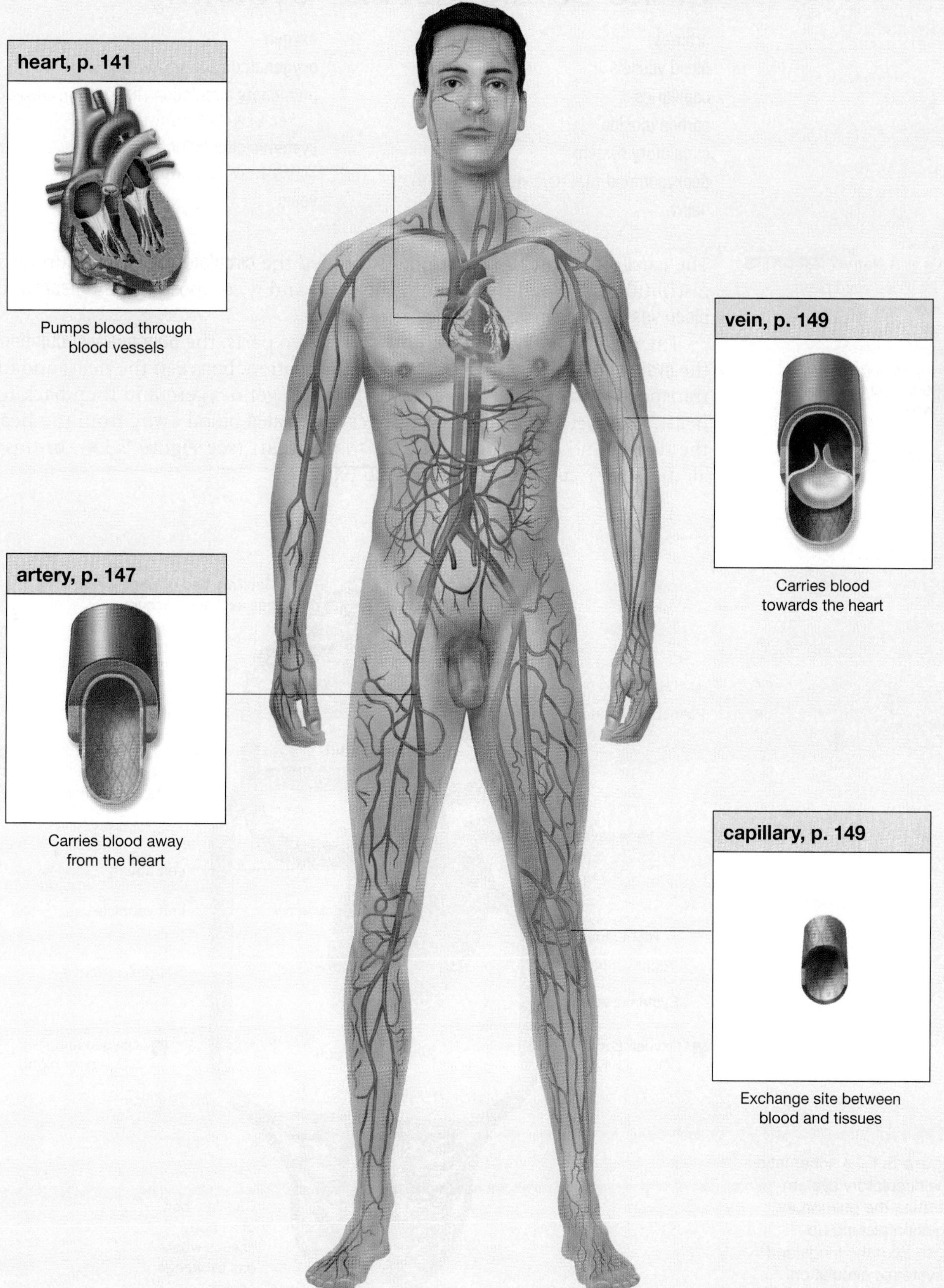

Anatomy and Physiology of the Cardiovascular System

arteries
blood vessels
capillaries
carbon dioxide
circulatory system
deoxygenated (dee-OK-sih-jen-ay-ted)
heart
oxygen
oxygenated (OK-sih-jen-ay-ted)
pulmonary circulation (PULL-mon-air-ee / ser-kew-LAY-shun)
systemic circulation (sis-TEM-ik / ser-kew-LAY-shun)
veins

What's In A Name?
Look for these word parts:
ox/o = oxygen
pulmon/o = lung
system/o = system
-ary = pertaining to
-ic = pertaining to
di- = two

The cardiovascular (CV) system, also called the **circulatory system**, maintains the distribution of blood throughout the body and is composed of the **heart** and the **blood vessels—arteries**, **capillaries**, and **veins**.

The circulatory system is composed of two parts: the **pulmonary circulation** and the **systemic circulation**. The pulmonary circulation, between the heart and lungs, transports **deoxygenated** blood to the lungs to get oxygen, and then back to the heart. The systemic circulation carries **oxygenated** blood away from the heart to the tissues and cells, and then back to the heart (see Figure 5.1 ■). In this way all the body's cells receive blood and oxygen.

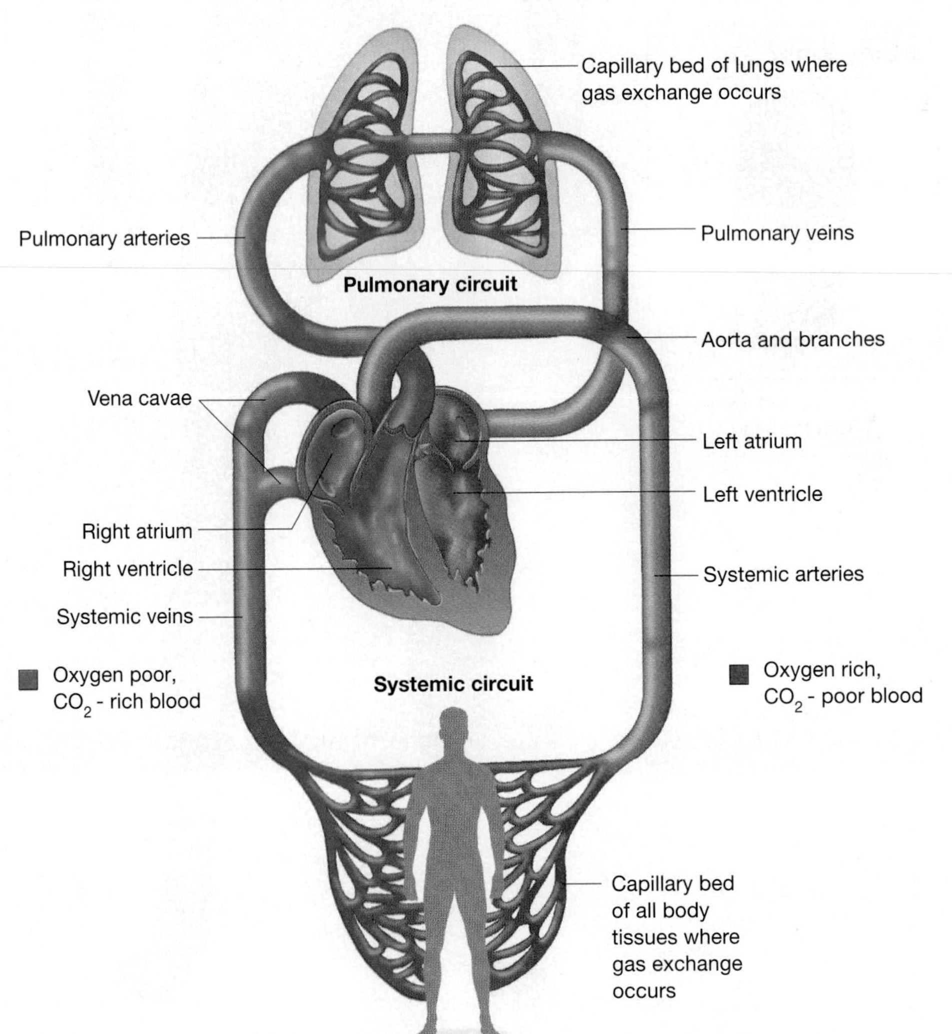

■ **Figure 5.1** A schematic of the circulatory system illustrating the pulmonary circulation picking up oxygen from the lungs and the systemic circulation delivering oxygen to the body.

In addition to distributing **oxygen** and other nutrients, such as glucose and amino acids, the cardiovascular system also collects the waste products from the body's cells. **Carbon dioxide** and other waste products produced by metabolic reaction are transported by the cardiovascular system to the lungs, liver, and kidneys where they are eliminated from the body.

Heart

apex (AY-peks)

cardiac muscle (CAR-dee-ak)

The heart is a muscular pump made up of **cardiac muscle** fibers that could be considered a muscle rather than an organ. It has four chambers, or cavities, and beats an average of 60–100 beats per minute (bpm) or about 100,000 times in one day. Each time the cardiac muscle contracts, blood is ejected from the heart and pushed throughout the body within the blood vessels.

The heart is located in the mediastinum in the center of the chest cavity; however, it is not exactly centered; more of the heart is on the left side of the mediastinum than the right (see Figure 5.2 ■). At about the size of a fist and shaped like an upside-down pear, the heart lies directly behind the sternum. The tip of the heart at the lower edge is called the **apex**.

Med Term Tip

Your heart is approximately the size of your clenched fist and pumps 4,000 gallons of blood each day. It will beat at least three billion times during your lifetime.

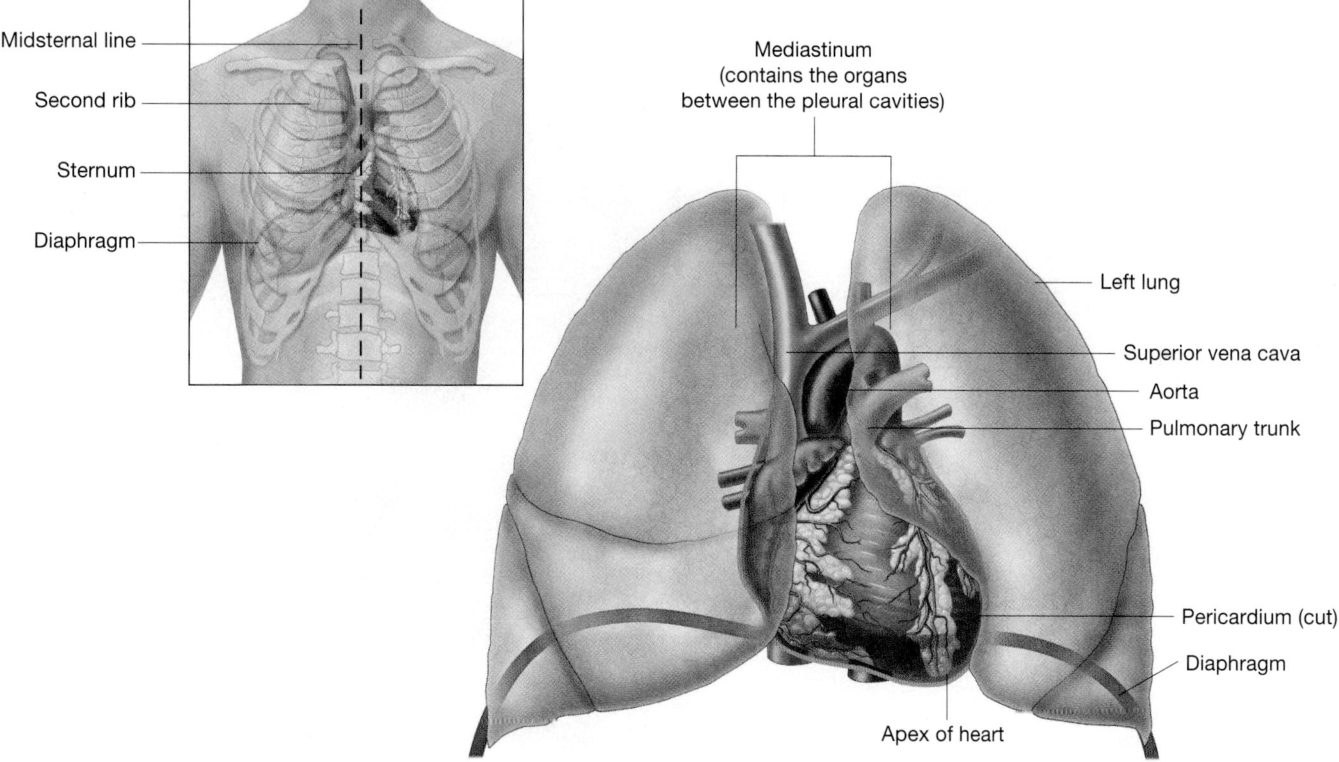

■ **Figure 5.2** Location of the heart within the mediastinum of the thoracic cavity.

What's In A Name?

Look for these word parts:
cardi/o = heart
pariet/o = cavity wall
viscer/o = internal organ
-al = pertaining to
epi- = above

Med Term Tip

These layers become important when studying the disease conditions affecting the heart. For instance, when the prefix *endo-* is added to *carditis*, forming *endocarditis*, we know that the inflammation is within the "inner layer of the heart." In discussing the muscular action of the heart, the combining form *my/o*, meaning "muscle," is added to *cardium* to form the word *myocardium.* The diagnosis *myocardial infarction* (MI), or heart attack, means that the patient has an infarct or "dead tissue in the muscle of the heart." The prefix *peri-*, meaning "around," when added to the word *cardium* refers to the sac "surrounding the heart." Therefore, *pericarditis* is an "inflammation of the outer sac of the heart."

Heart Layers

endocardium (en-doh-CAR-dee-um)
epicardium (ep-ih-CAR-dee-um)
myocardium (my-oh-CAR-dee-um)
parietal pericardium (pah-RYE-eh-tal / pair-ih-CAR-dee-um)
pericardium (pair-ih-CAR-dee-um)
visceral pericardium (VISS-er-al / pair-ih-CAR-dee-um)

The wall of the heart is quite thick and composed of three layers (see Figure 5.3■):

1. The **endocardium** is the inner layer of the heart lining the heart chambers. It is a very smooth, thin layer that serves to reduce friction as the blood passes through the heart chambers.
2. The **myocardium** is the thick, muscular middle layer of the heart. Contraction of this muscle layer develops the pressure required to pump blood through the blood vessels.
3. The **epicardium** is the outer layer of the heart. The heart is enclosed within a double-layered pleural sac, called the **pericardium**. The epicardium is the **visceral pericardium**, or inner layer of the sac. The outer layer of the sac is the **parietal pericardium**. Fluid between the two layers of the sac reduces friction as the heart beats.

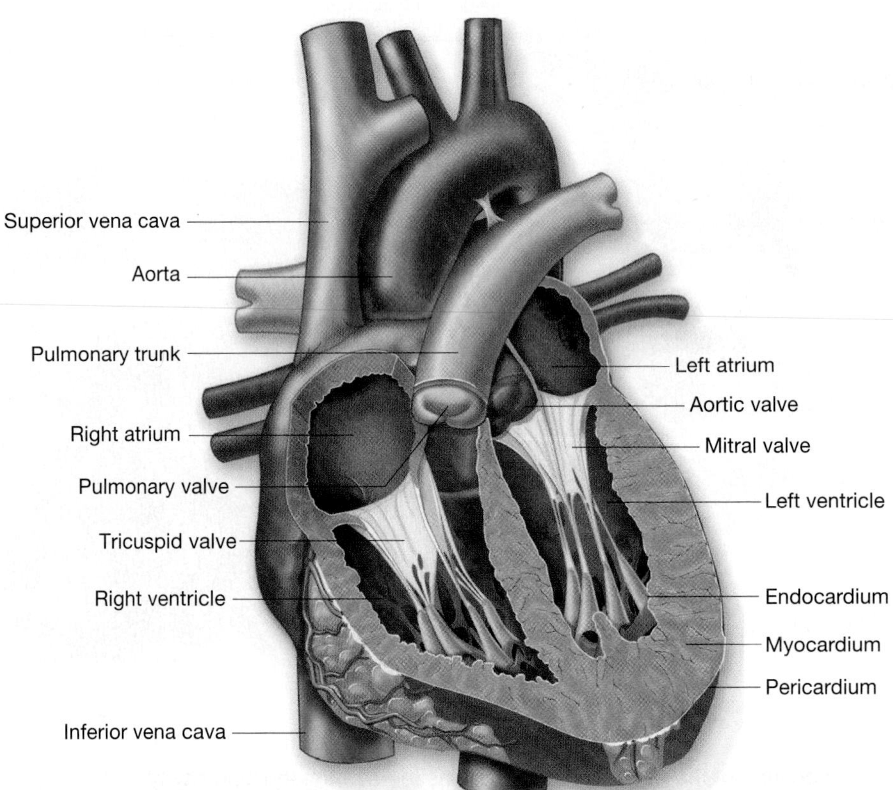

■ **Figure 5.3** Internal view of the heart illustrating the heart chambers, heart layers, and major blood vessels associated with the heart.

Heart Chambers

atria (AY-tree-ah)
interatrial septum (in-ter-AY-tree-al / SEP-tum)
interventricular septum (in-ter-ven-TRIK-yoo-lar / SEP-tum)
ventricles (VEN-trik-lz)

The heart is divided into four chambers or cavities (see Figures 5.3 and 5.4). There are two **atria**, or upper chambers, and two **ventricles**, or lower chambers. These chambers are divided into right and left sides by walls called the **interatrial septum** and the **interventricular septum**. The atria are the receiving chambers of the heart. Blood returning to the heart via veins first collects in the atria. The ventricles are the pumping chambers. They have a much thicker myocardium and their contraction ejects blood out of the heart and into the great arteries.

Med Term Tip

The term *ventricle* comes from the Latin term *venter*, which means "little belly." Although it originally referred to the abdomen and then the stomach, it came to stand for any hollow region inside an organ.

Heart Valves

aortic valve (ay-OR-tik)
atrioventricular valve (ay-tree-oh-ven-TRIK-yoo-lar)
bicuspid valve (bye-CUSS-pid)
cusps
mitral valve (MY-tral)
pulmonary valve (PULL-mon-air-ee)
semilunar valve (sem-ih-LOO-nar)
tricuspid valve (try-CUSS-pid)

Four valves act as restraining gates to control the direction of blood flow. They are situated at the entrances and exits to the ventricles (see Figure 5.4 ■). Properly functioning valves allow blood to flow only in the forward direction by blocking it from returning to the previous chamber.

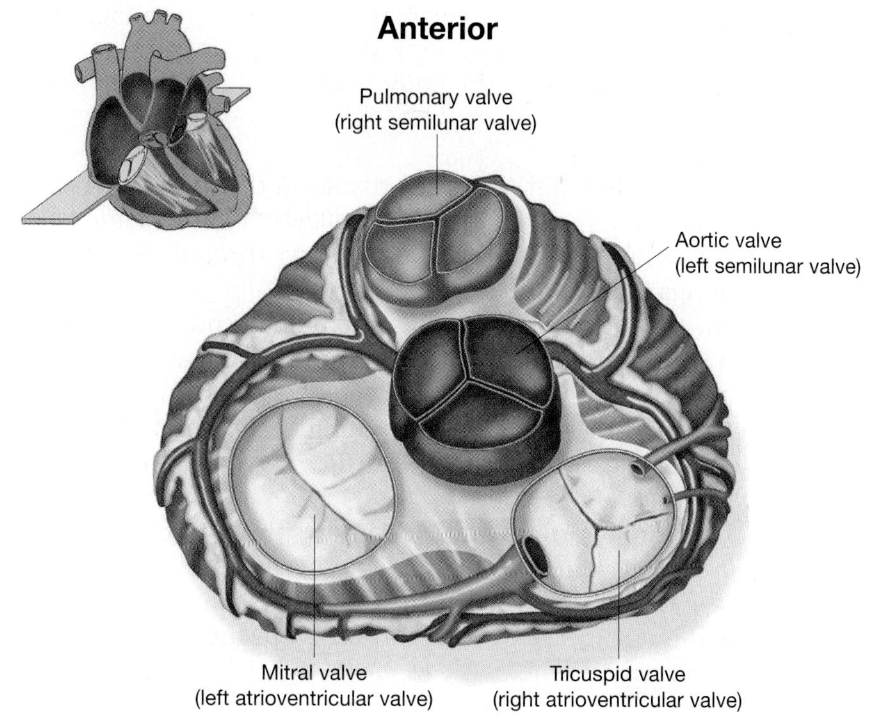

■ **Figure 5.4** Superior view of heart valves illustrating position, size, and shape of each valve.

What's In A Name?

Look for these word parts:
pulmon/o = lung
-al = pertaining to
-ar = pertaining to
bi- = two
semi- = partial
tri- = three

Med Term Tip

The heart makes two distinct sounds referred to as "lub-dupp." These sounds are produced by the forceful snapping shut of the heart valves. *Lub* is the closing of the atrioventricular valves. *Dupp* is the closing of the semilunar valves.

The four valves are as follows:

1. **Tricuspid valve**: an **atrioventricular valve** (AV), meaning that it controls the opening between the right atrium and the right ventricle. Once the blood enters the right ventricle, it cannot go back up into the atrium again. The prefix *tri-*, meaning three, indicates that this valve has three leaflets or **cusps**.
2. **Pulmonary valve**: a **semilunar valve**. The prefix *semi-*, meaning half, and the term **lunar**, meaning moon, indicate that this valve looks like a half moon. Located between the right ventricle and the pulmonary artery, this valve prevents blood that has been ejected into the pulmonary artery from returning to the right ventricle as it relaxes.
3. **Mitral valve**: also called the **bicuspid valve**, indicating that it has two cusps. Blood flows through this atrioventricular valve to the left ventricle and cannot go back up into the left atrium.
4. **Aortic valve**: a semilunar valve located between the left ventricle and the aorta. Blood leaves the left ventricle through this valve and cannot return to the left ventricle.

Blood Flow Through the Heart

aorta (ay-OR-tah)
diastole (dye-ASS-toe-lee)
inferior vena cava (VEE-nah / KAY-vah)
pulmonary artery (PULL-mon-air-ee)
pulmonary veins
superior vena cava
systole (SIS-toe-lee)

The flow of blood through the heart is very orderly (see Figure 5.5 ■). It progresses through the heart to the lungs, where it receives oxygen; then goes back to the heart; and then out to the body tissues and parts. The normal process of blood flow is:

What's In A Name?

Look for these word parts:
infer/o = below
pulmon/o = lung
super/o = above
-ary = pertaining to
-ior = pertaining to

1. Deoxygenated blood from all the tissues in the body enters a relaxed right atrium via two large veins called the **superior vena cava** and **inferior vena cava**.
2. The right atrium contracts and blood flows through the tricuspid valve into the relaxed right ventricle.
3. The right ventricle then contracts and blood is pumped through the pulmonary valve into the **pulmonary artery**, which carries it to the lungs for oxygenation.
4. The left atrium receives blood returning to the heart after being oxygenated by the lungs. This blood enters the relaxed left atrium from the four **pulmonary veins**.
5. The left atrium contracts and blood flows through the mitral valve into the relaxed left ventricle.
6. When the left ventricle contracts, the blood is pumped through the aortic valve and into the **aorta**, the largest artery in the body. The aorta carries blood to all parts of the body.

It can be seen that the heart chambers alternate between relaxing, in order to fill, and contracting to push blood forward. The period of time a chamber is relaxed is **diastole**. The contraction phase is **systole**.

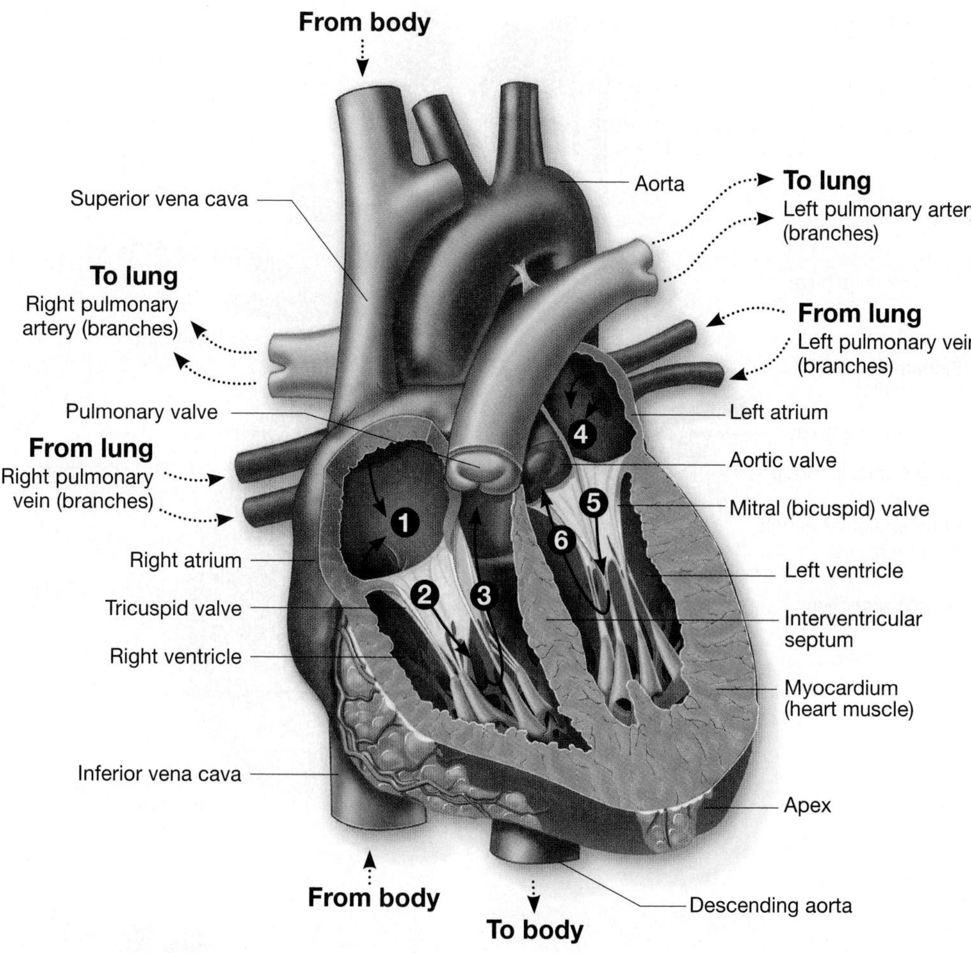

■ **Figure 5.5** The path of blood flow through the chambers of the left and right side of the heart, including the veins delivering blood to the heart and arteries receiving blood ejected from the heart.

Conduction System of the Heart

atrioventricular bundle
atrioventricular node
autonomic nervous system (aw-toh-NOM-ik / NER-vus / SIS-tem)
bundle branches
bundle of His
pacemaker
Purkinje fibers (per-KIN-gee)
sinoatrial node (sigh-noh-AY-tree-al)

The heart rate is regulated by the **autonomic nervous system**; therefore, we have no voluntary control over the beating of our heart. Special tissue within the heart is responsible for conducting an electrical impulse stimulating the different chambers to contract in the correct order.

The path that the impulses travel is as follows (see Figure 5.6 ■):

1. The **sinoatrial** (SA, S-A) **node**, or **pacemaker**, is where the electrical impulses begin. From the sinoatrial node a wave of electricity travels through the atria, causing them to contract, or go into systole.
2. The **atrioventricular node** is stimulated.
3. This node transfers the stimulation wave to the **atrioventricular bundle** (formerly called **bundle of His**).
4. The electrical signal next travels down the **bundle branches** within the interventricular septum.
5. The **Purkinje fibers** out in the ventricular myocardium are stimulated, resulting in ventricular systole.

What's In A Name?

Look for these word parts:
atri/o = atrium
-al = pertaining to
-ic = pertaining to
auto- = self

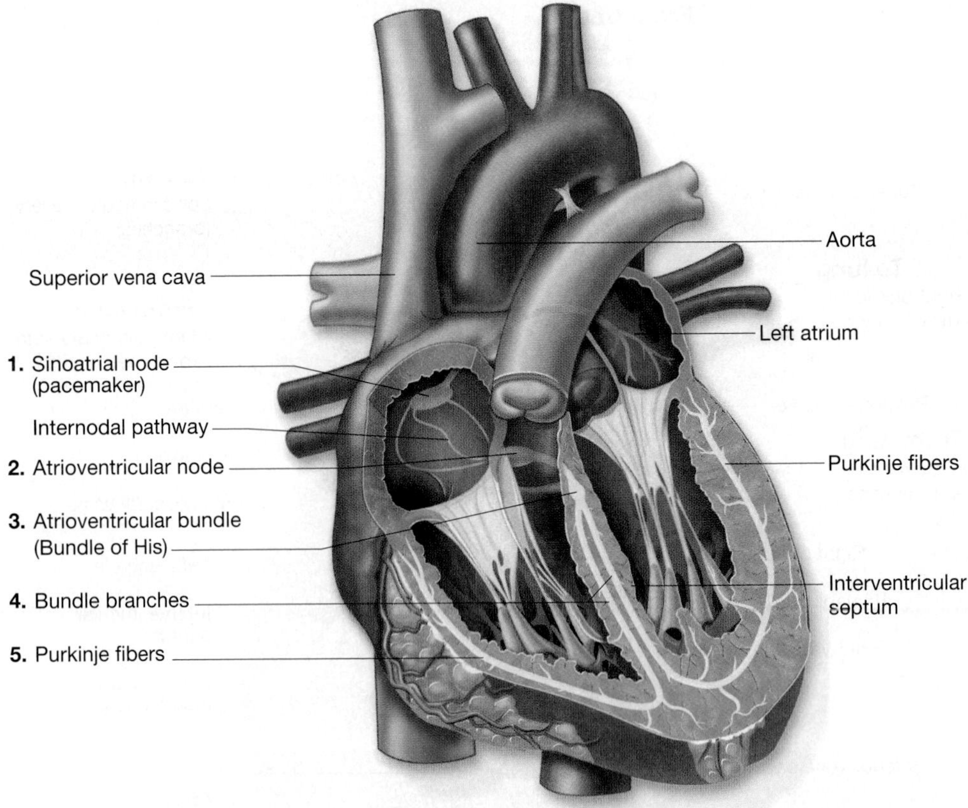

■ **Figure 5.6** The conduction system of the heart; traces the path of the electrical impulse that stimulates the heart chambers to contract in the correct sequence.

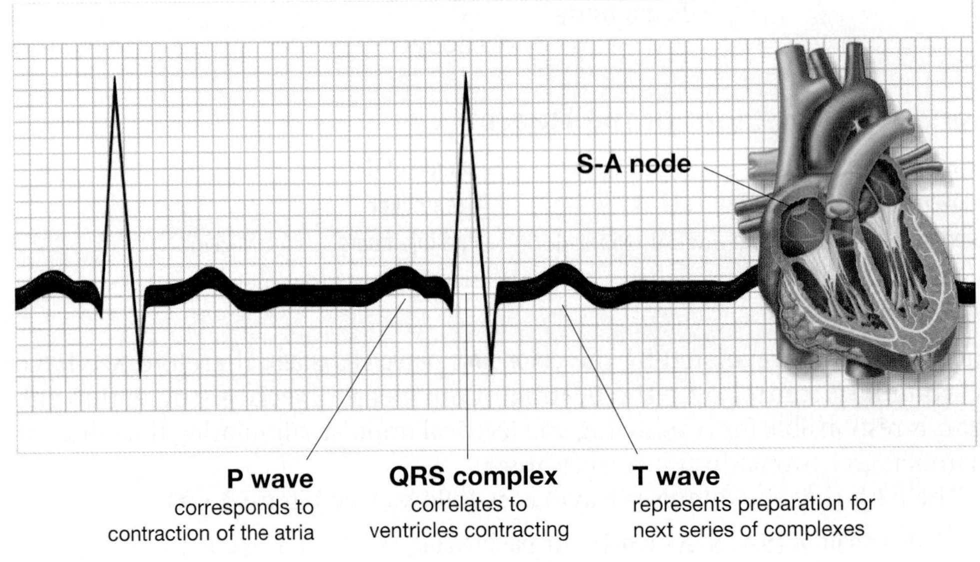

■ **Figure 5.7** An electrocardiogram (EKG) wave record of the electrical signal as it moves through the conduction system of the heart. This signal stimulates the chambers of the heart to contract and relax in the proper sequence.

Med Term Tip

The electrocardiogram, referred to as an EKG or ECG, is a measurement of the electrical activity of the heart (see Figure 5.7 ■). This can give the physician information about the health of the heart, especially the myocardium.

Blood Vessels

lumen (LOO-men)

There are three types of blood vessels: arteries, capillaries, and veins (see Figure 5.8 ■). These are the pipes that circulate blood throughout the body. The **lumen** is the channel within these vessels through which blood flows.

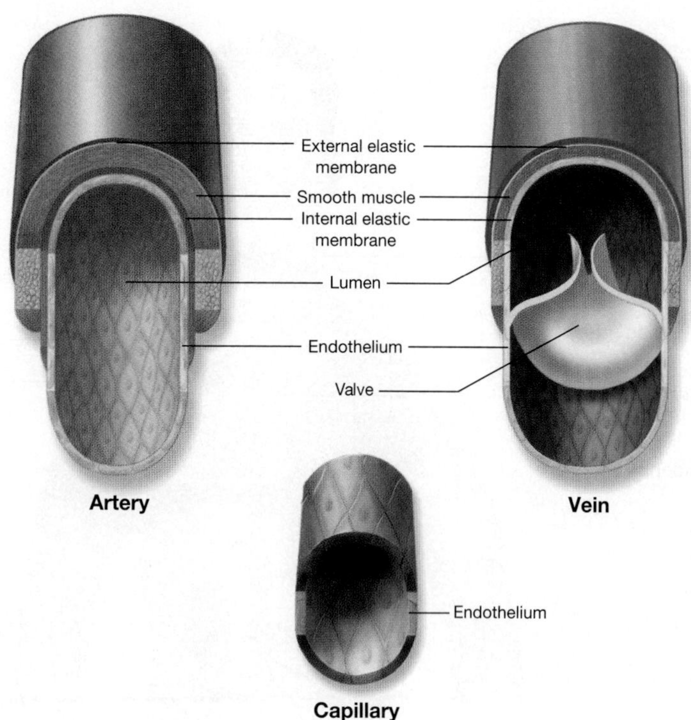

■ **Figure 5.8** Comparative structure of arteries, capillaries, and veins.

Arteries

arterioles (ar-TEE-ree-ohlz)

coronary arteries (KOR-ah-nair-ee / AR-te-reez)

The arteries are the large, thick-walled vessels that carry the blood away from the heart. The walls of arteries contain a thick layer of smooth muscle that can contract or relax to change the size of the arterial lumen. The pulmonary artery carries deoxygenated blood from the right ventricle to the lungs. The largest artery, the aorta, begins from the left ventricle of the heart and carries oxygenated blood to all the body systems. The **coronary arteries** then branch from the aorta and provide blood to the myocardium (see Figure 5.9 ■). As they travel through the body, the arteries branch into progressively smaller-sized arteries. The smallest of the arteries, called **arterioles**, deliver blood to the capillaries. Figure 5.10 ■ illustrates the major systemic arteries.

Med Term Tip

The term *coronary*, from the Latin word for crown, describes how the great vessels encircle the heart as they emerge from the top of the heart.

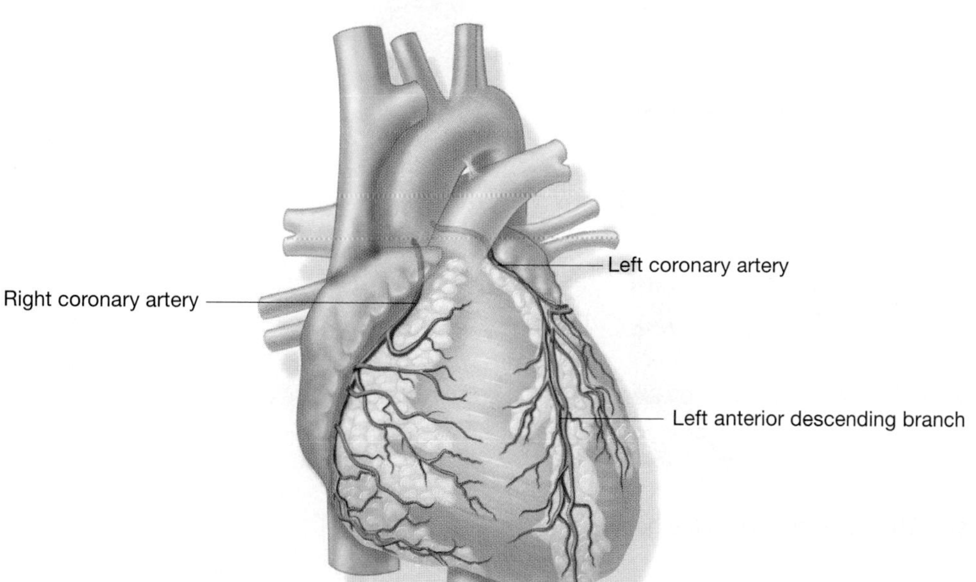

■ **Figure 5.9** The coronary arteries.

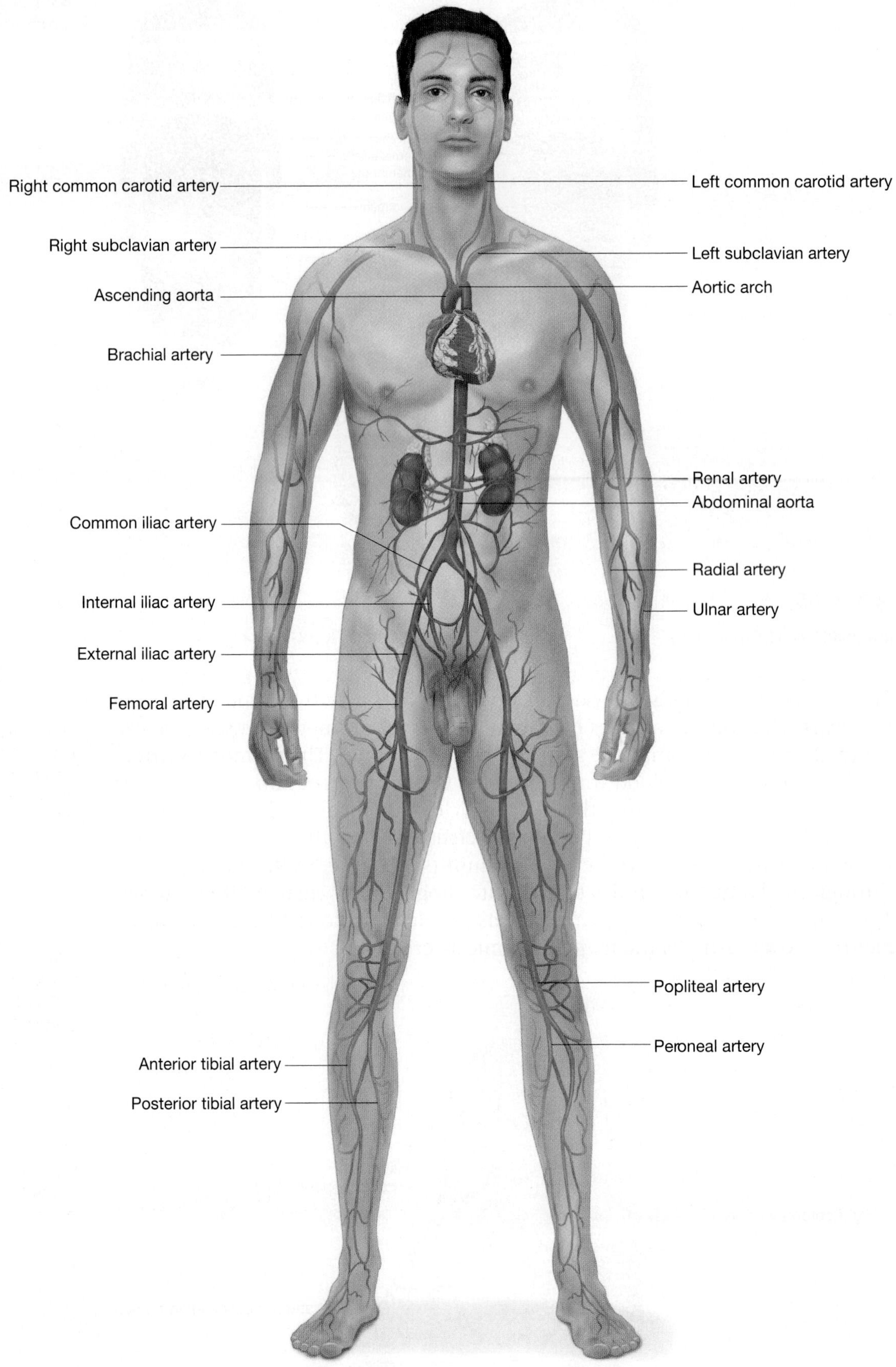
Right common carotid artery
Left common carotid artery
Right subclavian artery
Left subclavian artery
Ascending aorta
Aortic arch
Brachial artery
Renal artery
Abdominal aorta
Common iliac artery
Radial artery
Internal iliac artery
Ulnar artery
External iliac artery
Femoral artery
Popliteal artery
Peroneal artery
Anterior tibial artery
Posterior tibial artery

■ **Figure 5.10** The major arteries of the body.

Capillaries

capillary bed

Capillaries are a network of tiny blood vessels referred to as a **capillary bed**. Arterial blood flows into a capillary bed, and venous blood flows back out. Capillaries are very thin walled, allowing for the diffusion of the oxygen and nutrients from the blood into the body tissues (see Figure 5.8). Likewise, carbon dioxide and waste products are able to diffuse out of the body tissues and into the bloodstream to be carried away. Since the capillaries are so small in diameter, the blood will not flow as quickly through them as it does through the arteries and veins. This means that the blood has time for an exchange of nutrients, oxygen, and waste material to take place. As blood exits a capillary bed, it returns to the heart through a vein.

Veins

venules (VEN-yools)

The veins carry blood back to the heart (see Figure 5.8). Blood leaving capillaries first enters small **venules**, which then merge into larger veins. Veins have much thinner walls than arteries, causing them to collapse easily. The veins also have valves that allow the blood to move only toward the heart. These valves prevent blood from backflowing, ensuring that blood always flows toward the heart. The two large veins that enter the heart are the superior vena cava, which carries blood from the upper body, and the inferior vena cava, which carries blood from the lower body. Blood pressure in the veins is much lower than in the arteries. Muscular action against the veins and skeletal muscle contractions help in the movement of blood. Figure 5.11 ■ illustrates the major systemic veins.

Pulse and Blood Pressure

blood pressure (BP)
diastolic pressure (dye-ah-STOL-ik)
pulse
systolic pressure (sis-TOL-ik)

Blood pressure (BP) is a measurement of the force exerted by blood against the wall of a blood vessel. During ventricular systole, blood is under a lot of pressure from the ventricular contraction, giving the highest blood pressure reading—the **systolic pressure**. The **pulse** felt at the wrist or throat is the surge of blood caused by the heart contraction. This is why pulse rate is normally equal to heart rate. During ventricular diastole, blood is not being pushed by the heart at all and the blood pressure reading drops to its lowest point—the **diastolic pressure**. Therefore, to see the full range of what is occurring with blood pressure, both numbers are required. Blood pressure is also affected by several other characteristics of the blood and the blood vessels. These include the elasticity of the arteries, the diameter of the blood vessels, the viscosity of the blood, the volume of blood flowing through the vessels, and the amount of resistance to blood flow.

What's In A Name?

Look for these word parts:
-ic = pertaining to

Med Term Tip

The instrument used to measure blood pressure is called a *sphygmomanometer.* The combining form *sphygm/o* means "pulse" and the suffix *-manometer* means "instrument to measure pressure." A blood pressure reading is reported as two numbers, for example, 120/80. The 120 is the systolic pressure and the 80 is the diastolic pressure. There is no one "normal" blood pressure number. The normal blood pressure for an adult is a systolic pressure less than 120 and diastolic pressure less than 80.

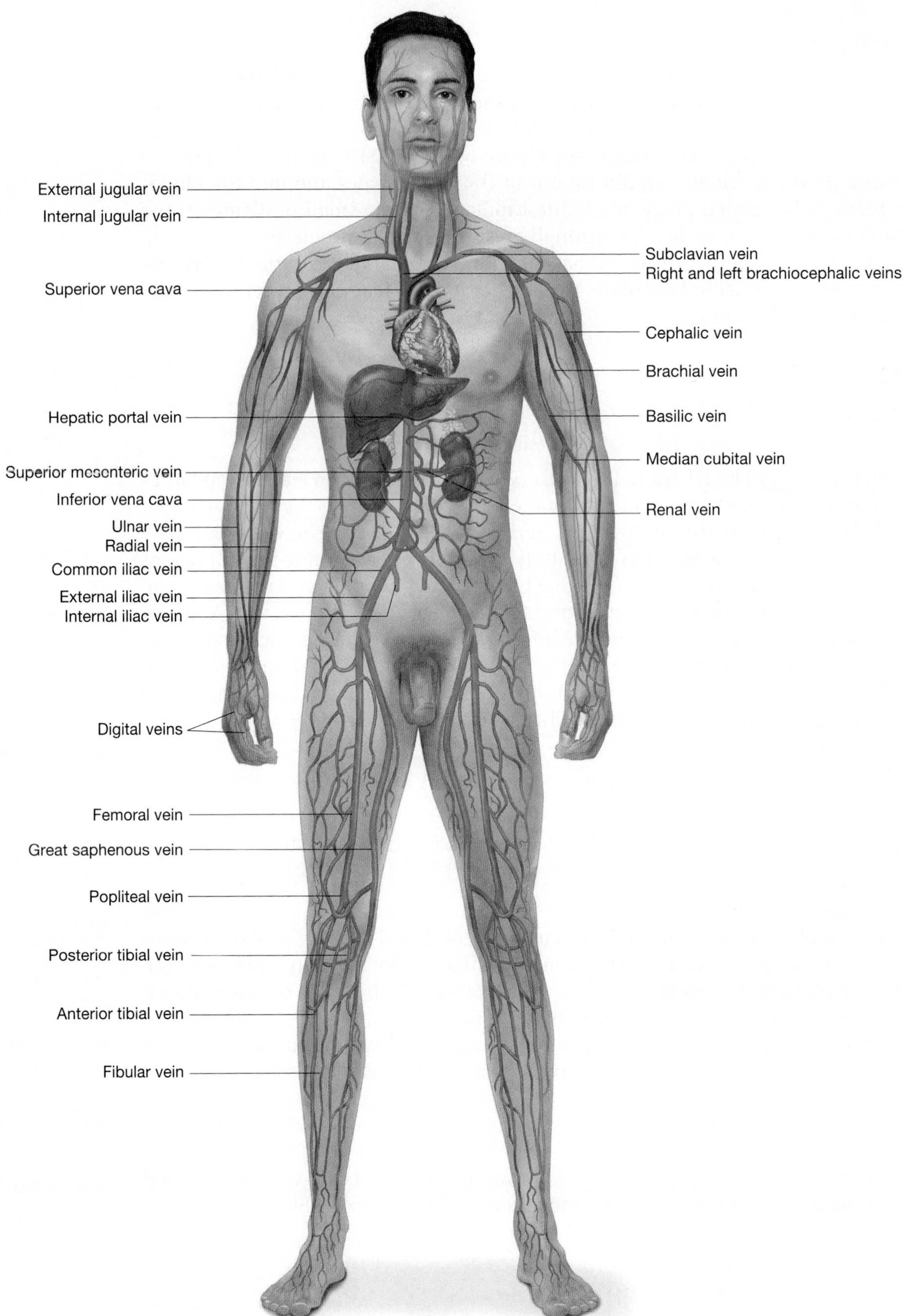
External jugular vein
Internal jugular vein
Superior vena cava
Hepatic portal vein
Superior mesenteric vein
Inferior vena cava
Ulnar vein
Radial vein
Common iliac vein
External iliac vein
Internal iliac vein
Digital veins
Femoral vein
Great saphenous vein
Popliteal vein
Posterior tibial vein
Anterior tibial vein
Fibular vein
Subclavian vein
Right and left brachiocephalic veins
Cephalic vein
Brachial vein
Basilic vein
Median cubital vein
Renal vein

■ **Figure 5.11** The major veins of the body.

Practice As You Go

A. Complete the Statement

1. The study of the heart is called ____________________.
2. The three layers of the heart are ____________________, ____________________, and ____________________.
3. The impulse for the heartbeat (the pacemaker) originates in the ____________________.
4. Arteries carry blood ____________________ the heart.
5. The four heart valves are ____________________, ____________________, ____________________, and ____________________.
6. The ____________________ are the receiving chambers of the heart and the ____________________ are the pumping chambers.
7. The ____________________ circulation carries blood to and from the lungs.
8. The pointed tip of the heart is called the ____________________.
9. The ____________________ divides the heart into left and right halves.
10. ____________________ is the contraction phase of the heartbeat and ____________________ is the relaxation phase.

Terminology

Word Parts Used to Build Cardiovascular System Terms

The following lists contain the combining forms, suffixes, and prefixes used to build terms in the remaining sections of this chapter.

Combining Forms

angi/o	vessel
aort/o	aorta
arteri/o	artery
ather/o	fatty substance
atri/o	atrium
cardi/o	heart
coron/o	heart
corpor/o	body
cutane/o	skin
cyan/o (see Chapter 7)	blue
duct/o	to bring
electr/o	electricity

embol/o	plug
hem/o (see Chapter 6)	blood
isch/o	to hold back
lip/o	fat
my/o	muscle
myocardi/o	heart muscle
orth/o	straight
pector/o	chest
peripher/o (see Chapter 12)	away from center
phleb/o	vein
pulmon/o	lung

sept/o	a wall
son/o	sound
sphygm/o	pulse
steth/o	chest
thromb/o	clot
valv/o	valve
valvul/o	valve
varic/o	dilated vein
vas/o	vessel
vascul/o	blood vessel
ven/o	vein
ventricul/o	ventricle

Suffixes

-ac	pertaining to
-al	pertaining to
-ar	pertaining to
-ary	pertaining to
-cardia	heart condition
-eal	pertaining to
-ectomy	surgical removal
-gram	record
-graphy	process of recording
-ia	condition
-ic	pertaining to

-itis	inflammation
-logy	study of
-lytic	destruction
-manometer	instrument to measure pressure
-megaly	enlarged
-ole	small
-oma	mass
-ose	pertaining to
-osis	abnormal condition
-ous	pertaining to
-pathy	disease

-plasty	surgical repair
-rrhexis	rupture
-sclerosis	hardening
-scope	instrument for viewing
-spasm	involuntary muscle contraction
-stenosis	narrowing
-tension	pressure
-tic	pertaining to
-tonic	pertaining to tone
-ule	small

Prefixes

a-	without
anti-	against
brady-	slow
de-	without
endo-	inner
extra-	outside of

hyper-	excessive
hypo-	insufficient
inter-	between
intra-	within
per-	through
peri-	around

poly-	many
re-	again
tachy-	fast
tetra-	four
trans-	across
ultra-	beyond

Adjective Forms of Anatomical Terms

Term	Word Parts	Definition
aortic (ay-OR-tik)	aort/o = aorta -ic = pertaining to	Pertaining to the aorta.
arterial (ar-TEE-ree-al)	arteri/o = artery -al = pertaining to	Pertaining to an artery.
arteriole (ar-TEE-ree-ohl)	arteri/o = artery -ole = small	A small (narrow in diameter) artery.
atrial (AY-tree-al)	atri/o = atrium -al = pertaining to	Pertaining to the atrium.
atrioventricular (AV, A-V) (AY-tree-oh-ven-TRIK-yoo-lar)	atri/o = atrium ventricul/o = ventricle -ar = pertaining to	Pertaining to the atrium and ventricle.
cardiac (CAR-dee-ak)	cardi/o = heart -ac = pertaining to	Pertaining to the heart.
coronary (KOR-ah-nair-ee)	coron/o = heart -ary = pertaining to	Pertaining to the heart.

Adjective Forms of Anatomical Terms (continued)

Term	Word Parts	Definition
interatrial (in-ter-AY-tree-al)	inter- = between atri/o = atrium -al = pertaining to	Pertaining to between the atria.
interventricular (in-ter-ven-TRIK-yoo-lar)	inter- = between ventricul/o = ventricle -ar = pertaining to	Pertaining to between the ventricles.
myocardial (my-oh-CAR-dee-al)	myocardi/o = heart muscle -al = pertaining to	Pertaining to heart muscle.
valvular (VAL-view-lar)	valvul/o = valve -ar = pertaining to	Pertaining to a valve.
vascular (VAS-kwee-lar)	vascul/o = blood vessel -ar = pertaining to	Pertaining to a blood vessel.
venous (VEE-nus)	ven/o = vein -ous = pertaining to	Pertaining to a vein.
ventricular (ven-TRIK-yoo-lar)	ventricul/o = ventricle -ar = pertaining to	Pertaining to a ventricle.
venule (VEN-yool)	ven/o = vein -ule = small	A small (narrow in diameter) vein.

Practice As You Go

B. Give the adjective form for each anatomical structure

1. The heart ____________________
2. Between the ventricles ____________________
3. An artery ____________________
4. A small vein ____________________
5. The heart muscle ____________________
6. An atrium ____________________

Pathology

Term	Word Parts	Definition
Medical Specialties		
cardiology (car-dee-ALL-oh-jee)	cardi/o = heart -logy = study of	The branch of medicine involving diagnosis and treatment of conditions and diseases of the cardiovascular system. Physician is a *cardiologist.*

Pathology (continued)

Term	Word Parts	Definition
cardiovascular technologist/ technician	**cardi/o** = heart **vascul/o** = blood vessel **-ar** = pertaining to	Healthcare professional trained to perform a variety of diagnostic and therapeutic procedures including electrocardiography, echocardiography, and exercise stress tests.
Signs and Symptoms		
angiitis (an-jee-EYE-tis)	**angi/o** = vessel **-itis** = inflammation	Inflammation of a vessel.
angiospasm (AN-jee-oh-spazm)	**angi/o** = vessel **-spasm** = involuntary muscle contraction	An involuntary muscle contraction of the smooth muscle in the wall of a vessel; narrows the vessel.
angiostenosis (an-jee-oh-sten-OH-sis)	**angi/o** = vessel **-stenosis** = narrowing	The narrowing of a vessel.
bradycardia (brad-ee-CAR-dee-ah)	**brady-** = slow **-cardia** = heart condition	The condition of having a slow heart rate, typically less than 60 beats/minute; highly trained aerobic persons may normally have a slow heart rate.
embolus (EM-boh-lus)	**embol/o** = plug	The obstruction of a blood vessel by a blood clot that has broken off from a thrombus somewhere else in the body and traveled to the point of obstruction. If it occurs in a coronary artery, it may result in a myocardial infarction. ■ **Figure 5.12** Illustration of an embolus floating in an artery. The embolus will become lodged in a blood vessel that is smaller than it is, resulting in occlusion of that artery.
infarct (IN-farkt)		An area of tissue within an organ or part that undergoes necrosis (death) following the loss of its blood supply.
ischemia (ih-SKEE-mee-uh)	**isch/o** = to hold back **hem/o** = blood **-ia** = condition	The localized and temporary deficiency of blood supply due to an obstruction to the circulation.
murmur (MUR-mur)		A sound, in addition to the normal heart sounds, arising from blood flowing through the heart. This extra sound may or may not indicate a heart abnormality.
orthostatic hypotension (or-thoh-STAT-ik)	**orth/o** = straight **hypo-** = insufficient **-tension** = pressure	The sudden drop in blood pressure a person experiences when standing straight up suddenly.
palpitations (pal-pih-TAY-shunz)		Pounding, racing heartbeats.

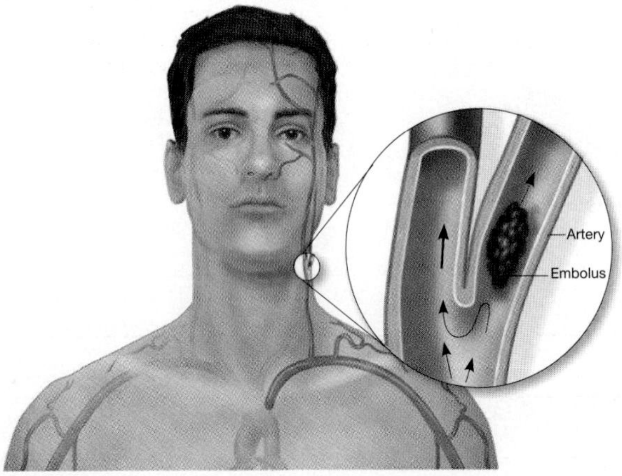

Pathology (continued)

Term	Word Parts	Definition
plaque (plak)		A yellow, fatty deposit of lipids in an artery that is the hallmark of atherosclerosis. Also called an *atheroma.*
regurgitation (re-ger-gih-TAY-shun)	re- = again	To flow backward. In the cardiovascular system this refers to the backflow of blood through a valve.
tachycardia (tak-ee-CAR-dee-ah)	tachy- = fast -cardia = heart condition	The condition of having a fast heart rate, typically more than 100 beats/minute while at rest.
thrombus (THROM-bus)	thromb/o = clot	A blood clot forming within a blood vessel. May partially or completely occlude the blood vessel.

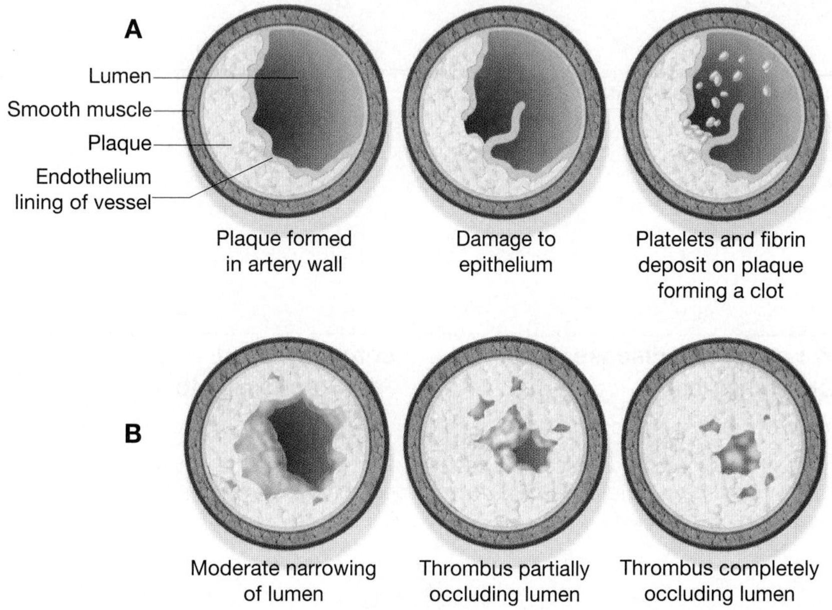

■ **Figure 5.13** Development of an atherosclerotic plaque that progressively narrows the lumen of an artery to the point that a thrombus fully occludes the lumen.

Term	Word Parts	Definition
Heart		
angina pectoris (an-JYE-nah / PECK-tor-is)	pector/o = chest	Condition in which there is severe pain with a sensation of constriction around the heart. Caused by a deficiency of oxygen to the heart muscle. Commonly called *chest pain* (CP).
arrhythmia (ah-RITH-mee-ah)	a- = without -ia = condition	Irregularity in the heartbeat or action. Comes in many different forms; some are not serious, while others are life-threatening.
bundle branch block (BBB)		Occurs when the electrical impulse is blocked from traveling down the bundle of His or bundle branches. Results in the ventricles beating at a different rate than the atria. Also called a *heart block.*

Pathology (continued)

Term	Word Parts	Definition
cardiac arrest	cardi/o = heart -ac = pertaining to	Complete stopping of heart activity.
cardiomegaly (car-dee-oh-MEG-ah-lee)	cardi/o = heart -megaly = enlarged	An enlarged heart.
cardiomyopathy (car-dee-oh-my-OP-ah-thee)	cardi/o = heart my/o = muscle -pathy = disease	General term for a disease of the myocardium. Can be caused by alcohol abuse, parasites, viral infection, and congestive heart failure. One of the most common reasons a patient may require a heart transplant.
congenital septal defect (CSD)	sept/o = a wall -al = pertaining to	A hole, present at birth, in the septum between two heart chambers; results in a mixture of oxygenated and deoxygenated blood. There can be an *atrial septal defect* (ASD) and a *ventricular septal defect* (VSD).
congestive heart failure (CHF) (kon-JESS-tiv)		Pathological condition of the heart in which there is a reduced outflow of blood from the left side of the heart because the left ventricle myocardium has become too weak to efficiently pump blood. Results in weakness, breathlessness, and edema.
coronary artery disease (CAD) (KOR-ah-nair-ee)	coron/o = heart -ary = pertaining to	Insufficient blood supply to the heart muscle due to an obstruction of one or more coronary arteries. May be caused by atherosclerosis and may cause angina pectoris and myocardial infarction.

Med Term Tip

All types of cardiovascular disease have been the number one killer of Americans since the 19th century. This disease kills more people annually than the next six causes of death combined.

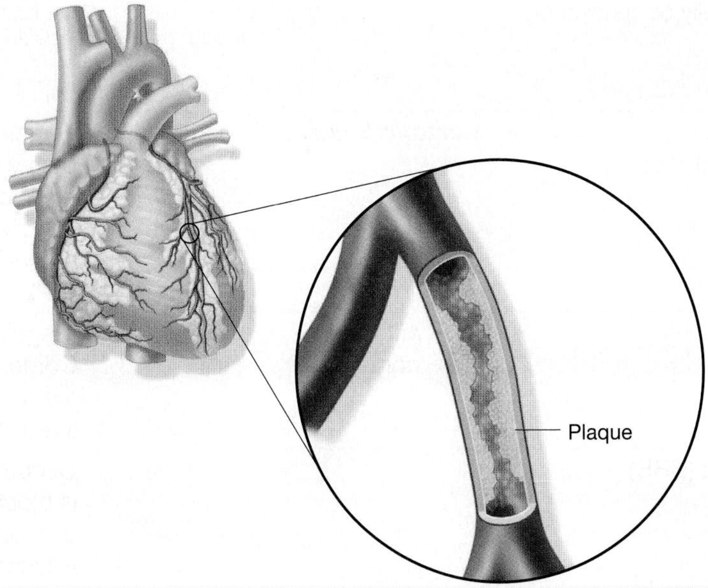

■ Figure 5.14 Formation of an atherosclerotic plaque within a coronary artery; may lead to coronary artery disease, angina pectoris, and myocardial infarction.

Pathology (continued)

Term	Word Parts	Definition
endocarditis (en-doh-car-DYE-tis)	endo- = inner **cardi/o** = heart -itis = inflammation	Inflammation of the lining membranes of the heart. May be due to bacteria or to an abnormal immunological response. In bacterial endocarditis, the mass of bacteria that forms is referred to as *vegetation.*
fibrillation (fih-brill-AY-shun)		An extremely serious arrhythmia characterized by an abnormal quivering or contraction of heart fibers. When this occurs in the ventricles, cardiac arrest and death can occur. Emergency equipment to defibrillate, or convert the heart to a normal beat, is necessary.
flutter		An arrhythmia in which the atria beat too rapidly, but in a regular pattern.
heart valve prolapse (PROH-laps)		Condition in which the cusps or flaps of the heart valve are too loose and fail to shut tightly, allowing blood to flow backward through the valve when the heart chamber contracts. Most commonly occurs in the mitral valve, but may affect any of the heart valves.
heart valve stenosis (steh-NOH-sis)	-stenosis = narrowing	Condition in which the cusps or flaps of the heart valve are too stiff and are unable to open fully (making it difficult for blood to flow through) or shut tightly (allowing blood to flow backward). This condition may affect any of the heart valves.
myocardial infarction (MI) (my-oh-CAR-dee-al / in-FARC-shun)	**myocardi/o** = heart muscle -al = pertaining to	Condition caused by the partial or complete occlusion or closing of one or more of the coronary arteries. Symptoms include a squeezing pain or heavy pressure in the middle of the chest (angina pectoris). A delay in treatment could result in death. Also referred to as a *heart attack.* See Figure 5.15 ■.

Pathology (continued)

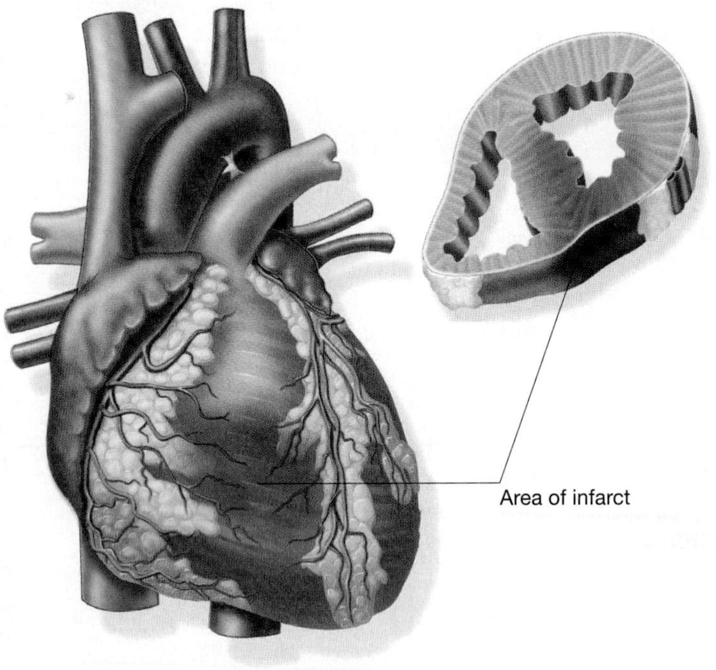

■ **Figure 5.15** External and cross-sectional view of an infarct caused by a myocardial infarction.

Term	Word Parts	Definition
myocarditis (my-oh-car-DYE-tis)	**myocardi/o** = heart muscle **-itis** = inflammation	Inflammation of the muscle layer of the heart wall.
pericarditis (pair-ih-car-DYE-tis)	peri- = around **cardi/o** = heart **-itis** = inflammation	Inflammation of the pericardial sac around the heart.
tetralogy of Fallot (teh-TRALL-oh-jee / fal-LOH)	tetra- = four **-logy** = study of	Combination of four congenital anomalies: pulmonary stenosis, an interventricular septal defect, improper placement of the aorta, and hypertrophy of the right ventricle. Needs immediate surgery to correct.
valvulitis (val-view-LYE-tis)	**valvul/o** = valve **-itis** = inflammation	The inflammation of a heart valve.
Blood Vessels		
aneurysm (AN-yoo-rizm)		Weakness in the wall of an artery resulting in localized widening of the artery. Although an aneurysm may develop in any artery, common sites include the aorta in the abdomen and the cerebral arteries in the brain. See Figure 5.16 ■.

Pathology (continued)

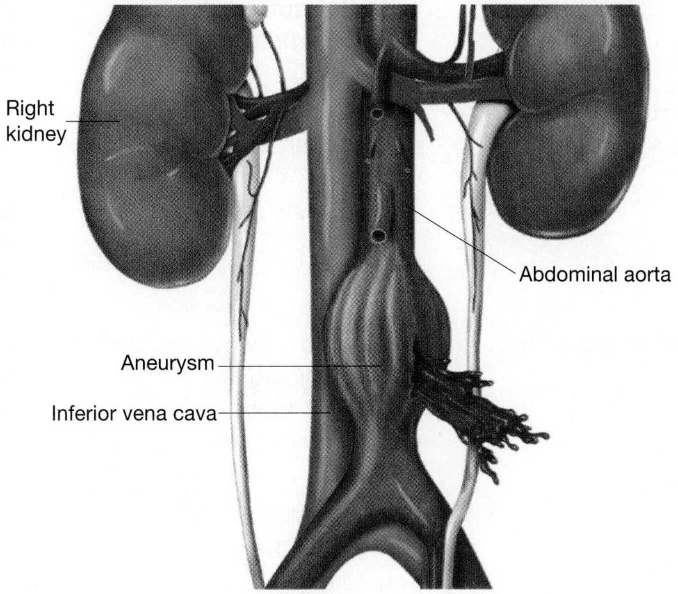

Term	Word Parts	Definition
Figure 5.16 Illustration of a large aneurysm in the abdominal aorta that has ruptured.		
arteriorrhexis (ar-tee-ree-oh-REK-sis)	arteri/o = artery -rrhexis = rupture	A ruptured artery; may occur if an aneurysm ruptures an arterial wall.
arteriosclerosis (ar-tee-ree-oh-skleh-ROH-sis)	arteri/o = artery -sclerosis = hardening	Thickening, hardening, and loss of elasticity of the walls of the arteries. Most often due to atherosclerosis.
atheroma (ath-er-OH-mah)	ather/o = fatty substance -oma = mass	A deposit of fatty substance in the wall of an artery that bulges into and narrows the lumen of the artery; a characteristic of atherosclerosis. Also called a *plaque*.
atherosclerosis (ath-er-oh-skleh-ROH-sis)	ather/o = fatty substance -sclerosis = hardening	The most common form of arteriosclerosis. Caused by the formation of yellowish plaques of cholesterol on the inner walls of arteries (see again Figures 5.13 and 5.14).
coarctation of the aorta (CoA) (koh-ark-TAY-shun)		Severe congenital narrowing of the aorta.
deep vein thrombosis (DVT) (THROM-boh-sis)	thromb/o = clot	The formation of a blood clot in a vein deep in the body, most commonly the legs. An embolus breaking off from this thrombosis would travel to the lungs and block blood flow through the lungs.
hemorrhoid (HEM-oh-royd)	hem/o = blood	Varicose veins in the anal region.
hypertension (HTN) (high-per-TEN-shun)	hyper- = excessive -tension = pressure	Blood pressure (BP) above the normal range. *Essential* or *primary hypertension* occurs directly from cardiovascular disease. *Secondary hypertension* refers to high blood pressure resulting from another disease such as kidney disease.

Pathology (continued)

Term	Word Parts	Definition
hypotension (high-poh-TEN-shun)	hypo- = insufficient -tension = pressure	Decrease in blood pressure (BP). Can occur in shock, infection, cancer, anemia, or as death approaches.
patent ductus arteriosus (PDA) (PAY-tent / DUCK-tus / ar-tee-ree-OH-sis)	duct/o = to bring arteri/o = artery	Congenital heart anomaly in which the fetal connection between the pulmonary artery and the aorta fails to close at birth. This condition may be treated with medication and resolve with time. However, in some cases surgery is required.
peripheral vascular disease (PVD)	peripher/o = away from center -al = pertaining to vascul/o = blood vessel -ar = pertaining to	Any abnormal condition affecting blood vessels outside the heart. Symptoms may include pain, pallor, numbness, and loss of circulation and pulses.
phlebitis (fleh-BYE-tis)	phleb/o = vein -itis = inflammation	The inflammation of a vein.
polyarteritis (pol-ee-ar-ter-EYE-tis)	poly- = many arteri/o = artery -itis = inflammation	Inflammation of several arteries.
Raynaud's phenomenon (ray-NOZ)		Periodic ischemic attacks affecting the extremities of the body, especially the fingers, toes, ears, and nose. The affected extremities become cyanotic and very painful. These attacks are brought on by arterial constriction due to extreme cold or emotional stress.
thrombophlebitis (throm-boh-fleh-BYE-tis)	thromb/o = clot phleb/o = vein -itis = inflammation	Inflammation of a vein resulting in the formation of blood clots within the vein.
varicose veins (VAIR-ih-kohs)	varic/o = dilated vein -ose = pertaining to	Swollen and distended veins, usually in the legs.

Practice As You Go

C. Terminology Matching

Match each term to its definition.

1. ________ arrhythmia
2. ________ thrombus
3. ________ bradycardia
4. ________ murmur
5. ________ phlebitis

a. swollen, distended veins
b. inflammation of vein
c. serious congenital anomaly
d. slow heart rate
e. cusps are too loose

6. ________ hypotension	f. irregular heartbeat
7. ________ varicose vein	g. an extra heart sound
8. ________ tetralogy of Fallot	h. clot in blood vessel
9. ________ valve prolapse	i. low blood pressure
10. ________ plaque	j. fatty deposit in artery

Diagnostic Procedures

Term	Word Parts	Definition
Medical Procedures		
auscultation (oss-kul-TAY-shun)		Process of listening to the sounds within the body by using a stethoscope.
sphygmomanometer (sfig-moh-mah-NOM-eh-ter)	sphygm/o = pulse -manometer = instrument to measure pressure	Instrument for measuring blood pressure (BP). Also referred to as a *blood pressure cuff.*
■ **Figure 5.17** Using a sphygmomanometer to measure blood pressure. *(Michal Heron, Pearson Education)*		
stethoscope (STETH-oh-scope)	steth/o = chest -scope = instrument for viewing	Instrument for listening to body sounds (auscultation), such as the chest, heart, or intestines.
Clinical Laboratory Tests		
cardiac enzymes (CAR-dee-ak / EN-zyms)	cardi/o = heart -ac = pertaining to	Blood test to determine the level of enzymes specific to heart muscles in the blood. An increase in the enzymes may indicate heart muscle damage such as a myocardial infarction. These enzymes include creatine phosphokinase (CPK), lactate dehydrogenase (LDH), and glutamic oxaloacetic transaminase (GOT).
serum lipoprotein level (SEE-rum / lip-oh-PROH-teen)	lip/o = fat	Blood test to measure the amount of cholesterol and triglycerides in the blood. An indicator of atherosclerosis risk.

Diagnostic Procedures (continued)

Term	Word Parts	Definition
Diagnostic Imaging		
angiogram (AN-jee-oh-gram)	angi/o = vessel -gram = record	X-ray record of a vessel taken during angiography.
angiography (an-jee-OG-rah-fee)	angi/o = vessel -graphy = process of recording	X-rays taken after the injection of an opaque material into a blood vessel. Can be performed on the aorta as an aortic angiography, on the heart as angiocardiography, and on the brain as a cerebral angiography.
cardiac scan	cardi/o = heart -ac = pertaining to	Patient is given radioactive thallium intravenously and then scanning equipment is used to visualize the heart. It is especially useful in determining myocardial damage.
Doppler ultrasonography (DOP-ler / ul-trah-son-OG-rah-fee)	ultra- = beyond son/o = sound -graphy = process of recording	Measurement of sound-wave echoes as they bounce off tissues and organs to produce an image. This procedure is used to measure velocity of blood moving through blood vessels to look for blood clots or deep vein thromboses.
echocardiography (ECHO) (ek-oh-car-dee-OG-rah-fee)	cardi/o = artery -graphy = process of recording	Noninvasive diagnostic procedure using ultrasound to visualize internal cardiac structures. Cardiac valve activity can be evaluated using this method.
Cardiac Function Tests		
catheter (KATH-eh-ter)		Flexible tube inserted into the body for the purpose of moving fluids into or out of the body. In the cardiovascular system a catheter is used to place dye into blood vessels so they may be visualized on X-rays.
cardiac catheterization (CC, cath) (CAR-dee-ak / cath-eh-ter-ih-ZAY-shun)	cardi/o = heart -ac = pertaining to	Passage of a thin-tube catheter through a blood vessel leading to the heart. Done to detect abnormalities, to collect cardiac blood samples, and to determine the blood pressure within the heart.
electrocardiogram (ECG, EKG) (ee-lek-tro-CAR-dee-oh-gram)	electr/o = electricity cardi/o = heart -gram = record	Hardcopy record produced by electrocardiography.
electrocardiography (ECG, EKG) (ee-lek-troh-car-dee-OG-rah-fee)	electr/o = electricity cardi/o = heart -graphy = process of recording	Process of recording the electrical activity of the heart. Useful in the diagnosis of abnormal cardiac rhythm and heart muscle (myocardium) damage.
Holter monitor		Portable ECG monitor worn by a patient for a period of a few hours to a few days to assess the heart and pulse activity as the person goes through the activities of daily living. Used to assess a patient who experiences chest pain and unusual heart activity during exercise and normal activities.

Diagnostic Procedures (continued)

Term	Word Parts	Definition
stress testing ■ **Figure 5.18** Man undergoing a stress test on a treadmill while physician monitors his condition. *(Jonathan Nourok/ PhotoEdit Inc.)*	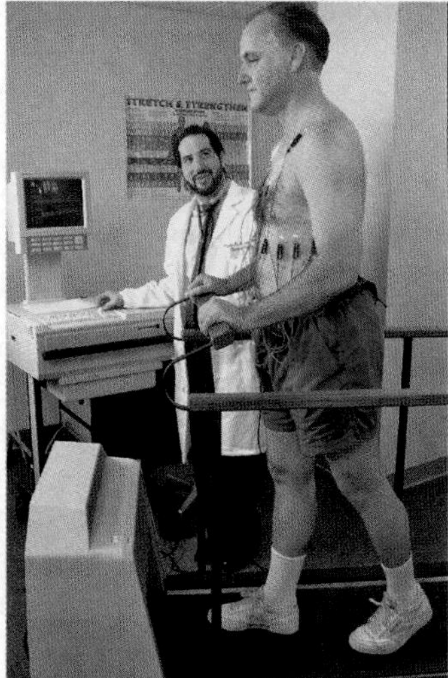	Method for evaluating cardiovascular fitness. The patient is placed on a treadmill or a bicycle and then subjected to steadily increasing levels of work. An EKG and oxygen levels are taken while the patient exercises. The test is stopped if abnormalities occur on the EKG. Also called an *exercise test* or a *treadmill test.*

Therapeutic Procedures

Term	Word Parts	Definition
Medical Procedures		
cardiopulmonary resuscitation (CPR) (car-dee-oh-PULL-mon-air-ee / ree-suss-ih-TAY-shun)	cardi/o = heart pulmon/o = lung -ary = pertaining to	Procedure to restore cardiac output and oxygenated air to the lungs for a person in cardiac arrest. A combination of chest compressions (to push blood out of the heart) and artificial respiration (to blow air into the lungs) is performed by one or two CPR-trained rescuers.
defibrillation (dee-fib-rih-LAY-shun)	de- = without	Procedure that converts serious irregular heartbeats, such as fibrillation, by giving electric shocks to the heart using an instrument called a defibrillator. Also called *cardioversion.* Automated external defibrillators (AED) are portable devices that automatically detect life-threatening arrhythmias and deliver the appropriate electrical shock. They are designed to be used by nonmedical personnel and are found in public places such as shopping malls and schools.

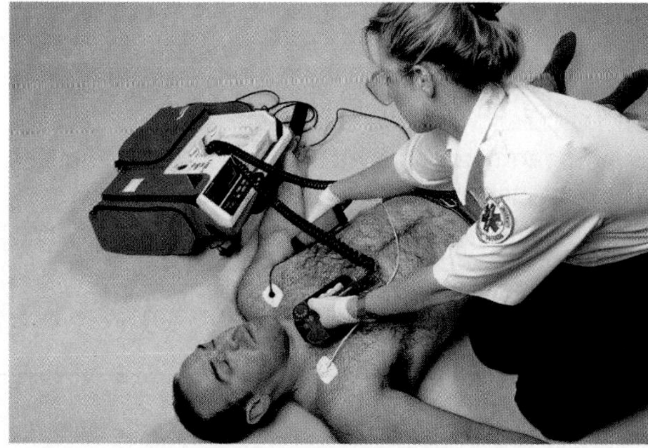

■ **Figure 5.19** An emergency medical technician positions defibrillator paddles on the chest of a supine male patient. *(Floyd Jackson, Pearson Education)*

Therapeutic Procedures (continued)

Term	Word Parts	Definition
extracorporeal circulation (ECC) (EX-tra-core-poor-EE-al)	extra- = outside of corpor/o = body -eal = pertaining to	During open-heart surgery, the routing of blood to a heart-lung machine so it can be oxygenated and pumped to the rest of the body.
implantable cardioverter-defibrillator (ICD) (CAR-dee-oh-ver-ter / de-FIB-rih-lay-tor)	cardi/o = heart de- = without	Device implanted in the heart that delivers an electrical shock to restore a normal heart rhythm. Particularly useful for persons who experience ventricular fibrillation.
pacemaker implantation		Electrical device that substitutes for the natural pacemaker of the heart. It controls the beating of the heart by a series of rhythmic electrical impulses. An external pacemaker has the electrodes on the outside of the body. An internal pacemaker has the electrodes surgically implanted within the chest wall. ■ **Figure 5.20** Color enhanced X-ray showing a pacemaker implanted in the left side of the chest and the electrode wires running to the heart muscle. *(UHB Trust/Getty Images)*
thrombolytic therapy (throm-boh-LIT-ik / THAIR-ah-pee)	thromb/o = clot -lytic = destruction	Process in which drugs, such as streptokinase (SK) or tissue plasminogen activator (tPA), are injected into a blood vessel to dissolve clots and restore blood flow.
Surgical Procedures		
aneurysmectomy (an-yoo-riz-MEK-toh-mee)	-ectomy = surgical removal	Surgical removal of the sac of an aneurysm.
arterial anastomosis (ar-TEE-ree-all / ah-nas-toe-MOE-sis)	arteri/o = artery -al = pertaining to	Surgical joining together of two arteries. Performed if an artery is severed or if a damaged section of an artery is removed.
atherectomy (ath-er-EK-toh-mee)	ather/o = fatty substance -ectomy = surgical removal	Surgical procedure to remove a deposit of fatty substance, an atheroma, from an artery.
coronary artery bypass graft (CABG) (KOR-ah-nair-ee)	coron/o = heart -ary = pertaining to	Open-heart surgery in which a blood vessel from another location in the body (often a leg vein) is grafted to route blood around a blocked coronary artery.
embolectomy (em-boh-LEK-toh-mee)	embol/o = plug -ectomy = surgical removal	Removal of an embolus or clot from a blood vessel.

Therapeutic Procedures (continued)

Term	Word Parts	Definition
endarterectomy (end-ar-teh-REK-toh-mee)	endo- = inner arteri/o = artery -ectomy = surgical removal	Removal of the diseased or damaged inner lining of an artery. Usually performed to remove atherosclerotic plaques.
heart transplantation		Replacement of a diseased or malfunctioning heart with a donor's heart.
intracoronary artery stent (in-trah-KOR-ah-nair-ee / AR-ter-ee)	intra- = within coron/o = heart -ary = pertaining to	Placement of a stent within a coronary artery to treat coronary ischemia due to atherosclerosis.
■ **Figure 5.21** The process of placing a stent in a blood vessel. A) A catheter is used to place a collapsed stent next to an atherosclerotic plaque; B) stent is expanded; C) catheter is removed, leaving the expanded stent behind.		
ligation and stripping (lye-GAY-shun)		Surgical treatment for varicose veins. The damaged vein is tied off (ligation) and removed (stripping).
percutaneous transluminal coronary angioplasty (PTCA) (per-kyoo-TAY-nee-us / trans-LOO-mih-nal / KOR-ah-nair-ee / AN-jee-oh-plas-tee)	per- = through cutane/o = skin -ous = pertaining to trans- = across -al = pertaining to angi/o = vessel -plasty = surgical repair	Method for treating localized coronary artery narrowing. A balloon catheter is inserted through the skin into the coronary artery and inflated to dilate the narrow blood vessel.
■ **Figure 5.22** Balloon angioplasty: A) deflated balloon catheter is approaching an atherosclerotic plaque; B) plaque is compressed by inflated balloon; C) plaque remains compressed after balloon catheter is removed.		

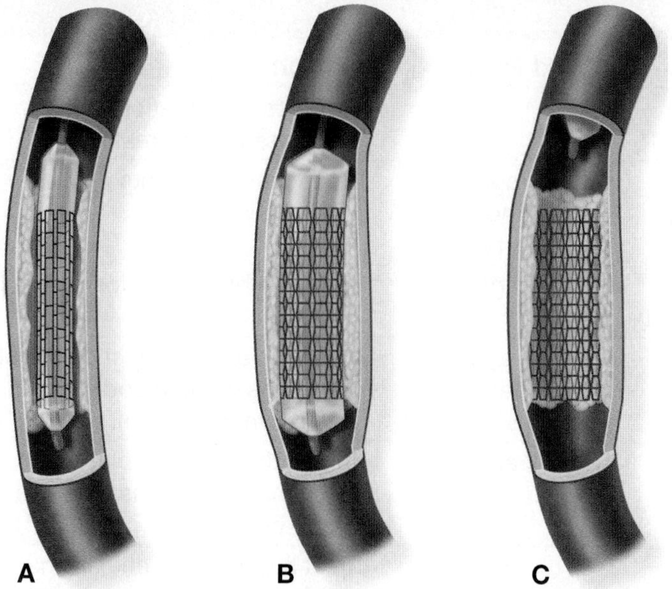

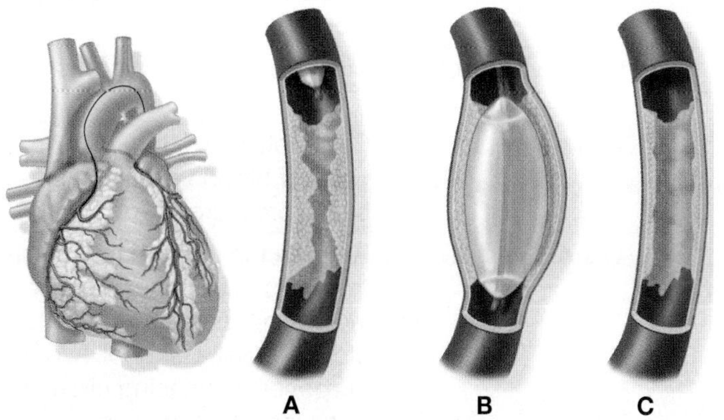

Therapeutic Procedures (continued)

Term	Word Parts	Definition
stent		Stainless steel tube placed within a blood vessel or a duct to widen the lumen (see again Figure 5.21 ■).
valve replacement		Removal of a diseased heart valve and replacement with an artificial valve.
valvoplasty (VAL-voh-plas-tee)	valv/o = valve -plasty = surgical repair	Surgical procedure to repair a heart valve.

Pharmacology

Classification	Word Parts	Action	Examples
ACE inhibitor drugs		Produce vasodilation and decrease blood pressure.	benazepril, Lotensin; catopril, Capoten
antiarrhythmic (an-tye-a-RHYTH-mik)	anti- = against a- = without -ic = pertaining to	Reduces or prevents cardiac arrhythmias.	flecainide, Tambocor; ibutilide, Corvert
anticoagulant (an-tye-koh-AG-you-lant)	anti- = against	Prevents blood clot formation.	heparin; warfarin, Coumadin
antilipidemic (an-tye-lip-ih-DEM-ik)	anti- = against lip/o = fat -ic = pertaining to	Reduces amount of cholesterol and lipids in the bloodstream; treats hyperlipidemia.	atorvastatin, Lipitor; simvastatin, Zocor
antiplatelet agents	anti- = against	Inhibit the ability of platelets to clump together as part of a blood clot.	clopidogrel, Plavix; aspirin; ticlopidine, Ticlid
beta-blocker drugs		Treat hypertension and angina pectoris by lowering the heart rate.	metoprolol, Lopressor; propranolol, Inderal
calcium channel blocker drugs		Treat hypertension, angina pectoris, and congestive heart failure by causing the heart to beat less forcefully and less often.	diltiazem, Cardizem; nifedipine, Procardia
cardiotonic (card-ee-oh-TAHN-ik)	cardi/o = heart -tonic = pertaining to tone	Increases the force of cardiac muscle contraction; treats congestive heart failure.	digoxin, Lanoxin
diuretic (dye-you-RET-ik)	-tic = pertaining to	Increases urine production by the kidneys, which works to reduce plasma and therefore blood volume, resulting in lower blood pressure.	furosemide, Lasix
thrombolytic (throm-boh-LIT-ik)	thromb/o = clot -lytic = destruction	Dissolves existing blood clots.	tissue plasminogen activator (tPA); alteplase, Activase
vasoconstrictor (vaz-oh-kon-STRICK-tor)	vas/o = vessel	Contracts smooth muscle in walls of blood vessels; raises blood pressure.	metaraminol, Aramine
vasodilator (vaz-oh-DYE-late-or)	vas/o = vessel	Relaxes the smooth muscle in the walls of arteries, thereby increasing diameter of the blood vessel. Used for two main purposes: increasing circulation to an ischemic area and reducing blood pressure.	nitroglycerine, Nitro-Dur; isoxsuprine, Vasodilan

Practice As You Go

D. Procedure Matching

Match each procedure to its definition.

1. ________ cardiac enzymes
2. ________ Doppler ultrasound
3. ________ Holter monitor
4. ________ cardiac scan
5. ________ stress testing
6. ________ echocardiography
7. ________ extracorporeal circulation
8. ________ ligation and stripping
9. ________ thrombolytic therapy
10. ________ PTAC

a. visualizes heart after patient is given radioactive thallium
b. uses ultrasound to visualize heart beating
c. blood test that indicates heart muscle damage
d. uses treadmill to evaluate cardiac fitness
e. removes varicose veins
f. clot-dissolving drugs
g. measures velocity of blood moving through blood vessels
h. balloon angioplasty
i. use of a heart-lung machine
j. portable EKG monitor

Abbreviations

AED	automated external defibrillator	**CP**	chest pain
AF	atrial fibrillation	**CPR**	cardiopulmonary resuscitation
AMI	acute myocardial infarction	**CSD**	congenital septal defect
AS	arteriosclerosis	**CV**	cardiovascular
ASD	atrial septal defect	**DVT**	deep vein thrombosis
ASHD	arteriosclerotic heart disease	**ECC**	extracorporeal circulation
AV, A-V	atrioventricular	**ECG, EKG**	electrocardiogram
BBB	bundle branch block (L for left; R for right)	**ECHO**	echocardiogram
BP	blood pressure	**GOT**	glutamic oxaloacetic transaminase
bpm	beats per minute	**HTN**	hypertension
CABG	coronary artery bypass graft	**ICD**	implantable cardioverter-defibrillator
CAD	coronary artery disease	**ICU**	intensive care unit
cath	catheterization	**IV**	intravenous
CC	cardiac catheterization, chief complaint	**LVH**	left ventricular hypertrophy
CCU	coronary care unit	**MI**	myocardial infarction, mitral insufficiency
CHF	congestive heart failure	**mm Hg**	millimeters of mercury
CoA	coarctation of the aorta	**MR**	mitral regurgitation

Abbreviations (continued)

MS	mitral stenosis **Word Watch** Be careful using the abbreviation *MS*, which can mean either "mitral stenosis" or "multiple sclerosis."	**S1** **S2**	first heart sound second heart sound
MVP	mitral valve prolapse	**SA, S-A**	sinoatrial
P	pulse	**SK**	streptokinase
PAC	premature atrial contraction	**tPA**	tissue plasminogen activator
PDA	patent ductus arteriosus	**V fib**	ventricular fibrillation
PTCA	percutaneous transluminal coronary angioplasty	**VSD**	ventricular septal defect
PVC	premature ventricular contraction	**VT**	ventricular tachycardia

Practice As You Go

E. What's the Abbreviation?

1. mitral valve prolapse ______________________________
2. ventricular septal defect ______________________________
3. percutaneous transluminal coronary angioplasty ______________________________
4. ventricular fibrillation ______________________________
5. deep vein thrombosis ______________________________
6. lactate dehydrogenase ______________________________
7. coarctation of the aorta ______________________________
8. tissue plasminogen activator ______________________________
9. cardiovascular ______________________________
10. extracorporeal circulation ______________________________

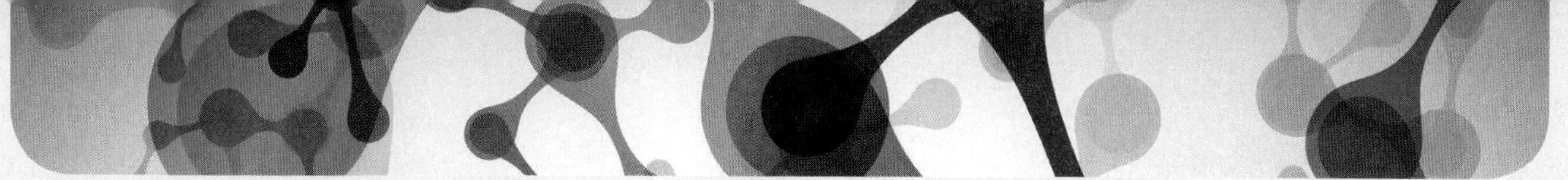

Chapter Review

Real-World Applications

Medical Record Analysis

This Discharge Summary contains 12 medical terms. Underline each term and write it in the list below the report. Then define each term.

Date: 6/1/2015

Patient: Jorge Johnson

Patient complaint: Severe pain in the right ankle with any movement of lower limb.

Discharge Summary

Admitting Diagnosis:	Difficulty breathing, hypertension, tachycardia
Final Diagnosis:	CHF secondary to mitral valve prolapse
History of Present Illness:	Patient was brought to the Emergency Room by her family because of difficulty breathing and palpitations. Patient reports that she has experienced these symptoms for the past six months, but this episode is more severe than any previous. Upon admission in the ER, heart rate was 120 beats per minute and blood pressure was 180/110. The results of an EKG and cardiac enzyme blood tests were normal. She was admitted for a complete workup for tachycardia and hypertension.
Summary of Hospital Course:	Patient underwent a full battery of diagnostic tests. A prolapsed mitral valve was observed by echocardiography. A stress test had to be stopped early due to onset of severe difficulty in breathing. Angiocardiography failed to demonstrate significant CAD. Blood pressure and tachycardia were controlled with medications. At discharge, HR was 88 beats per minute and blood pressure was 165/98.
Discharge Plans:	There was no evidence of a myocardial infarction or significant CAD. Patient was placed on a low-salt and low-cholesterol diet. She received instructions on beginning a carefully graded exercise program. She is to continue her medications. If symptoms are not controlled by these measures, a mitral valve replacement will be considered.

	Term	Definition
1.	______________	______________
2.	______________	______________
3.	______________	______________
4.	______________	______________
5.	______________	______________
6.	______________	______________
7.	______________	______________
8.	______________	______________
9.	______________	______________
10.	______________	______________
11.	______________	______________
12.	______________	______________

Chart Note Transcription

The chart note below contains 11 phrases that can be reworded with a medical term that you learned in this chapter. Each phrase is identified with an underline. Determine the medical term and write your answers in the space provided.

Pearson General Hospital Coronary Care Unit

Task Edit View Time Scale Options Help Download Archive Date: 17 May 2015

Current Complaint:	A 56-year-old male was admitted to the Cardiac Care Unit from the Emergency Room with left arm pain, severe pain around the heart, **1** an abnormally slow heartbeat, **2** nausea, and vomiting.
Past History:	Patient reports no heart problems prior to this episode. He has taken medication for high blood pressure **3** for the past five years. His family history is significant for a father and brother who both died in their 50s from death of heart muscle. **4**
Signs and Symptoms:	Patient reports severe pain around the heart that radiates into his left jaw and arm. A record of the heart's electrical activity **5** and a blood test to determine the amount of heart damage **6** were abnormal.
Diagnosis:	An acute death of heart muscle **4** resulting from insufficient blood flow to heart muscle due to obstruction of coronary artery. **7**
Treatment:	First, provide supportive care during the acute phase. Second, evaluate heart damage by passing a thin tube through a blood vessel into the heart to detect abnormalities **8** and evaluate heart fitness by having patient exercise on a treadmill. **9** Finally, perform surgical intervention by either inflating a balloon catheter to dilate a narrow vessel **10** or by open heart surgery to create a shunt around a blocked vessel. **11**

1. ____________________
2. ____________________
3. ____________________
4. ____________________
5. ____________________
6. ____________________
7. ____________________
8. ____________________
9. ____________________
10. ____________________
11. ____________________

Case Study

Below is a case study presentation of a patient with a condition covered by this chapter. Read the case study and answer the questions below. Some questions will ask for information not included within this chapter. Use your text, a medical dictionary, or any other reference material you choose to answer these questions.

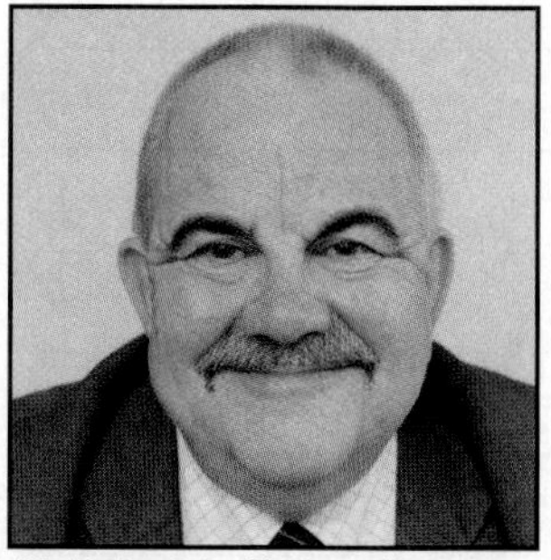

(Christopher Oates/Shutterstock)

Mr. Thomas is a 62-year-old man who has been diagnosed with an acute myocardial infarction with the following symptoms and history. His chief complaint is a persistent, crushing chest pain that radiates to his left arm, jaw, neck, and shoulder blade. He describes the pain, which he has had for the past 12 hours, as a "squeezing" sensation around his heart. He has also suffered nausea, dyspnea, and diaphoresis. He has a low-grade temperature and his blood pressure is within a normal range at 130/82. He states that he smokes two packs of cigarettes a day, is overweight by 50 pounds, and has a family history of hypertension and coronary artery disease. He leads a relatively sedentary lifestyle.

Questions

1. What is the common name for Mr. Thomas's acute condition? Look this condition up in a reference source and include a short description of it.

 ____

 ____

2. What do you think the phrase "chief complaint" means?

 ____

 ____

3. What is the medical term for this patient's chief complaint? Define this term.

 ____

 ____

4. List and define each of the patient's additional symptoms in your own words. (These terms appear in other chapters of the book or use a medical dictionary.)

 ____

 ____

5. Using your text as a resource, name and describe three diagnostic tests that may be performed to determine the extent of the patient's heart damage.

 ____

 ____

6. What risk factors for developing heart disease does Mr. Thomas have? What changes should he make?

 ____

 ____

Practice Exercises

A. Word Building Practice

The combining form **cardi/o** refers to the heart. Use it to write a term that means:

1. pertaining to the heart ______________________
2. disease of the heart muscle ______________________
3. enlargement of the heart ______________________
4. fast heart condition ______________________
5. slow heart condition ______________________
6. record of heart electricity ______________________

The combining form **angi/o** refers to the vessel. Use it to write a term that means:

7. vessel narrowing ______________________
8. vessel inflammation ______________________
9. involuntary muscle contraction of a vessel ______________________

The combining form **arteri/o** refers to the artery. Use it to write a term that means:

10. pertaining to an artery ______________________
11. hardening of an artery ______________________
12. small artery ______________________

Add the appropriate prefix to **carditis** to form the term that matches each definition:

13. inflammation of the inner lining of the heart ______________________
14. inflammation of the outer layer of the heart ______________________
15. inflammation of the muscle of the heart ______________________

B. Define the Combining Form

	Definition	Example from Chapter
1. **cardi/o**		
2. **valvul/o**		
3. **steth/o**		
4. **arteri/o**		
5. **phleb/o**		
6. **angi/o**		
7. **ventricul/o**		
8. **thromb/o**		
9. **atri/o**		
10. **ather/o**		

C. Name That Term

1. pertaining to a vein ____________________
2. study of the heart ____________________
3. record of a vein ____________________
4. process of recording electrical activity of the heart ____________________
5. high blood pressure ____________________
6. low blood pressure ____________________
7. surgical repair of valve ____________________
8. pertaining to between ventricles ____________________
9. removal of fatty substance ____________________
10. narrowing of the arteries ____________________

D. Name That Suffix

	Suffix	Example from Chapter
1. pressure		
2. abnormal narrowing		
3. instrument to measure pressure		
4. small		
5. hardening		

E. What Does it Stand For?

1. BP ______
2. CHF ______
3. MI ______
4. CCU ______
5. PVC ______
6. CPR ______
7. CAD ______
8. CP ______
9. EKG ______
10. S1 ______

F. Define the Term

1. catheter ______
2. infarct ______
3. thrombus ______
4. palpitation ______
5. regurgitation ______
6. aneurysm ______
7. cardiac arrest ______
8. fibrillation ______
9. myocardial infarction ______
10. hemorrhoid ______

G. Fill in the Blank

angiography	murmur	varicose veins	echocardiogram
pacemaker	CHF	defibrillation	angina pectoris
Holter monitor	hypertension	MI	CCU

1. Tiffany was born with a congenital condition resulting in an abnormal heart sound called a(n) ______.
2. Joseph suffered an arrhythmia resulting in cardiac arrest. The emergency team used an instrument to give electric shocks to the heart to create a normal heart rhythm. This procedure is called ______.
3. Marguerite has been placed on a low-sodium diet and medication to bring her blood pressure down to a normal range. She suffers from ______.

4. Tony has had an artificial device called a(n) ______________________ inserted to control the beating of his heart by producing rhythmic electrical impulses.

5. Derrick's physician determined that he had ______________________ after examining his legs and finding swollen, tortuous veins.

6. Laura has persistent chest pains that require medication. The term for the pain is ______________________.

7. La Tonya will be admitted to what hospital unit after surgery to correct her heart condition? ______________________.

8. Stephen is going to have a coronary artery bypass graft to correct the blockage in his coronary arteries. He recently suffered a heart attack as a result of this occlusion. His attack is called a(n) ______________________.

9. Stephen's physician scheduled a(n) ______________, an X-ray to determine the extent of his blood vessel damage.

10. Maria is scheduled to have a diagnostic procedure that uses ultrasound to produce an image of the heart valves is going to have a(n) ______________________.

11. Eric must wear a device for 24 hours that will keep track of his heart activity as he performs his normal daily routine. This device is called a(n) ______________________.

12. Lydia is 82 years old and is suffering from a heart condition that causes weakness, edema, and breathlessness. Her heart failure is the cause of her lung congestion. This condition is called ______________________.

H. Pharmacology Challenge

Fill in the classification for each drug description, then match the brand name.

	Drug Description	Classification	Brand Name
1.	________ prevents arrhythmia	______________	a. tPA
2.	________ reduces cholesterol	______________	b. Coumadin
3.	________ increases force of heart contraction	______________	c. Cardizem
4.	________ increases urine production	______________	d. Nitro-Dur
5.	________ prevents blood clots	______________	e. Tambocor
6.	________ dissolves blood clots	______________	f. Lanoxin
7.	________ relaxes smooth muscle in artery wall	______________	g. Lipitor
8.	________ cause heart to beat less forcefully	______________	h. Lasix

MyMedicalTerminologyLab™

MyMedicalTerminologyLab is a premium online homework management system that includes a host of features to help you study. Registered users will find:

- Learning activities and homework assignments
- Fun games and activities built within a virtual hospital
- Powerful tools that track and analyze your results—allowing you to create a personalized learning experience
- Videos, flashcards, and audio pronunciations to help enrich your progress
- Streaming lesson presentations and self-paced learning modules
- A space where you and your instructors can view and manage your assignments

Labeling Exercise

Image A

Write the labels for this figure on the numbered lines provided.

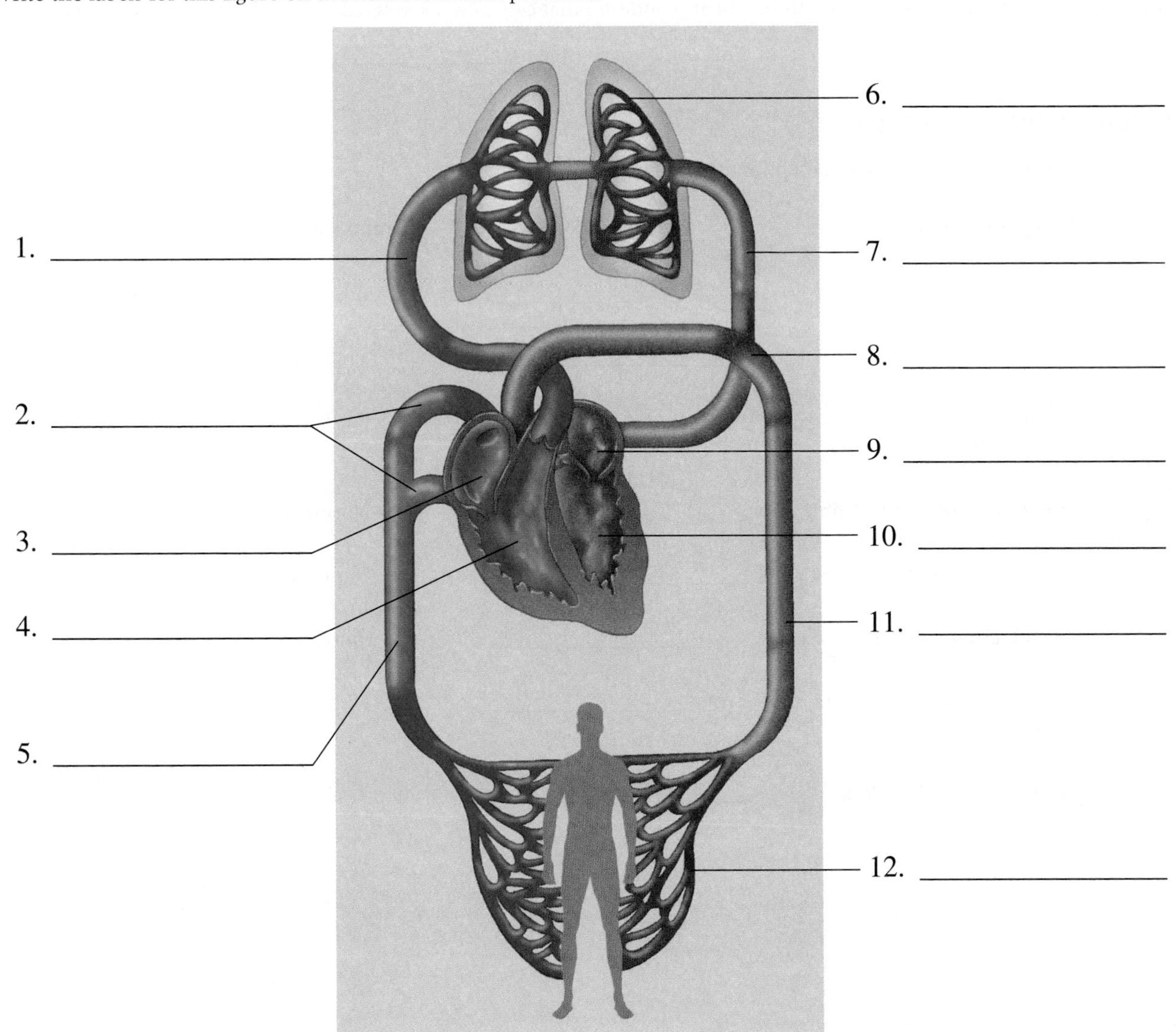

Image B

Write the labels for this figure on the numbered lines provided.

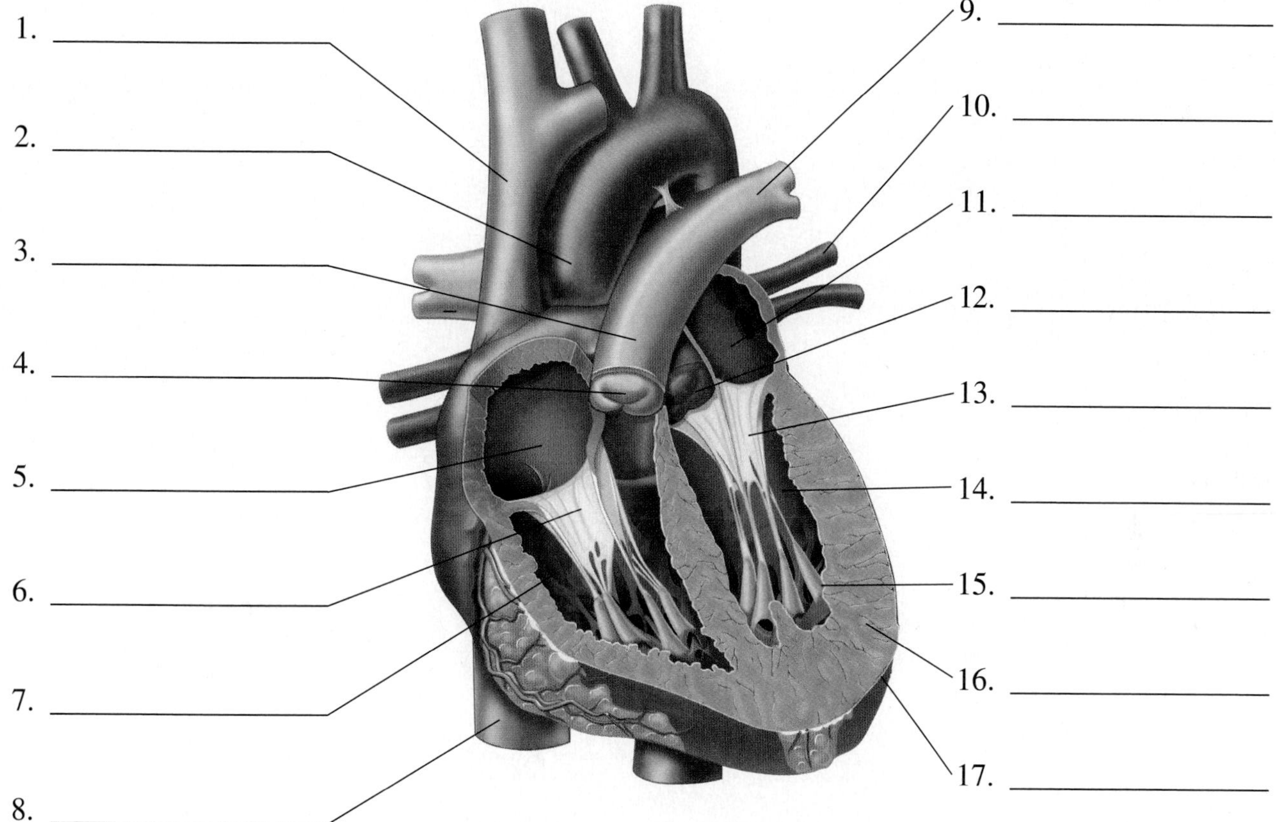

6

Blood and the Lymphatic and Immune Systems

Learning Objectives

Upon completion of this chapter, you will be able to

- Identify and define the combining forms and suffixes introduced in this chapter.
- Gain the ability to pronounce medical terms and major anatomical structures.
- List the major components, structures, and organs of the blood and lymphatic and immune systems and their functions.
- Describe the blood typing systems.
- Discuss immunity, the immune response, and standard precautions.
- Identify and define blood and lymphatic and immune system anatomical terms.
- Identify and define selected blood and lymphatic and immune system pathology terms.
- Identify and define selected blood and lymphatic and immune system diagnostic procedures.
- Identify and define selected blood and lymphatic and immune system therapeutic procedures.
- Identify and define selected medications associated with blood and the lymphatic and immune systems.
- Define selected abbreviations associated with blood and the lymphatic and immune systems.

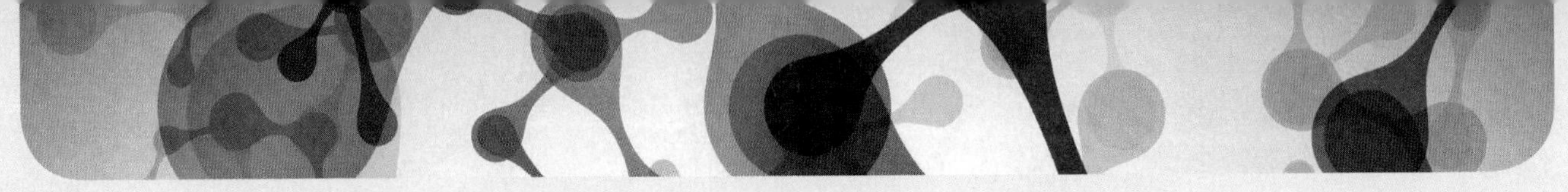

Section I: Blood at a Glance

Function

Blood transports gases, nutrients, and wastes to all areas of the body either attached to red blood cells or dissolved in the plasma. White blood cells fight infection and disease, and platelets initiate the blood clotting process.

Organs

Here are the primary components that comprise blood:

formed elements

- **erythrocytes**
- **leukocytes**
- **platelets**

plasma

Word Parts

Here are the most common word parts (with their meanings) used to build blood terms. For a more comprehensive list, refer to the Terminology section of this chapter.

Combining Forms

agglutin/o	clumping
bas/o	base
chrom/o	color
coagul/o	clotting
eosin/o	rosy red
fibrin/o	fibers
fus/o	pouring
granul/o	granules
hem/o	blood
hemat/o	blood
morph/o	shape
neutr/o	neutral
phag/o	eat, swallow
sanguin/o	blood
septic/o	infection

Suffixes

-apheresis	removal, carry away
-crit	separation of
-cytic	pertaining to cells
-cytosis	more than the normal number of cells
-emia	blood condition
-globin	protein
-penia	abnormal decrease, too few
-phil	attracted to
-philia	condition of being attracted to
-philic	pertaining to being attracted to
-plastic	pertaining to formation
-plastin	formation
-poiesis	formation
-rrhagic	pertaining to abnormal flow
-stasis	standing still

Blood Illustrated

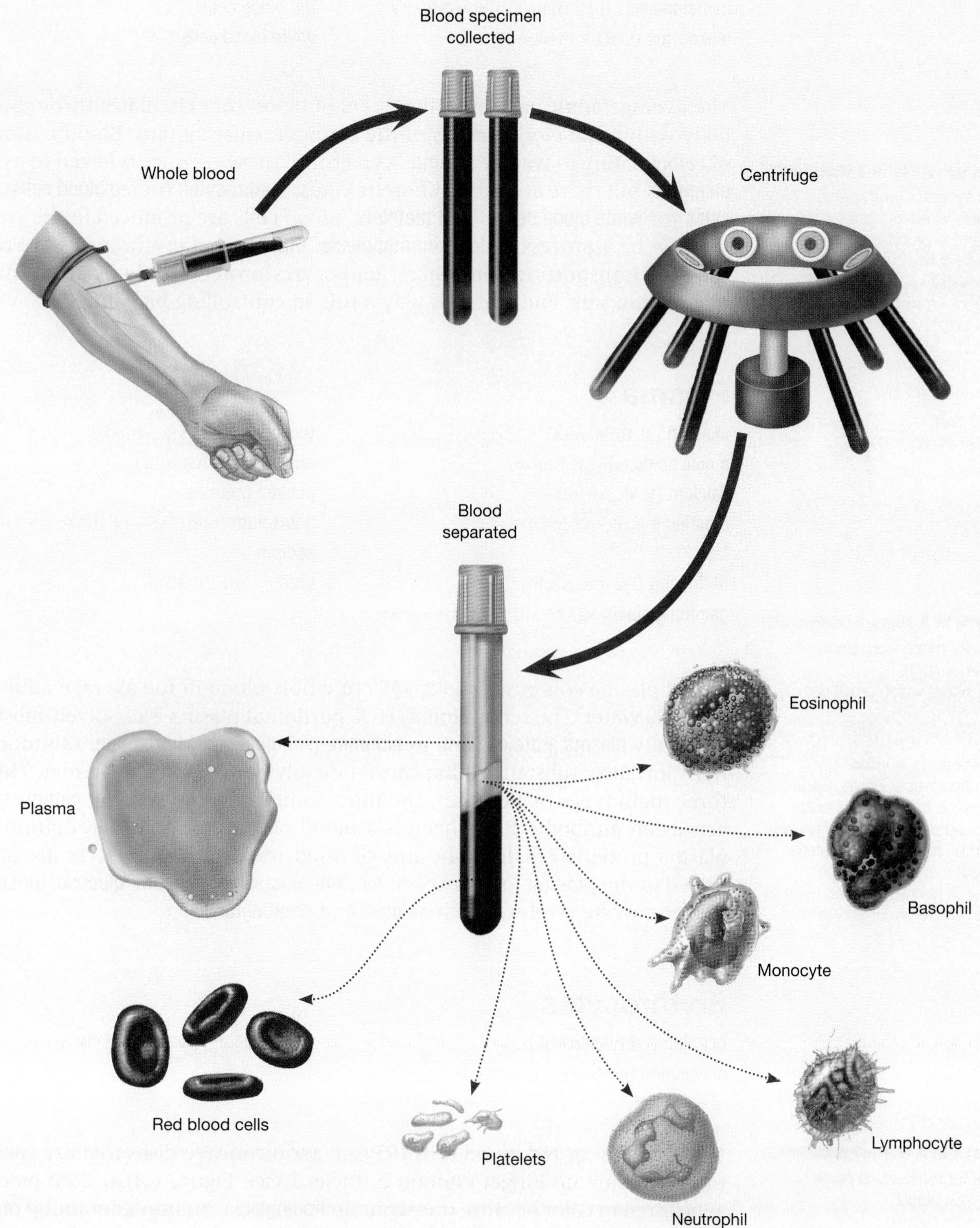

Anatomy and Physiology of Blood

erythrocytes (eh-RITH-roh-sights)
formed elements
hematopoiesis (hee-mah-toh-poy-EE-sis)
leukocytes (LOO-koh-sights)
plasma (PLAZ-mah)
platelets (PLAYT-lets)
red blood cells
white blood cells

What's In A Name?
Look for these word parts:
erythr/o = red
hemat/o = blood
leuk/o = white
-cyte = cell
-poiesis = formation

The average adult has about five liters of blood that circulates throughout the body within the blood vessels of the cardiovascular system. Blood is a mixture of cells floating in watery **plasma**. As a group, these cells are referred to as **formed elements**, but there are three different kinds: **erythrocytes** (or **red blood cells**), **leukocytes** (or **white blood cells**), and **platelets**. Blood cells are produced in the red bone marrow by a process called **hematopoiesis**. Plasma and erythrocytes are responsible for transporting substances, leukocytes protect the body from invading microorganisms, and platelets play a role in controlling bleeding.

Plasma

albumin (al-BEW-min)
amino acids (ah-MEE-noh)
calcium (KAL-see-um)
creatinine (kree-AT-in-in)
fats
fibrinogen (fye-BRIN-oh-jen)
gamma globulin (GAM-ah / GLOB-yoo-lin)
globulins (GLOB-yew-lenz)
glucose (GLOO-kohs)
plasma proteins
potassium (poh-TASS-ee-um)
sodium
urea (yoo-REE-ah)

What's In A Name?
Look for these word parts:
fibrin/o = fibers
-gen = that which produces

Word Watch
Plasma and *serum* are not interchangeable words. Serum is plasma, but with fibrinogen removed or inactivated. This way it can be handled and tested without it clotting. The term *serum* is also sometimes used to mean antiserum or antitoxin.

Liquid plasma composes about 55% of whole blood in the average adult and is 90–92% water. The remaining 8–10% portion of plasma is dissolved substances, especially **plasma proteins** such as **albumin**, **globulins**, and **fibrinogen**. Albumin helps transport fatty substances that cannot dissolve in the watery plasma. There are three main types of globulins; the most commonly known one, **gamma globulin**, acts as an antibody. Fibrinogen is a blood-clotting protein. In addition to the plasma proteins, smaller amounts of other important substances are also dissolved in the plasma for transport: **calcium**, **potassium**, **sodium**, **glucose**, **amino acids**, **fats**, and waste products such as **urea** and **creatinine**.

Erythrocytes

bilirubin (bil-ly-ROO-bin)
enucleated (ee-NEW-klee-ate-ed)
hemoglobin (hee-moh-GLOH-bin)

What's In A Name?
Look for these word parts:
hem/o = blood
-globin = protein

Erythrocytes, or red blood cells (RBCs), are biconcave disks that are **enucleated**, meaning they no longer contain a nucleus (see Figure 6.1 ■). Red blood cells appear red in color because they contain **hemoglobin**, an iron-containing pigment. Hemoglobin is the part of the red blood cell that picks up oxygen from the lungs and delivers it to the tissues of the body.

There are about five million erythrocytes per cubic millimeter of blood. The total number in an average-sized adult is 35 trillion, with males having more red blood cells than females. Erythrocytes have an average lifespan of 120 days,

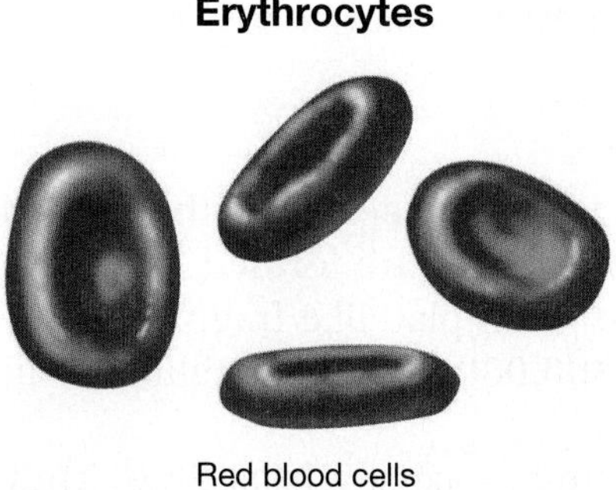

■ **Figure 6.1** The biconcave disk shape of erythrocytes (red blood cells).

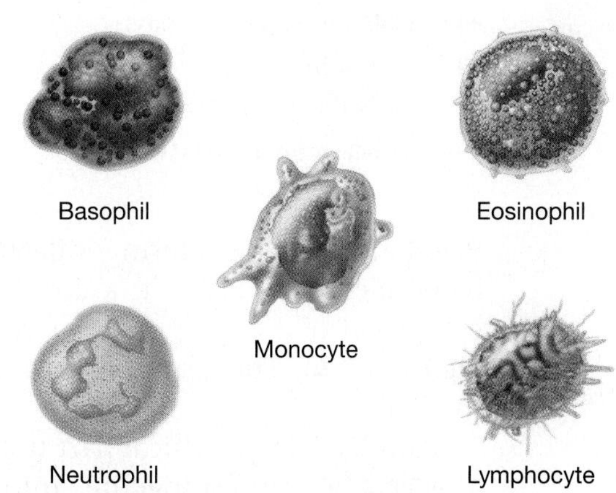

■ **Figure 6.2** The five different types of leukocytes (white blood cells).

and then the spleen removes the wornout and damaged ones from circulation. Much of the red blood cell, such as the iron, can be reused, but one portion, **bilirubin**, is a waste product disposed of by the liver.

Leukocytes

agranulocytes (ah-GRAN-yew-loh-sights)
granulocytes (GRAN-yew-loh-sights)
pathogens (PATH-oh-ginz)

Leukocytes, also referred to as white blood cells (WBCs), provide protection against the invasion of **pathogens** such as bacteria, viruses, and other foreign material. In general, white blood cells have a spherical shape with a large nucleus, and there are about 8,000 per cubic millimeter of blood (see Figure 6.2 ■). There are five different types of white blood cells, each with its own strategy for protecting the body. The five can be subdivided into two categories: **granulocytes** (with granules in the cytoplasm) and **agranulocytes** (without granules in the cytoplasm). The name and function of each type is presented in Table 6.1 ■.

Table 6.1 Leukocyte Classification

Leukocyte	Function
Granulocytes	
Basophils (basos) (BAY-soh-fillz)	Release histamine and heparin to damaged tissues
Eosinophils (eosins, eos) (ee-oh-SIN-oh-fillz)	Destroy parasites and increase during allergic reactions
Neutrophils (NOO-troh-fillz)	Engulfs foreign and damaged cells (phagocytosis); most numerous of the leukocytes
Agranulocytes	
Monocytes (monos) (MON-oh-sights)	Engulfs foreign and damaged cells (phagocytosis)
Lymphocytes (lymphs) (LIM-foh-sights)	Plays several different roles in immune response

Med Term Tip

Your body makes about two million erythrocytes every second. Of course, it must then destroy two million every second to maintain a relatively constant 30 trillion red blood cells.

What's In A Name?

Look for these word parts:
bas/o = base
eosin/o = rosy red
granul/o = granules
lymph/o = lymph
neutr/o = neutral
path/o = disease
-cyte = cell
-gen = that which produces
-phil = attracted to
a- = without
mono- = one

Med Term Tip

A *phagocyte* is a cell that has the ability to ingest (**phag/o** = eat; **-cyte** = cell) and digest bacteria and other foreign particles. This process, *phagocytosis*, is critical for the control of bacteria within the body.

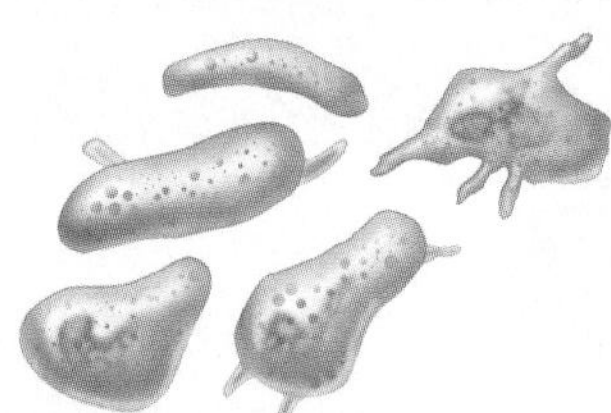

■ **Figure 6.3** Platelet structure.

What's In A Name?

Look for these word parts:
agglutin/o = clumping
hem/o = blood
thromb/o = clot
-cyte = cell
-plastin = formation
-stasis = standing still
pro- = before

Platelets

agglutinate (ah-GLOO-tih-nayt)
fibrin (FYE-brin)
hemostasis (hee-moh-STAY-sis)
prothrombin (proh-THROM-bin)
thrombin (THROM-bin)
thrombocyte (THROM-boh-sight)
thromboplastin (throm-boh-PLAS-tin)

Platelet, the modern term for **thrombocyte**, refers to the smallest of all the formed blood elements. Platelets are not whole cells, but rather are formed when the cytoplasm of a large precursor cell shatters into small platelike fragments (see Figure 6.3 ■). There are between 200,000 and 300,000 per cubic millimeter in the body.

Platelets play a critical part in the blood-clotting process or **hemostasis**. They **agglutinate** or clump together into small clusters when a blood vessel is cut or damaged. Platelets also release a substance called **thromboplastin**, which, in the presence of calcium, reacts with **prothrombin** (a clotting protein in the blood) to form **thrombin**. Then thrombin, in turn, works to convert fibrinogen to **fibrin**, which eventually becomes the meshlike blood clot.

Blood Typing

ABO system
blood typing
Rh factor

Each person's blood is different due to the presence of antigens or markers on the surface of erythrocytes. Before a person receives a blood transfusion, it is important to do **blood typing**. This laboratory test determines if the donated blood is compatible with the recipient's blood. There are many different subgroups of blood markers, but the two most important ones are the **ABO system** and **Rh factor**.

ABO System

type A
type AB
type B
type O
universal donor
universal recipient

In the ABO blood system there are two possible red blood cell markers, A and B. A marker is one method by which cells identify themselves. A person with an A marker is said to have **type A** blood. Type A blood produces anti-B antibodies that will attack type B blood. The presence of a B marker gives **type B** blood and anti-A antibodies (that will attack type A blood). If both markers are present, the blood is **type AB** and does not contain any antibodies. Therefore, type AB blood will not attack any other blood type. The absence of either an A or a B marker results in **type O** blood, which contains both anti-A and anti-B antibodies. Type O blood will attack all other blood types (A, B, and AB). For further information on antibodies, refer to the lymphatic section later in this chapter.

Because type O blood does not have either marker A or B, it will not react with anti-A or anti-B antibodies. For this reason, a person with type O blood is referred to as a **universal donor**. In extreme cases, type O blood may be given to a person with any of the other blood types. Similarly, type AB blood is the **universal recipient**. A person with type AB blood has no antibodies against the other blood types and, therefore, in extreme cases, can receive any type of blood.

Rh Factor

Rh-negative **Rh-positive**

Rh factor is not as difficult to understand as the ABO system. A person with the Rh factor on his or her red blood cells is said to be **Rh-positive** (Rh+). Since this person has the factor, he or she will not make anti-Rh antibodies. A person without the Rh factor is **Rh-negative** (Rh−) and will produce anti-Rh antibodies. Therefore, an Rh+ person may receive both an Rh+ and an Rh− transfusion, but an Rh− person can receive only Rh− blood.

Practice As You Go

A. Complete the Statement

1. The study of the blood is called ____________________.
2. The process whereby cells ingest and destroy bacteria within the body is ____________________.
3. The formed elements of blood are the ____________________, ____________________, and ____________________.
4. The fluid portion of blood is called ____________________.
5. The medical term for blood clotting is ____________________.

Terminology

Word Parts Used to Build Blood Terms

The following lists contain the combining forms, suffixes, and prefixes used to build terms in the remaining sections of this chapter.

Combining Forms

bas/o	base
chrom/o	color
coagul/o	clotting
cyt/o	cell
eosin/o	rosy red
erythr/o	red
fibrin/o	fibers

fus/o	pouring
hem/o	blood
hemat/o	blood
leuk/o	white
lip/o	fat
lymph/o	lymph
morph/o	shape

neutr/o	neutral
phleb/o	vein
sanguin/o	blood
septic/o	infection
thromb/o	clot

Suffixes

-apheresis	removal, carry away
-crit	separation of
-cyte	cell
-cytic	pertaining to cells

-cytosis	more than the normal number of cells
-emia	blood condition
-globin	protein

-ia	condition
-ic	pertaining to
-ion	action
-logy	study of

Suffixes (continued)

-lytic	destruction
-oma	mass
-otomy	cutting into
-ous	pertaining to
-penia	too few

-phil	attracted to
-philia	condition of being attracted to
-philic	pertaining to being attracted to

-plastic	pertaining to formation
-rrhage	abnormal flow
-rrhagic	pertaining to abnormal flow

Prefixes

a-	without
an-	without
anti-	against
auto-	self

dys-	abnormal
homo-	same
hyper-	excessive
hypo-	insufficient

mono-	one
pan-	all
poly-	many
trans-	across

Adjective Forms of Anatomical Terms

Term	Word Parts	Definition
basophilic (bay-soh-FILL-ik)	bas/o = base -philic = pertaining to being attracted to	A granulocytic leukocyte that attracts a basic pH stain.
eosinophilic (ee-oh-sin-oh-FILL-ik)	eosin/o = rosy red -philic = pertaining to being attracted to	A granulocytic leukocyte that attracts a rosy red stain.
erythrocytic (eh-rith-roh-SIT-ik)	erythr/o = red -cytic = pertaining to cells	A red blood cell.
fibrinous (fye-brin-us)	fibrin/o = fibers -ous = pertaining to	Pertaining to fibers.
hematic (hee-MAT-ik)	hemat/o = blood -ic = pertaining to	Pertaining to blood.
leukocytic (loo-koh-SIT-ik)	leuk/o = white -cytic = pertaining to cells	A white blood cell.
lymphocytic (lim-foh-SIT-ik)	lymph/o = lymph -cytic = pertaining to cells	An agranulocytic leukocyte formed in lymphatic tissue.
monocytic (mon-oh-SIT-ik)	mono- = one -cytic = pertaining to cells	An agranulocytic leukocyte with a single, large nucleus.
neutrophilic (noo-troh-FILL-ik)	neutr/o = neutral -philic = pertaining to being attracted to	A granulocytic leukocyte that attracts a neutral pH stain.
sanguinous (SANG-gwih-nus)	sanguin/o = blood -ous = pertaining to	Pertaining to blood.
thrombocytic (throm-boh-SIT-ik)	thromb/o = clot -cytic = pertaining to cells	A clotting cell; a platelet.

Practice As You Go

B. Give the adjective form for each anatomical structure

1. Blood ______________________ or ______________________
2. White cell ______________________
3. Clotting cell ______________________
4. Fibers ______________________
5. Red cell ______________________

Pathology

Term	Word Parts	Definition
Medical Specialties		
hematology (hee-mah-TALL-oh-jee)	hemat/o = blood -logy = study of	The branch of medicine specializing in treatment of diseases and conditions of the blood. Physician is a *hematologist.*
Signs and Symptoms		
blood clot ■ **Figure 6.4** Electronmicrograph showing a blood clot composed of fibrin, red blood cells, and tissue debris. *(Eye of Science/Science Source)*	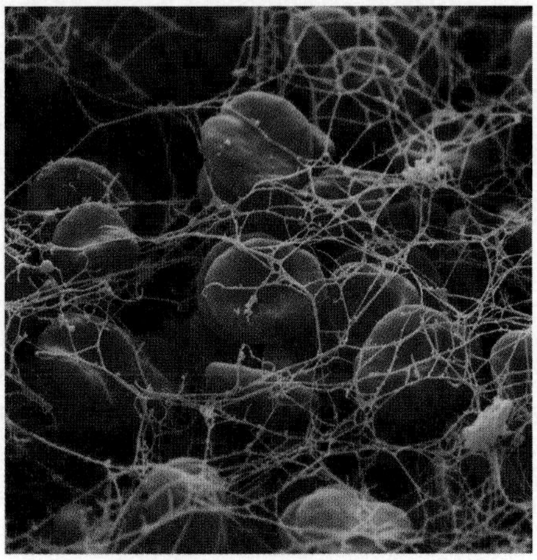	The hard collection of fibrin, blood cells, and tissue debris that is the end result of hemostasis or the blood-clotting process.
coagulate (koh-ag-YOO-late)	coagul/o = clotting	To convert from a liquid to a gel or solid, as in blood coagulation.
dyscrasia (dis-CRAZ-ee-ah)	dys- = abnormal -ia = condition	A general term indicating the presence of a disease affecting blood.
hematoma (hee-mah-TOH-mah)	hemat/o = blood -oma = mass	The collection of blood under the skin as the result of blood escaping into the tissue from damaged blood vessels. Commonly referred to as a *bruise.*

Word Watch

The term *hematoma* is confusing. Its simple translation is "blood mass." However, it is used to refer to blood that has leaked out of a blood vessel and has pooled in the tissues causing swelling.

Pathology (continued)

Term	Word Parts	Definition
hemorrhage (HEM-er-rij)	hem/o = blood -rrhage = abnormal flow	Blood flowing out of a blood vessel (i.e., bleeding).
Blood		
hemophilia (hee-moh-FILL-ee-ah)	hem/o = blood -philia = condition of being attracted to	Hereditary blood disease in which blood-clotting time is prolonged due to a lack of one vital clotting factor. It is transmitted by a sex-linked trait from females to males, appearing almost exclusively in males.
hyperlipidemia (HYE-per-lip-id-ee-mee-ah)	hyper- = excessive lip/o = fat -emia = blood condition	Condition of having too high a level of lipids such as cholesterol in the bloodstream. A risk factor for developing atherosclerosis and coronary artery disease.
pancytopenia (pan-sigh-toe-PEN-ee-ah)	pan- = all cyt/o = cell -penia = too few	Having too few of all cells.
septicemia (sep-tih-SEE-mee-ah)	septic/o = infection -emia = blood condition	Having bacteria or their toxins in the bloodstream. *Sepsis* is a term that means putrefaction or infection. Commonly referred to as *blood poisoning.*
Erythrocytes		
anemia (an-NEE-mee-ah)	an- = without -emia = blood condition	A large group of conditions characterized by a reduction in the number of red blood cells or the amount of hemoglobin in the blood; results in less oxygen reaching the tissues.
aplastic anemia (a-PLAS-tik / an-NEE-mee-ah)	a- = without -plastic = pertaining to formation an- = without -emia = blood condition	Severe form of anemia that develops as a consequence of loss of functioning red bone marrow. Results in a decrease in the number of all the formed elements. Treatment may eventually require a bone marrow transplant.
erythrocytosis (ee-RITH-row-sigh-toe-sis)	erythr/o = red -cytosis = more than normal number of cells	The condition of having too many red blood cells.
erythropenia (ee-RITH-row-pen-ee-ah)	erythr/o = red -penia = too few	The condition of having too few red blood cells.
hemolytic anemia (hee-moh-LIT-ik / an-NEE-mee-ah)	hem/o = blood -lytic = destruction an- = without -emia = blood condition	An anemia that develops as the result of the destruction of erythrocytes.
hemolytic reaction (hee-moh-LIT-ik)	hem/o = blood -lytic = destruction	The destruction of a patient's erythrocytes that occurs when receiving a transfusion of an incompatible blood type. Also called a *transfusion reaction.*

Pathology (continued)

Term	Word Parts	Definition
hypochromic anemia (hi-poe-CHROME-ik / an-NEE-mee-ah)	hypo- = insufficient **chrom/o** = color -ic = pertaining to an- = without -emia = blood condition	Anemia resulting from having insufficient hemoglobin in the erythrocytes. Named because the hemoglobin molecule is responsible for the dark red color of the erythrocytes.
iron-deficiency anemia	an- = without -emia = blood condition	Anemia resulting from not having sufficient iron to manufacture hemoglobin.
pernicious anemia (PA) (per-NISH-us / an-NEE-mee-ah)	an- = without -emia = blood condition	Anemia associated with insufficient absorption of vitamin B_{12} by the digestive system. Vitamin B_{12} is necessary for erythrocyte production.
polycythemia vera (pol-ee-sigh-THEE-mee-ah / VAIR-rah)	poly- = many **cyt/o** = cell **hem/o** = blood -ia = condition	Production of too many red blood cells by the bone marrow. Blood becomes too thick to easily flow through the blood vessels.
sickle cell anemia	an- = without -emia = blood condition	A genetic disorder in which erythrocytes take on an abnormal curved or "sickle" shape. These cells are fragile and are easily damaged, leading to hemolytic anemia.

Normal red blood cells

Sickled cells

■ **Figure 6.5** Comparison of normal-shaped erythrocytes and the abnormal sickle shape noted in patients with sickle cell anemia.

Term	Word Parts	Definition
thalassemia (thal-ah-SEE-mee-ah)	-emia = blood condition	A genetic disorder in which the body is unable to make functioning hemoglobin, resulting in anemia.
Leukocytes		
leukemia (loo-KEE-mee-ah)	**leuk/o** = white -emia = blood condition	Cancer of the white blood cell–forming red bone marrow resulting in a large number of abnormal and immature white blood cells circulating in the blood.
leukocytosis (LOO-koh-sigh-toh-sis)	**leuk/o** = white **-cytosis** = more than normal number of cells	The condition of having too many white blood cells.
leukopenia (LOO-koh-pen-ee-ah)	**leuk/o** = white -penia = too few	The condition of having too few white blood cells.

Pathology (continued)

Term	Word Parts	Definition
Platelets		
thrombocytosis (throm-boh-sigh-TOH-sis)	thromb/o = clot -cytosis = more than normal number of cells	The condition of having too many platelets.
thrombopenia (THROM-boh-pen-ee-ah)	thromb/o = clot -penia = too few	The condition of having too few platelets.

Practice As You Go

C. Terminology Matching

Match each term to its definition.

1. ________ thalassemia
2. ________ dyscrasia
3. ________ hematoma
4. ________ anemia
5. ________ hemophilia

a. disease in which blood does not clot

b. condition with reduced number of RBCs

c. mass of blood

d. type of anemia

e. general term for blood disorders

Diagnostic Procedures

Term	Word Parts	Definition
Clinical Laboratory Tests		
blood culture and sensitivity (C&S)		Sample of blood is incubated in the laboratory to check for bacterial growth. If bacteria are present, they are identified and tested to determine which antibiotics they are sensitive to.
complete blood count (CBC)		Combination of blood tests including red blood cell count (RBC), white blood cell count (WBC), hemoglobin (Hgb), hematocrit (Hct), white blood cell differential, and platelet count.
erythrocyte sedimentation rate (ESR, SR, sed rate) (eh-RITH-roh-sight / sed-ih-men-TAY-shun)	erythr/o = red -cyte = cell	Blood test to determine the rate at which mature red blood cells settle out of the blood after the addition of an anticoagulant. This is an indicator of the presence of an inflammatory disease.
hematocrit (HCT, Hct, crit) (hee-MAT-oh-krit)	hemat/o = blood -crit = separation of	Blood test to measure the volume of red blood cells (erythrocytes) within the total volume of blood.
hemoglobin (Hgb, hb, HGB) (hee-moh-GLOH-bin)	hem/o = blood -globin = protein	A blood test to measure the amount of hemoglobin present in a given volume of blood.

Diagnostic Procedures (continued)

Term	Word Parts	Definition
platelet count (PLAYT-let)		Blood test to determine the number of platelets in a given volume of blood.
prothrombin time (pro-time, PT) (proh-THROM-bin)	thromb/o = clot	A measure of the blood's coagulation abilities by measuring how long it takes for a clot to form after prothrombin has been activated.
red blood cell count (RBC)		Blood test to determine the number of erythrocytes in a volume of blood. A decrease in red blood cells may indicate anemia; an increase may indicate polycythemia.
red blood cell morphology	morph/o = shape -logy = study of	Examination of a specimen of blood for abnormalities in the shape (morphology) of the erythrocytes. Used to determine diseases such as sickle cell anemia.
sequential multiple analyzer computer (SMAC)		Machine for doing multiple blood chemistry tests automatically.
white blood cell count (WBC)		Blood test to measure the number of leukocytes in a volume of blood. An increase may indicate the presence of infection or a disease such as leukemia. A decrease in white blood cells may be caused by radiation therapy or chemotherapy.
white blood cell differential (diff) (diff-er-EN-shal)		Blood test to determine the number of each variety of leukocytes.
Medical Procedures		
bone marrow aspiration (as-pih-RAY-shun)		Sample of bone marrow is removed by aspiration with a needle and examined for diseases such as leukemia or aplastic anemia.
phlebotomy (fleh-BOT-oh-me)	phleb/o = vein -otomy = cutting into	Incision into a vein in order to remove blood for a diagnostic test. Also called *venipuncture.*

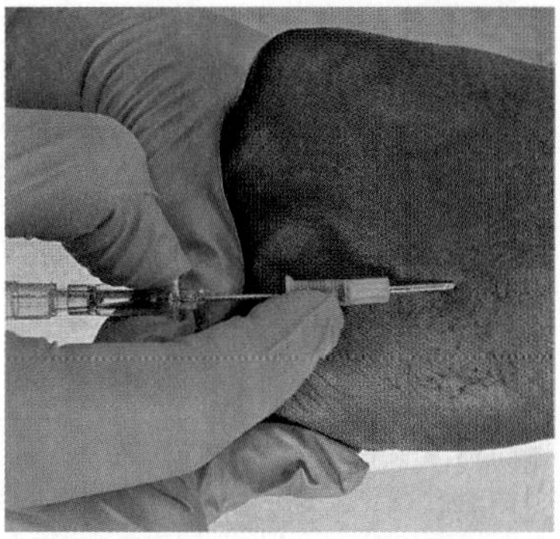

■ **Figure 6.6** Phlebotomist using a needle to withdraw blood. *(Michal Heron, Pearson Education)*

Therapeutic Procedures

Term	Word Parts	Definition
Medical Procedures		
autologous transfusion (aw-TALL-oh-gus / trans-FYOO-zhun)	auto- = self	Procedure for collecting and storing a patient's own blood several weeks prior to the actual need. It can then be used to replace blood lost during a surgical procedure.
blood transfusion (trans-FYOO-zhun)	trans- = across fus/o = pouring -ion = action	Artificial transfer of blood into the bloodstream. **Med Term Tip** Before a patient receives a blood transfusion, the laboratory performs a **type and cross-match**. This test first double-checks the blood type of both the donor's and recipient's blood. Then a cross-match is performed. This process mixes together small samples of both bloods and observes the mixture for adverse reactions.
bone marrow transplant (BMT)		Patient receives red bone marrow from a donor after the patient's own bone marrow has been destroyed by radiation or chemotherapy.
homologous transfusion (hoh-MALL-oh-gus / trans-FYOO-zhun)	homo- = same	Replacement of blood by transfusion of blood received from another person.
packed red cells		A transfusion in which most of the plasma, leukocytes, and platelets have been removed, leaving only erythrocytes.
plasmapheresis (plaz-mah-fah-REE-sis)	-apheresis = removal, carry away	Method of removing plasma from the body without depleting the formed elements. Whole blood is removed and the cells and plasma are separated. The cells are returned to the patient along with a donor plasma transfusion.
whole blood		Refers to the mixture of both plasma and formed elements.

Pharmacology

Classification	Word Parts	Action	Examples
anticoagulant (an-tih-koh-AG-yoo-lant)	anti- = against coagul/o = clotting	Substance that prevents blood clot formation. Commonly referred to as a *blood thinner.*	heparin, HepLock; warfarin, Coumadin
antihemorrhagic (an-tih-hem-er-RAJ-ik)	anti- = against hem/o = blood -rrhagic = pertaining to abnormal flow	Substance that prevents or stops hemorrhaging; a *hemostatic agent.*	aminocaproic acid, Amicar; vitamin K
antiplatelet agents (an-tih-PLATE-let)	anti- = against	Substance that interferes with the action of platelets. Prolongs bleeding time. Used to prevent heart attacks and strokes.	clopidogrel, Plavix; ticlopidine, Ticlid
hematinic (hee-mah-TIN-ik)	hemat/o = blood -ic = pertaining to	Substance that increases the number of erythrocytes or the amount of hemoglobin in the blood.	epoetin alfa, Procrit; darbepoetin alfa, Aranesp
thrombolytic (throm-boh-LIT-ik)	thromb/o = clot -lytic = destruction	Term meaning able to dissolve existing blood clots.	alteplase, Activase; streptokinase, Streptase

Practice As You Go

D. Match each procedure term with its definition

1. ________ phlebotomy
2. ________ SMAC
3. ________ plasmapheresis
4. ________ whole blood
5. ________ culture and sensitivity

a. method of removing plasma from the body
b. mixture of plasma and formed elements
c. removal of blood from a vein
d. test for bacterial growth
e. machine to conduct blood chemistry tests

Abbreviations

ALL	acute lymphocytic leukemia	**lymphs**	lymphocytes
AML	acute myelogenous leukemia	**monos**	monocytes
basos	basophils	**PA**	pernicious anemia
BMT	bone marrow transplant	**PCV**	packed cell volume
CBC	complete blood count	**PMN, polys**	polymorphonuclear neutrophil
CLL	chronic lymphocytic leukemia	**PT, pro-time**	prothrombin time
CML	chronic myelogenous leukemia	**RBC**	red blood cell
diff	differential	**Rh+**	Rh-positive
eosins, eos	eosinophils	**Rh–**	Rh-negative
ESR, SR, sed rate	erythrocyte sedimentation rate	**segs**	segmented neutrophils
HCT, Hct, crit	hematocrit	**SMAC**	sequential multiple analyzer computer
Hgb, Hb, HGB	hemoglobin	**WBC**	white blood cell

Practice As You Go

E. What's the Abbreviation?

1. acute lymphocytic leukemia ________________
2. bone marrow transplant ________________
3. eosinophils ________________
4. hematocrit ________________
5. pernicious anemia ________________
6. complete blood count ________________
7. differential ________________
8. white blood cell ________________

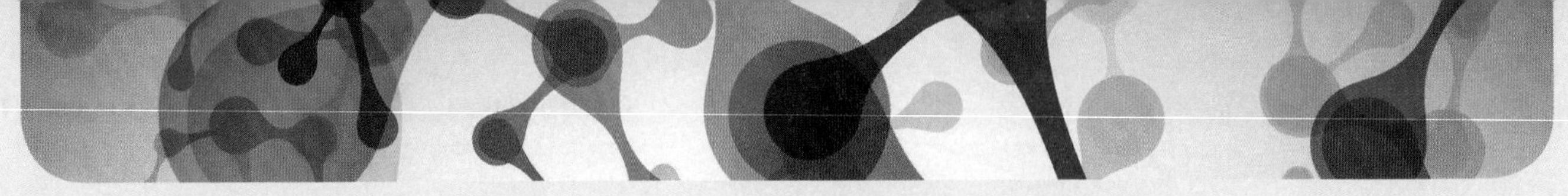

Section II: The Lymphatic and Immune Systems at a Glance

Function

The lymphatic system consists of a network of lymph vessels that pick up excess tissue fluid, cleanse it, and return it to the circulatory system. It also picks up fats that have been absorbed by the digestive system. The immune system fights disease and infections.

Organs

Here are the primary structures that comprise the lymphatic and immune systems:

lymph nodes
lymphatic vessels
spleen
thymus gland
tonsils

Word Parts

Here are the most common word parts (with their meanings) used to build lymphatic and immune system terms. For a more comprehensive list, refer to the Terminology section of this chapter.

Combining Forms

adenoid/o	adenoids
axill/o	axilla (underarm)
immun/o	protection
inguin/o	groin region
lymph/o	lymph
lymphaden/o	lymph node
lymphangi/o	lymph vessel
nucle/o	nucleus
splen/o	spleen
thym/o	thymus gland
tonsill/o	tonsils

Suffixes

-edema	swelling
-globulin	protein
-phage	to eat
-toxic	pertaining to poison

The Lymphatic and Immune Systems Illustrated

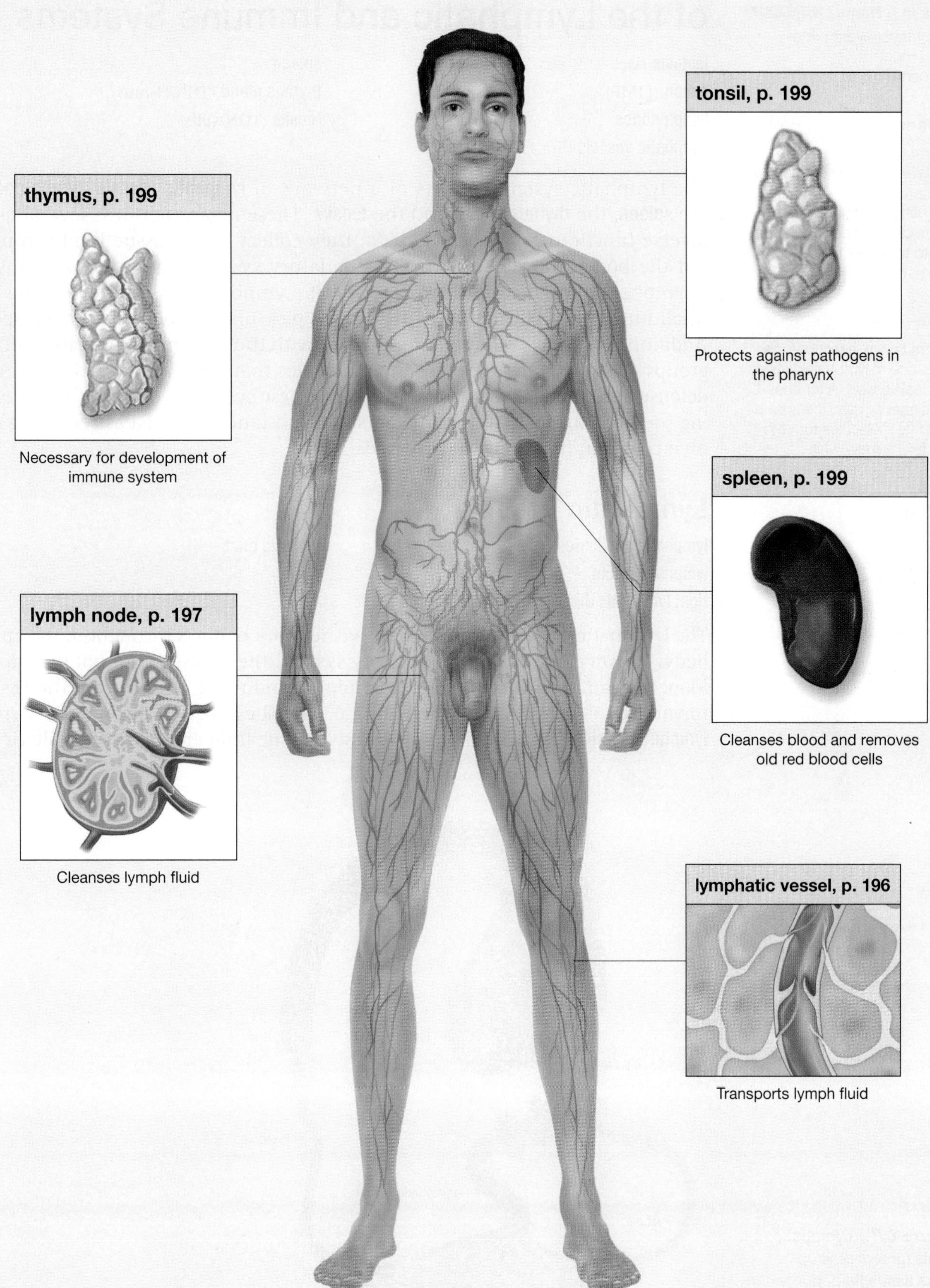

Anatomy and Physiology of the Lymphatic and Immune Systems

What's In A Name?
Look for these word parts:
lact/o = milk
-eal = pertaining to

Med Term Tip
The term *lymph* comes from the Latin word *lympha* meaning "clear spring water." Although a very pale, clear yellow, lymph appears crystal clear when compared to the other body fluid, blood.

Med Term Tip
The term *lacteal* describes the appearance of lymph fluid inside the lacteal vessels. After absorbing fats from a meal, the suspended fat molecules turn the lymph fluid a milky white.

lacteals (lack-TEE-als)
lymph (LIMF)
lymph nodes
lymphatic vessels (lim-FAT-ik)
spleen
thymus gland (THIGH-mus)
tonsils (TON-sulls)

The lymphatic system consists of a network of **lymphatic vessels**, **lymph nodes**, the **spleen**, the **thymus gland**, and the **tonsils**. These organs perform several quite diverse functions for the body. First, they collect excess tissue fluid throughout the body and return it to the circulatory system. The fluid, once inside a lymphatic vessel, is referred to as **lymph**. Lymph vessels located around the small intestines, called **lacteals**, are able to pick up absorbed fats for transport. Additionally, the lymphatic system works with the immune system to form the groups of cells, tissues, organs, and molecules that serve as the body's primary defense against the invasion of pathogens. These systems work together defending the body against foreign invaders and substances, as well as removing our own cells that have become diseased.

Lymphatic Vessels

lymphatic capillaries (CAP-ih-lair-eez)
lymphatic ducts
right lymphatic duct
thoracic duct
valves

The lymphatic vessels form an extensive network of ducts throughout the entire body. However, unlike the circulatory system, these vessels are not in a closed loop. Instead, they serve as one-way pipes conducting lymph from the tissues toward the thoracic cavity (see Figure 6.7 ■). These vessels begin as very small **lymphatic capillaries** in the tissues. Excessive tissue fluid enters these capillaries to

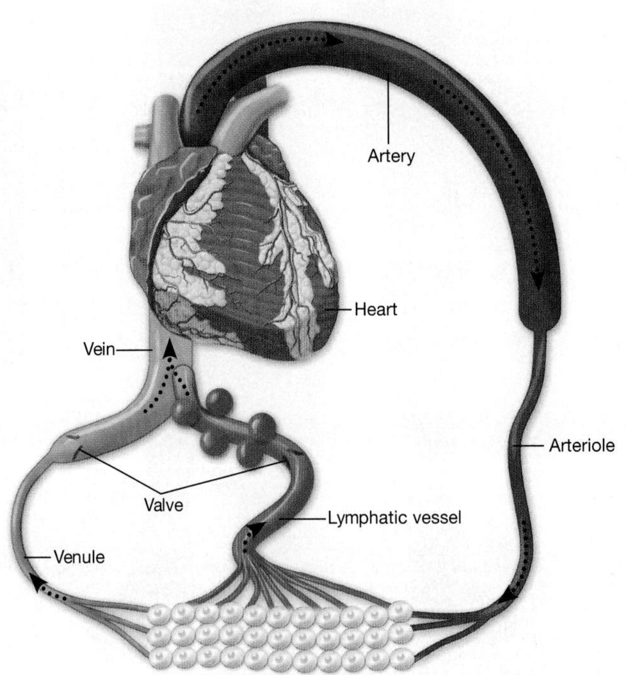

■ **Figure 6.7** Lymphatic vessels (green) pick up excess tissue fluid, purify it in lymph nodes, and return it to the circulatory system.

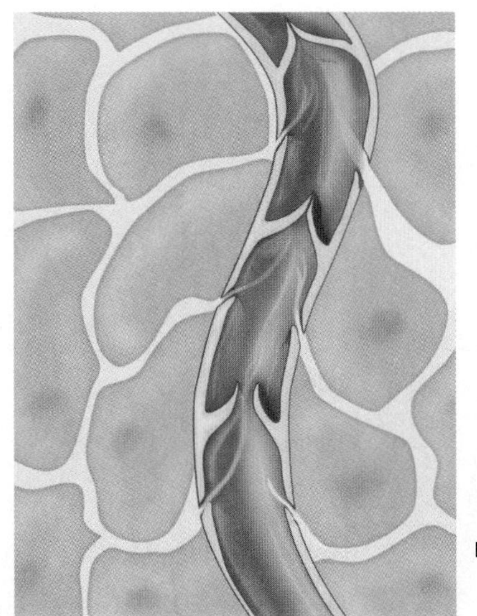

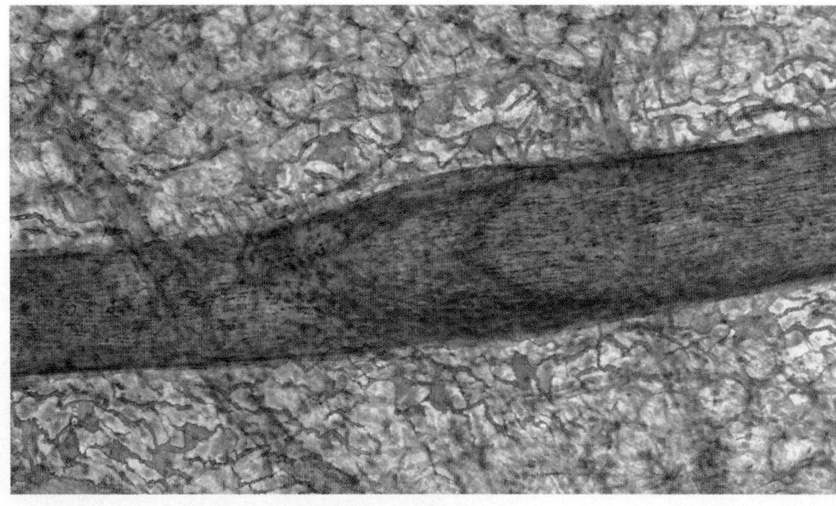

■ **Figure 6.8** A - Lymphatic vessel with valves within tissue cells; B - Photomicrograph of lymphatic vessel with valve clearly visible. *(Michael Abbey/Photo Researchers, Inc.)*

begin the trip back to the circulatory system. The capillaries merge into larger lymphatic vessels. This is a very low-pressure system, so these vessels have **valves** along their length to ensure that lymph can only move forward toward the thoracic cavity (see Figure 6.8■). These vessels finally drain into one of two large **lymphatic ducts**, the **right lymphatic duct** or the **thoracic duct**. The smaller right lymphatic duct drains the right arm and the right side of the head, neck, and chest. This duct empties lymph into the right subclavian vein. The larger thoracic duct drains lymph from the rest of the body and empties into the left subclavian vein (see Figure 6.9■).

What's In A Name?

Look for these word parts:
thorac/o = chest
-ic = pertaining to

Med Term Tip

The term *capillary* is also used to describe the minute blood vessels within the circulatory system. This is one of several general medical terms, such as valves, cilia, and hair, that are used in several systems.

Lymph Nodes

lymph glands

Lymph nodes are small organs composed of lymphatic tissue located along the route of the lymphatic vessels. These nodes, also referred to as **lymph glands**, house lymphocytes and antibodies and therefore work to remove pathogens and cell debris as lymph passes through them on its way back to the thoracic cavity (see Figure 6.10■). Lymph nodes also serve to trap and destroy cells from cancerous tumors. Although found throughout the body, lymph nodes are particularly concentrated in several regions. For example, lymph nodes concentrated in the neck region drain lymph from the head. See again Figure 6.9 and Table 6.2■ for a description of some of the most important sites for lymph nodes.

Med Term Tip

In surgical procedures to remove a malignancy from an organ, such as a breast, the adjacent lymph nodes are also tested for cancer. If cancerous cells are found in the tested lymph nodes, the disease is said to have spread or *metastasized.* Tumor cells may then spread to other parts of the body by means of the lymphatic system.

Table 6.2 Sites for Lymph Nodes

Name	Location	Function
axillary (AK-sih-lair-ee)	armpits	Drain arms and shoulder region; cancer cells from breasts may be present
cervical (SER-vih-kal)	neck	Drain head and neck; may be enlarged during upper respiratory infections
inguinal (ING-gwih-nal)	groin	Drain legs and lower pelvis
mediastinal (mee-dee-ass-TYE-nal)	chest	Drain chest cavity

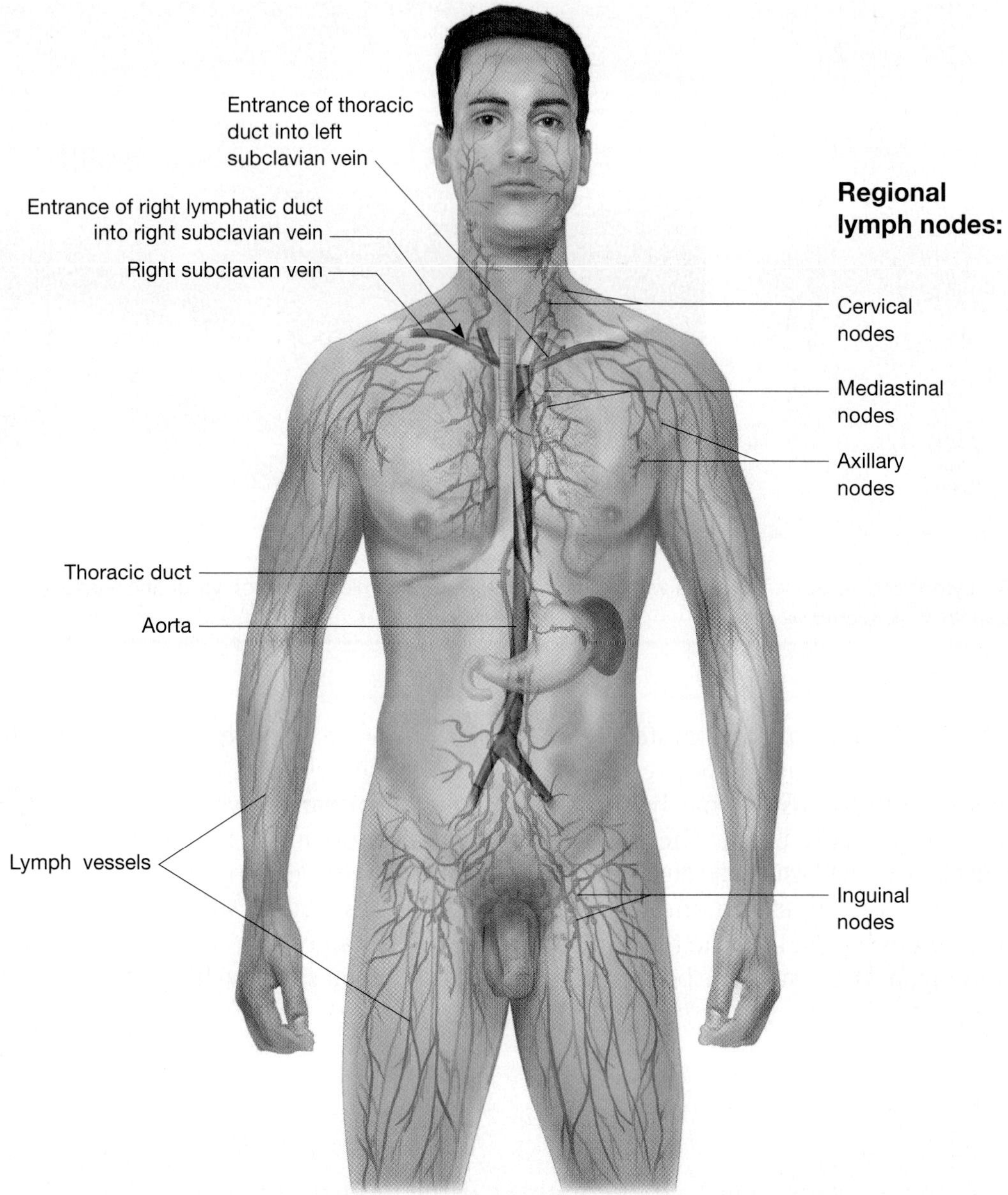

■ **Figure 6.9** Location of lymph vessels, lymphatic ducts, and areas of lymph node concentrations.

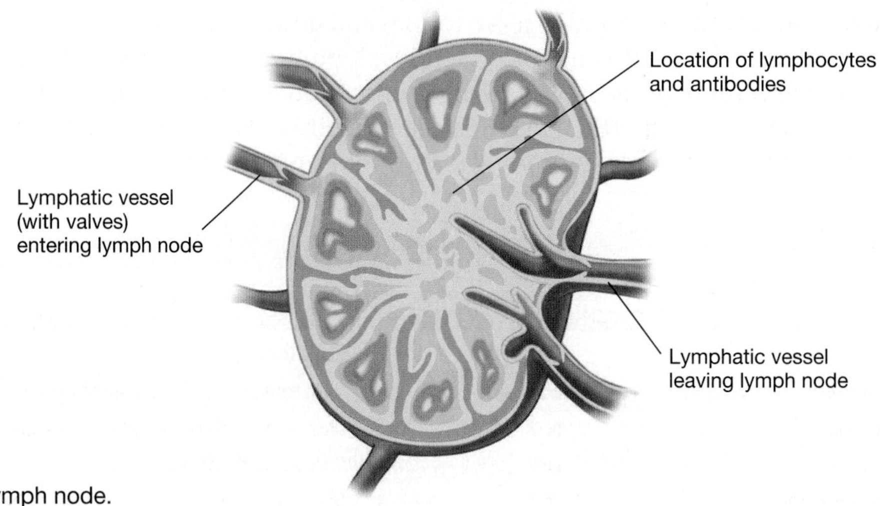

■ **Figure 6.10** Structure of a lymph node.

Tonsils

adenoids (ADD-eh-noydz)
lingual tonsils (LING-gwal)
palatine tonsils (PAL-ah-tyne)
pharyngeal tonsils (fair-IN-jee-al)
pharynx (FAIR-inks)

The tonsils are collections of lymphatic tissue located on each side of the throat or **pharynx** (see Figure 6.11 ■). There are three sets of tonsils: **palatine tonsils, pharyngeal tonsils** (commonly referred to as the **adenoids**), and **lingual tonsils.** All tonsils contain a large number of leukocytes and act as filters to protect the body from the invasion of pathogens through the digestive or respiratory systems. Tonsils are not vital organs and can safely be removed if they become a continuous site of infection.

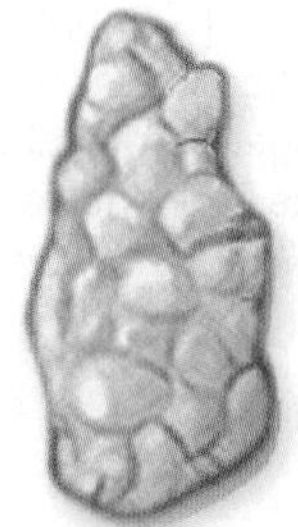

■ **Figure 6.11** The shape of a tonsil.

What's In A Name?

Look for these word parts:
lingu/o = tongue
palat/o = palate
pharyng/o = pharynx
-al = pertaining to
-eal = pertaining to
-ine = pertaining to

Spleen

blood sinuses
macrophages (MACK-roh-fayj-ez)

The spleen, located in the upper left quadrant of the abdomen, consists of lymphatic tissue that is highly infiltrated with blood vessels (see Figure 6.12 ■). These vessels spread out into slow-moving **blood sinuses.** The spleen filters out and destroys old red blood cells, recycles the iron, and also stores some of the blood supply for the body. Phagocytic **macrophages** line the blood sinuses in the spleen to engulf and remove pathogens. Because the blood is moving through the organ slowly, the macrophages have time to carefully identify pathogens and wornout red blood cells. The spleen is also not a vital organ and can be removed due to injury or disease. However, without the spleen, a person's susceptibility to a bloodstream infection may be increased.

What's In A Name?

Look for these word parts:
macro- = large
-phage = to eat

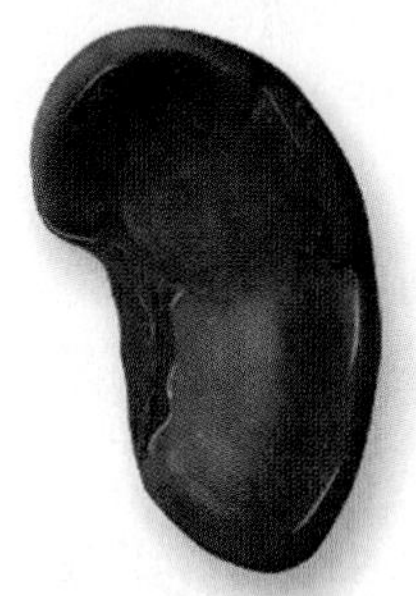

■ **Figure 6.12** The shape of the spleen.

Thymus Gland

T cells
T lymphocytes
thymosin (thigh-MOH-sin)

The thymus gland, located in the upper portion of the mediastinum, is essential for the proper development of the immune system (see Figure 6.13 ■). It assists the body with the immune function and the development of antibodies. This organ's hormone, **thymosin**, changes lymphocytes to **T lymphocytes** (simply called **T cells**), which play an important role in the immune response. The thymus is active in the unborn child and throughout childhood until adolescence, when it begins to shrink in size.

What's In A Name?

Look for these word parts:
lymph/o = lymph
-cyte = cell

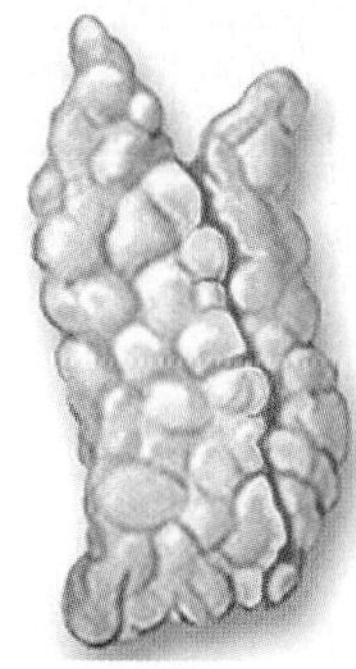

■ **Figure 6.13** The shape of the thymus gland.

Immunity

acquired immunity
active acquired immunity
bacteria (bak-TEE-ree-ah)
cancerous tumors
fungi (FUN-jee)
immune response
immunity (im-YOO-nih-tee)
immunizations (im-yoo-nih-ZAY-shuns)
natural immunity
passive acquired immunity
protozoans (proh-toh-ZOH-anz)
toxins
vaccinations (vak-sih-NAY-shuns)
viruses

Immunity is the body's ability to defend itself against pathogens, such as **bacteria, viruses, fungi, protozoans, toxins,** and **cancerous tumors.** Immunity comes in two forms: **natural immunity** and **acquired immunity.** Natural immunity, also called

What's In A Name?

Look for this word part:
-ous = pertaining to

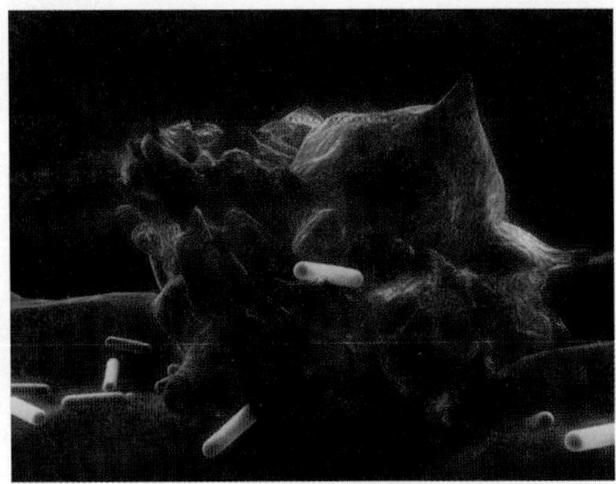

■ **Figure 6.14** Enhanced photomicrograph showing a macrophage (purple) attacking bacillus Escherichia coli (green). *(Sebastian Kaulitzki/Shutterstock)*

innate immunity, is not specific to a particular disease and does not require prior exposure to the pathogenic agent. A good example of natural immunity is the macrophage. These leukocytes are present throughout all the tissues of the body, but are concentrated in areas of high exposure to invading bacteria, like the lungs and digestive system. They are very active phagocytic cells, ingesting and digesting any pathogen they encounter (see Figure 6.14■).

Acquired immunity is the body's response to a specific pathogen and may be established either passively or actively. **Passive acquired immunity** results when a person receives protective substances produced by another human or animal. This may take the form of maternal antibodies crossing the placenta to a baby or an antitoxin or gamma globulin injection. **Active acquired immunity** develops following direct exposure to the pathogenic agent. The agent stimulates the body's **immune response**, a series of different mechanisms all geared to neutralize the agent. For example, a person typically can catch chickenpox only once because once the body has successfully fought the virus, it will be able to more quickly recognize and kill it in the future. **Immunizations** or **vaccinations** are special types of active acquired immunity. Instead of actually being exposed to the infectious agent and having the disease, a person is exposed to a modified or weakened pathogen that is still capable of stimulating the immune response but not actually causing the disease.

Immune Response

antibody (AN-tih-bod-ee)
antibody-mediated immunity
antigen–antibody complex
antigens (AN-tih-jens)
B cells
B lymphocytes
cell-mediated immunity
cellular immunity
cytotoxic (sigh-toh-TOK-sik)
humoral immunity (HYOO-mor-al)
immunoglobulin (Ig) (im-yoo-noh-GLOB-yoo-lin)
natural killer (NK) cells
pathogenic (path-oh-JEN-ik)

What's In A Name?

Look for these word parts:
cyt/o = cell
immun/o = protection
lymph/o = lymph
path/o = disease
-al = pertaining to
-ar = pertaining to
-cyte = cell
-gen = that which produces
-genic = producing
-globulin = protein
-toxic = pertaining to poison
anti- = against

Disease-causing, or **pathogenic**, agents are recognized as being foreign because they display proteins that are different from a person's own natural proteins. Those foreign proteins, called **antigens**, stimulate the immune response. The immune response consists of two distinct and different processes: **humoral immunity** (also called **antibody-mediated immunity**) and **cellular immunity** (also called **cell-mediated immunity**).

Med Term Tip

The term *humoral* comes from the Latin word for "liquid." It is the old-fashioned term to refer to the fluids of the body.

Humoral immunity refers to the production of **B lymphocytes**, also called **B cells**, which respond to antigens by producing a protective protein, called an **antibody** (also called an **immunoglobulin**). Antibodies combine with the antigen to form an **antigen–antibody complex**. This complex either targets the foreign substance for phagocytosis or prevents the infectious agent from damaging healthy cells.

Cellular immunity involves the production of T cells and **natural killer** (NK) **cells**. These defense cells are **cytotoxic**, meaning that they physically attack and destroy pathogenic cells.

Standard Precautions

cross-infection
nosocomial infection (no-so-KOH-mee-all)
Occupational Safety and Health Administration (OSHA)
reinfection
self-inoculation

Hospitals and other healthcare settings contain a large number of infective pathogens. Patients and healthcare workers are exposed to each other's pathogens and sometimes become infected. An infection acquired in this manner, as a result of hospital exposure, is referred to as a **nosocomial infection**. Nosocomial infections can spread in several ways. **Cross-infection** occurs when a person, either a patient or healthcare worker, acquires a pathogen from another patient or healthcare worker. **Reinfection** takes place when a patient becomes infected again with the same pathogen that originally brought him or her to the hospital. **Self-inoculation** occurs when a person becomes infected in a different part of the body by a pathogen from another part of his or her own body—such as intestinal bacteria spreading to the urethra.

What's In A Name?

Look for these word parts:
-al = pertaining to
re- = again

Med Term Tip

The term *nosocomial* comes from the Greek word *nosokomeion*, meaning hospital.

With the appearance of the hepatitis B virus (HBV) in the mid-1960s and the human immunodeficiency virus (HIV) in the mid-1980s, the fight against spreading infections took on even greater significance. In 1987 the **Occupational Safety and Health Administration** (OSHA) issued mandatory guidelines to ensure that all employees at risk of exposure to body fluids are provided with personal protective equipment. These guidelines state that all human blood, tissue, and body fluids must be treated as if they were infected with HIV, HBV, or other bloodborne pathogens. These guidelines were expanded in 1992 and 1996 to encourage the fight against not just bloodborne pathogens, but all nosocomial infections spread by contact with blood, mucous membranes, nonintact skin, and all body fluids (including amniotic fluid, vaginal secretions, pleural fluid, cerebrospinal fluid, peritoneal fluid, pericardial fluid, and semen). These guidelines are commonly referred to as the Standard Precautions:

1. Wash hands before putting on and after removing gloves and before and after working with each patient or patient equipment.
2. Wear gloves when in contact with any body fluid, mucous membrane, or nonintact skin or if you have chapped hands, a rash, or open sores.
3. Wear a nonpermeable gown or apron during procedures that are likely to expose you to any body fluid, mucous membrane, or nonintact skin.
4. Wear a mask and protective equipment or a face shield when patients are coughing often or if body fluid droplets or splashes are likely.
5. Wear a facemask and eyewear that seal close to the face during procedures that cause body tissues to be vaporized.
6. Remove for proper cleaning any shared equipment—such as a thermometer, stethoscope, or blood pressure cuff—that has come into contact with body fluids, mucous membrane, or nonintact skin.

Med Term Tip

The simple act of thoroughly washing your hands is the most effective method of preventing the spread of infectious diseases.

Practice As You Go

F. Complete the Statement

1. The organs of the lymphatic system other than lymphatic vessels and lymph nodes are the ____________________, ____________________, and ____________________.
2. The two lymph ducts are the ____________________ and ____________________.
3. The primary concentrations of lymph nodes are the ____________________, ____________________, ____________________, and ____________________ regions.
4. ____________________ immunity develops following direct exposure to a pathogen.
5. Humoral immunity is also referred to as ____________________ immunity.

Terminology

Word Parts Used to Build Lymphatic and Immune System Terms

The following lists contain the combining forms, suffixes, and prefixes used to build terms in the remaining sections of this chapter.

Combining Forms

adenoid/o	adenoids
axill/o	axilla, underarm
cortic/o	outer layer
immun/o	protection
inguin/o	groin
lymph/o	lymph

lymphaden/o	lymph node
lymphangi/o	lymph vessel
nucle/o	nucleus
path/o	disease
pneumon/o (see Chapter 7)	lung

sarc/o	flesh
splen/o	spleen
thym/o	thymus gland
tonsill/o	tonsils

Suffixes

-al	pertaining to
-ar	pertaining to
-ary	pertaining to
-atic	pertaining to
-ectomy	surgical removal
-edema	swelling
-gram	record
-graphy	process of recording

-ia	condition
-iasis	abnormal condition
-ic	pertaining to
-itis	inflammation
-logy	study of
-megaly	enlarged
-oma	tumor

-osis	abnormal condition
-pathy	disease
-therapy	treatment

Prefixes

anti-	against

auto-	self

mono-	one

Adjective Form of Anatomical Terms

Term	Word Parts	Definition
axillary (AK-sih-lair-ee)	axill/o = axilla, underarm -ary = pertaining to	Pertaining to the underarm region.
inguinal (ING-gwih-nal)	inguin/o = groin -al = pertaining to	Pertaining to the groin region.
lymphangial (lim-FAN-gee-al)	lymphangi/o = lymph vessel -al = pertaining to	Pertaining to lymph vessels.
lymphatic (lim-FAT-ik)	lymph/o = lymph -atic = pertaining to	Pertaining to lymph.
splenic (SPLEN-ik)	splen/o = spleen -ic = pertaining to	Pertaining to the spleen.
thymic (THIGH-mik)	thym/o = thymus gland -ic = pertaining to	Pertaining to the thymus gland.
tonsillar (ton-sih-lar)	tonsill/o = tonsils -ar = pertaining to	Pertaining to the tonsils.

Practice As You Go

G. Give the adjective form for each anatomical structure

1. Spleen ____________________
2. Lymph ____________________
3. Tonsil ____________________
4. Thymus gland ____________________
5. Lymph vessel ____________________

Pathology

Term	Word Parts	Definition
Medical Specialties		
allergist (AL-er-jist)		A physician who specializes in testing for and treating allergies.
immunology (im-yoo-NALL-oh-jee)	immun/o = protection -logy = study of	A branch of medicine concerned with diagnosis and treatment of infectious diseases and other disorders of the immune system. Physician is an *immunologist.*
pathology (path-OL-oh-gee)	path/o = disease -logy = study of	A branch of medicine concerned with determining the underlying causes and development of diseases. Physician is a *pathologist.*

Pathology (continued)

Term	Word Parts	Definition
Signs and Symptoms		
hives		Appearance of wheals as part of an allergic reaction.
inflammation (in-flah-MAY-shun) ■ **Figure 6.15** Inflammation as illustrated by cellulitis of the nose. Note that the area is red and swollen. It is also painful and hot to touch. *(ARENA Creative/Shutterstock)*		The tissues' response to injury from pathogens or physical agents. Characterized by redness, pain, swelling, and feeling hot to touch. **Word Watch** The terms *inflammation* and *inflammatory* are spelled with two *m*'s, while *inflame* and *inflamed* each have only one *m*. These may be the most commonly misspelled terms by medical terminology students.
lymphedema (limf-eh-DEE-mah)	lymph/o = lymph -edema = swelling	Edema appearing in the extremities due to an obstruction of the lymph flow through the lymphatic vessels.
splenomegaly (splee-noh-MEG-ah-lee)	splen/o = spleen -megaly = enlarged	An enlarged spleen.
urticaria (er-tih-KAY-ree-ah)		Severe itching associated with hives, usually linked to food allergy, stress, or drug reactions.
Allergic Reactions		
allergy (AL-er-jee)		Hypersensitivity to a common substance in the environment or to a medication. The substance causing the allergic reaction is called an *allergen.*
anaphylactic shock (an-ah-fih-LAK-tik)		Life-threatening condition resulting from a severe allergic reaction. Examples of instances that may trigger this reaction include bee stings, medications, or the ingestion of foods. Circulatory and respiratory problems occur, including respiratory distress, hypotension, edema, tachycardia, and convulsions. Also called **anaphylaxis**.
Lymphatic System		
adenoiditis (add-eh-noyd-EYE-tis)	adenoid/o = adenoids -itis = inflammation	Inflammation of the adenoids.
autoimmune disease	auto- = self	A disease resulting from the body's immune system attacking its own cells as if they were pathogens. Examples include systemic lupus erythematosus, rheumatoid arthritis, and multiple sclerosis.

Pathology (continued)

Term	Word Parts	Definition
elephantiasis (el-eh-fan-TYE-ah-sis)	-iasis = abnormal condition	Inflammation, obstruction, and destruction of the lymph vessels resulting in enlarged tissues due to edema.
Hodgkin's disease (HD) (HOJ-kins)		Also called *Hodgkin's lymphoma.* Cancer of the lymphatic cells found in concentration in the lymph nodes. Named after Thomas Hodgkin, a British physician, who first described it.
lymphadenitis (lim-fad-en-EYE-tis)	lymphaden/o = lymph node -itis = inflammation	Inflammation of the lymph nodes. Referred to as *swollen glands.*
lymphadenopathy (lim-fad-eh-NOP-ah-thee)	lymphaden/o = lymph node -pathy = disease	A general term for lymph node diseases.
lymphangioma (lim-fan-jee-OH-mah)	lymphangi/o = lymph vessel -oma = tumor	A tumor in a lymphatic vessel.
lymphoma (lim-FOH-mah)	lymph/o = lymph -oma = tumor	A tumor in lymphatic tissue.
mononucleosis (mono) (mon-oh-nook-lee-OH-sis)	mono- = one nucle/o = nucleus -osis = abnormal condition Med Term Tip Mononuclear is a term occasionally used to describe any cell that has a large, single, round nucleus, including lymphocytes and monocytes. This is opposed to having a lobed nucleus like the other white blood cells.	Acute infectious disease with a large number of abnormal mononuclear lymphocytes. Caused by the Epstein–Barr virus. Abnormal liver function may occur.
non-Hodgkin's lymphoma (NHL) ■ **Figure 6.16** Photo of the neck of a patient with non-Hodgkin's lymphoma showing swelling associated with enlarged lymph nodes. *(Dr. P. Marazzi/Science Source)*	lymph/o = lymph -oma = tumor	Cancer of the lymphatic tissues other than Hodgkin's lymphoma.
thymoma (thigh-MOH-mah)	thym/o = thymus gland -oma = tumor	A tumor of the thymus gland.
tonsillitis (ton-sil-EYE-tis)	tonsill/o = tonsils -itis = inflammation	Inflammation of the tonsils.
Immune System		
acquired immunodeficiency syndrome (AIDS) (ac-quired / im-you-noh-dee-FIH-shen-see / SIN-drohm)	immun/o = protection	Disease involving a defect in the cell-mediated immunity system. A syndrome of opportunistic infections occurring in the final stages of infection with the human immunodeficiency virus (HIV). This virus attacks T4 lymphocytes and destroys them, reducing the person's ability to fight infection.

Pathology (continued)

Term	Word Parts	Definition
AIDS-related complex (ARC)		Early stage of AIDS. There is a positive test for the virus, but only mild symptoms of weight loss, fatigue, skin rash, and anorexia.
graft versus host disease (GVHD)		Serious complication of bone marrow transplant (graft). Immune cells from the donor bone marrow attack the recipient's (host's) tissues.
human immunodeficiency virus (HIV) (im-yoo-noh-dee-FIH-shen-see) ■ **Figure 6.17** Color enhanced scanning electron micrograph of HIV virus (red) infecting T-helper cells (green). *(NIBSC/Science Photo Library/ Science Source)*	immun/o = protection	Virus that causes AIDS; also known as a **retrovirus**.
immunocompromised (im-you-noh-KOM-pro-mized)	immun/o = protection	Having an immune system that is unable to respond properly to pathogens. Also called *immunodeficiency disorder.*
Kaposi's sarcoma (KS) (KAP-oh-seez / sar-KOH-mah)	sarc/o = flesh -oma= tumor	Form of skin cancer frequently seen in patients with AIDS. It consists of brownish-purple papules that spread from the skin and metastasize to internal organs. Named for dermatologist Moritz Kaposi.
opportunistic infections		Infectious diseases associated with patients who have compromised immune systems and therefore a lowered resistance to infections and parasites. May be the result of HIV infection.
pneumocystis pneumonia (PCP) (noo-moh-SIS-tis / noo-MOH-nee-ah)	pneumon/o = lung -ia = condition	Pneumonia common in patients with weakened immune systems, such as AIDS patients, caused by the *Pneumocystis jiroveci* fungus.
sarcoidosis (sar-koyd-OH-sis)	-osis = abnormal condition	Disease of unknown cause that forms fibrous lesions commonly appearing in the lymph nodes, liver, skin, lungs, spleen, eyes, and small bones of the hands and feet.
severe combined immunodeficiency syndrome (SCIDS)	immun/o = protection	Disease seen in children born with a nonfunctioning immune system. Often these children are forced to live in sealed sterile rooms.

Practice As You Go

H. Terminology Matching

Match each term to its definition.

1. ________ allergy
2. ________ hives
3. ________ Hodgkin's disease
4. ________ sarcoidosis
5. ________ graft vs. host disease

a. seen in an allergic reaction
b. complication of bone marrow transplant
c. a hypersensitivity reaction
d. a type of cancer
e. autoimmune disease

Diagnostic Procedures

Term	Word Parts	Definition
Clinical Laboratory Tests		
enzyme-linked immunosorbent assay (ELISA) (EN-zym / LINKT / im-yoo-noh-sor-bent / ASS-say)	immun/o = protection	Blood test for an antibody to the HIV virus. A positive test means that the person has been exposed to the virus. There may be a false-positive reading, and then the Western blot test would be used to verify the results.
Western blot		Test used as a backup to the ELISA blood test to detect the presence of the antibody to HIV (AIDS virus) in the blood.
Diagnostic Imaging		
lymphangiogram (lim-FAN-jee-oh-gram)	lymphangi/o = lymph vessel -gram = record	X-ray record of the lymphatic vessels produced by lymphangiography.
lymphangiography (lim-FAN-jee-oh-graf-ee)	lymphangi/o = lymph vessel -graphy = process of recording	X-ray taken of the lymph vessels after the injection of dye into the foot. The lymph flow through the chest is traced.
Additional Diagnostic Procedures		
Monospot		Blood test for infectious mononucleosis.
scratch test		Form of allergy testing in which the body is exposed to an allergen through a light scratch on the skin. See Figure 6.18 ■.

Diagnostic Procedures (continued)

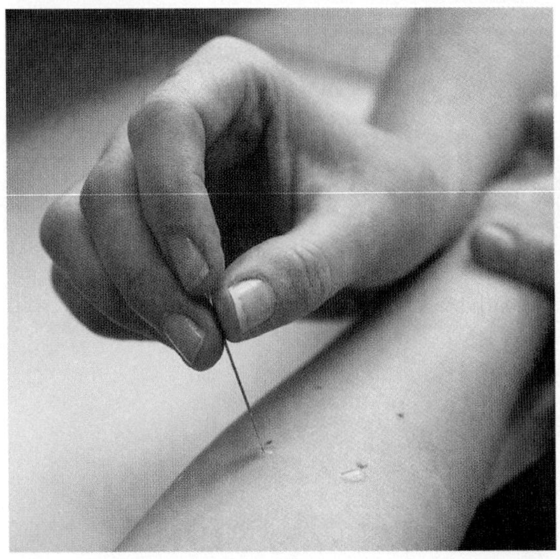

A

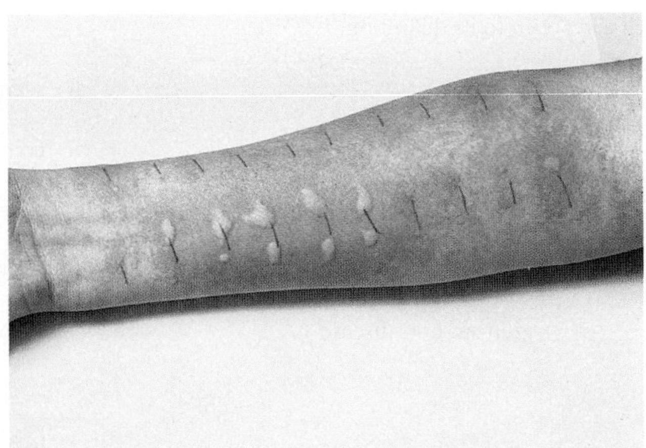

B

■ **Figure 6.18** A - Scratch test; patient is exposed to allergens through light scratch in the skin. B - Positive scratch test results. Inflammation indicates person is allergic to that substance. *(A - James King-Holmes/Science Photo Library/Science Source.; B - Southern Illinois University/Science Source.)*

Therapeutic Procedures

Term	Word Parts	Definition
Medical Procedures		
immunotherapy (IM-yoo-noh-thair-ah-pee)	immun/o = protection -therapy = treatment	Giving a patient an injection of immunoglobulins or antibodies in order to treat a disease. The antibodies may be produced by another person or animal, for example, antivenom for snake bites. More recent developments include treatments to boost the activity of the immune system, especially to treat cancer and AIDS.
vaccination (vak-sih-NAY-shun)		Exposure to a weakened pathogen that stimulates the immune response and antibody production in order to confer protection against the full-blown disease. Also called *immunization.*
Surgical Procedures		
adenoidectomy (add-eh-noyd-EK-toh-mee)	adenoid/o = adenoids -ectomy = surgical removal	Surgical removal of the adenoids.
lymphadenectomy (lim-fad-eh-NEK-toh-mee)	lymphaden/o = lymph node -ectomy = surgical removal	Removal of a lymph node. This is usually done to test for malignancy.
splenectomy (splee-NEK-toh-mee)	splen/o = spleen -ectomy = surgical removal	Surgical removal of the spleen.
thymectomy (thigh-MEK-toh-mee)	thym/o = thymus gland -ectomy = surgical removal	Surgical removal of the thymus gland.
tonsillectomy (ton-sih-LEK-toh-mee)	tonsill/o = tonsils -ectomy = surgical removal	Surgical removal of the tonsils.

Pharmacology

Classification		Action	Examples
antihistamine (an-tih-HIST-ah-meen)	anti- = against	Blocks the effects of histamine released by the body during an allergic reaction.	cetirizine, Zyrtec; diphenhydramine, Benadryl
corticosteroids (core-tih-koh-STARE-royds)	cortic/o = outer layer	A hormone produced by the adrenal cortex that has very strong anti-inflammatory properties. Particularly useful in treating autoimmune diseases.	prednisone; methylprednisolone, Solu-Medrol
immunosuppressants (im-yoo-noh-sue-PRESS-antz)	immun/o = protection	Block certain actions of the immune system. Required to prevent rejection of a transplanted organ.	mycophenolate mofetil, CellCept; cyclosporine, Neoral
protease inhibitor drugs (PROH-tee-ace)		Inhibit protease, an enzyme viruses need to reproduce.	indinavir, Crixivan; saquinavir, Fortovase
reverse transcriptase inhibitor drugs (trans-KRIP-tays)		Inhibit reverse transcriptase, an enzyme needed by viruses to reproduce.	lamivudine, Epivir; zidovudine, Retrovir

Practice As You Go

I. Match each procedure term with its definition

1. ________ ELISA
2. ________ vaccination
3. ________ scratch test
4. ________ Monospot
5. ________ lymphangiography

a. test for mononucleosis
b. an X-ray
c. immunization
d. allergy testing
e. blood test for antibody to HIV virus

Abbreviations

AIDS	acquired immunodeficiency syndrome	**KS**	Kaposi's sarcoma
ARC	AIDS-related complex	**mono**	mononucleosis
ELISA	enzyme-linked immunosorbent assay	**NHL**	non-Hodgkin's lymphoma
GVHD	graft versus host disease	**NK**	natural killer cells
HD	Hodgkin's disease	**PCP**	pneumocystis pneumonia
HIV	human immunodeficiency virus	**SCIDS**	severe combined immunodeficiency syndrome
Ig	immunoglobulins (IgA, IgD, IgE, IgG, IgM)		

Practice As You Go

J. What's the Abbreviation?

1. acquired immunodeficiency syndrome ______________________
2. AIDS-related complex ______________________
3. human immunodeficiency virus ______________________
4. mononucleosis ______________________
5. Kaposi's sarcoma ______________________
6. immunoglobulin ______________________
7. severe combined immunodeficiency syndrome ______________________
8. pneumocystis pneumonia ______________________

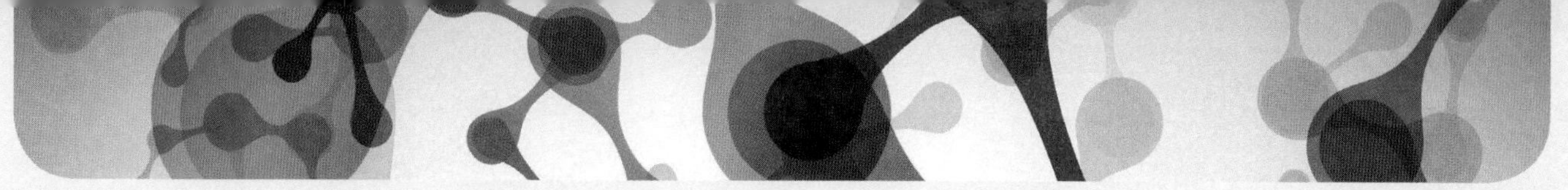

Chapter Review

Real-World Applications

Medical Record Analysis

This Discharge Summary contains 11 medical terms. Underline each term and write it in the list below the report. Then define each term. Note: Some terms are defined in other chapters; use your glossary-index to locate and define these terms.

Discharge Summary

Admitting Diagnosis:	Splenomegaly, weight loss, diarrhea, fatigue, chronic cough
Final Diagnosis:	Non-Hodgkin's lymphoma of spleen; splenectomy
History of Present Illness:	Patient is a 36-year-old businessman who was first seen in the office with complaints of feeling generally "rundown," intermittent diarrhea, weight loss, and, more recently, a dry cough. He states he has been aware of these symptoms for approximately six months. Monospot and ELISA are both negative. In spite of a 35-pound weight loss, he has abdominal swelling and splenomegaly was detected. He was admitted to the hospital for further evaluation and treatment.
Summary of Hospital Course:	Full-body MRI confirmed splenomegaly and located a 3-cm encapsulated tumor in the spleen. Biopsies taken from the splenic tumor confirmed the diagnosis of non-Hodgkin's lymphoma. The patient underwent splenectomy for removal of the tumor.
Discharge Plans:	Patient was discharged home following recovery from the splenectomy. The abdominal swelling and diarrhea were resolved, but the dry cough persisted. He was referred to an oncologist for evaluation and surveillance for metastases.

	Term	Definition
1.	______________	______________
2.	______________	______________
3.	______________	______________
4.	______________	______________
5.	______________	______________
6.	______________	______________
7.	______________	______________
8.	______________	______________
9.	______________	______________
10.	______________	______________
11.	______________	______________

Chart Note Transcription

The chart note below contains 10 phrases that can be reworded with a medical term that you learned in this chapter. Each phrase is identified with an underline. Determine the medical term and write your answers in the space provided.

Pearson General Hospital Consultation Report

Task Edit View Time Scale Options Help Download Archive Date: 17 May 2015

Current Complaint:	Patient is a 22-year-old female referred to the specialist in treating blood disorders **1** by her internist. Her complaints include fatigue, weight loss, and easy bruising.
Past History:	Patient had normal childhood diseases. She is a college student and was feeling well until symptoms gradually appeared starting approximately three months ago.
Signs and Symptoms:	An immunoassay test for HIV exposure **2** was normal. The measure of the blood's coagulation abilities **3** indicated that the blood took too long to form a clot. A blood test to count all the blood cells **4** reported too few red blood cells **5** and too few clotting cells. **6** There were too many white blood cells, **7** but they were immature and abnormal. A sample of bone marrow obtained for microscopic examination **8** found an excessive number of immature white blood cells.
Diagnosis:	Cancer of the white blood cell–forming bone marrow. **9**
Treatment:	Aggressive chemotherapy for the cancer of the white blood cell–forming bone marrow **9** and replacement blood from another person **10** to replace the erythrocytes and platelets.

1. ______________________________
2. ______________________________
3. ______________________________
4. ______________________________
5. ______________________________
6. ______________________________
7. ______________________________
8. ______________________________
9. ______________________________
10. ______________________________

Case Study

Below is a case study presentation of a patient with a condition covered in this chapter. Read the case study and answer the questions below. Some questions will ask for information not included within this chapter. Use your text, a medical dictionary, or any other reference material you choose to answer these questions.

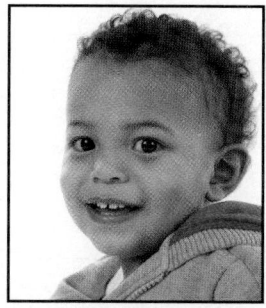

(Flashon Studio/Shutterstock)

A two-year-old boy is being seen by a hematologist. The child's symptoms include the sudden onset of high fevers, thrombopenia, epistaxis, gingival bleeding, petechiae, and ecchymoses after minor traumas. The physician has ordered a bone marrow aspiration to confirm the clinical diagnosis of acute lymphocytic leukemia. If the diagnosis is positive, the child will be placed immediately on intensive chemotherapy. The physician has informed the parents that treatment produces remission in 90% of children with ALL, especially those between the ages of two and eight.

Questions

1. What pathological condition does the hematologist suspect? Look this condition up in a reference source and include a short description of it.

   ____

   ____

2. List and define each of the patient's presenting symptoms in your own words.

   ____

   ____

3. What diagnostic test did the physician perform? Describe it in your own words.

   ____

   ____

4. Explain the phrase "clinical diagnosis" in your own words.

   ____

   ____

5. If the suspected diagnosis is correct, explain the treatment that will begin.

   ____

   ____

6. What do you think the term "remission" means?

   ____

   ____

Practice Exercises

A. Word Building Practice

The combining form **splen/o** refers to the spleen. Use it to write a term that means:

1. enlargement of the spleen ______________________
2. surgical removal of the spleen ______________________
3. cutting into the spleen ______________________

The combining form **lymph/o** refers to the lymph. Use it to write a term that means:

4. lymph cells ______________________
5. tumor of the lymph system ______________________

The combining form **lymphaden/o** refers to the lymph nodes. Use it to write a term that means:

6. disease of a lymph gland ______________________
7. tumor of a lymph gland ______________________
8. inflammation of a lymph gland ______________________

The combining form **immun/o** refers to the immune system. Use it to write a term that means:

9. specialist in the study of the immune system ______________________
10. immune protein ______________________
11. study of the immune system ______________________

The combining form **hemat/o** refers to blood. Use it to write a term that means:

12. relating to the blood ______________________
13. blood tumor or mass ______________________
14. blood formation ______________________

The combining form **hem/o** refers to blood. Use it to write a term that means:

15. blood destruction ______________________
16. blood protein ______________________

The suffix **-penia** refers to too few (cells). Use it to write a term that means:

17. too few white (cells) ______________________
18. too few red (cells) ______________________
19. too few of all cells ______________________

The suffix **-cytosis** refers to more than the normal number of cells. Use it to write a term that means:

20. more than the normal number of white cells ____________________
21. more than the normal number of red cells ____________________
22. more than the normal number of clotting cells ____________________

The suffix **-cyte** refers to cells. Use it to write a term that means:

23. red cell ____________________
24. white cell ____________________
25. lymph cell ____________________

B. What Does it Stand For?

1. basos ____________________
2. CBC ____________________
3. Hgb ____________________
4. PT ____________________
5. GVHD ____________________
6. RBC ____________________
7. PCV ____________________
8. ESR ____________________
9. diff ____________________
10. lymphs ____________________

C. Identify the Combining Form

	Combining Form	Example from Chapter
1. lymph node	______________	______________
2. clot	______________	______________
3. blood	______________	______________
4. tonsil	______________	______________
5. eat/swallow	______________	______________
6. lymph vessel	______________	______________
7. disease	______________	______________
8. spleen	______________	______________
9. lymph	______________	______________

D. Fill in the Blank

Kaposi's sarcoma	mononucleosis	Hodgkin's disease	aplastic
polycythemia vera	anaphylactic shock	AIDS	pernicious
pneumocystis	HIV		

1. The condition characterized by the production of too many red blood cells is called ______________________.
2. The Epstein–Barr virus is thought to be responsible for what infectious disease? ______________________.
3. A life-threatening allergic reaction is ______________________.
4. The virus responsible for causing AIDS is ______________________.
5. A cancer that is seen frequently in AIDS patients is ______________________.
6. An ELISA is used to test for ______________________.
7. Malignant tumors concentrate in lymph nodes with this disease: ______________________.
8. A type of pneumonia seen in AIDS patients is ______________________ pneumonia.
9. ______________________ anemia is a severe form of anemia caused by nonfunctioning red bone marrow.
10. ______________________ anemia is the result of a vitamin B_{12} deficiency.

E. Pharmacology Challenge

Fill in the classification for each drug description, then match the brand name.

Drug Description	Classification	Brand Name
1. _______ inhibits enzyme needed for viral reproduction	______________	a. HepLock
2. _______ prevents blood clot formation	______________	b. Activase
3. _______ stops bleeding	______________	c. Solu-Medrol
4. _______ blocks effects of histamine	______________	d. Amicar
5. _______ prevents rejection of a transplanted organ	______________	e. Epivir
6. _______ dissolves existing blood clots	______________	f. CellCept
7. _______ increases number of erythrocytes	______________	g. Procrit
8. _______ strong anti-inflammatory properties	______________	h. Zyrtec
9. _______ interferes with action of platelets	______________	i. Plavix

F. Terminology Matching

Match each term to its definition.

1. _______ culture and sensitivity
2. _______ hematocrit
3. _______ complete blood count
4. _______ erythrocyte sedimentation rate
5. _______ prothrombin time
6. _______ white cell differential
7. _______ red cell morphology

a. measure of blood's clotting ability
b. counts number of each type of blood cell
c. examines cells for abnormal shape
d. checks blood for bacterial growth and best antibiotic to use
e. determines number of each type of white blood cell
f. measures percent of whole blood that is red blood cells
g. an indicator of the presence of an inflammatory condition

G. Define the Term

1. immunotherapy ______________________________
2. Western blot ______________________________
3. opportunistic infection ______________________________
4. urticaria ______________________________
5. inflammation ______________________________
6. homologous transfusion ______________________________
7. pernicious anemia ______________________________
8. leukemia ______________________________
9. hemorrhage ______________________________
10. septicemia ______________________________

Labeling Exercise

Image A

Write the labels for this figure on the numbered lines provided.

1. ________________

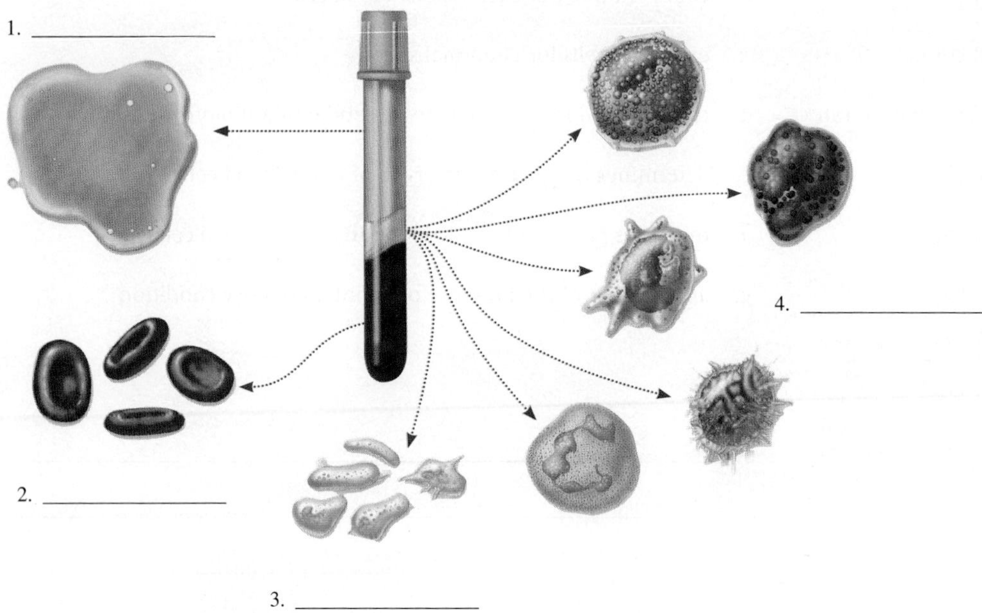

4. ________________

2. ________________

3. ________________

Image B

Write the labels for this figure on the numbered lines provided.

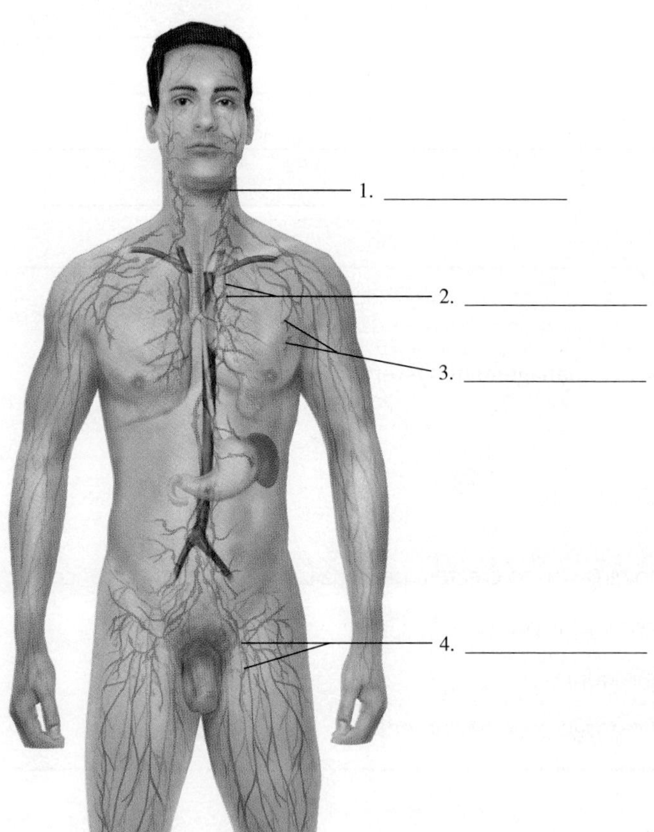

1. ________________

2. ________________

3. ________________

4. ________________

Image C

Write the labels for this figure on the numbered lines provided.

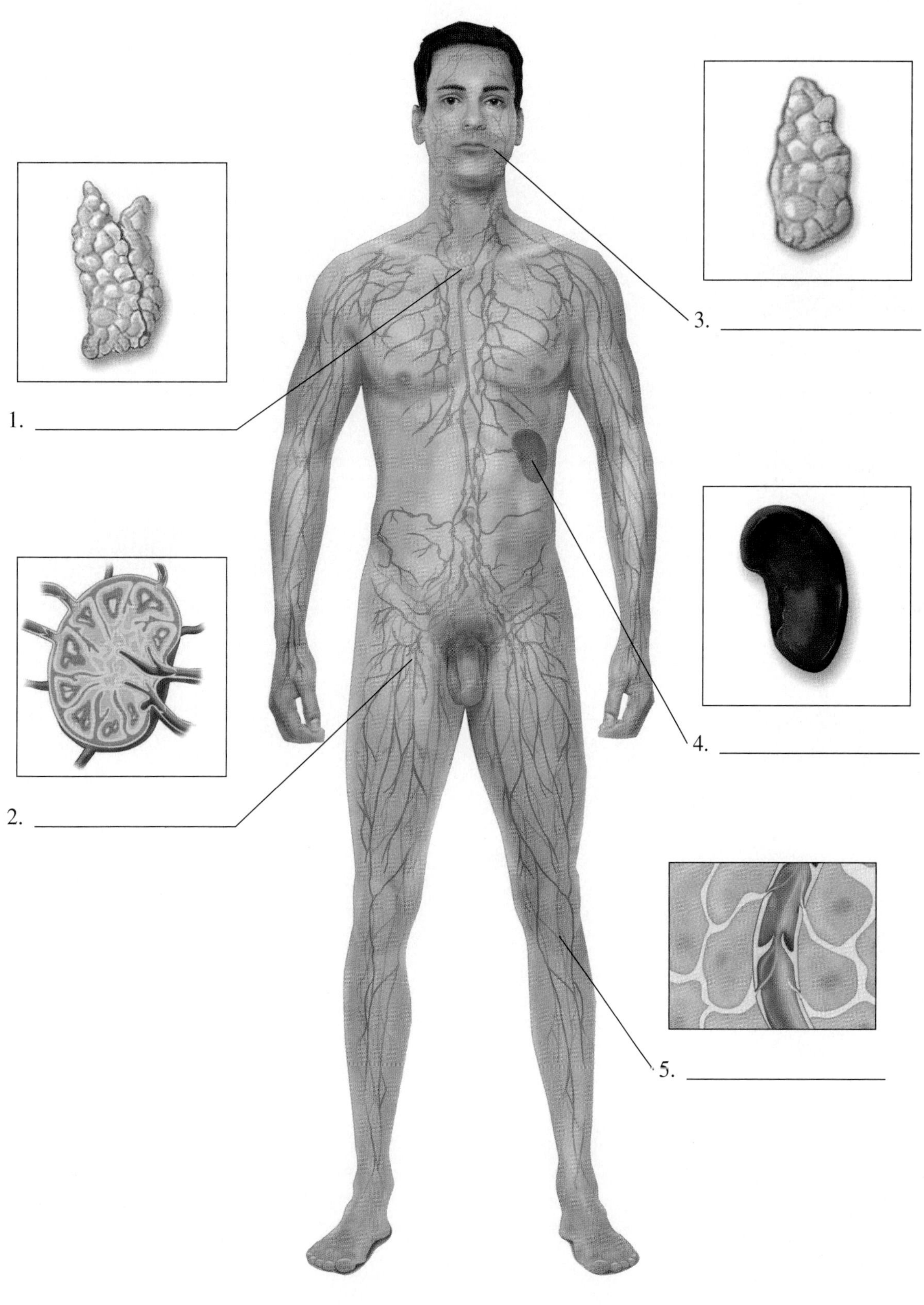

7

Respiratory System

Learning Objectives

Upon completion of this chapter, you will be able to

- Identify and define the combining forms and suffixes introduced in this chapter.
- Correctly spell and pronounce medical terms and major anatomical structures relating to the respiratory system.
- Locate and describe the major organs of the respiratory system and their functions.
- List and describe the lung volumes and capacities.
- Describe the process of respiration.
- Identify and define respiratory system anatomical terms.
- Identify and define selected respiratory system pathology terms.
- Identify and define selected respiratory system diagnostic procedures.
- Identify and define selected respiratory system therapeutic procedures.
- Identify and define selected medications relating to the respiratory system.
- Define selected abbreviations associated with the respiratory system.

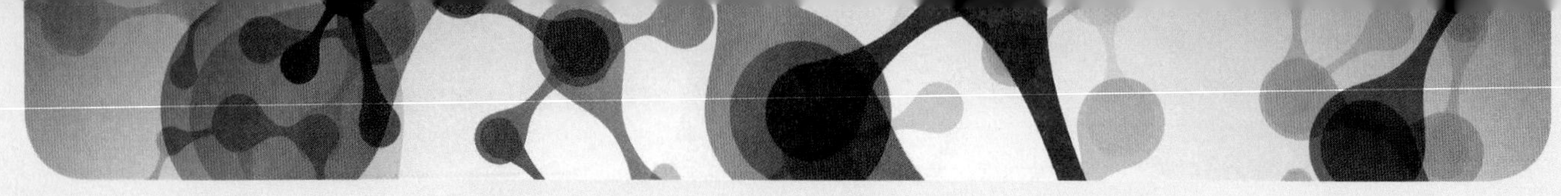

Respiratory System at a Glance

Function

The organs of the respiratory system are responsible for bringing fresh air into the lungs, exchanging oxygen for carbon dioxide between the air sacs of the lungs and the bloodstream, and exhaling the stale air.

Organs

Here are the primary structures that comprise the respiratory system:

nasal cavity
pharynx
larynx
trachea
bronchial tubes
lungs

Word Parts

Here are the most common word parts (with their meanings) used to build respiratory system terms. For a more comprehensive list, refer to the Terminology section of this chapter.

Combining Forms

aer/o	air
alveol/o	alveolus
anthrac/o	coal
atel/o	incomplete
bronch/o	bronchus
bronchi/o	bronchus
bronchiol/o	bronchiole
coni/o	dust
cyan/o	blue
cyst/o	sac
diaphragmat/o	diaphragm
epiglott/o	epiglottis
hal/o	to breathe
laryng/o	larynx
lob/o	lobe
muc/o	mucus
nas/o	nose
ox/o, ox/i	oxygen
pharyng/o	pharynx
pleur/o	pleura
pneum/o	lung, air
pneumon/o	lung, air
pulmon/o	lung
rhin/o	nose
sept/o	wall
sinus/o	sinus
somn/o	sleep
spir/o	breathing
trache/o	trachea
tuss/o	cough

Suffixes

-capnia	carbon dioxide
-osmia	smell
-phonia	voice
-pnea	breathing
-ptysis	spitting
-thorax	chest

Respiratory System Illustrated

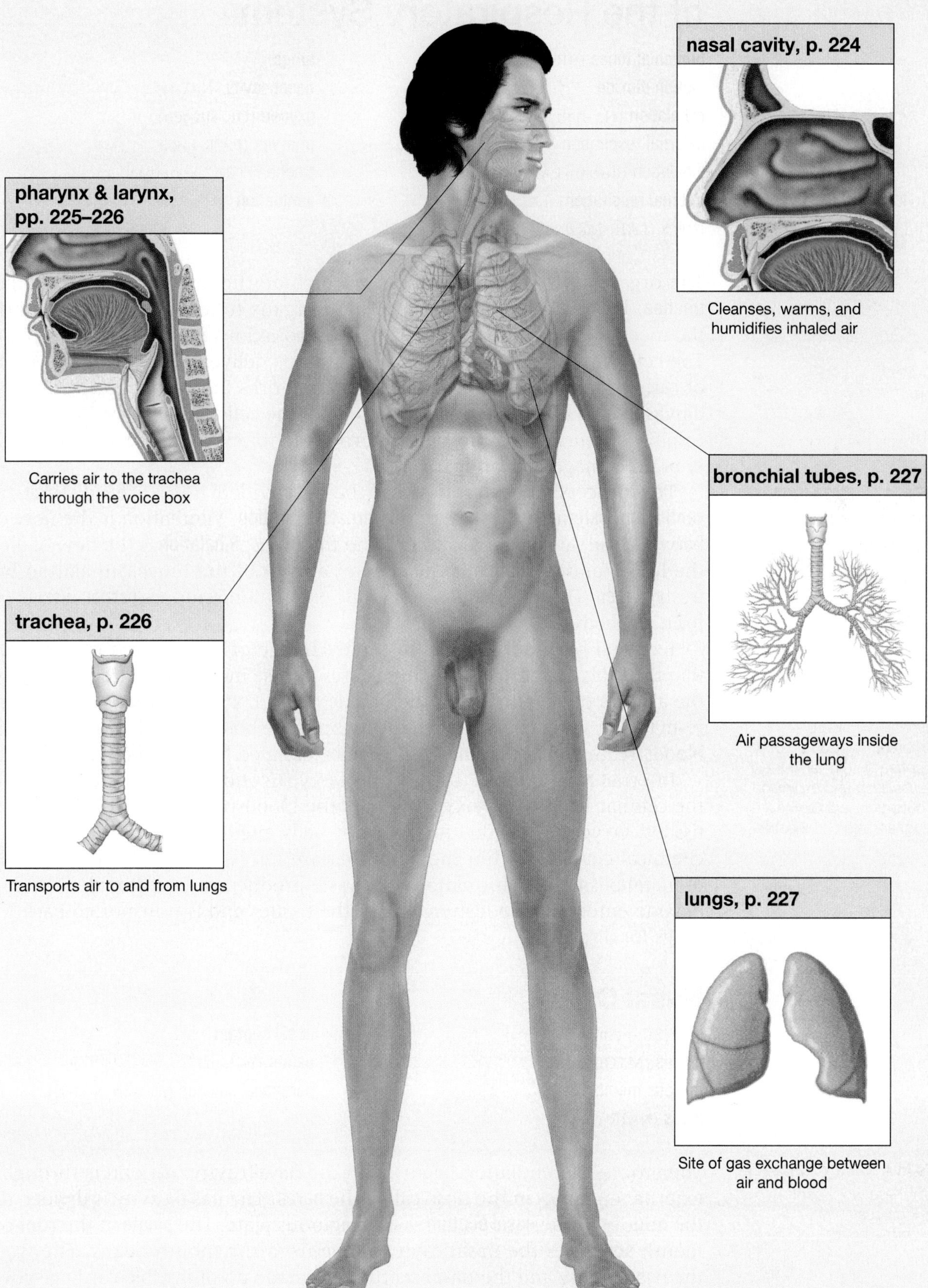

Anatomy and Physiology of the Respiratory System

bronchial tubes (BRONG-key-all)
carbon dioxide
exhalation (eks-hah-LAY-shun)
external respiration
inhalation (in-hah-LAY-shun)
internal respiration
larynx (LAIR-inks)
lungs
nasal cavity (NAY-zl)
oxygen (OK-sih-jen)
pharynx (FAIR-inks)
trachea (TRAY-kee-ah)
ventilation

The organs of the respiratory system include the **nasal cavity**, **pharynx**, **larynx**, **trachea**, **bronchial tubes**, and **lungs**. These organs function together to perform the mechanical and, for the most part, unconscious mechanism of respiration. The cells of the body require the continuous delivery of oxygen and removal of carbon dioxide. The respiratory system works in conjunction with the cardiovascular system to deliver oxygen to all the cells of the body. The process of respiration must be continuous; interruption for even a few minutes can result in brain damage and/or death.

What's In A Name?
Look for these word parts:
hal/o = to breathe
ox/i = oxygen
-al = pertaining to
di- = two
ex- = outward
in- = inward

Word Watch
The terms *inhalation* and *inspiration* (in- = inward + spir/o = breathing) can be used interchangeably. Similarly, the terms *exhalation* and *expiration* (ex- = outward + spir/o = breathing) are interchangeable.

The process of respiration can be subdivided into three distinct parts: **ventilation**, **external respiration**, and **internal respiration**. Ventilation is the flow of air between the outside environment and the lungs. **Inhalation** is the flow of air into the lungs, and **exhalation** is the flow of air out of the lungs. Inhalation brings fresh **oxygen** (O_2) into the air sacs, while exhalation removes **carbon dioxide** (CO_2) from the body.

External respiration refers to the exchange of oxygen and carbon dioxide that takes place in the lungs. These gases diffuse in opposite directions between the air sacs of the lungs and the bloodstream. Oxygen enters the bloodstream from the air sacs to be delivered throughout the body. Carbon dioxide leaves the bloodstream and enters the air sacs to be exhaled from the body.

Internal respiration is the process of oxygen and carbon dioxide exchange at the cellular level when oxygen leaves the bloodstream and is delivered to the tissues. Oxygen is needed for the body cells' metabolism, all the physical and chemical changes within the body that are necessary for life. The by-product of metabolism is the formation of a waste product, carbon dioxide. The carbon dioxide enters the bloodstream from the tissues and is transported back to the lungs for disposal.

Nasal Cavity

cilia (SIL-ee-ah)
mucus (MYOO-kus)
mucous membrane
nares (NAIR-eez)
nasal septum
palate (PAL-at)
paranasal sinuses (pair-ah-NAY-zl)

What's In A Name?
Look for these word parts:
muc/o = mucus
-ous = pertaining to

The process of ventilation begins with the nasal cavity. Air enters through two external openings in the nose called the **nares**. The nasal cavity is divided down the middle by the **nasal septum**, a cartilaginous plate. The **palate** in the roof of the mouth separates the nasal cavity above from the mouth below. The walls of the nasal cavity and the nasal septum are made up of flexible cartilage covered with **mucous membrane** (see Figure 7.1 ■). In fact, much of the respiratory tract is covered with mucous membrane, which secretes a sticky fluid, **mucus**, to help

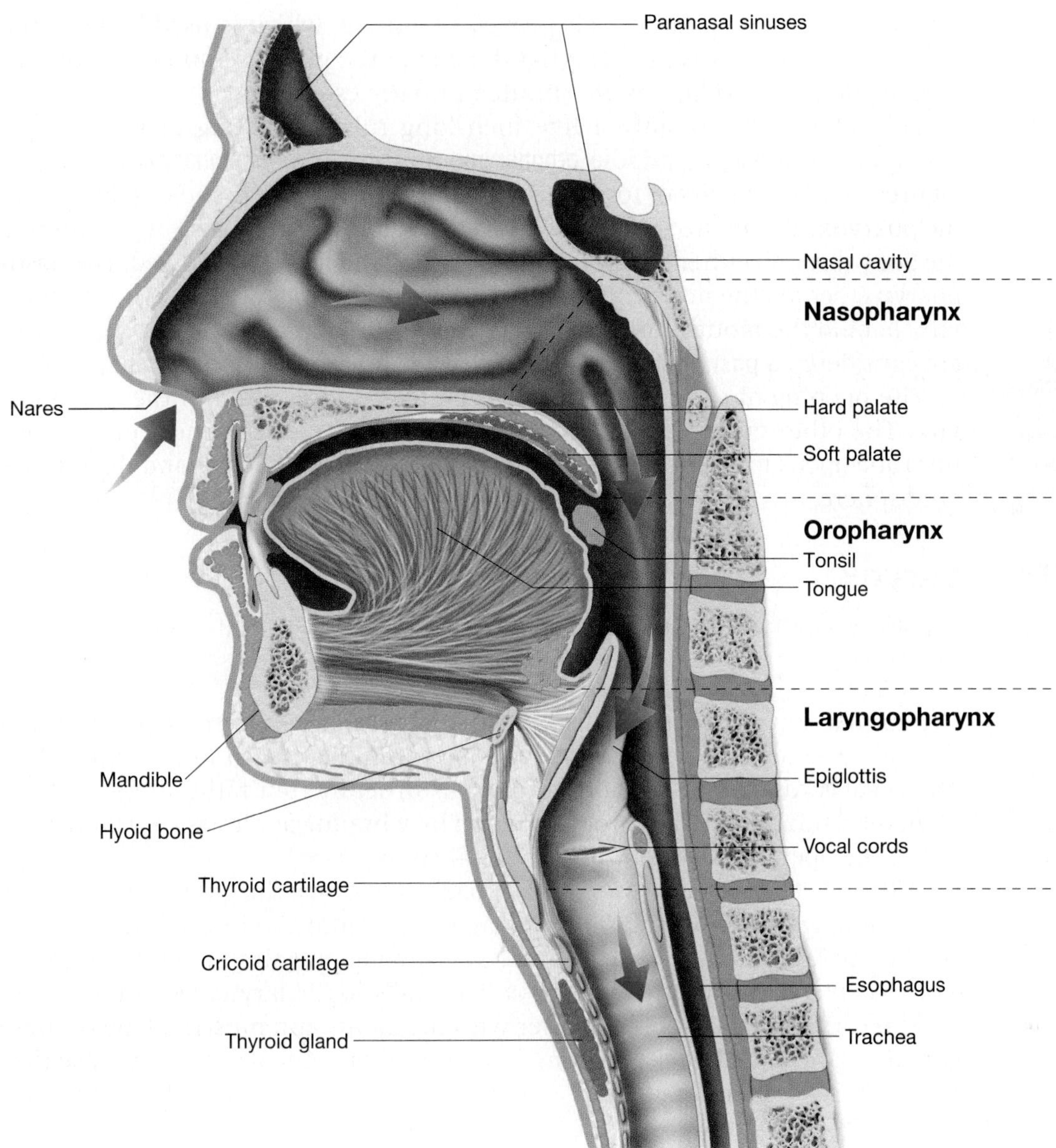

■ **Figure 7.1** Sagittal section of upper respiratory system illustrating the internal anatomy of the nasal cavity, pharynx, larynx, and trachea.

cleanse the air by trapping dust and bacteria. Since this membrane is also wet, it moisturizes inhaled air as it passes by the surface of the cavity. Very small hairs or **cilia** line the opening to the nose (as well as much of the airways), and filter out large dirt particles before they can enter the lungs. Capillaries in the mucous membranes warm inhaled air as it passes through the airways. Additionally, several **paranasal sinuses**, or air-filled cavities, are located within the facial bones. The sinuses act as an echo chamber during sound production and give resonance to the voice.

Med Term Tip

Anyone who has experienced a nosebleed, or *epistaxis*, is aware of the plentiful supply of blood vessels in the nose.

Word Watch

The term *cilia* means hair, and there are other body systems that have cilia or cilialike processes. For example, when discussing the eye, *cilia* means eyelashes.

Pharynx

adenoids (ADD-eh-noydz)
auditory tube
eustachian tube (yoo-STAY-she-en)
laryngopharynx (lair-ring-goh-FAIR-inks)
lingual tonsils (LING-gwal)
nasopharynx (nay-zoh-FAIR-inks)
oropharynx (or-oh-FAIR-inks)
palatine tonsils (PAL-ah-tine)
pharyngeal tonsils (fair-IN-jee-al)

What's In A Name?

Look for these word parts:
audit/o = hearing
lingu/o = tongue
-al = pertaining to
-ory = pertaining to

Med Term Tip

In the early 1970s it was common practice to remove the tonsils and adenoids in children suffering from repeated infections. However, it is now understood how important these organs are to remove pathogens from the air we breathe and the food we eat. Antibiotic treatment has also reduced the severity of infections.

Air next enters the pharynx, also called the *throat*, which is used by both the respiratory and digestive systems. At the end of the pharynx, air enters the trachea while food and liquids are shunted into the esophagus.

The pharynx is roughly a five inch-long tube consisting of three parts: the upper **nasopharynx**, middle **oropharynx**, and lower **laryngopharynx** (see again Figure 7.1). Three pairs of tonsils (collections of lymphatic tissue) are located in the pharynx. Tonsils are strategically placed to help keep pathogens from entering the body through either the air breathed or food and liquid swallowed. The nasopharynx, behind the nose, contains the **adenoids** or **pharyngeal tonsils.** The oropharynx, behind the mouth, contains the **palatine tonsils** and the **lingual tonsils**. Tonsils are considered a part of the lymphatic system and are discussed in Chapter 6.

The opening of the **eustachian** or **auditory tube** is also found in the nasopharynx. The other end of this tube is in the middle ear. Each time you swallow, this tube opens to equalize air pressure between the middle ear and the outside atmosphere.

What's In A Name?

Look for these word parts:
epi- = above

Med Term Tip

Stuttering may actually result from faulty neuromuscular control of the larynx. Some stutterers can sing or whisper without difficulty. Both singing and whispering involve movements of the larynx that differ from those required for regular speech.

Med Term Tip

The term *Adam's apple* is thought to come from a fable that when Adam realized he had sinned in the Garden of Eden, he was unable to swallow the apple in his throat.

Larynx

epiglottis (ep-ih-GLOT-iss)
glottis (GLOT-iss)
thyroid cartilage (THIGH-royd / CAR-tih-lij)
vocal cords

The larynx, or *voice box*, is a muscular structure located between the pharynx and the trachea and contains the **vocal cords** (see again Figure 7.1 and Figure 7.2 ■). The vocal cords are not actually cordlike in structure, but rather they are folds of membranous tissue that produce sound by vibrating as air passes through the **glottis**, the opening between the two vocal cords.

A flap of cartilaginous tissue, the **epiglottis**, sits above the glottis and provides protection against food and liquid being inhaled into the lungs. The epiglottis covers the larynx and trachea during swallowing and shunts food and liquid from the pharynx into the esophagus. The walls of the larynx are composed of several cartilage plates held together with ligaments and muscles. One of these cartilages, the **thyroid cartilage**, forms what is known as the *Adam's apple*. The thyroid cartilage is generally larger in males than in females and helps to produce the deeper male voice.

Trachea

The trachea, also called the *windpipe*, is the passageway for air that extends from the pharynx and larynx down to the main bronchi (see Figure 7.3 ■). Measuring approximately four inches in length, it is composed of smooth muscle and

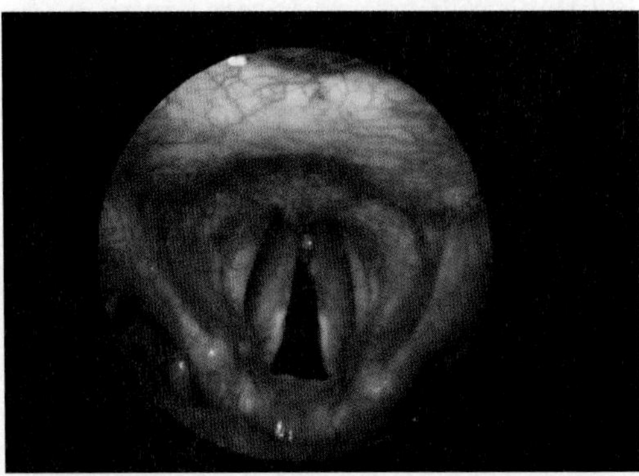

■ **Figure 7.2** The vocal cords within the larynx, superior view from the pharynx. *(CNRI/Science Source)*

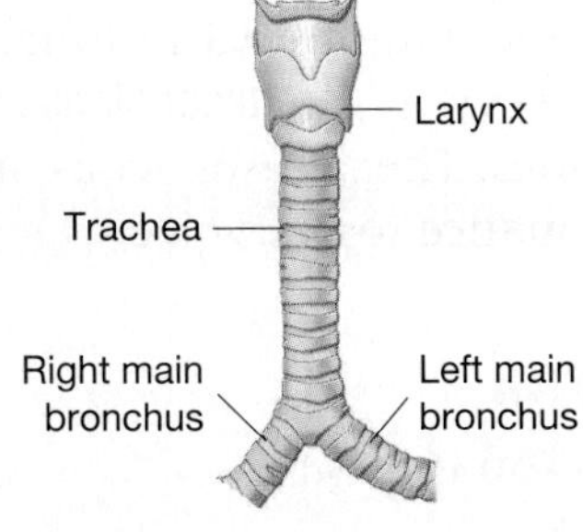

■ **Figure 7.3** Structure of the trachea which extends from the larynx above to the main bronchi below.

cartilage rings and is lined by mucous membrane and cilia. Therefore, it also assists in cleansing, warming, and moisturizing air as it travels to the lungs.

What's In A Name?

Look for these word parts:
bronchi/o = bronchus
-ole = small

Bronchial Tubes

alveoli (al-VEE-oh-lye)
bronchioles (BRONG-key-ohlz)
bronchus (BRONG-kus)
pulmonary capillaries
respiratory membrane

Med Term Tip

The respiratory system can be thought of as an upside-down tree and its branches. The trunk of the tree consists of the pharynx, larynx, and trachea. The trachea then divides into two branches, the bronchi. Each bronchus divides into smaller and smaller branches. In fact, this branching system of tubes is referred to as the *bronchial tree.*

The distal end of the trachea divides to form the left and right main (primary) bronchi. Each **bronchus** enters one of the lungs and branches repeatedly to form secondary and tertiary bronchi. Each branch becomes narrower until the narrowest branches, the **bronchioles**, are formed (see Figure 7.4■). Each bronchiole terminates in a small group of air sacs, called **alveoli**. Each lung has approximately 150 million alveoli. The walls of alveoli are elastic, giving them the ability to expand to hold air and then recoil to their original size. A network of **pulmonary capillaries** from the pulmonary blood vessels tightly encases each alveolus (see Figure 7.5■). In fact, the walls of the alveoli and capillaries are so tightly associated with each other they are referred to as a single unit, the **respiratory membrane**. The exchange of oxygen and carbon dioxide between the air within the alveolus and the blood inside the capillaries takes place across the respiratory membrane.

Lungs

apex
base
hilum (HYE-lum)
lobes
mediastinum (mee-dee-ass-TYE-num)
parietal pleura (pah-RYE-eh-tal)
pleura (PLOO-rah)
pleural cavity
serous fluid (SEER-us)
visceral pleura (VISS-er-al)

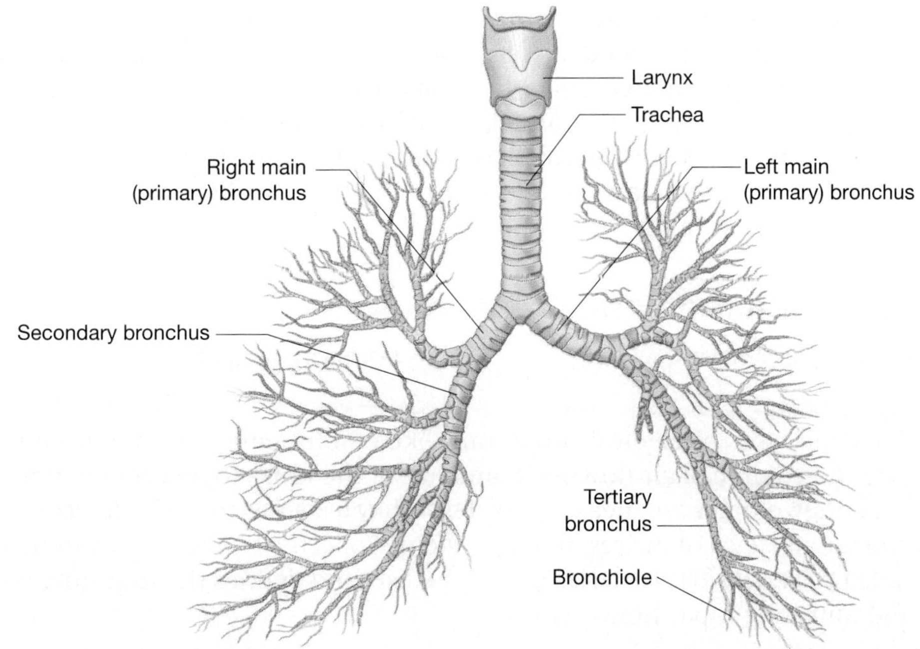

■ **Figure 7.4** The bronchial tree, note how each main bronchus enters a lung and then branches into smaller and smaller primary bronchi, secondary bronchi, and bronchioles.

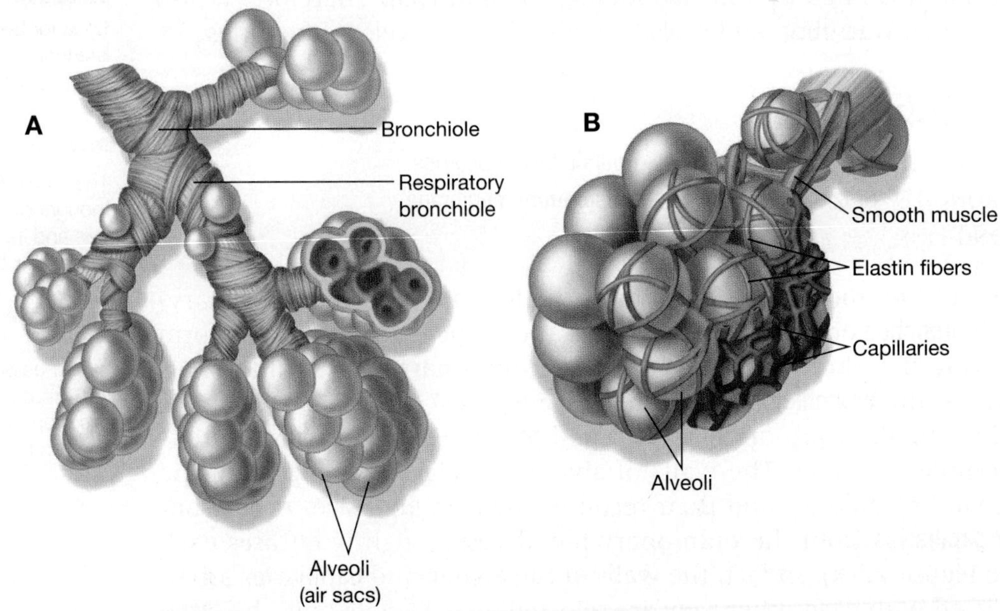

■ **Figure 7.5** A) Each bronchiole terminates in an alveolar sac, a group of alveoli. B) Alveoli encased by network capillaries, forming the respiratory membrane.

What's In A Name?
Look for these word parts:
pariet/o = cavity wall
viscer/o = internal organs
-al = pertaining to
-ous = pertaining to

Each lung is the total collection of the bronchi, bronchioles, and alveoli. They are spongy to the touch because they contain air. The lungs are protected by a double membrane called the **pleura**. The pleura's outer membrane is the **parietal pleura**, which also lines the wall of the chest cavity. The inner membrane, or **visceral pleura**, adheres to the surface of the lungs. The pleural membrane is folded in such a way that it forms a sac around each lung, referred to as the **pleural cavity**. There is normally slippery, watery **serous fluid** between the two layers of the pleura that reduces friction when the two layers rub together as the lungs repeatedly expand and contract.

Med Term Tip
Some of the abnormal lung sounds heard with a stethoscope, such as crackling and rubbing, are made when the parietal and/or visceral pleura become inflamed and rub against one another.

The lungs contain divisions or **lobes**. There are three lobes in the larger right lung (right upper, right middle, and right lower lobes) and two in the left lung (left upper and left lower lobes). The pointed superior portion of each lung is the **apex**, while the broader lower area is the **base**. Entry of structures like the bronchi, pulmonary blood vessels, and nerves into each lung occurs along its medial border in an area called the **hilum**. The lungs within the thoracic cavity are protected from puncture and damage by the ribs. The area between the right and left lung is called the **mediastinum** and contains the heart, aorta, esophagus, thymus gland, and trachea. See Figure 7.6 ■ for an illustration of the lungs within the chest cavity.

Lung Volumes and Capacities

pulmonary function test **respiratory therapist**

What's In A Name?
Look for these word parts:
spir/o = breathing
-ory = pertaining to
re- = again

For some types of medical conditions, like emphysema, it is important to measure the volume of air flowing in and out of the lungs to determine lung capacity. Lung volumes are measured by **respiratory therapists** to aid in determining the functioning level of the respiratory system. Collectively, these measurements are called **pulmonary function tests**. Table 7.1 ■ lists and defines the four lung volumes and four lung capacities.

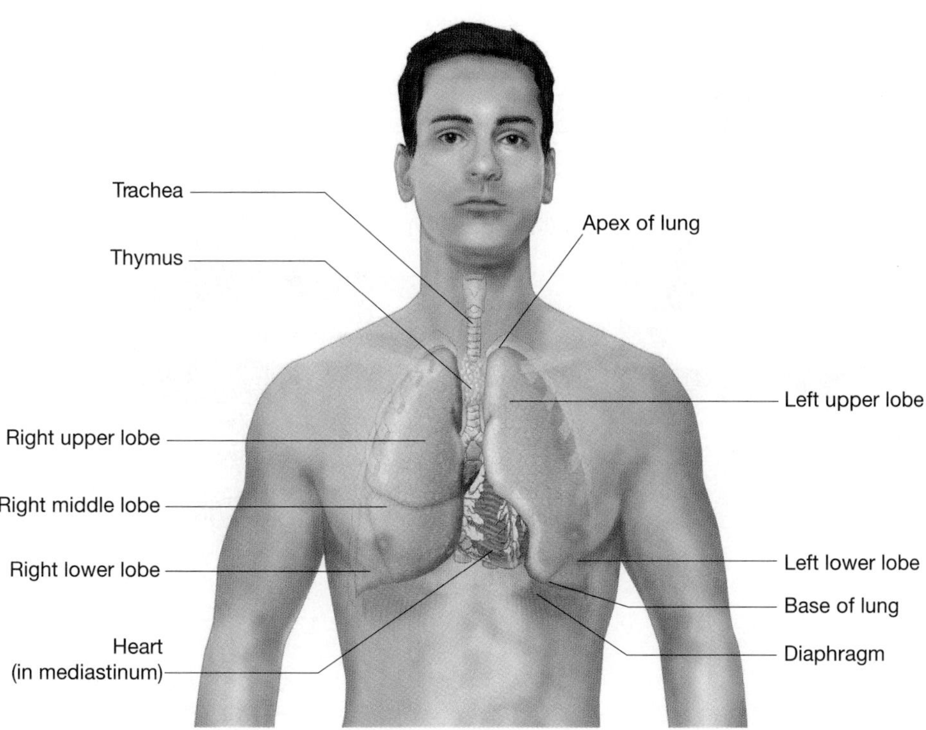

■ **Figure 7.6** Position of the lungs within the thoracic cavity, anterior view illustrating regions of the lungs and their relationship to other thoracic organs.

Respiratory Muscles

diaphragm

intercostal muscles (in-ter-KOS-tal)

Air moves in and out of the lungs due to the difference between the atmospheric pressure and the pressure within the chest cavity. The **diaphragm**, the muscle separating the abdomen from the thoracic cavity, produces this difference in pressure. To do this, the diaphragm contracts and moves downward. This increase in thoracic cavity volume causes a decrease in pressure, or negative thoracic pressure, within the chest cavity. Air then flows into the lungs (inhalation) to equalize the pressure. The **intercostal muscles** between the ribs assist in inhalation by raising the rib cage to further enlarge the thoracic cavity. See Figure 7.7■ for

What's In A Name?
Look for these word parts:
cost/o = ribs
-al = pertaining to
inter- = between

Table 7.1 Lung Volumes and Capacities

Term	Definition
Tidal volume (TV)	The amount of air that enters the lungs in a single inhalation or leaves the lungs in a single exhalation of quiet breathing. In an adult this is normally 500 mL.*
Inspiratory reserve volume (IRV)	The amount of air that can be forcibly inhaled after a normal inspiration. Also called complemental air; generally measures around 3,000 mL.*
Expiratory reserve volume (ERV)	The amount of air that can be forcibly exhaled after a normal quiet exhalation. This is also called supplemental air; approximately 1,000 mL.*
Residual volume (RV)	The air remaining in the lungs after a forced exhalation; about 1,500 mL* in an adult.
Inspiratory capacity (IC)	The volume of air inhaled after a normal exhale.
Functional residual capacity (FRC)	The air that remains in the lungs after a normal exhalation has taken place.
Vital capacity (VC)	The total volume of air that can be exhaled after a maximum inhalation. This amount will be equal to the sum of TV, IRV, and ERV.
Total lung capacity (TLC)	The volume of air in the lungs after a maximal inhalation.

* There is a normal range for measurements of the volume of air exchanged. The numbers given are for the average measurement.

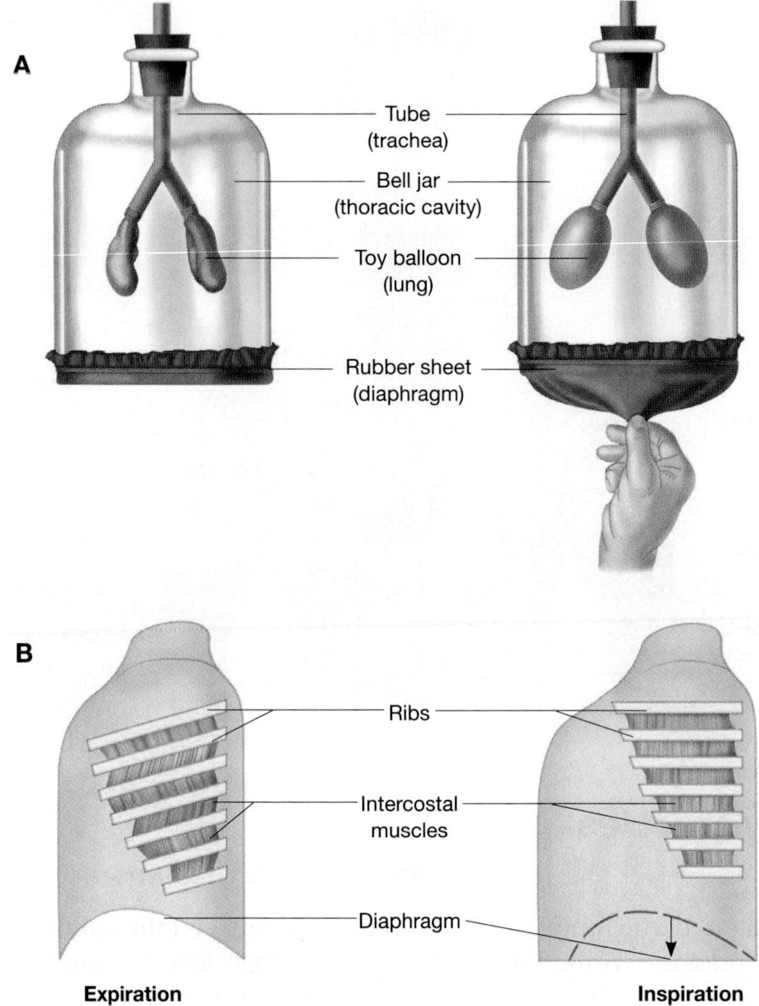

■ **Figure 7.7** A) Bell jar apparatus demonstrating how downward movement of the diaphragm results in air flowing into the lungs.
B) Action of the intercostal muscles lifts the ribs to assist the diaphragm in enlarging the volume of the thoracic cavity.

Med Term Tip

Diaphragmatic breathing is taught to singers and public speakers. You can practice this type of breathing by allowing your abdomen to expand during inhalation and contract during exhalation while your shoulders remain motionless.

an illustration of the role of the diaphragm in inhalation. Similarly, when the diaphragm and intercostal muscles relax, the thoracic cavity becomes smaller. This produces an increase in pressure within the cavity, or positive thoracic pressure, and air flows out of the lungs, resulting in exhalation. Therefore, a quiet, unforced exhalation is a passive process since it does not require any muscle contraction. When a forceful inhalation or exhalation is required, additional chest and neck muscles become active to create larger changes in thoracic pressure.

Respiratory Rate

vital signs

Respiratory rate (measured in breaths per minute) is one of our **vital signs** (VS), along with heart rate, temperature, and blood pressure. The respiratory rate is normally regulated by the level of CO_2 in the blood. When the CO_2 level is high, we breathe more rapidly to expel the excess. Likewise, when CO_2 levels drop, our respiratory rate will also drop.

When the respiratory rate falls outside the range of normal, it may indicate an illness or medical condition. For example, when a patient is running an elevated temperature and has shortness of breath (SOB) due to pneumonia, the respiratory rate may increase dramatically. Or a brain injury or some medications, such as those for pain, can cause a decrease in the respiratory rate. See Table 7.2 ■ for normal respiratory rate ranges for different age groups.

Table 7.2 Respiratory Rates for Different Age Groups

Age	Respirations Per Minute
Newborn	30–60
1-year-old	18–30
16-year-old	16–20
Adult	12–20

Practice As You Go

A. Complete the Statement

1. The organs of the respiratory system are ________, ________, ________, ________, ________, and ________.
2. The passageway for food, liquids, and air is the ________.
3. The ________ helps to keep food out of the respiratory tract.
4. The muscle that divides the thoracic cavity from the abdominal cavity is the ________.
5. The right lung has ________ lobes; the left lung has ________ lobes.
6. The air sacs at the ends of the bronchial tree are called ________.
7. The term for the double membrane around the lungs is ________.
8. The small branches of the bronchi are the ________ and the air sacs are the ________.

Terminology

Word Parts Used to Build Respiratory System Terms

The following lists contain the combining forms, suffixes, and prefixes used to build terms in the remaining sections of this chapter.

Combining Forms

aer/o	air
alveol/o	alveolus
angi/o	vessel
anthrac/o	coal
arteri/o	artery
atel/o	incomplete
bi/o	life
bronch/o	bronchus
bronchi/o	bronchus
bronchiol/o	bronchiole

carcin/o	cancer
cardi/o	heart
coni/o	dust
cortic/o	outer layer
cyan/o	blue
cyst/o	sac
cyt/o	cell
diaphragmat/o	diaphragm
embol/o	plug

epiglott/o	epiglottis
fibr/o	fibers
hem/o	blood
hist/o	tissue
laryng/o	larynx
lob/o	lobe
muc/o	mucus
myc/o	fungus
nas/o	nose
orth/o	straight

Combining Forms (continued)

ot/o	ear
ox/i	oxygen
ox/o	oxygen
pharyng/o	pharynx
pleur/o	pleura
pneum/o	air

pneumon/o	lung
pulmon/o	lung
py/o	pus
rhin/o	nose
sept/o	wall
sinus/o	sinus

somn/o	sleep
spir/o	breathing
thorac/o	chest
trache/o	trachea
tuss/o	cough

Suffixes

-al	pertaining to
-algia	pain
-ar	pertaining to
-ary	pertaining to
-capnia	carbon dioxide
-centesis	puncture to withdraw fluid
-dynia	pain
-eal	pertaining to
-ectasis	dilation
-ectomy	surgical removal
-emia	blood condition
-genic	produced by
-gram	record
-graphy	process of recording
-ia	condition
-ic	pertaining to

-ism	state of
-itis	inflammation
-logy	study of
-lytic	destruction
-meter	instrument to measure
-metry	process of measuring
-oma	tumor
-ory	pertaining to
-osis	abnormal condition
-osmia	smell
-ostomy	surgically create an opening
-otomy	cutting into
-phonia	voice
-plasm	formation

-plasty	surgical repair
-plegia	paralysis
-pnea	breathing
-ptysis	spitting
-rrhagia	abnormal flow condition
-rrhea	discharge
-scope	instrument for viewing
-scopy	process of visually examining
-spasm	involuntary muscle contraction
-stenosis	narrowing
-thorax	chest
-tic	pertaining to

Prefixes

a-	without
an-	without
anti-	against
brady-	slow
de-	without

dys-	difficult, abnormal
endo-	within
eu-	normal
hyper-	excessive
hypo-	insufficient

pan-	all
para-	beside
poly-	many
re-	again
tachy-	fast

Adjective Forms of Anatomical Terms

Term	Word Parts	Definition
alveolar (al-VEE-oh-lar)	alveol/o = alveolus -ar = pertaining to	Pertaining to the alveoli.
bronchial (BRONG-ee-all)	bronchi/o = bronchus -al = pertaining to	Pertaining to a bronchus.
bronchiolar (brong-KEY-oh-lar)	bronchiol/o = bronchiole -ar = pertaining to	Pertaining to a bronchiole.
diaphragmatic (dye-ah-frag-MAT-ik)	diaphragmat/o = diaphragm -ic = pertaining to	Pertaining to the diaphragm.
epiglottic (ep-ih-GLOT-ik)	epiglott/o = epiglottis -ic = pertaining to	Pertaining to the epiglottis.
laryngeal (lair-in-GEE-all)	laryng/o = larynx -eal = pertaining to	Pertaining to the larynx.
nasal (NAY-zal)	nas/o = nose -al = pertaining to	Pertaining to the nose or nasal cavity.
nasopharyngeal (NAY-zoh-fah-RIN-gee-all)	nas/o = nose pharyng/o = pharynx -eal = pertaining to	Pertaining to the nose and pharynx.
paranasal (pair-ah-NAY-zal)	para- = beside nas/o = nose -al = pertaining to	Pertaining to beside the nose.
pharyngeal (fair-in-GEE-all)	pharyng/o = pharynx -eal = pertaining to	Pertaining to the pharynx.
pleural (PLOO-ral)	pleur/o = pleura -al = pertaining to	Pertaining to the pleura.
pulmonary (PULL-mon-air-ee)	pulmon/o = lung -ary = pertaining to	Pertaining to the lung.
septal (SEP-tal)	sept/o = wall -al = pertaining to	Pertaining to the nasal septum.
thoracic (tho-RASS-ik)	thorac/o = chest -ic = pertaining to	Pertaining to the chest.
tracheal (TRAY-key-al)	trache/o = trachea -al = pertaining to	Pertaining to the trachea.

Practice As You Go

B. Give the adjective form for each anatomical structure

1. The larynx ______________________
2. The lung ______________________
3. Beside the sinuses ______________________
4. An alveolus ______________________
5. The nose ______________________
6. The diaphragm ______________________

Pathology

Term	Word Parts	Definition
Medical Specialties		
internal medicine		Branch of medicine involving the diagnosis and treatment of diseases and conditions of internal organs such as the respiratory system. The physician is an *internist*.
otorhinolaryngology (ENT) (oh-toh-rye-noh-lair-in-GOL-oh-jee)	ot/o = ear rhin/o = nose laryng/o = larynx -logy = study of	Branch of medicine involving the diagnosis and treatment of conditions and diseases of the ear, nose, and throat region. The physician is an *otorhinolaryngologist*. This medical specialty may also be referred to as *otolaryngology*.
pulmonology (pull-mon-ALL-oh-jee)	pulmon/o = lung -logy = study of	Branch of medicine involved in the diagnosis and treatment of diseases and disorders of the respiratory system. Physician is a *pulmonologist*.
respiratory therapy	re- = again spir/o = breathing -ory = pertaining to	Allied health specialty that assists patients with respiratory and cardiopulmonary disorders. Duties of a *respiratory therapist* include conducting pulmonary function tests, monitoring oxygen and carbon dioxide levels in the blood, administering breathing treatments, and ventilator management.
thoracic surgery (tho-RASS-ik)	thorac/o = chest -ic = pertaining to	Branch of medicine involving the diagnosis and treatment of conditions and diseases of the respiratory system by surgical means. Physician is a *thoracic surgeon*.

Pathology (continued)

Term	Word Parts	Definition
Signs and Symptoms		
anosmia (ah-NOZ-mee-ah)	an- = without -osmia = smell	Lack of the sense of smell.
anoxia (ah-NOK-see-ah)	an- = without ox/o = oxygen -ia = condition	Condition of receiving almost no oxygen from inhaled air.
aphonia (a-FOH-nee-ah)	a- = without -phonia = voice	Condition of being unable to produce sounds.
apnea (AP-nee-ah)	a- = without -pnea = breathing	Not breathing.
asphyxia (as-FIK-see-ah)	a- = without -ia = condition	Lack of oxygen that can lead to unconsciousness and death if not corrected immediately; also called *asphyxiation* or *suffocation*. Common causes include drowning, foreign body in the respiratory tract, poisoning, and electric shock.
aspiration (as-peer-RAY-shun)	spir/o = breathing	Refers to withdrawing fluid from a body cavity using suction. For example, using a long needle and syringe to withdraw fluid from the pleural cavity, or using a vacuum pump to remove phlegm from a patient's airway. Additionally, it refers to inhaling food, liquid, or a foreign object into the airways, which may lead to the development of pneumonia.
bradypnea (bray-DIP-nee-ah)	brady- = slow -pnea = breathing	Breathing too slowly; a low respiratory rate.
bronchiectasis (brong-key-EK-tah-sis)	bronchi/o = bronchus -ectasis = dilation	Dilated bronchus.
bronchospasm (BRONG-koh-spazm)	bronch/o = bronchus -spasm = involuntary muscle contraction	Involuntary muscle spasm of the smooth muscle in the wall of the bronchus.
Cheyne–Stokes respiration (CHAIN / STOHKS / res-pir-AY-shun)	re- = again spir/o = breathing	Abnormal breathing pattern in which there are long periods (10–60 seconds) of apnea followed by deeper, more rapid breathing. Named for John Cheyne, a Scottish physician, and Sir William Stokes, an Irish surgeon.
clubbing		Abnormal widening and thickening of the ends of the fingers and toes associated with chronic oxygen deficiency. Seen in patients with chronic respiratory conditions or circulatory problems.
crackles		Abnormal crackling or bubbling sound made during inspiration. Usually indicates the presence of fluid or mucus in the small airways. Also called *rales*.

Pathology (continued)

Term	Word Parts	Definition
cyanosis (sigh-ah-NO-sis)	cyan/o = blue -osis = abnormal condition 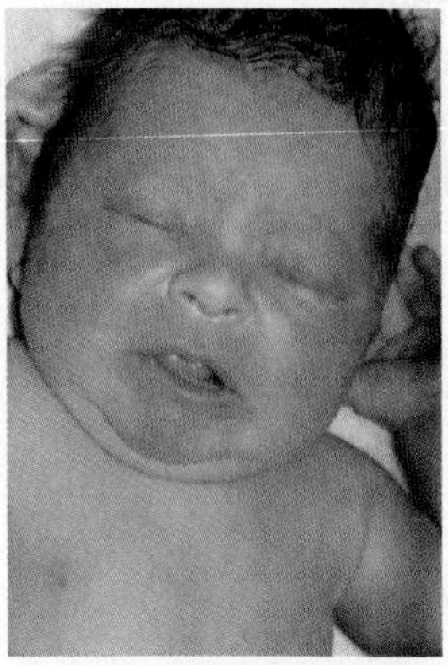	Refers to the bluish tint of skin that is receiving an insufficient amount of oxygen or circulation.
dysphonia (dis-FOH-nee-ah)	dys- = difficult, abnormal -phonia = voice	Condition of having difficulty producing sounds or producing abnormal sounds.
dyspnea (DISP-nee-ah)	dys- = difficult -pnea = breathing	Term describing difficult or labored breathing.
epistaxis (ep-ih-STAKS-is)		Nosebleed.
eupnea (yoop-NEE-ah)	eu- = normal -pnea = breathing	Normal breathing and respiratory rate.
hemoptysis (hee-MOP-tih-sis)	hem/o = blood -ptysis = spitting	To cough up blood or blood-stained sputum.
hemothorax (hee-moh-THOH-raks)	hem/o = blood -thorax = chest	Presence of blood in the chest cavity.
hypercapnia (high-per-CAP-nee-ah)	hyper- = excessive -capnia = carbon dioxide	Condition of having excessive carbon dioxide in the body.
hyperpnea (high-per-NEE-ah)	hyper- = excessive -pnea = breathing	Taking deep breaths.
hyperventilation (HYE-per-vent-ill-a-shun)	hyper- = excessive	Breathing both too fast (tachypnea) and too deep (hyperpnea).
hypocapnia (high-poh-CAP-nee-ah)	hypo- = insufficient -capnia = carbon dioxide	An insufficient level of carbon dioxide in the body; a very serious problem because it is the presence of carbon dioxide that stimulates respiration, not the absence of oxygen. Therefore, a person with low carbon dioxide levels would respond with an increased respiratory rate.
hypopnea (high-POP-nee-ah)	hypo- = insufficient -pnea = breathing	Taking shallow breaths.

■ **Figure 7.8** A cyanotic infant. Note the bluish tinge to the skin around the lips, chin, and nose. *(St Bartholomew's Hospital, London/Science Source)*

Med Term Tip

When divers wish to hold their breath longer, they first hyperventilate (breathe faster and deeper) in order to get rid of as much CO_2 as possible. This will hold off the urge to breathe, allowing a diver to stay submerged longer.

Pathology (continued)

Term	Word Parts	Definition
hypoventilation (HYE-poh-vent-ill-a-shun)	hypo- = insufficient	Breathing both too slow (bradypnea) and too shallow (hypopnea).
hypoxemia (high-pox-EE-mee-ah)	hypo- = insufficient ox/o = oxygen -emia = blood condition	Condition of having an insufficient amount of oxygen in the bloodstream.
hypoxia (high-POX-ee-ah)	hypo- = insufficient ox/o = oxygen -ia = condition	Condition of receiving an insufficient amount of oxygen from inhaled air.
laryngoplegia (lair-RING-goh-plee-gee-ah)	laryng/o = larynx -plegia = paralysis	Paralysis of the muscles controlling the larynx.
orthopnea (or-THOP-nee-ah)	orth/o = straight -pnea = breathing	Term describing dyspnea that is worsened by lying flat. The patient feels able to breathe easier while sitting straight up; a common occurrence in those with pulmonary disease.
pansinusitis (pan-sigh-nus-EYE-tis)	pan- = all sinus/o = sinus -itis = inflammation	Inflammation of all the paranasal sinuses.
patent (PAY-tent)		Open or unblocked, such as a patent airway.
phlegm (FLEM)		Thick mucus secreted by the membranes lining the respiratory tract. When phlegm is coughed through the mouth, it is called *sputum*. Phlegm is examined for color, odor, and consistency and tested for the presence of bacteria, viruses, and fungi.
pleural rub (PLOO-ral)	pleur/o = pleura -al = pertaining to	Grating sound made when the two layers of the pleura rub together during respiration. It is caused when one of the surfaces becomes thicker as a result of inflammation or other disease conditions. This rub can be felt through the fingertips when placed on the chest wall or heard through a stethoscope.
pleurodynia (ploor-oh-DIN-ee-ah)	pleur/o = pleura -dynia = pain	Pleural pain.
pyothorax (pye-oh-THOH-raks)	py/o = pus -thorax = chest	Presence of pus in the chest cavity; indicates a bacterial infection.
rhinitis (rye-NYE-tis)	rhin/o = nose -itis = inflammation	Inflammation of the nasal cavity.
rhinorrhagia (rye-noh-RAH-jee-ah)	rhin/o = nose -rrhagia = abnormal flow condition	Rapid flow of blood from the nose.
rhinorrhea (rye-noh-REE-ah)	rhin/o = nose -rrhea = discharge	Discharge from the nose; commonly called a *runny nose*.

Pathology (continued)

Term	Word Parts	Definition
rhonchi (RONG-kigh)		Somewhat musical sound during expiration, often found in asthma or infection. Caused by spasms of the bronchial tubes. Also called *wheezing*.
shortness of breath (SOB)		Term used to indicate that a patient is having some difficulty breathing; also called *dyspnea*. The causes can range from mild SOB after exercise to SOB associated with heart disease.
sputum (SPEW-tum)		Mucus or phlegm coughed up from the lining of the respiratory tract.
	Med Term Tip The term *sputum*, from the Latin word meaning "to spit," now refers to the material coughed up and spit out from the respiratory system.	
stridor (STRIGH-dor)		Harsh, high-pitched, noisy breathing sound made when there is an obstruction of the bronchus or larynx. Found in conditions such as croup in children.
tachypnea (tak-ip-NEE-ah)	tachy- = fast -pnea = breathing	Breathing fast; a high respiratory rate.
thoracalgia (thor-ah-KAL-jee-ah)	thorac/o = chest -algia = pain	Chest pain. Does not refer to angina pectoris.
tracheostenosis (tray-kee-ohsteh-NOH-sis)	trache/o = trachea -stenosis = narrowing	Narrowing of the trachea.
Upper Respiratory System		
croup (KROOP)		Acute respiratory condition found in infants and children characterized by a barking type of cough or stridor.
diphtheria (dif-THEAR-ee-ah)	-ia = condition	Bacterial upper respiratory infection characterized by the formation of a thick membranous film across the throat and a high mortality rate. Rare now due to the childhood diphtheria, pertussis, tetanus (DPT) vaccine.
laryngitis (lair-in-JYE-tis)	laryng/o = larynx -itis = inflammation	Inflammation of the larynx.
nasopharyngitis (nay-zoh-fair-in-JYE-tis)	nas/o = nose pharyng/o = pharynx -itis = inflammation	Inflammation of the nasal cavity and pharynx; commonly called the *common cold*.
pertussis (per-TUH-sis)	tuss/o = cough	Commonly called *whooping cough*, due to the whoop sound made when coughing. An infectious bacterial disease of the upper respiratory system that children receive immunization against as part of their DPT shots.
pharyngitis (fair-in-JYE-tis)	pharyng/o = pharynx -itis = inflammation	Inflammation of the pharynx; commonly called a *sore throat*.

Pathology (continued)

Term	Word Parts	Definition
rhinomycosis (rye-noh-my-KOH-sis)	rhin/o = nose myc/o = fungus -osis = abnormal condition	Fungal infection of the nasal cavity.
Bronchial Tubes		
asthma (AZ-mah) Med Term Tip The term *asthma*, from the Greek word meaning "panting," describes the breathing pattern of a person having an asthma attack.		Disease caused by various conditions, like allergens, and resulting in constriction of the bronchial airways, dyspnea, coughing, and wheezing. Can cause violent spasms of the bronchi (bronchospasms) but is generally not a life-threatening condition. Medication can be very effective.
bronchiectasis (brong-key-EK-tah-sis)	bronchi/o = bronchus -ectasis = dilation	Abnormal enlargement of bronchi; may be the result of a lung infection. This condition can be irreversible and result in destruction of the bronchial walls. Major symptoms include coughing up a large amount of purulent sputum, crackles, and hemoptysis.
bronchitis (brong-KIGH-tis)	bronch/o = bronchus -itis = inflammation	Inflammation of a bronchus.
bronchogenic carcinoma (brong-koh-JEN-ik / car-sin-OH-mah)	bronch/o = bronchus -genic = produced by carcin/o = cancer -oma = tumor	Malignant tumor originating in the bronchi. Usually associated with a history of cigarette smoking.

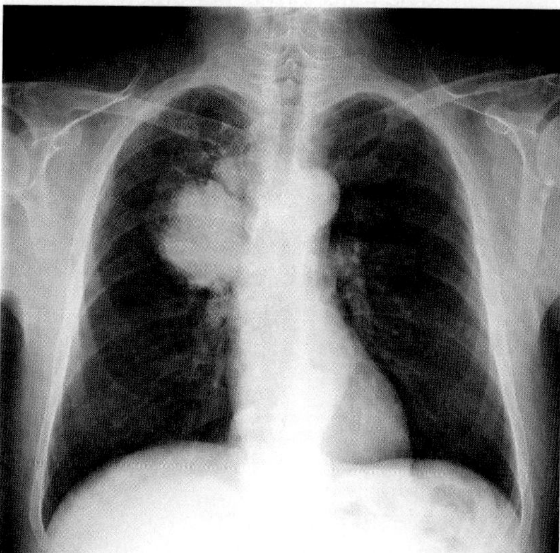

■ **Figure 7.9** Color enhanced X-ray of large malignant tumor in the right lung. *(Du Cane Medical Imaging Ltd./Science Source)*

Term	Word Parts	Definition
Lungs		
adult respiratory distress syndrome (ARDS)	re- = again spir/o = breathing -ory = pertaining to	Acute respiratory failure in adults characterized by tachypnea, dyspnea, cyanosis, tachycardia, and hypoxemia. May follow trauma, pneumonia, or septic infections. Also called *acute respiratory distress syndrome*.

Pathology (continued)

Term	Word Parts	Definition
anthracosis (an-thra-KOH-sis)	anthrac/o = coal -osis = abnormal condition	Type of pneumoconiosis that develops from the collection of coal dust in the lung. Also called *black lung* or *miner's lung*.
asbestosis (az-bes-TOH-sis)	-osis = abnormal condition	Type of pneumoconiosis that develops from collection of asbestos fibers in the lungs. May lead to the development of lung cancer.
atelectasis (at-eh-LEK-tah-sis)	atel/o = incomplete -ectasis = dilation	Condition in which the alveoli in a portion of the lung collapse, preventing the respiratory exchange of oxygen and carbon dioxide. Can be caused by a variety of conditions, including pressure on the lung from a tumor or other object. Term also used to describe the failure of a newborn's lungs to expand.
chronic obstructive pulmonary disease (COPD) (PULL-mon-air-ee)	pulmon/o = lung -ary = pertaining to	Progressive, chronic, and usually irreversible group of conditions, like emphysema, in which the lungs have a diminished capacity for inspiration (inhalation) and expiration (exhalation). The person may have dyspnea upon exertion and a cough.
cystic fibrosis (CF) (SIS-tik / fye-BROH-sis) Med Term Tip Cystic fibrosis received its name from fibrotic cysts that are visible in the pancreas as scarred areas.	cyst/o = sac -ic = pertaining to fibr/o = fibers -osis = abnormal condition	Hereditary condition causing the exocrine glands to malfunction. The patient produces very thick mucus that causes severe congestion within the lungs, pancreas, and intestine. Through more advanced treatment, many children are now living into adulthood with this disease.
emphysema (em-fih-SEE-mah)		Pulmonary condition characterized by the destruction of the walls of the alveoli, resulting in fewer, overexpanded air sacs. Can occur as a result of long-term heavy smoking. Air pollution also worsens this disease. The patient may not be able to breathe except in a sitting or standing position.
histoplasmosis (his-toh-plaz-MOH-sis)	hist/o = tissue -plasm = formation -osis = abnormal condition	Pulmonary infection caused by the fungus *Histoplasma capsulatum*, found in dust and in the droppings of pigeons and chickens. The translation of the name of this condition reflects the microscopic appearance of the fungus.

Pathology (continued)

Term	Word Parts	Definition
infant respiratory distress syndrome (IRDS)	re- = again spir/o = breathing -ory = pertaining to	Lung condition most commonly found in premature infants that is characterized by tachypnea and respiratory grunting. The condition is caused by a lack of surfactant necessary to keep the lungs inflated. Also called *hyaline membrane disease* (HMD) and *respiratory distress syndrome of the newborn*.
influenza (flu) (in-floo-EN-za)		Viral infection of the respiratory system characterized by chills, fever, body aches, and fatigue. Commonly called the *flu*.
Legionnaires' disease (lee-jen-AYRZ)		Severe, often fatal bacterial infection characterized by pneumonia and liver and kidney damage. Named after people who came down with it at an American Legion convention in 1976.
***Mycoplasma* pneumonia** (MY-koh-plaz-ma)	myc/o = fungus -plasm = formation	Less severe but longer lasting form of pneumonia caused by the *Mycoplasma pneumoniae* bacteria. Also called *walking pneumonia*. The translation of the name of this condition reflects the microscopic appearance of the bacteria (in spite of its name, the pathologic agent is a bacterium).
pneumoconiosis (noo-moh-koh-nee-OH-sis)	pneum/o = lung coni/o = dust -osis = abnormal condition	Condition resulting from inhalation of environmental particles that become toxic. Can be the result of inhaling coal dust (anthracosis) or asbestos (asbestosis).
pneumonia (noo-MOH-nee-ah)	pneumon/o = lung -ia = condition	Inflammatory condition of the lung that can be caused by bacteria, viruses, fungi, and aspirated substances. Results in the filling of the alveoli and air spaces with fluid.
pulmonary edema (PULL-mon-air-ee / eh-DEE-mah)	pulmon/o = lung -ary = pertaining to	Condition in which lung tissue retains an excessive amount of fluid, especially in the alveoli. Results in dyspnea.
pulmonary embolism (EM-boh-lizm)	pulmon/o = lung -ary = pertaining to embol/o = plug -ism = state of	Obstruction of the pulmonary artery or one of its branches by an embolus (often a blood clot broken away from another area of the body). May cause an infarct in the lung tissue.
pulmonary fibrosis (figh-BROH-sis)	pulmon/o = lung -ary = pertaining to fibr/o = fibers -osis = abnormal condition	Formation of fibrous scar tissue in the lungs that leads to decreased ability to expand the lungs. May be caused by infections, pneumoconiosis, autoimmune diseases, and toxin exposure.

Pathology (continued)

Term	Word Parts	Definition
severe acute respiratory syndrome (SARS)	re- = again spir/o = breathing -ory = pertaining to	Acute viral respiratory infection that begins like the flu but quickly progresses to severe dyspnea; high fatality rate in persons over age 65. First appeared in China in 2003.
silicosis (sil-ih-KOH-sis)	-osis = abnormal condition	Type of pneumoconiosis that develops from the inhalation of silica (quartz) dust found in quarrying, glasswork, sandblasting, and ceramics.
sleep apnea (AP-nee-ah)	a- = without -pnea = breathing	Condition in which breathing stops repeatedly during sleep long enough to cause a drop in oxygen levels in the blood.
sudden infant death syndrome (SIDS)		Unexpected and unexplained death of an apparently well infant under one year of age. The child suddenly stops breathing for unknown reasons.
tuberculosis (TB) (too-ber-kyoo-LOH-sis)	-osis = abnormal condition	Infectious disease caused by the bacteria *Mycobacterium tuberculosis.* Most commonly affects the respiratory system and causes inflammation and calcification in the lungs. Tuberculosis incidence is on the increase and is seen in many patients with weakened immune systems. Multidrug-resistant tuberculosis is a particularly dangerous form of the disease because some bacteria have developed a resistance to the standard drug therapy.
Pleural Cavity		
empyema (em-pye-EE-mah)	py/o = pus	Pus within the pleural space usually associated with a bacterial infection. Also called *pyothorax*.
pleural effusion (PLOO-ral / eh-FYOO-zhun)	pleur/o = pleura -al = pertaining to	Abnormal accumulation of fluid in the pleural cavity preventing the lungs from fully expanding. Physicians can detect the presence of fluid by tapping the chest (percussion) or listening with a stethoscope (auscultation).
pleurisy (PLOOR-ih-see)	pleur/o = pleura	Inflammation of the pleura characterized by sharp chest pain with each breath. Also called *pleuritis*.

Pathology (continued)

Term	Word Parts	Definition
pneumothorax (noo-moh-THOH-raks)	pneum/o = air -thorax = chest	Collection of air or gas in the pleural cavity, which may result in collapse of the lung.

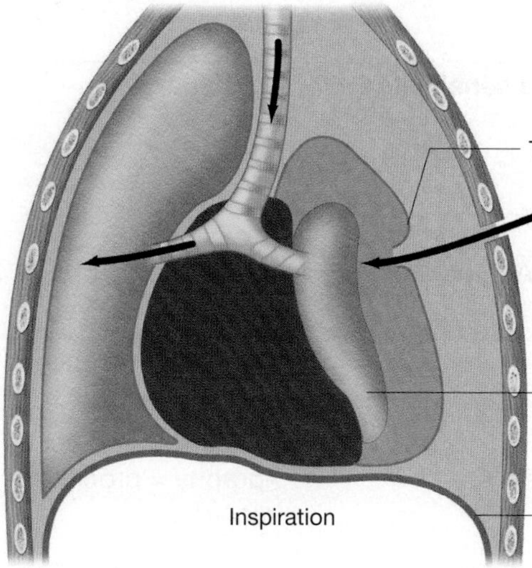

Torn pleura
Outside air entering pleural cavity
Left lung
Inspiration
Diaphragm

■ **Figure 7.10** Pneumothorax. Figure illustrates how puncture of thoracic wall and tearing of pleural membrane allows air into lung and results in collapsed lung.

Practice As You Go

C. Terminology Matching

Match each term to its definition.

1.	_______ inhaling environmental particles	a.	empyema
2.	_______ whooping cough	b.	blue tint to the skin
3.	_______ may result in collapsed lung	c.	caused by a fungus
4.	_______ pus in the pleural space	d.	epistaxis
5.	_______ respiratory tract mucus	e.	pneumoconiosis
6.	_______ nosebleed	f.	emphysema
7.	_______ cyanosis	g.	walking pneumonia
8.	_______ *Mycoplasma* pneumonia	h.	pneumothorax
9.	_______ disease with overexpanded air sacs	i.	pertussis
10.	_______ histoplasmosis	j.	phlegm

Diagnostic Procedures

Term	Word Parts	Definition
Clinical Laboratory Tests		
arterial blood gases (ABGs) (ar-TEE-ree-al)	arteri/o = artery -al = pertaining to	Testing for the gases present in the blood. Generally used to assist in determining the levels of oxygen (O_2) and carbon dioxide (CO_2) in the blood.
sputum culture and sensitivity (C&S) (SPEW-tum)		Testing sputum by placing it on a culture medium and observing any bacterial growth. The specimen is then tested to determine antibiotic effectiveness.
sputum cytology (SPEW-tum / sigh-TALL-oh-jee)	cyt/o = cell -logy = study of	Examining sputum for malignant cells.
Diagnostic Imaging		
bronchogram (BRONG-koh-gram)	bronch/o = bronchus -gram = record	X-ray record of the bronchus produced by bronchography.
bronchography (brong-KOG-rah-fee)	bronch/o = bronchus -graphy = process of recording	X-ray of the lung after a radiopaque substance has been inserted into the trachea or bronchial tube. Resulting X-ray is called a *bronchogram*.
chest X-ray (CXR)		Taking a radiographic picture of the lungs and heart from the back and sides.
pulmonary angiography (PULL-mon-air-ee / an-jee-OG-rah-fee)	pulmon/o = lung -ary = pertaining to angi/o = vessel -graphy = process of recording	Injecting dye into a blood vessel for the purpose of taking an X-ray of the arteries and veins of the lungs.
ventilation-perfusion scan (per-FUSE-shun)		Nuclear medicine diagnostic test that is especially useful in identifying pulmonary emboli. Radioactive air is inhaled for the ventilation portion to determine if air is filling the entire lung. Radioactive intravenous injection shows if blood is flowing to all parts of the lung.
Endoscopic Procedures		
bronchoscope (BRONG-koh-scope)	bronch/o = bronchus -scope = instrument for viewing	Instrument used to view inside a bronchus during a *bronchoscopy*.
bronchoscopy (Bronch) (brong-KOSS-koh-pee)	bronch/o = bronchus -scopy = process of visually examining	Visual examination of the inside of the bronchi; uses an instrument called a *bronchoscope* (see Figure 7.11 ■).
laryngoscope (lair-RING-go-scope)	laryng/o = larynx -scope = instrument for viewing	Instrument used to view inside the larynx during a *laryngoscopy*.
laryngoscopy (lair-in-GOSS-koh-pee)	laryng/o = larynx -scopy = process of visually examining	Examination of the interior of the larynx with a lighted instrument called a *laryngoscope*.

Diagnostic Procedures (continued)

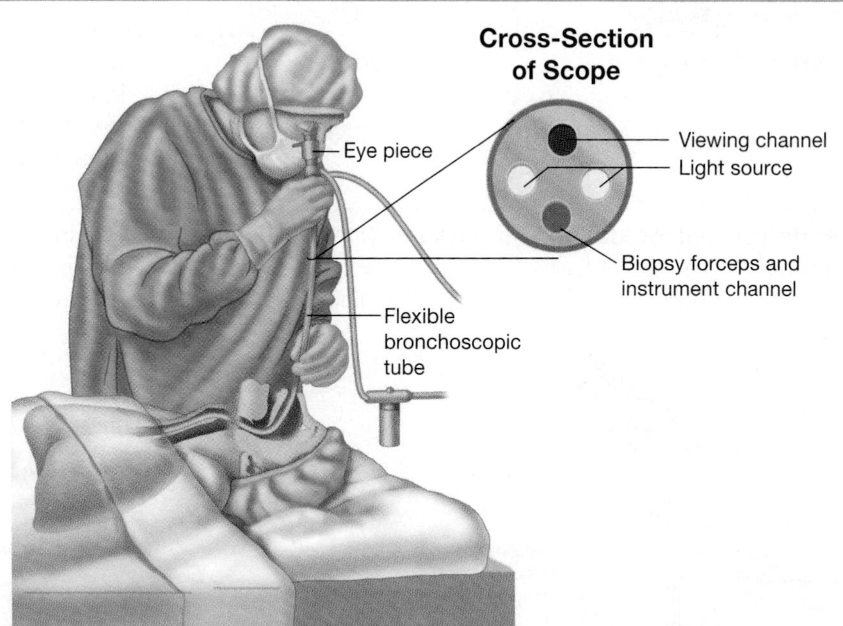

■ **Figure 7.11** Bronchoscopy. Figure illustrates physician using a bronchoscope to inspect the patient's bronchial tubes. Advances in technology include using a videoscope which projects the internal view of the bronchus onto a video screen.

Term	Word Parts	Definition
Pulmonary Function Tests		
oximeter (ox-IM-eh-ter)	**ox/i** = oxygen **-meter** = instrument to measure	Instrument that measures the amount of oxygen in the bloodstream.
oximetry (ox-IM-eh-tree)	**ox/i** = oxygen **-metry** = process of measuring	Procedure to measure the oxygen level in the blood using a device, an *oximeter*, placed on the patient's fingertip or earlobe.
pulmonary function test (PFT) (PULL-mon-air-ee)	**pulmon/o** = lung **-ary** = pertaining to	Group of diagnostic tests that give information regarding air flow in and out of the lungs, lung volumes, and gas exchange between the lungs and bloodstream.
spirometer (spy-ROM-eh-ter)	**spir/o** = breathing **-meter** = instrument to measure	Instrument to measure lung capacity used for *spirometry*.
spirometry (spy-ROM-eh-tree)	**spir/o** = breathing **-metry** = process of measuring	Procedure to measure lung capacity using a *spirometer*.
Additional Diagnostic Procedures		
polysomnography (polly-som-NOG-rah-fee)	**poly-** = many **somn/o** = sleep **-graphy** = process of recording	Monitoring a patient while sleeping to identify sleep apnea. Also called *sleep apnea study*.
sweat test		Test for cystic fibrosis. Patients with this disease have an abnormally large amount of salt in their sweat.
tuberculin skin test (TB test) (too-BER-kyoo-lin)		Procedure in which tuberculin purified protein derivative (PPD) is applied under the surface of the skin to determine if the patient has been exposed to tuberculosis. Also called a *Mantoux test*.

Therapeutic Procedures

Term	Word Parts	Definition
Respiratory Therapy		
aerosol therapy (AIR-oh-sol)	aer/o = air	Medication suspended in a mist intended for inhalation. Delivered by a *nebulizer*, which provides the mist for a period of time while the patient breathes, or a *metered-dose inhaler* (MDI), which delivers a single puff of mist.
endotracheal intubation (en-doh-TRAY-kee-al / in-too-BAY-shun)	endo- = within trache/o = trachea -al = pertaining to	Placing of a tube through the mouth, through the glottis, and into the trachea to create a patent airway.

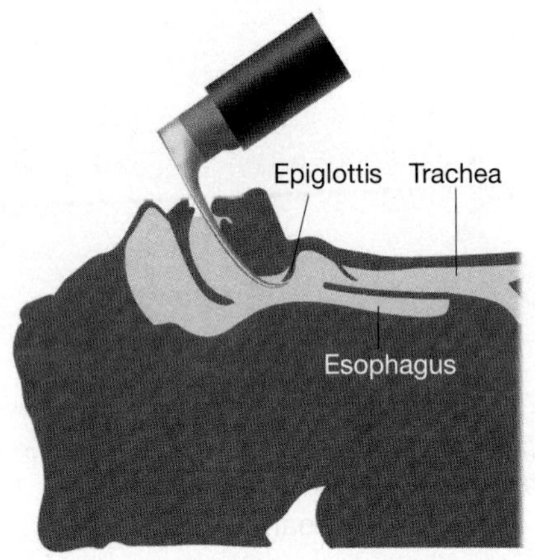

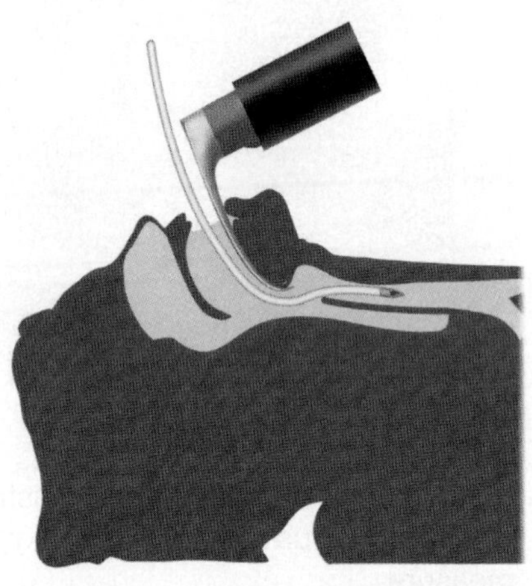
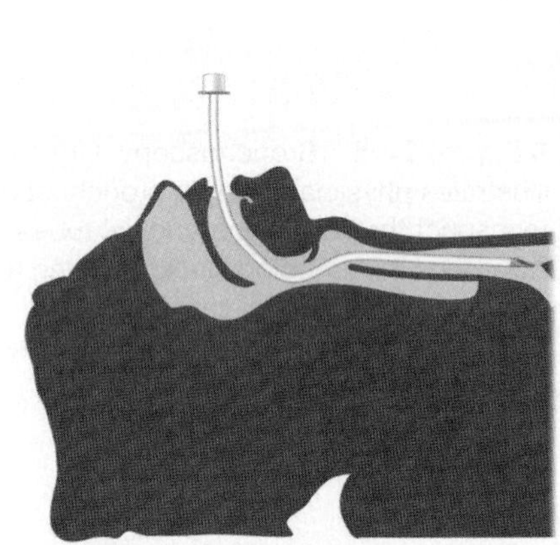

■ **Figure 7.12** Endotracheal intubation. First, a lighted scope is used to identify the trachea from the esophagus. Next, the tube is placed through the pharynx and into the trachea. Finally, the scope is removed, leaving the tube in place.

Term	Word Parts	Definition
intermittent positive pressure breathing (IPPB)		Method for assisting patients in breathing using a mask connected to a machine that produces an increased positive thoracic pressure.
nasal cannula (CAN-you-lah)	nas/o = nose -al = pertaining to	Two-pronged plastic device for delivering oxygen into the nose; one prong is inserted into each naris.
postural drainage	-al = pertaining to	Drainage of secretions from the bronchi by placing the patient in a position that uses gravity to promote drainage. Used for the treatment of cystic fibrosis and bronchiectasis.
supplemental oxygen therapy	-al = pertaining to	Providing a patient with additional concentration of oxygen to improve oxygen levels in the bloodstream. Oxygen may be provided by a mask or nasal cannula.
ventilator (VENT-ih-later)		Machine that provides artificial ventilation for a patient unable to breathe on his or her own. Also called a *respirator*.
Surgical Procedures		
bronchoplasty (BRONG-koh-plas-tee)	bronch/o = bronchus -plasty = surgical repair	Surgical repair of a bronchus.
laryngectomy (lair-in-JEK-toh-mee)	laryng/o = larynx -ectomy = surgical removal	Surgical removal of the larynx.
laryngoplasty (lair-RING-goh-plas-tee)	laryng/o = larynx -plasty = surgical repair	Surgical repair of the larynx.

Therapeutic Procedures (continued)

Term	Word Parts	Definition
lobectomy (loh-BEK-toh-mee)	lob/o = lobe -ectomy = surgical removal	Surgical removal of a lobe of a lung.
pleurectomy (ploor-EK-toh-mee)	pleur/o = pleura -ectomy = surgical removal	Surgical removal of the pleura.
pleurocentesis (ploor-oh-sen-TEE-sis)	pleur/o = pleura -centesis = puncture to withdraw fluid	Procedure involving insertion of a needle into the pleural space to withdraw fluid; may be a treatment for excess fluid accumulating or to obtain fluid for diagnostic examination.
pneumonectomy (NOO-moh-NEK-toh-mee)	pneum/o = lung -ectomy = surgical removal	Surgical removal of an entire lung.
rhinoplasty (RYE-noh-plas-tee)	rhin/o = nose -plasty = surgical repair	Surgical repair of the nose.
thoracentesis (thor-ah-sen-TEE-sis)	thorac/o = chest -centesis = puncture to withdraw fluid	Surgical puncture of the chest wall for the removal of fluids. Also called *thoracocentesis*.

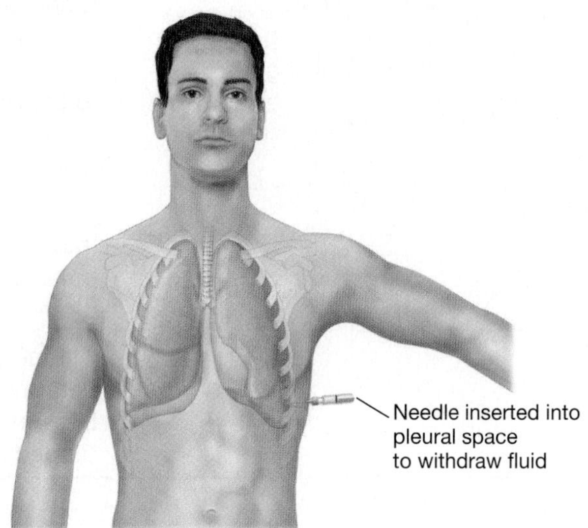

■ **Figure 7.13** Thoracentesis. The needle is inserted between the ribs to withdraw fluid from the pleural sac at the base of the left lung.

Term	Word Parts	Definition
thoracostomy (thor-ah-KOS-toh-mee)	thorac/o = chest -ostomy = surgically create an opening	Insertion of a tube into the chest cavity for the purpose of draining off fluid or air. Also called *chest tube*.
thoracotomy (thor-ah-KOT-oh-mee)	thorac/o = chest -otomy = cutting into	To cut into the chest cavity.
tracheotomy (tray-kee-OTT-oh-mee)	trache/o = trachea -otomy = cutting into	Surgical procedure often performed in an emergency that creates an opening directly into the trachea to allow the patient to breathe easier; also called *tracheostomy* (see Figure 7.14■).

Therapeutic Procedures (continued)

■ **Figure 7.14** A tracheotomy tube in place, inserted through an opening in the front of the neck and anchored within the trachea.

Term	Word Parts	Definition
Additional Procedures		
cardiopulmonary resuscitation (CPR) (car-dee-oh-PULL-mon-air-ee / ree-suss-ih-TAY-shun)	cardi/o = heart pulmon/o = lung -ary = pertaining to	Emergency treatment provided by persons trained in CPR and given to patients when their respirations and heart stop. CPR provides oxygen to the brain, heart, and other vital organs until medical treatment can restore normal heart and pulmonary function.
Heimlich maneuver (HYME-lik)		Technique for removing a foreign body from the trachea or pharynx by exerting diaphragmatic pressure. Named for Henry Heimlich, a U.S. thoracic surgeon.
percussion (per-KUH-shun)		Use of the fingertips to tap on a surface to determine the condition beneath the surface. Determined in part by the feel of the surface as it is tapped and the sound generated.

Practice As You Go

D. Terminology Matching

Match each term to its definition.

1. ________ sweat test
2. ________ measures oxygen levels in blood
3. ________ ventilator
4. ________ test to identify sleep apnea
5. ________ thoracentesis
6. ________ tuberculin test

a. polysomnography
b. Mantoux test
c. oximetry
d. puncture chest wall to remove fluid
e. respirator
f. test for cystic fibrosis

Pharmacology

Classification	Word Parts	Action	Examples
antibiotic (an-tih-bye-AW-tic)	anti- = against bi/o = life -tic = pertaining to	Kills bacteria causing respiratory infections.	ampicillin; amoxicillin, Amoxil; ciprofloxacin, Cipro
antihistamine (an-tih-HIST-ah-meen)	anti- = against	Blocks the effects of histamine that has been released by the body during an allergy attack.	fexofenadine, Allegra; loratadine, Claritin; diphenhydramine, Benadryl
antitussive (an-tih-TUSS-ive)	anti- = without tuss/o = cough	Relieves the urge to cough.	hydrocodon, Hycodan; dextromethorphan, Vicks Formula 44
bronchodilator (BRONG-koh-dye-late-or)	bronch/o = bronchus	Relaxes muscle spasms in bronchial tubes. Used to treat asthma.	albuterol, Proventil, Ventolin; theophyllin, Theo-Dur
corticosteroids (core-tih-koh-STAIR-ryods)	cortic/o = outer layer, cortex	Reduces inflammation and swelling in the respiratory tract.	fluticasone, Flonase; mometasone, Nasonex; triamcinolone, Azmacort
decongestant (dee-kon-JES-tant)	de- = without	Reduces stuffiness and congestion throughout the respiratory system.	oxymetazoline, Afrin, Dristan, Sinex; pseudoephedrine, Drixoral, Sudafed
expectorant (ek-SPEK-toh-rant)		Improves the ability to cough up mucus from the respiratory tract.	guaifenesin, Robitussin, Mucinex
mucolytic (myoo-koh-LIT-ik)	muc/o = mucus -lytic = destruction	Liquefies mucus so it is easier to cough and clear it from the respiratory tract.	N-acetyl-cysteine, Mucomyst

Abbreviations

ABGs	arterial blood gases	**IC**	inspiratory capacity
ARDS	adult (or acute) respiratory distress syndrome	**IPPB**	intermittent positive pressure breathing
Bronch	bronchoscopy	**IRDS**	infant respiratory distress syndrome
CF	cystic fibrosis	**IRV**	inspiratory reserve volume
CO_2	carbon dioxide	**LLL**	left lower lobe
COPD	chronic obstructive pulmonary disease	**LUL**	left upper lobe
CPR	cardiopulmonary resuscitation	**MDI**	metered-dose inhaler
C&S	culture and sensitivity	**O_2**	oxygen
CTA	clear to auscultation	**PFT**	pulmonary function test
CXR	chest X-ray	**PPD**	purified protein derivative
DOE	dyspnea on exertion	**R**	respiration
DPT	diphtheria, pertussis, tetanus injection	**RA**	room air
ENT	ear, nose, and throat	**RDS**	respiratory distress syndrome
ERV	expiratory reserve volume	**RLL**	right lower lobe
flu	influenza	**RML**	right middle lobe
FRC	functional residual capacity	**RRT**	registered respiratory therapist
HMD	hyaline membrane disease	**RUL**	right upper lobe

Abbreviations (continued)

RV	reserve volume	**TLC**	total lung capacity
SARS	severe acute respiratory syndrome	**TPR**	temperature, pulse, and respiration
SIDS	sudden infant death syndrome	**TV**	tidal volume
SOB	shortness of breath	**URI**	upper respiratory infection
TB	tuberculosis	**VC**	vital capacity

Practice As You Go

E. What's the Abbreviation?

1. upper respiratory infection ______________________________
2. pulmonary function test ______________________________
3. oxygen ______________________________
4. carbon dioxide ______________________________
5. chronic obstructive pulmonary disease ______________________________
6. bronchoscopy ______________________________
7. tuberculosis ______________________________
8. infant respiratory distress syndrome ______________________________

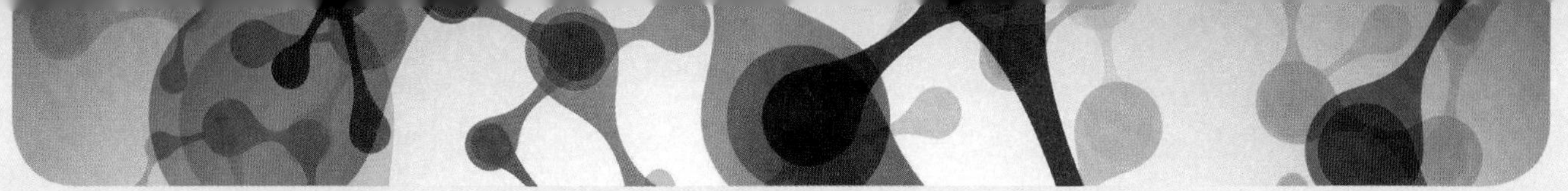

Chapter Review

Real-World Applications

Medical Record Analysis

This Pulmonology Consultation Report contains 12 medical terms. Underline each term and write it in the list below the report. Then define each term.

Pulmonology Consultation Report

Reason for Consultation:	Evaluation of increasingly severe asthma.
History of Present Illness:	Patient is a 10-year-old male who first presented to the Emergency Room with dyspnea, coughing, and wheezing at seven years of age. Attacks are increasing in frequency, and there do not appear to be any precipitating factors such as exercise. No other family members are asthmatics.
Results of Physical Examination:	Patient is currently in the ER with marked dyspnea, cyanosis around the lips, prolonged expiration, and a hacking cough producing thick phlegm. Auscultation revealed rhonchi throughout lungs. ABGs indicate hypoxemia. Spirometry reveals moderately severe airway obstruction during expiration. This patient responded to Proventil and he is beginning to cough less and breathe with less effort.
Assessment:	Acute asthma attack with severe airway obstruction. There is no evidence of infection. In view of increasing severity and frequency of attacks, all his medications should be reevaluated for effectiveness and all attempts to identify precipitating factors should be made.
Recommendations:	Patient is to continue to use Proventil for relief of bronchospasms. Instructions for taking medications and controlling severity of asthma attacks were carefully reviewed with the patient and his family.

	Term	Definition
1.	______________	______________________________
2.	______________	______________________________
3.	______________	______________________________
4.	______________	______________________________
5.	______________	______________________________
6.	______________	______________________________
7.	______________	______________________________
8.	______________	______________________________
9.	______________	______________________________
10.	______________	______________________________
11.	______________	______________________________
12.	______________	______________________________

Chart Note Transcription

The chart note below contains 11 phrases that can be reworded with a medical term that you learned in this chapter. Each phrase is identified with an underline. Determine the medical term and write your answers in the space provided.

Pearson General Hospital Emergency Room Record

Task Edit View Time Scale Options Help Download Archive Date: 17 May 2015

Current Complaint:	A 43-year-old female was brought to the Emergency Room by her family. She complained of painful and labored breathing, **1** rapid breathing, **2** and fever. Symptoms began three days ago, but have become much worse during the past 12 hours.
Past History:	Patient is a mother of three and a business executive. She has had no surgeries or previous serious illnesses.
Signs and Symptoms:	Temperature is 103°F, respiratory rate is 20 breaths/minute, blood pressure is 165/98, and heart rate is 90 bpm. A blood test to measure the levels of oxygen in the blood **3** indicates a marked low level of oxygen in the blood. **4** The process of listening to body sounds **5** of the lungs revealed abnormal crackling sounds **6** over the left lower chest. She is producing large amounts of pus-filled **7** mucus coughed up from the respiratory tract **8** and a chest X-ray **9** shows a large cloudy patch in the lower lobe of the left lung.
Diagnosis:	Left lower lobe inflammatory condition of the lungs caused by bacterial infection. **10**
Treatment:	Patient was started on intravenous antibiotics. She also required a tube placed through the mouth to create an airway **11** for three days.

1. ______________________________
2. ______________________________
3. ______________________________
4. ______________________________
5. ______________________________
6. ______________________________
7. ______________________________
8. ______________________________
9. ______________________________
10. ______________________________
11. ______________________________

Case Study

Below is a case study presentation of a patient with a condition discussed in this chapter. Read the case study and answer the questions below. Some questions will ask for information not included within this chapter. Use your text, a medical dictionary, or any other reference material you choose to answer these questions.

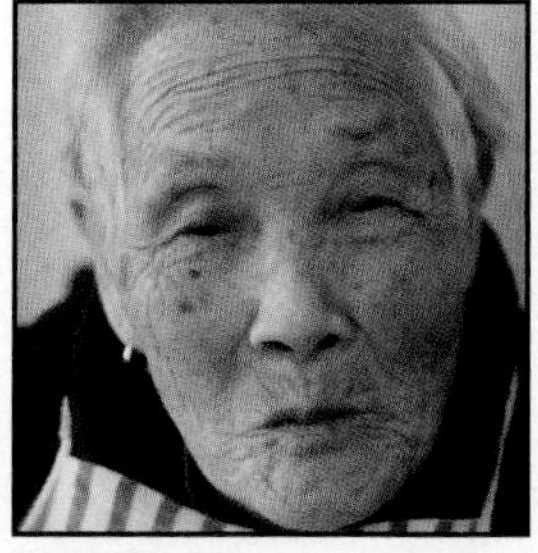

(Ni Qin/Getty Images)

An 88-year-old female was seen in the physician's office complaining of dyspnea, dizziness, orthopnea, elevated temperature, and a cough. Lung auscultation revealed crackles over the right bronchus. CXR revealed fluid in the RUL. The patient was sent to the hospital with an admitting diagnosis of pneumonia. Vital signs upon admission were temperature 102°F, pulse 100 BPM and rapid, respirations 24 breaths/min and labored, blood pressure 180/110. She was treated with IV antibiotics and IPPB. She responded well to treatment and was released home to her family with oral antibiotics on the third day.

Questions

1. What was this patient's admitting diagnosis? Look this condition up in a reference source and include a short description of it.

____

____

2. List and define each of the patient's presenting symptoms in your own words.

____

____

3. Define auscultation and CXR. Describe what each revealed in your own words.

____

____

4. What does the term "vital signs" mean? Describe this patient's vital signs.

____

____

5. Describe the treatments this patient received while in the hospital in your own words.

____

____

6. Explain the change in the patient's medication when she was discharged home.

____

____

Practice Exercises

A. Complete the Statement

1. The primary function of the respiratory system is ____________________.
2. The movement of air in and out of the lungs is called ____________________.
3. Define external respiration ____________________.
4. Define internal respiration ____________________.

B. Define the Suffix

	Definition	Example from Chapter
1. **-ectasis**	____________________	____________________
2. **-capnia**	____________________	____________________
3. **-phonia**	____________________	____________________
4. **-thorax**	____________________	____________________
5. **-pnea**	____________________	____________________
6. **-ptysis**	____________________	____________________
7. **-osmia**	____________________	____________________

C. Word Building Practice

The combining form **rhin/o** refers to the nose. Use it to write a term that means:

1. inflammation of the nose ____________________
2. discharge from the nose ____________________
3. surgical repair of the nose ____________________

The combining form **laryng/o** refers to the larynx or voice box. Use it to write a term that means:

4. inflammation of the larynx ____________________
5. spasm of the larynx ____________________
6. visual examination of the larynx ____________________
7. pertaining to the larynx ____________________
8. removal of the larynx ____________________
9. surgical repair of the larynx ____________________
10. paralysis of the larynx ____________________

The combining form **bronch/o** refers to the bronchus. Use it to write a term that means:

11. pertaining to bronchus ______
12. inflammation of the bronchus ______
13. visually examine the interior of the bronchus ______
14. produced by bronchus ______
15. spasm of the bronchus ______

The combining form **thorac/o** refers to the chest. Use it to write a term that means:

16. cutting into the chest ______
17. chest pain ______
18. pertaining to chest ______

The combining form **trache/o** refers to the trachea. Use it to write a term that means:

19. cutting into the trachea ______
20. narrowing of the trachea ______
21. pertaining to inside the trachea ______

The suffix **-pnea** means breathing. Use this suffix to write a medical term that means:

22. difficult or labored breathing ______
23. rapid breathing ______
24. can breathe only in an upright position ______
25. lack of breathing ______

D. Define the Combining Form

	Definition	Example from Chapter
1. **trache/o**	______	______
2. **laryng/o**	______	______
3. **bronch/o**	______	______
4. **spir/o**	______	______
5. **pneum/o**	______	______
6. **rhin/o**	______	______
7. **coni/o**	______	______
8. **pleur/o**	______	______
9. **epiglott/o**	______	______
10. **alveol/o**	______	______

	Definition	Example from Chapter
11. **pulmon/o**	__________	__________
12. **ox/o**	__________	__________
13. **sinus/o**	__________	__________
14. **lob/o**	__________	__________
15. **nas/o**	__________	__________

E. Name That Term

1. the process of breathing in __________
2. spitting up of blood __________
3. blood clot in the pulmonary artery __________
4. inflammation of a sinus __________
5. sore throat __________
6. air in the pleural cavity __________
7. whooping cough __________
8. cutting into the pleura __________
9. pain in the pleural region __________
10. common cold __________

F. What Does it Stand For?

1. CXR __________
2. TV __________
3. TPR __________
4. ABGs __________
5. DOE __________
6. RUL __________
7. SIDS __________
8. TLC __________
9. ARDS __________
10. MDI __________
11. CTA __________
12. SARS __________

G. Define the Term

1. total lung capacity ______
2. tidal volume ______
3. residual volume ______

H. Fill in the Blank

anthracosis	sputum cytology	cardiopulmonary resuscitation	patent
thoracentesis	respirator	ventilation-perfusion scan	rhonchi
supplemental oxygen	hyperventilation		

1. When the patient's breathing and heart stopped, the paramedics began ______.
2. The physician performed a ______ to remove fluid from the chest.
3. A ______ is also called a ventilator.
4. The patient received ______ through a nasal cannula.
5. An endotracheal intubation was performed to establish a ______ airway.
6. A ______ is a particularly useful test to identify a pulmonary embolus.
7. The result of the ______ was negative for cancer.
8. ______ involves tachypnea and hyperpnea.
9. ______ are wheezing lung sounds.
10. Miners are at risk of developing ______.

I. Pharmacology Challenge

Fill in the classification for each drug description, then match the brand name.

	Drug Description	Classification	Brand Name
1.	______ Reduces stuffiness and congestion	______	a. Hycodan
2.	______ Relieves the urge to cough	______	b. Flonase
3.	______ Kills bacteria	______	c. Cipro
4.	______ Improves ability to cough up mucus	______	d. Ventolin
5.	______ Liquefies mucus	______	e. Allegra
6.	______ Relaxes bronchial muscle spasms	______	f. Afrin
7.	______ Blocks allergy attack	______	g. Robitussin
8.	______ Reduces inflammation and swelling	______	h. Mucomyst

MyMedicalTerminologyLab™

MyMedicalTerminologyLab is a premium online homework management system that includes a host of features to help you study. Registered users will find:

- Learning activities and homework assignments
- Fun games and activities built within a virtual hospital
- Powerful tools that track and analyze your results—allowing you to create a personalized learning experience
- Videos, flashcards, and audio pronunciations to help enrich your progress
- Streaming lesson presentations and self-paced learning modules
- A space where you and your instructors can view and manage your assignments

Labeling Exercise

Image A

Write the labels for this figure on the numbered lines provided.

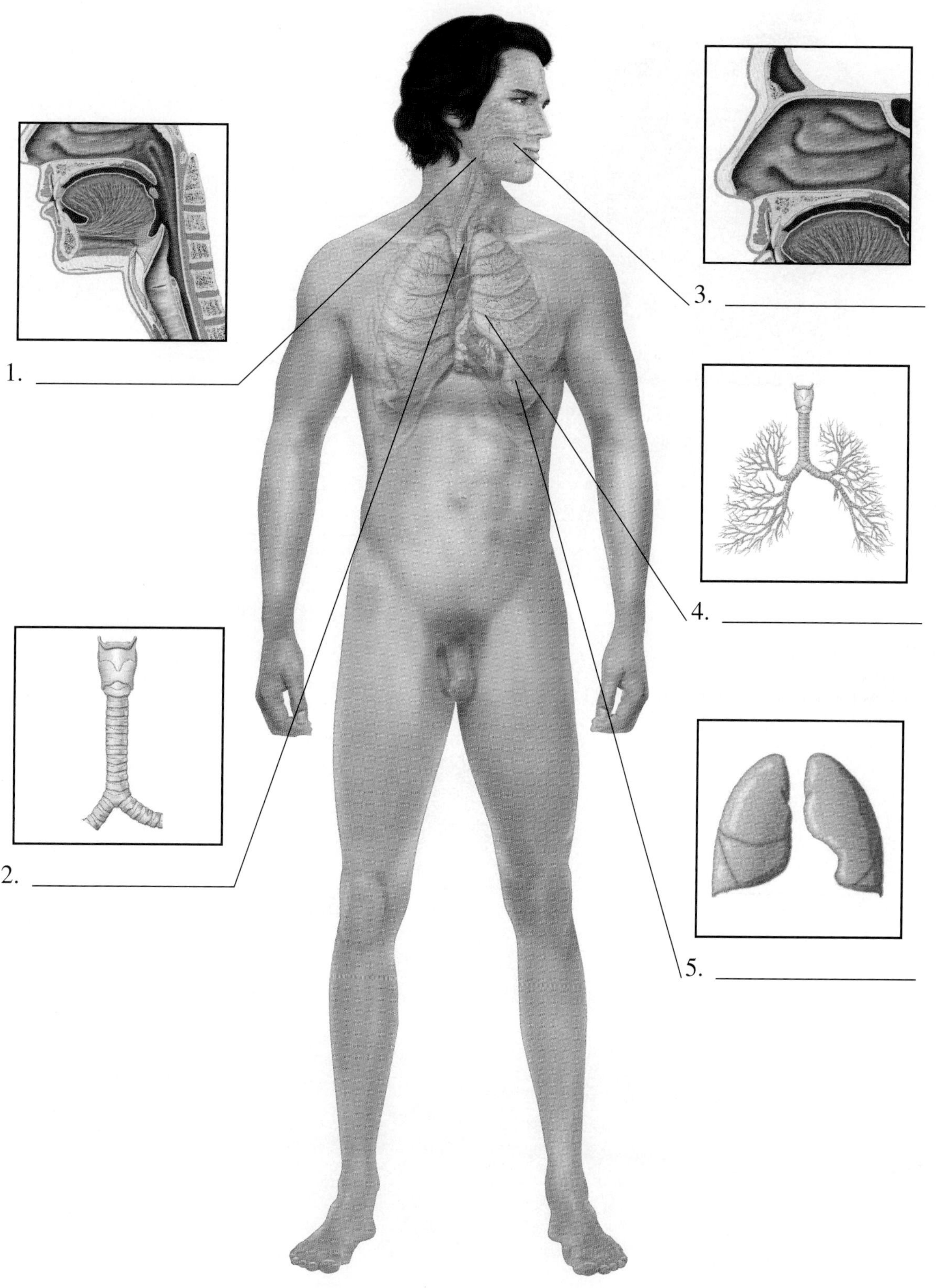

Image B

Write the labels for this figure on the numbered lines provided.

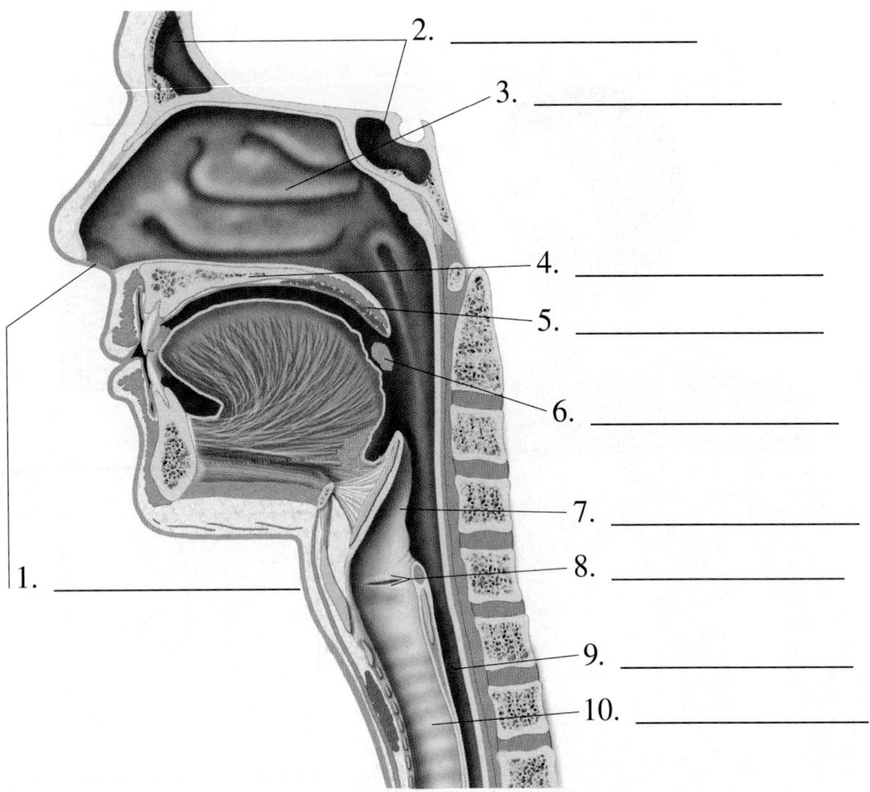

Image C

Write the labels for this figure on the numbered lines provided.

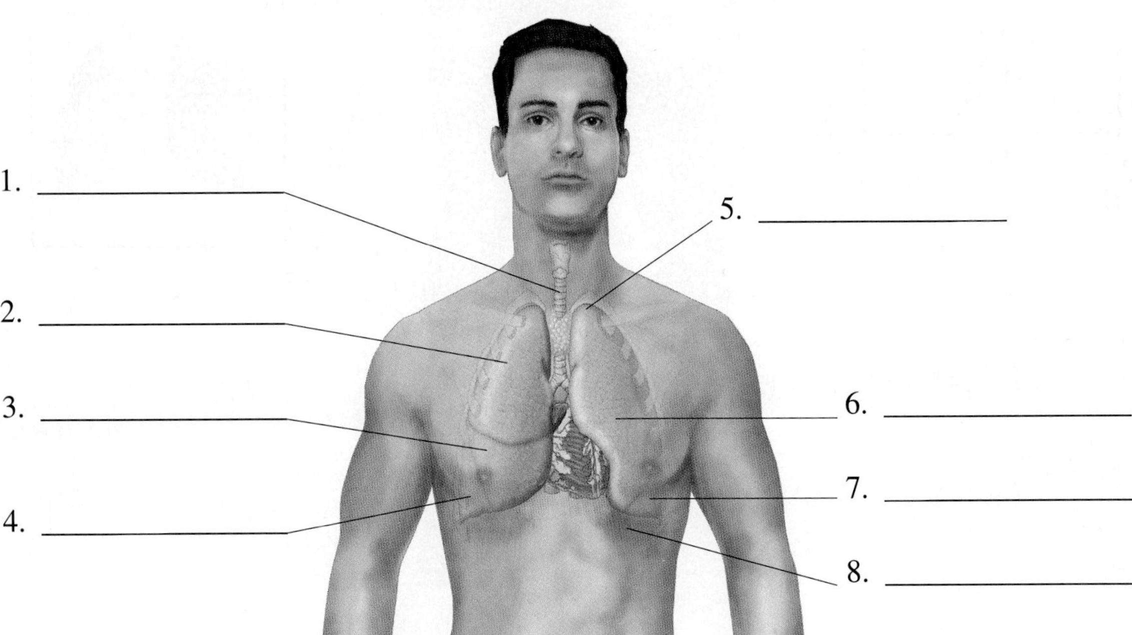

8

Digestive System

Learning Objectives

Upon completion of this chapter, you will be able to

- Identify and define the combining forms and suffixes introduced in this chapter.
- Correctly spell and pronounce medical terms and major anatomical structures relating to the digestive system.
- Locate and describe the major organs of the digestive system and their functions.
- Identify the shape and function of each type of tooth.
- Describe the function of the accessory organs of the digestive system.
- Identify and define digestive system anatomical terms.
- Identify and define selected digestive system pathology terms.
- Identify and define selected digestive system diagnostic procedures.
- Identify and define selected digestive system therapeutic procedures.
- Identify and define selected medications relating to the digestive system.
- Define selected abbreviations associated with the digestive system.

Digestive System at a Glance

Function

The digestive system begins breaking down food through mechanical and chemical digestion. After being digested, nutrient molecules are absorbed into the body and enter the bloodstream; any food not digested or absorbed is eliminated as solid waste.

Organs

Here are the primary structures that comprise the digestive system:

anus
esophagus
gallbladder (GB)
large intestine
liver
oral cavity
pancreas
pharynx
salivary glands
small intestine
stomach

Word Parts

Here are the most common word parts (with their meanings) used to build digestive system terms. For a more comprehensive list, refer to the Terminology section of this chapter.

Combining Forms

an/o	anus
append/o	appendix
appendic/o	appendix
bar/o	weight
bucc/o	cheek
cec/o	cecum
cholangi/o	bile duct
chol/e	bile, gall
cholecyst/o	gallbladder
choledoch/o	common bile duct
cirrh/o	yellow
col/o	colon
colon/o	colon
dent/o	tooth
diverticul/o	pouch
duoden/o	duodenum
enter/o	small intestine
esophag/o	esophagus
gastr/o	stomach
gingiv/o	gums
gloss/o	tongue
hepat/o	liver
ile/o	ileum
jejun/o	jejunum
labi/o	lip
lapar/o	abdomen
lingu/o	tongue
lith/o	stone
odont/o	tooth
or/o	mouth
palat/o	palate
pancreat/o	pancreas
pharyng/o	pharynx
polyp/o	polyp
proct/o	anus and rectum
pylor/o	pylorus
pyr/o	fire
rect/o	rectum
sialaden/o	salivary gland
sigmoid/o	sigmoid colon

(*continued on page 264*)

Digestive System Illustrated

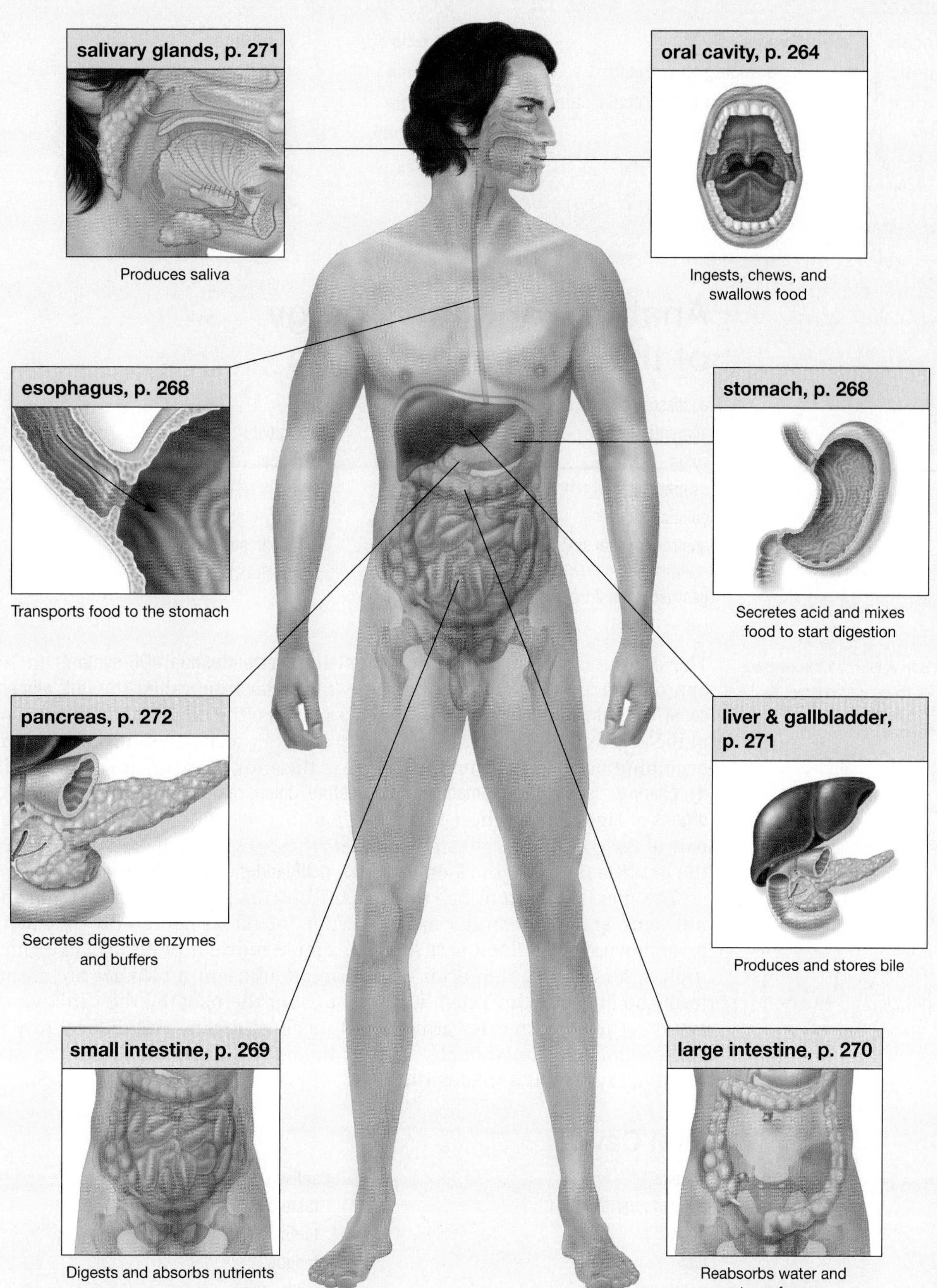

salivary glands, p. 271
Produces saliva
oral cavity, p. 264
Ingests, chews, and swallows food
esophagus, p. 268
Transports food to the stomach
stomach, p. 268
Secretes acid and mixes food to start digestion
pancreas, p. 272
Secretes digestive enzymes and buffers
liver & gallbladder, p. 271
Produces and stores bile
small intestine, p. 269
Digests and absorbs nutrients
large intestine, p. 270
Reabsorbs water and stores feces

Suffixes

-emesis	vomit	**-orexia**	appetite
-emetic	pertaining to vomiting	**-pepsia**	digestion
-iatric	pertaining to medical treatment	**-phagia**	eat, swallow
-istry	specialty of	**-prandial**	pertaining to a meal
-lithiasis	condition of stones	**-tripsy**	surgical crushing

Anatomy and Physiology of the Digestive System

accessory organs
alimentary canal (al-ih-MEN-tar-ree)
colon (COH-lon)
esophagus (eh-SOFF-ah-gus)
gallbladder
gastrointestinal system (gas-troh-in-TESS-tih-nal)
gastrointestinal tract
gut
liver
oral cavity
pancreas (PAN-kree-ass)
pharynx (FAIR-inks)
salivary glands (SAL-ih-vair-ee)
small intestine
stomach (STUM-ak)

What's In A Name?
Look for these word parts:
-ary = pertaining to
-ory = pertaining to

Med Term Tip
The term *alimentary* comes from the Latin term *alimentum* meaning "nourishment."

The digestive system, also known as the **gastrointestinal (GI) system**, includes approximately 30 feet of a continuous muscular tube called the **gut**, **alimentary canal**, or **gastrointestinal tract** that stretches between the mouth and the anus. Most of the organs in this system are actually different sections of this tube. In order, beginning at the mouth and continuing to the anus, these organs are the **oral cavity**, **pharynx**, **esophagus**, **stomach**, **small intestine**, **colon**, **rectum**, and **anus.** The **accessory organs** of digestion are those that participate in the digestion process, but are not part of the continuous alimentary canal. These organs, which are connected to the gut by a duct, are the **liver**, **pancreas**, **gallbladder**, and **salivary glands.**

The digestive system has three main functions: digesting food, absorbing nutrients, and eliminating waste. Digestion includes the physical and chemical breakdown of large food particles into simple nutrient molecules like glucose, triglycerides, and amino acids. These simple nutrient molecules are absorbed from the intestines and circulated throughout the body by the cardiovascular system. They are used for growth and repair of organs and tissues. Any food that cannot be digested or absorbed by the body is eliminated from the gastrointestinal system as a solid waste.

Oral Cavity

cheeks
gingiva (JIN-jih-vah)
gums
lips
palate (PAL-at)
saliva (suh-LYE-vah)
taste buds
teeth
tongue
uvula (YU-vyu-lah)

Digestion begins when food enters the mouth and is mechanically broken up by the chewing movements of the **teeth**. The muscular **tongue** moves the food within the mouth and mixes it with **saliva** (see Figure 8.1 ■). Saliva contains digestive enzymes to break down carbohydrates and slippery lubricants to make food easier to swallow. **Taste buds**, found on the surface of the tongue, can distinguish the bitter, sweet, sour, salty, and umami (savory) flavors in our food. The roof of the oral cavity is known as the **palate** and is subdivided into the hard palate (the bony anterior portion) and the soft palate (the flexible posterior portion). Hanging down from the posterior edge of the soft palate is the **uvula**. The uvula serves two important functions. First, it has a role in speech production and, second, it is the location of the gag reflex. This reflex is stimulated when food enters the throat without swallowing (e.g., laughing with food in your mouth). It is important because swallowing also results in the epiglottis covering the larynx to prevent food from entering the lungs (see Figure 8.2 ■). The **cheeks** form the lateral walls of this cavity and the **lips** are the anterior opening. The entire oral cavity is lined with mucous membrane, a portion of which forms the **gums**, or **gingiva**, that combine with connective tissue to cover the jaw bone and seal off the teeth in their bony sockets.

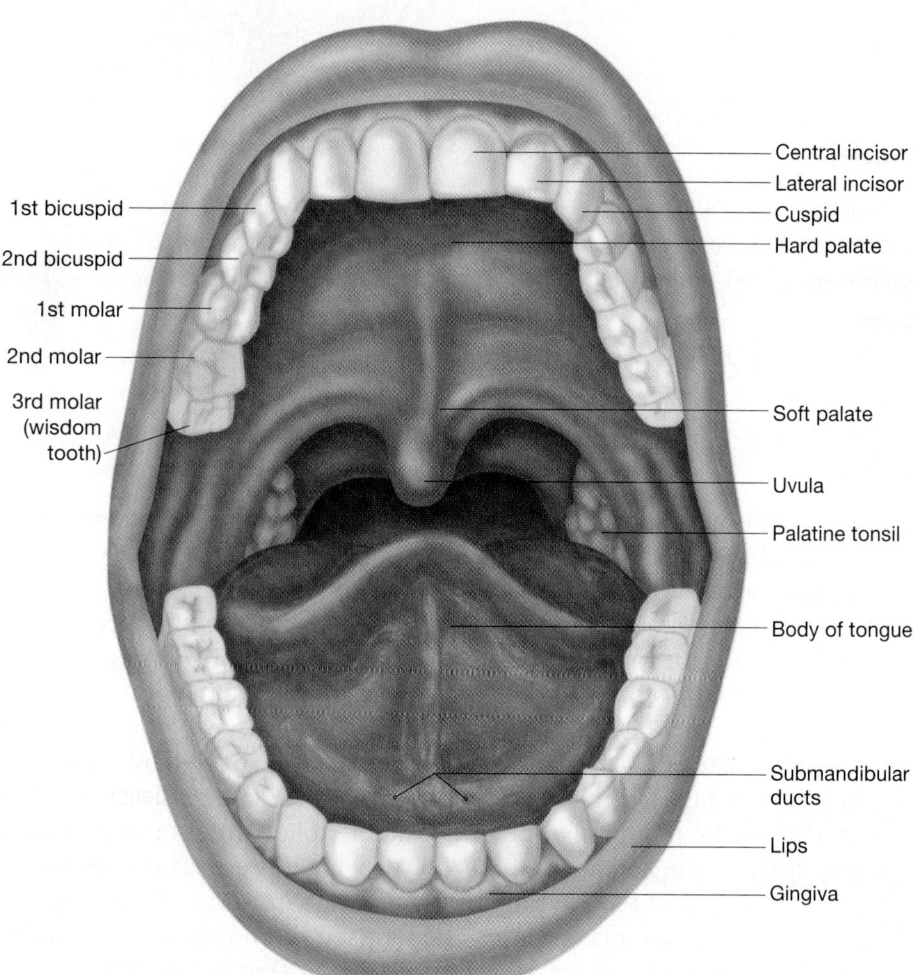

■ **Figure 8.1** Anatomy of structures of the oral cavity.

■ **Figure 8.2** Structures of the oral cavity, and pharynx, and esophagus.

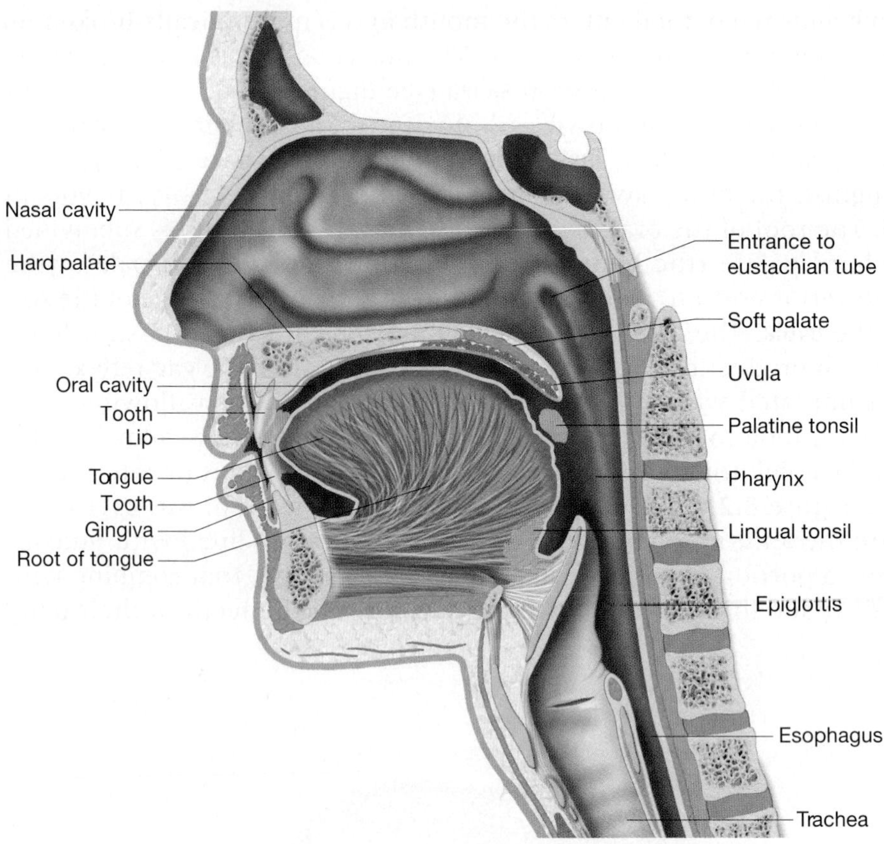

What's In A Name?

Look for these word parts:
cis/o = to cut
bi- = two
in- = inward
pre- = before

Med Term Tip

There are three different molars, simply referred to as the first, second, or third molars. However, the third molar has a more common name, the wisdom tooth. Not every person forms all four wisdom teeth. Unfortunately, most people do not have enough room in their jaws for the third molars to properly erupt through the gum, a condition requiring surgical removal of the third molar, referred to as an *impacted wisdom tooth*.

Med Term Tip

The combining form *dent/o* means teeth. Hence we have terms such as dentist and dentistry. The combining form *odont/o* also means teeth and when combined with *orth/o*, which means straight, we have the specialty of *orthodontics*, or straightening teeth.

Teeth

bicuspids (bye-CUSS-pids)
canines (KAY-nines)
cementum (see-MEN-tum)
crown
cuspids (CUSS-pids)
deciduous teeth (dee-SID-yoo-us)
dentin (DEN-tin)
enamel
incisors (in-SIGH-zors)
molars (MOH-lars)
periodontal ligaments (pair-ee-on-DON-tal)
permanent teeth
premolars (pree-MOH-lars)
pulp cavity
root
root canal

Teeth are an important part of the first stage of digestion. The teeth in the front of the mouth bite, tear, or cut food into small pieces. These cutting teeth include the **cuspids** (or **canines**) and the **incisors** (see Figure 8.3■). The remaining posterior teeth grind and crush food into even finer pieces. These grinding teeth include the **bicuspids** (or **premolars**) and the **molars**. A tooth can be subdivided into the **crown** and the **root**. The crown is that part of the tooth visible above the gum line; the root is below the gum line. The root is anchored in the bony socket of the jaw by **cementum** and tiny **periodontal ligaments**. The crown of the tooth is covered by a layer of **enamel**, the hardest substance in the body. Under the enamel layer is **dentin**, the substance that makes up the main bulk of the tooth. The hollow interior of a tooth is called the **pulp cavity** in the crown and the **root canal** in the root. These cavities contain soft tissue made up of blood vessels, nerves, and lymph vessels (see Figure 8.4■).

Humans have two sets of teeth. The first set, often referred to as baby teeth, are **deciduous teeth**. There are 20 teeth in this set that erupt through the gums between the ages of six and 28 months. At approximately six years of age, these teeth begin to fall out and are replaced by the 32 **permanent teeth**. This replacement process continues until about 18–20 years of age.

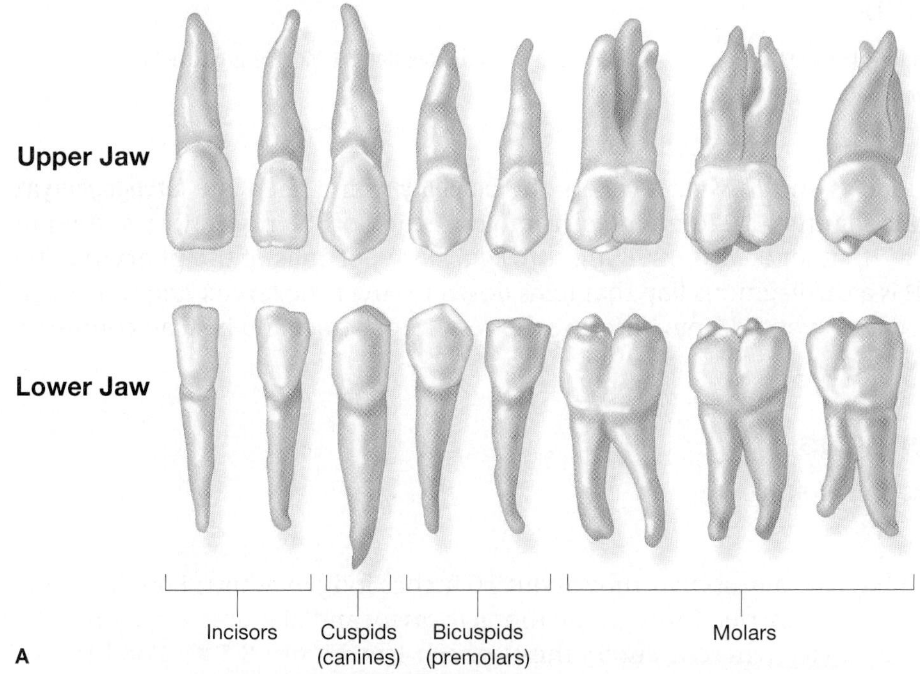

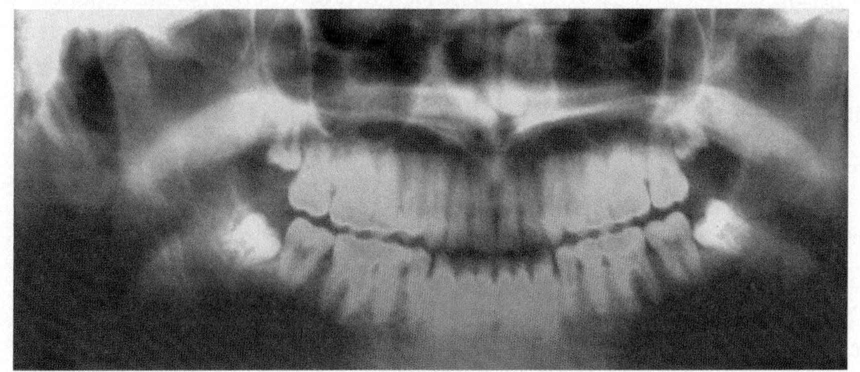

■ Figure 8.3 A) The name and shape of the adult teeth. These teeth represent those found in the right side of the mouth. Those of the left side would be a mirror image. The incisors and cuspids are cutting teeth. The bicuspids and molars are grinding teeth. B) Color enhanced X-ray of all teeth. Note the four wisdom teeth (3rd molars) that have not erupted. *(Science Source)*

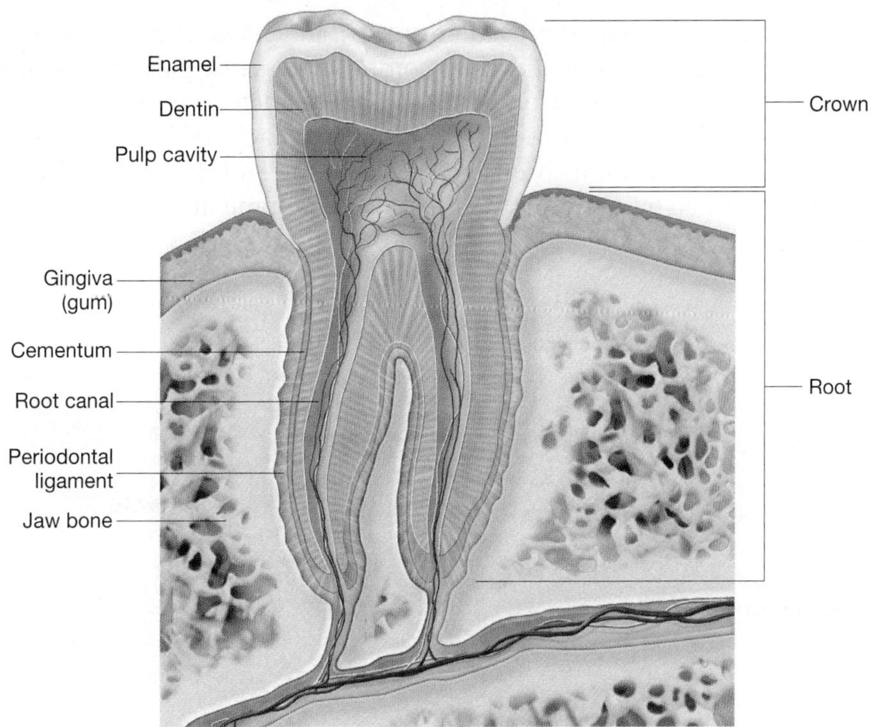

■ Figure 8.4 An adult tooth, longitudinal view showing internal structures of the crown and root.

Pharynx

epiglottis (ep-ih-GLOT-iss)
oropharynx
laryngopharynx (lair-ring-goh-FAIR-inks)

What's In A Name?
Look for these word parts:
laryng/o = larynx
or/o = mouth
epi- = above

When food is swallowed, it enters the **oropharynx** and then the **laryngopharynx** (see again Figure 8.2). Remember from your study of the respiratory system in Chapter 7 that air is also traveling through these portions of the pharynx. The **epiglottis** is a cartilaginous flap that folds down to cover the larynx and trachea so that food is prevented from entering the respiratory tract and instead continues into the esophagus.

Esophagus

peristalsis (pair-ih-STALL-sis)

Med Term Tip
It takes about 10 seconds for swallowed food to reach the stomach.

The esophagus is a muscular tube about 10 inches long in adults. Food entering the esophagus is carried through the thoracic cavity and diaphragm and into the abdominal cavity where it enters the stomach (see Figure 8.5 ■). Food is propelled along the esophagus by wavelike muscular contractions called **peristalsis**. In fact, peristalsis works to push food through the entire gastrointestinal tract.

Stomach

antrum (AN-trum)
body
cardiac sphincter (CAR-dee-ak / SFINGK-ter)
chyme (KIGHM)
fundus (FUN-dus)
hydrochloric acid
lower esophageal sphincter (eh-soff-ah-JEE-al / SFINGK-ter)
pyloric sphincter (pigh-LOR-ik / SFINGK-ter)
rugae (ROO-gay)
sphincters (SFINGK-ters)

The stomach, a J-shaped muscular organ that acts as a bag or sac to collect and churn food with digestive juices, is composed of three parts: the **fundus** or upper region, the **body** or main portion, and the **antrum** or lower region (see again Figure 8.5). The folds in the lining of the stomach are called **rugae**. When the stomach fills with food, the rugae stretch out and disappear. **Hydrochloric acid** (HCl) is secreted by glands in the mucous membrane lining of the stomach. Food

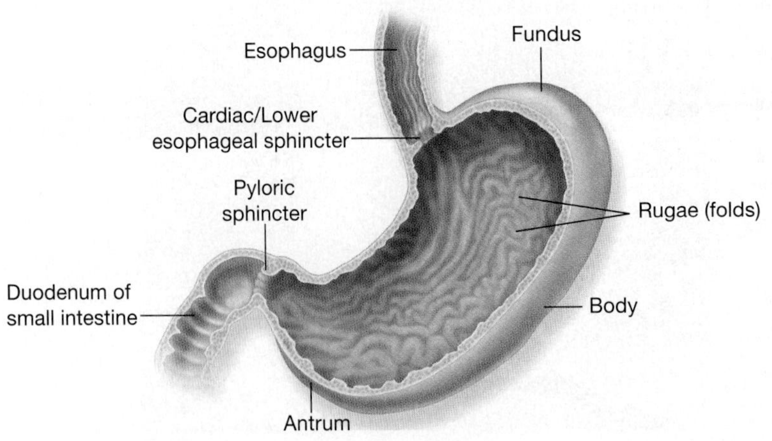

■ **Figure 8.5** The stomach, longitudinal view, showing regions and internal structures.

mixes with hydrochloric acid and other gastric juices to form a liquid mixture called **chyme**, which then passes through the remaining portion of the digestive system.

Entry into and exit from the stomach is controlled by muscular valves called **sphincters**. These valves open and close to ensure that food can only move forward down the gut tube. The **cardiac sphincter**, named for its proximity to the heart, is located between the esophagus and the fundus; also called the **lower esophageal sphincter** (LES), it keeps food from flowing backward into the esophagus.

The antrum tapers off into the **pyloric sphincter**, which regulates the passage of food into the small intestine. Only a small amount of the chyme is allowed to enter the small intestine with each opening of the sphincter for two important reasons. First, the small intestine is much narrower than the stomach and cannot hold as much as the stomach can. Second, the chyme is highly acidic and must be thoroughly neutralized as it leaves the stomach.

What's In A Name?

Look for these word parts:
cardi/o = heart
hydr/o = water
-ac = pertaining to
-ic = pertaining to

Med Term Tip

It is easier to remember the function of the pyloric sphincter when you note that *pylor/o* means "gatekeeper." This gatekeeper controls the forward movement of food. Sphincters are rings of muscle that can be opened and closed to control entry and exit from hollow organs like the stomach, colon, and bladder.

Small Intestine

duodenum (doo-oh-DEE-num / doo-OD-eh-num)
ileocecal valve (ill-ee-oh-SEE-kal)
ileum (ILL-ee-um)
jejunum (jih-JOO-num)

The small intestine, or small bowel, is the major site of digestion and absorption of nutrients from food. It is located between the pyloric sphincter and the colon (see Figure 8.6 ■). Because the small intestine is concerned with absorption of food products, an abnormality in this organ can cause malnutrition. The small intestine, with an average length of 20 feet, is the longest portion of the alimentary canal and has three sections: the **duodenum**, the **jejunum**, and the **ileum**.

- The duodenum extends from the pyloric sphincter to the jejunum, and is about 10–12 inches long. Digestion is completed in the duodenum after the liquid chyme from the stomach is mixed with digestive juices from the pancreas and gallbladder.
- The jejunum, or middle portion, extends from the duodenum to the ileum and is about eight feet long.

Word Watch

Be careful not to confuse the word root *ile/o* meaning "ileum," a portion of the small intestine and *ili/o* meaning "ilium," a pelvic bone.

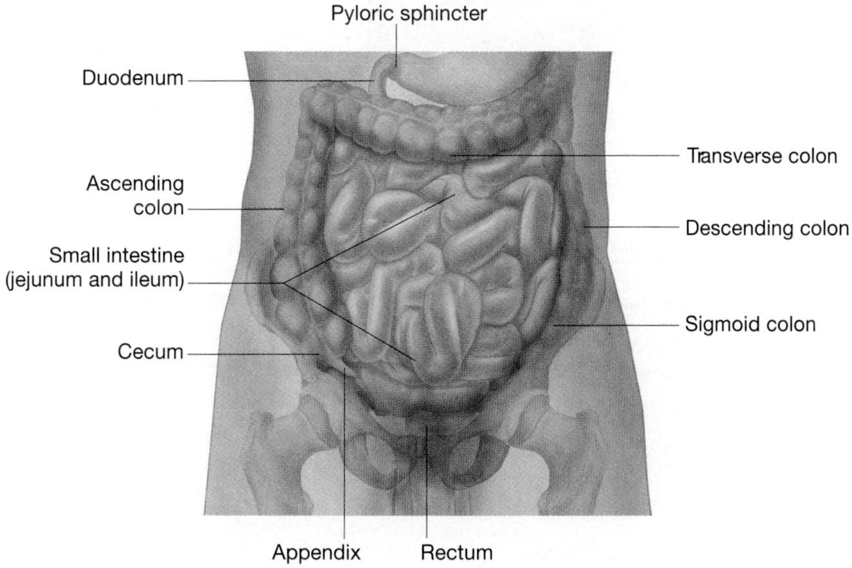

■ **Figure 8.6** The small intestine. Anterior view of the abdominopelvic cavity illustrating how the three sections of small intestine—duodenum, jejunum, ileum—begin at the pyloric sphincter and end at the colon, but are not arranged in an orderly fashion.

Med Term Tip

We can survive without a portion of the small intestine. For example, in cases of cancer, much of the small intestine and/or colon may have to be removed. The surgeon then creates an opening between the remaining intestine and the abdominal wall. The combining form for the section of intestine connected to the abdominal wall and the suffix *-ostomy* are used to describe this procedure. For example, if a person has a *jejunostomy*, the jejunum is connected to the abdominal wall and the ileum (and remainder of the gut tube) has been removed.

- The ileum is the last portion of the small intestine and extends from the jejunum to the colon. At 12 feet in length, it is the longest portion of the small intestine. The ileum connects to the colon with a sphincter called the **ileocecal valve.**

Large Intestine

anal sphincter (AY-nal / SFINGK-ter)
anus (AY-nus)
ascending colon
cecum (SEE-kum)
defecation
descending colon
feces (FEE-seez)
rectum (REK-tum)
sigmoid colon (SIG-moyd)
transverse colon
vermiform appendix (VER-mih-form / ah-PEN-diks)

Fluid that remains after the complete digestion and absorption of nutrients in the small intestine enters the large intestine (see Figure 8.7 ■). Most of this fluid is water that is reabsorbed into the body. The material that remains after absorption is solid waste called **feces** (or stool). This is the product evacuated in bowel movements (BM).

Word Watch

The term *colon* refers to only a portion of the large intestine. However, you should be aware that many people use it incorrectly as a general term referring to the entire intestinal system, both small and large intestines.

Med Term Tip

The term *defecation* comes from the Latin word meaning "to remove the dregs."

The large intestine is approximately 5 feet long and extends from the **ileocecal valve** to the **anus**; this includes the cecum, colon, and rectum. The cecum is a pouch or saclike area in the first 2–3 inches at the beginning of the colon. The **vermiform appendix** is a small worm-shaped outgrowth at the end of the cecum. The colon consists of the **ascending colon**, **transverse colon**, **descending colon**, and **sigmoid colon**. The ascending colon on the right side extends from the cecum to the lower border of the liver. The transverse colon moves horizontally across the upper abdomen toward the spleen. The descending colon then travels down the left side of the body to where the sigmoid colon begins. The sigmoid colon curves in an S-shape back to the midline of the body and ends at the **rectum**. The rectum, where feces are stored, leads into the anus, which contains the **anal sphincter**. This sphincter consists of rings of voluntary and involuntary muscles to control the evacuation of feces or **defecation**.

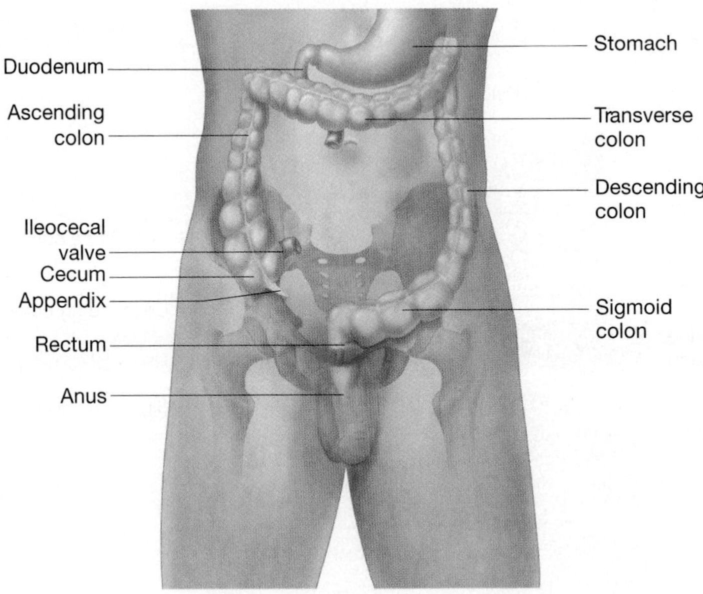

■ **Figure 8.7** The regions of the colon beginning with the cecum and ending at the anus.

Accessory Organs of the Digestive System

As described earlier, the accessory organs of the digestive system are the salivary glands, the liver, the pancreas, and the gallbladder. In general, these organs function by producing much of the digestive fluids and enzymes necessary for the chemical breakdown of food. Each is attached to the gut tube by a duct.

Med Term Tip

In anatomy the term *accessory* generally means that the structure is auxiliary to a more important structure. This is not true for these organs. Digestion would not be possible without the digestive juices produced by these organs.

Salivary Glands

amylase (AM-ill-ace)
bolus
parotid glands (pah-ROT-id)
sublingual glands (sub-LING-gwal)
submandibular glands (sub-man-DIB-yoo-lar)

Salivary glands in the oral cavity produce saliva. This very watery and slick fluid allows food to be swallowed with less danger of choking. Saliva mixed with food in the mouth forms a **bolus**, chewed food that is ready to swallow. Saliva also contains the digestive enzyme **amylase** that begins the digestion of carbohydrates. There are three pairs of salivary glands. The **parotid glands** are in front of the ears, and the **submandibular glands** and **sublingual glands** are in the floor of the mouth (see Figure 8.8 ■).

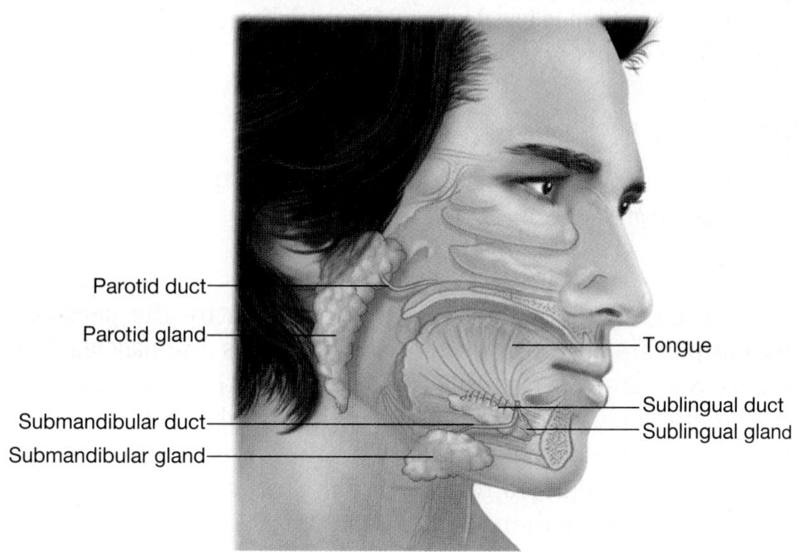

■ **Figure 8.8** The salivary glands: parotid, sublingual, and submandibular. This image shows the position of each gland and its duct emptying into the oral cavity.

Liver

bile (BYE-al)
emulsification (ee-mull-sih-fih-KAY-shun)

The liver, a large organ located in the right upper quadrant of the abdomen, has several functions including processing the nutrients absorbed by the intestines, detoxifying harmful substances in the body, and producing **bile** (see Figure 8.9 ■). Bile is important for the digestion of fats and lipids because it breaks up large fat globules into much smaller droplets, making them easier to digest in the watery environment inside the intestines. The process is called **emulsification**.

Med Term Tip

The liver weighs about four pounds and has so many important functions that people cannot live without it. It has become a major transplant organ. The liver is also able to regenerate itself. You can lose more than half of your liver, and it will regrow.

Gallbladder

common bile duct
cystic duct (SIS-tik)
hepatic duct (hep-PAT-tik)

Bile produced by the liver is stored in the gallbladder (GB). As the liver produces bile, it travels down the **hepatic duct** and up the **cystic duct** into the gallbladder

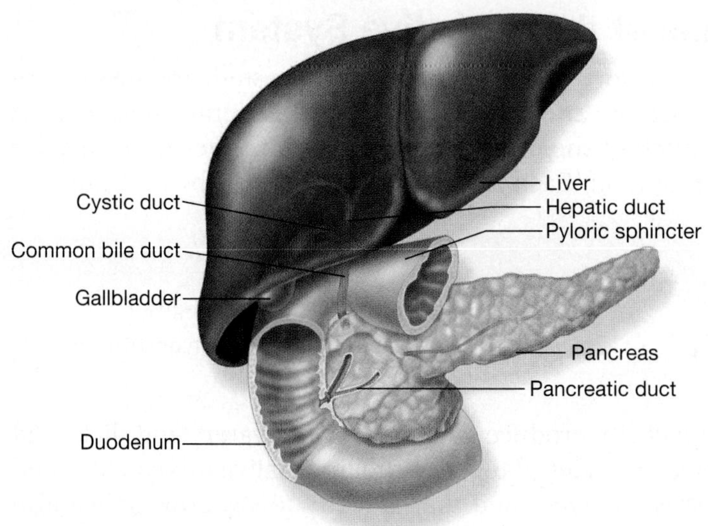

■ Figure 8.9 The liver, gallbladder, and pancreas. Image shows the relationship of these three organs and their ducts to the duodenum.

(see again Figure 8.9). In response to the presence of fat in the chyme, the muscular wall of the gallbladder contracts and sends bile back down the cystic duct and into the **common bile duct** (CBD), which carries bile to the duodenum where it is able to emulsify the fat in chyme.

Pancreas

buffers

pancreatic enzymes (pan-kree-AT-ik / EN-zimes)

pancreatic duct (pan-kree-AT-ik)

The pancreas, connected to the duodenum by the **pancreatic duct**, produces two important secretions for digestion: **buffers** and **pancreatic enzymes** (see again Figure 8.9). Buffers neutralize acidic chyme that has just left the stomach, and pancreatic enzymes chemically digest carbohydrates, fats, and proteins. The pancreas is also an endocrine gland that produces the hormones insulin and glucagon, which play a role in regulating the level of glucose in the blood and are discussed in further detail in Chapter 11.

Practice As You Go

A. Complete the Statement

1. The digestive system is also known as the ____________________ system.
2. The continuous muscular tube of the digestive system is called the ____________________ or ____________________ and stretches between the ____________________ and ____________________.
3. The accessory organs of the digestive system are the ____________________, ____________________, ____________________, and ____________________.

4. The three main functions of the digestive system are ____________________, ____________________, and ____________________.

5. The incisors are examples of ____________________ teeth and the molars are examples of ____________________ teeth.

6. Food is propelled through the gut by wavelike muscular contractions called ____________________.

7. Food in the stomach is mixed with ____________________ and other gastric juices to form a watery mixture called ____________________.

8. The three sections of small intestine in order are the ____________________, ____________________, and ____________________.

9. The S-shaped section of colon that curves back toward the rectum is called the ____________________ colon.

10. ____________________ produced by the liver is responsible for the ____________________ of fats. It is stored in the ____________________.

Terminology

Word Parts Used to Build Digestive System Terms

The following lists contain the combining forms, suffixes, and prefixes used to build terms in the remaining sections of this chapter.

Combining Forms

an/o	anus
append/o	appendix
appendic/o	appendix
bar/o	weight
bucc/o	cheek
carcin/o	cancer
cec/o	cecum
chol/e	bile
cholangi/o	bile duct
cholecyst/o	gallbladder
choledoch/o	common bile duct
cirrh/o	yellow
col/o	colon
colon/o	colon
cutane/o	skin
cyst/o	sac
dent/o	tooth

diverticul/o	pouch
duoden/o	duodenum
enter/o	small intestine
esophag/o	esophagus
gastr/o	stomach
gingiv/o	gums
gloss/o	tongue
hem/o	blood
hemat/o	blood
hepat/o	liver
ile/o	ileum
inguin/o	groin
jejun/o	jejunum
labi/o	lip
lapar/o	abdomen
lingu/o	tongue
lith/o	stone

nas/o	nose
odont/o	tooth
or/o	mouth
orth/o	straight
palat/o	palate
pancreat/o	pancreas
pharyng/o	pharynx
polyp/o	polyp
proct/o	anus and rectum
pylor/o	pylorus
pyr/o	fire
rect/o	rectum
sialaden/o	salivary gland
sigmoid/o	sigmoid colon
ven/o	vein

Suffixes

-al	pertaining to
-algia	pain
-centesis	process of removing fluid
-eal	pertaining to
-ectomy	surgical removal
-emesis	vomiting
-emetic	pertaining to vomiting
-gram	record
-graphy	process of recording
-iatric	pertaining to medical treatment

-ic	pertaining to
-istry	specialty of
-itis	inflammation
-lithiasis	condition of stones
-logy	study of
-oma	tumor
-orexia	appetite
-osis	abnormal condition
-ostomy	surgically create an opening
-otomy	cutting into
-ous	pertaining to
-pepsia	digestion

-pexy	surgical fixation
-phagia	eat, swallow
-plasty	surgical repair
-plegia	paralysis
-prandial	pertaining to a meal
-ptosis	drooping
-scope	instrument to view
-scopic	pertaining to visually examining
-scopy	process of viewing
-tic	pertaining to
-tripsy	surgical crushing

Prefixes

a-	without
an-	without
anti-	against
brady-	slow
dys-	abnormal, painful, difficult
endo-	within
ex-	outward

hyper-	excessive
hypo-	below
in-	inward
intra-	within
per-	through
peri-	around

poly-	many
post-	after
re-	again
retro-	backward
sub-	under
trans-	across

Adjective Forms of Anatomical Terms

Term	Word Parts	Definition
anal	an/o = anus -al = pertaining to **Word Watch** Be careful when using the combining form *an/o* meaning "anus" and the prefix *an-* meaning "none."	Pertaining to the anus.
buccal (BYOO-kal)	bucc/o = cheek -al = pertaining to	Pertaining to the cheeks.
buccolabial (BYOO-koh-labe-ee-all)	bucc/o = cheek labi/o = lip -al = pertaining to	Pertaining to the cheeks and lips.
cecal (SEE-kal)	cec/o = cecum -al = pertaining to	Pertaining to the cecum.
cholecystic (koh-lee-SIS-tik)	cholecyst/o = gallbladder -ic = pertaining to	Pertaining to the gallbladder.

Adjective Forms of Anatomical Terms (continued)

Term	Word Parts	Definition
colonic (koh-LON-ik)	colon/o = colon -ic = pertaining to	Pertaining to the colon.
colorectal (kohl-oh-REK-tall)	col/o = colon rect/o = rectum -al = pertaining to	Pertaining to the colon and rectum.
cystic (SIS-tik)	cyst/o = sac -ic = pertaining to	Pertaining to the gallbladder. The combining form **cyst/o** is referring to the sac-like shape of the gallbladder.
dental (DENT-all)	dent/o = tooth -al = pertaining to	Pertaining to the teeth.
duodenal (duo-DEEN-all / do-ODD-in-all)	duoden/o = duodenum -al = pertaining to	Pertaining to the duodenum.
enteric (en-TARE-ik)	enter/o = small intestine -ic = pertaining to	Pertaining to the small intestine.
esophageal (eh-soff-ah-JEE-al)	esophag/o = esophagus -eal = pertaining to	Pertaining to the esophagus.
gastric (GAS-trik)	gastr/o = stomach -ic = pertaining to	Pertaining to the stomach.
gastrointestinal (GI) (gas-troh-in-TESS-tih-nal)	gastr/o = stomach -al = pertaining to	Pertaining to the stomach and intestines.
gingival (JIN-jih-vul)	gingiv/o = gums -al = pertaining to	Pertaining to the gums.
glossal (GLOSS-all)	gloss/o = tongue -al = pertaining to	Pertaining to the tongue.
hepatic (hep-AT-ik)	hepat/o = liver -ic = pertaining to	Pertaining to the liver.
hypoglossal (high-poe-GLOSS-all)	hypo- = under gloss/o = tongue -al = pertaining to	Pertaining to under the tongue.
ileal (ILL-ee-all)	ile/o = ileum -al = pertaining to	Pertaining to the ileum.
ileocecal (ill-ee-oh-SEE-kal)	ile/o = ileum cec/o = cecum -al = pertaining to	Pertaining to the ileum and cecum.
jejunal (jih-JUNE-all)	jejun/o = jejunum -al = pertaining to	Pertaining to the jejunum.
nasogastric (nay-zoh-GAS-trik)	nas/o = nose gastr/o = stomach -ic = pertaining to	Pertaining to the nose and stomach.
oral (OR-ral)	or/o = mouth -al = pertaining to	Pertaining to the mouth.
pancreatic (pan-kree-AT-ik)	pancreat/o = pancreas -ic = pertaining to	Pertaining to the pancreas.

Adjective Forms of Anatomical Terms (continued)

Term	Word Parts	Definition
periodontal (pair-ee-oh-DON-tal)	peri- = around odont/o = tooth -al = pertaining to	Pertaining to around the teeth.
pharyngeal (fair-in-JEE-all)	pharyng/o = pharynx -eal = pertaining to	Pertaining to the pharynx.
pyloric (pie-LORE-ik)	pylor/o = pylorus -ic = pertaining to	Pertaining to the pylorus.
rectal (RECK-tall)	rect/o = rectum -al = pertaining to	Pertaining to the rectum.
sigmoidal (sig-MOYD-all)	sigmoid/o = sigmoid colon -al = pertaining to	Pertaining to the sigmoid colon.
sublingual (sub-LING-gwal)	sub- = under lingu/o = tongue -al = pertaining to	Pertaining to under the tongue.
submandibular (sub-man-DIB-yoo-lar)	sub- = under mandibul/o = mandible -ar = pertaining to	Pertaining to under the mandible.

Practice As You Go

B. Give the adjective form for each anatomical structure

1. The duodenum ____________________
2. Nose and stomach ____________________
3. The liver ____________________
4. The pancreas ____________________
5. The gallbladder ____________________ or ____________________
6. Under the tongue ____________________
7. The esophagus ____________________
8. The sigmoid colon ____________________

Pathology

Term	Word Parts	Definition
Medical Specialties		
dentistry	dent/o = tooth -istry = specialty of	Branch of healthcare involved with the prevention, diagnosis, and treatment of conditions involving the teeth, jaw, and mouth. Practitioner is a *dentist.*
gastroenterology (gas-troh-en-ter-ALL-oh-jee)	gastr/o = stomach enter/o = small intestine -logy = study of	Branch of medicine involved in diagnosis and treatment of diseases and disorders of the digestive system. Physician is a *gastroenterologist*.
oral surgery	or/o = mouth -al = pertaining to	Branch of dentistry that uses surgical means to treat dental conditions. Specialist is an *oral surgeon*.
orthodontics (or-thoh-DON-tiks)	orth/o = straight odont/o = tooth -ic = pertaining to	Branch of dentistry concerned with correction of problems with tooth alignment. Specialist is an *orthodontist*.
periodontics (pair-ee-oh-DON-tiks)	peri- = around odont/o = tooth -ic = pertaining to	Branch of dentistry concerned with treating conditions involving the gums and tissues surrounding the teeth. Specialist is a *periodontist*.
proctology (prok-TOL-oh-jee)	proct/o = anus and rectum -logy = study of	Branch of medicine involved in diagnosis and treatment of diseases and disorders of the anus and rectum. Physician is a *proctologist*.
Signs and Symptoms		
anorexia (an-oh-REK-see-ah)	an- = without -orexia = appetite	General term meaning loss of appetite that may accompany other conditions. Also used to refer to *anorexia nervosa*, which is characterized by severe weight loss from excessive dieting.
aphagia (ah-FAY-jee-ah)	a- = without -phagia = eat, swallow	Being unable to swallow or eat.
ascites (ah-SIGH-teez)		Collection or accumulation of fluid in the peritoneal cavity.
bradypepsia (brad-ee-PEP-see-ah)	brady- = slow -pepsia = digestion	Having a slow digestive system.
cachexia (ka-KEK-see-ah)		Loss of weight and generalized wasting that occurs during a chronic disease.
cholecystalgia (koh-lee-sis-TAL-jee-ah)	cholecyst/o = gallbladder -algia = pain	Having gallbladder pain.
constipation (kon-stih-PAY-shun)		Experiencing difficulty in defecation or infrequent defecation.
dentalgia (dent-AL-gee-ah)	dent/o = tooth -algia = pain	Tooth pain.

Pathology (continued)

Term	Word Parts	Definition
diarrhea (dye-ah-REE-ah)		Passing of frequent, watery, or bloody bowel movements. Usually accompanies gastrointestinal (GI) disorders.
dysorexia (dis-oh-REKS-ee-ah)	dys- = abnormal -orexia = appetite	Abnormal appetite; usually a diminished appetite.
dyspepsia (dis-PEP-see-ah)	dys- = painful -pepsia = digestion	"Upset stomach"; indigestion.
dysphagia (dis-FAY-jee-ah)	dys- = difficult -phagia = eat, swallow	Having difficulty swallowing or eating.
emesis (EM-eh-sis)	*Emesis* is the Latin term meaning "to vomit"	Vomiting.
gastralgia (gas-TRAL-jee-ah)	gastr/o = stomach -algia = pain	Stomach pain.
hematemesis (hee-mah-TEM-eh-sis)	hemat/o = blood -emesis = vomiting	Vomiting blood.
hematochezia (hee-mat-oh-KEY-zee-ah)	hemat/o = blood	Passing bright red blood in the stool.
hyperemesis (high-per-EM-eh-sis)	hyper- = excessive -emesis = vomiting	Excessive vomiting.
jaundice (JAWN-diss)		Yellow cast to the skin, mucous membranes, and the whites of the eyes caused by the deposit of bile pigment from too much bilirubin in the blood. Bilirubin is a waste product produced when worn-out red blood cells are broken down. May be a symptom of a disorder such as gallstones blocking the common bile duct or carcinoma of the liver. Also called *icterus*.
melena (me-LEE-nah)		Passage of dark tarry stool. Color is the result of digestive enzymes working on blood in the gastrointestinal tract.
nausea (NAW-see-ah)	Med Term Tip The term *nausea* comes from the Greek word for "seasickness."	Urge to vomit.
obesity		Body weight that is above a healthy level. A person whose weight interferes with normal activity and body function has *morbid obesity*.
polyphagia (pall-ee-FAY-jee-ah)	poly- = many -phagia = eat, swallow	Excessive eating; eating too much.
postprandial (post-PRAN-dee-all)	post- = after -prandial = pertaining to a meal	After a meal.
pyrosis (pie-ROW-sis)	pyr/o = fire -osis = abnormal condition	Pain and burning sensation usually caused by stomach acid splashing up into the esophagus. Commonly called *heartburn*.

Pathology (continued)

Term	Word Parts	Definition
regurgitation (ree-gur-jih-TAY-shun)	re- = again	Return of fluids and solids from the stomach into the mouth.
Oral Cavity		
aphthous ulcers (AF-thus)		Painful ulcers in the mouth of unknown cause. Commonly called *canker sores*.
cleft lip (CLEFT)		Congenital anomaly in which the upper lip and jaw bone fail to fuse in the midline, leaving an open gap. Often seen along with a cleft palate. Corrected with surgery.
cleft palate (CLEFT / PAL-at)		Congenital anomaly in which the roof of the mouth has a split or fissure. Corrected with surgery.
dental caries (KAIR-eez)	dent/o = tooth -al = pertaining to	Gradual decay and disintegration of teeth caused by bacteria; may lead to abscessed teeth. Commonly called a *tooth cavity*.
gingivitis (jin-jih-VIGH-tis)	gingiv/o = gums -itis = inflammation	Inflammation of the gums.
herpes labialis (HER-peez / lay-bee-AL-iz)	labi/o = lip	Infection of the lip by the herpes simplex virus type 1 (HSV-1). Also called *fever blisters* or *cold sores*.
periodontal disease (pair-ee-oh-DON-tal)	peri- = around odont/o = tooth -al = pertaining to	Disease of the supporting structures of the teeth, including the gums and bones; the most common cause of tooth loss.
sialadenitis (sigh-al-add-eh-NIGH-tis)	sialaden/o = salivary gland -itis = inflammation	Inflammation of a salivary gland.
Pharynx and Esophagus		
esophageal varices (eh-soff-ah-JEE-al / VAIR-ih-seez)	esophag/o = esophagus -eal = pertaining to	Enlarged and swollen varicose veins in the lower end of the esophagus. If these rupture, serious hemorrhage results; often related to liver disease.
gastroesophageal reflux disease (GERD) (gas-troh-ee-sof-ah-GEE-all / REE-fluks)	gastr/o = stomach esophag/o = esophagus -eal = pertaining to	Acid from the stomach flows backward up into the esophagus causing inflammation and pain.
pharyngoplegia (fair-in-goh-PLEE-jee-ah)	pharyng/o = pharynx -plegia = paralysis	Paralysis of the throat muscles.
Stomach		
gastric carcinoma (GAS-trik / car-si-NOH-mah)	gastr/o = stomach -ic = pertaining to	Cancerous tumor in the stomach.
gastritis (gas-TRY-tis)	gastr/o = stomach -itis = inflammation	Stomach inflammation.
gastroenteritis (gas-troh-en-ter-EYE-tis)	gastr/o = stomach enter/o = small intestine -itis = inflammation	Inflammation of the stomach and small intestine.

Pathology (continued)

Term	Word Parts	Definition
hiatal hernia (high-AY-tal / HER-nee-ah)	-al = pertaining to	Protrusion of the stomach through the diaphragm (also called a *diaphragmatocele*) and extending into the thoracic cavity; gastroesophageal reflux disease is a common symptom.

■ **Figure 8.10** A hiatal hernia or diaphragmatocele. A portion of the stomach protrudes through the diaphragm into the thoracic cavity.

Term	Word Parts	Definition
peptic ulcer disease (PUD) (PEP-tik / ULL-sir)	-ic = pertaining to	Ulcer occurring in the lower portion of the esophagus, stomach, and/or duodenum; thought to be caused by the acid of gastric juices. Initial damage to the protective lining of the stomach may be caused by a *Helicobacter pylori* (*H. pylori*) bacterial infection. If the ulcer extends all the way through the wall of the stomach, it is called a *perforated ulcer*, which requires immediate surgery to repair.

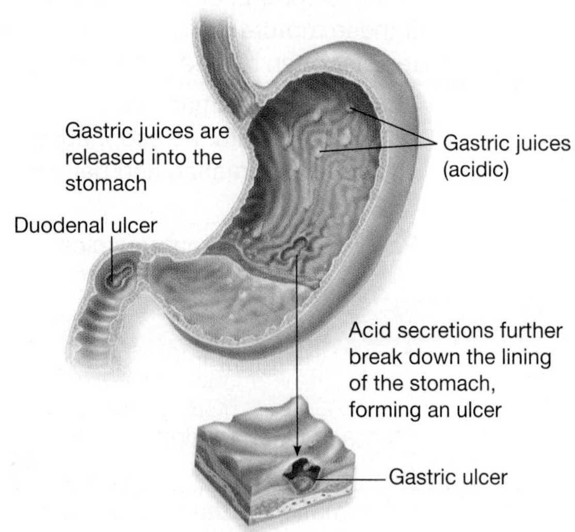

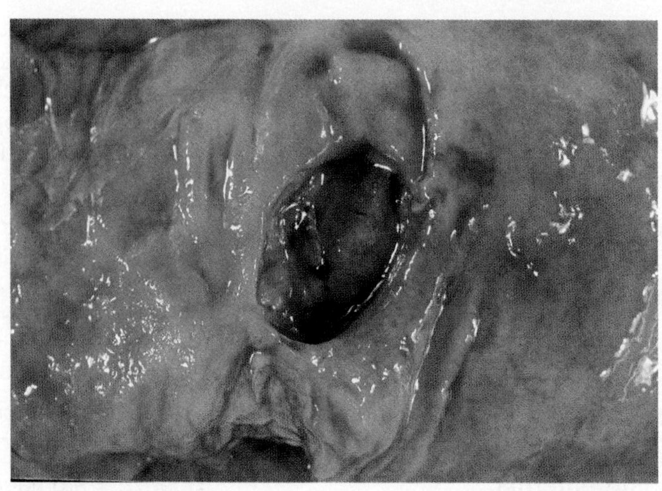

■ **Figure 8.11** A) Figure illustrating the location and appearance of a peptic ulcer in both the stomach and the duodenum. B) Photomicrograph illustrating a gastric ulcer. *(Dr. E. Walker/Science Photo Library/Science Source).*

Pathology (continued)

Term	Word Parts	Definition
Small Intestine and Large Intestine		
anal fistula (FIH-styoo-lah)	-al = pertaining to	Abnormal tube-like passage from the surface around the anal opening directly into the rectum.
appendicitis (ah-pen-dih-SIGH-tis)	appendic/o = appendix -itis = inflammation	Inflammation of the appendix; may require an *appendectomy*.
bowel incontinence (in-CON-tih-nence)		Inability to control defecation.
colorectal carcinoma (kohl-oh-REK-tall / car-si-NOH-mah)	col/o = colon rect/o = rectum -al = pertaining to carcin/o = cancer -oma = tumor	Cancerous tumor originating in the colon or rectum.
Crohn's disease (KROHNZ)		Form of chronic inflammatory bowel disease affecting primarily the ileum and/or colon. Also called *regional ileitis*. This autoimmune condition affects all the layers of the bowel wall and results in scarring and thickening of the gut wall.
diverticulitis (dye-ver-tik-yoo-LYE-tis)	diverticul/o = pouch -itis = inflammation	Inflammation of a *diverticulum* (an outpouching off the gut), especially in the colon. Inflammation often results when food becomes trapped within the pouch.

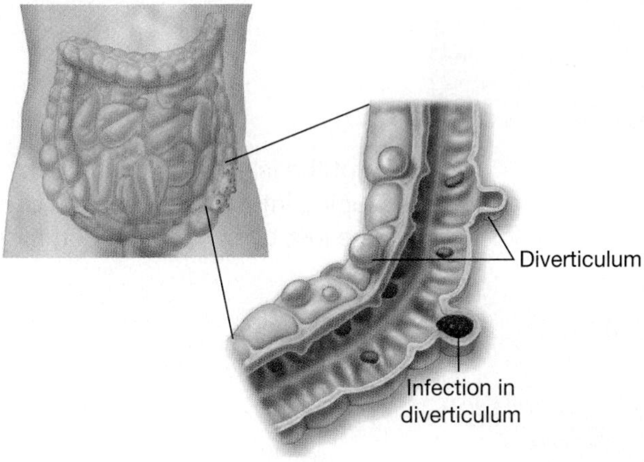

■ **Figure 8.12** Diverticulosis. Figure illustrates external and internal appearance of diverticula.

Term	Word Parts	Definition
diverticulosis (dye-ver-tik-yoo-LOW-sis)	diverticul/o = pouch -osis = abnormal condition	Condition of having diverticula (outpouches off the gut). May lead to *diverticulitis* if one becomes inflamed.
dysentery (dis-in-TARE-ee)		Disease characterized by diarrhea, often with mucus and blood; severe abdominal pain; fever; and dehydration. Caused by ingesting food or water contaminated by chemicals, bacteria, protozoans, or parasites.
enteritis (en-ter-EYE-tis)	enter/o = small intestine -itis = inflammation	Inflammation of the small intestine.
hemorrhoids (HEM-oh-roydz)	hem/o = blood	Varicose veins in the rectum and anus.

Pathology (continued)

Term	Word Parts	Definition
ileus (ILL-ee-us)		Severe abdominal pain, inability to pass stool, vomiting, and abdominal distension as a result of an intestinal blockage. The blockage can be a physical block such as a tumor or the failure of bowel contents to move forward due to loss of peristalsis (a nonmechanical blockage). May require surgery to reverse the blockage.
inguinal hernia (ING-gwih-nal / HER-nee-ah) Loop of intestine protruding through opening in abdominal muscles ■ **Figure 8.13** An inguinal hernia. A portion of the small intestine is protruding through the abdominal muscles into the groin region.	**inguin/o** = groin -al = pertaining to	Hernia or protrusion of a loop of small intestine into the inguinal (groin) region through a weak spot in the abdominal muscle wall that develops into a hole. May become *incarcerated* or *strangulated* if the muscle tightens down around the loop of intestine and cuts off its blood flow.
intussusception (in-tuh-suh-SEP-shun) 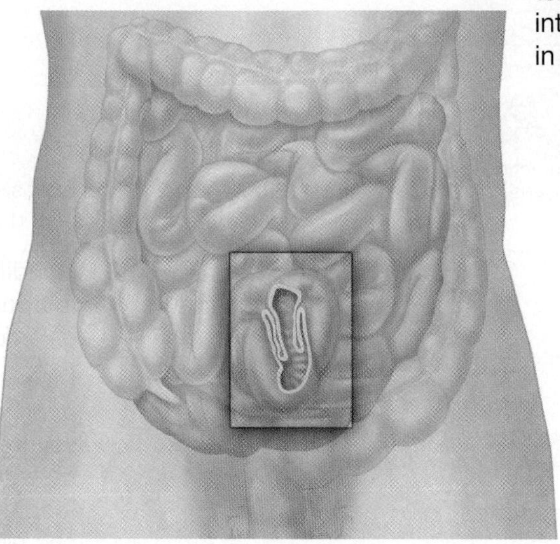 ■ **Figure 8.14** Intussusception. A short length of small intestine has telescoped into itself.	in- = inward	Result of the intestine slipping or telescoping into another section of intestine just below it. More common in children.
irritable bowel syndrome (IBS)		Disturbance in the functions of the intestine from unknown causes. Symptoms generally include abdominal discomfort and an alteration in bowel activity. Also called *spastic colon* or *functional bowel syndrome*.

Pathology (continued)

Term	Word Parts	Definition
polyposis (pall-ee-POH-sis)	polyp/o = polyp -osis = abnormal condition	Presence of small tumors, called **polyps**, containing a pedicle or stemlike attachment in the mucous membranes of the large intestine (colon); may be precancerous.
proctoptosis (prok-top-TOH-sis)	proct/o = rectum and anus -ptosis = drooping	proctoptosis definition, so it reads “Prolapsed or drooping rectum and anus.
ulcerative colitis (ULL-sir-ah-tiv / koh-LYE-tis)	col/o = colon -itis = inflammation	Chronic inflammatory condition resulting in numerous ulcers formed on the mucous membrane lining of the colon; the cause is unknown. Also known as *inflammatory bowel disease* (IBD).
volvulus (VOL-vyoo-lus)		Condition in which the bowel twists upon itself causing an obstruction; painful and requires immediate surgery.

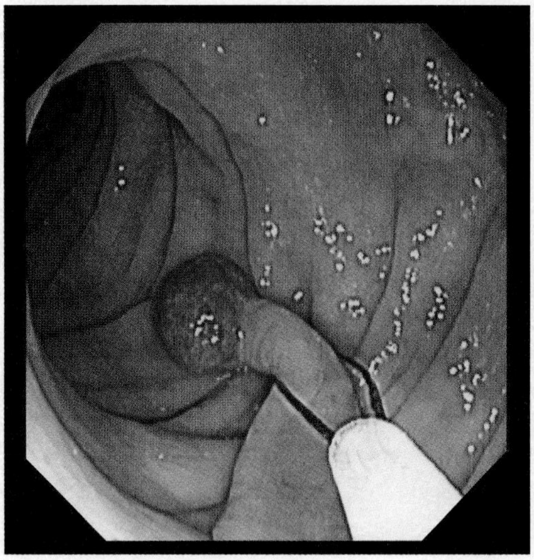

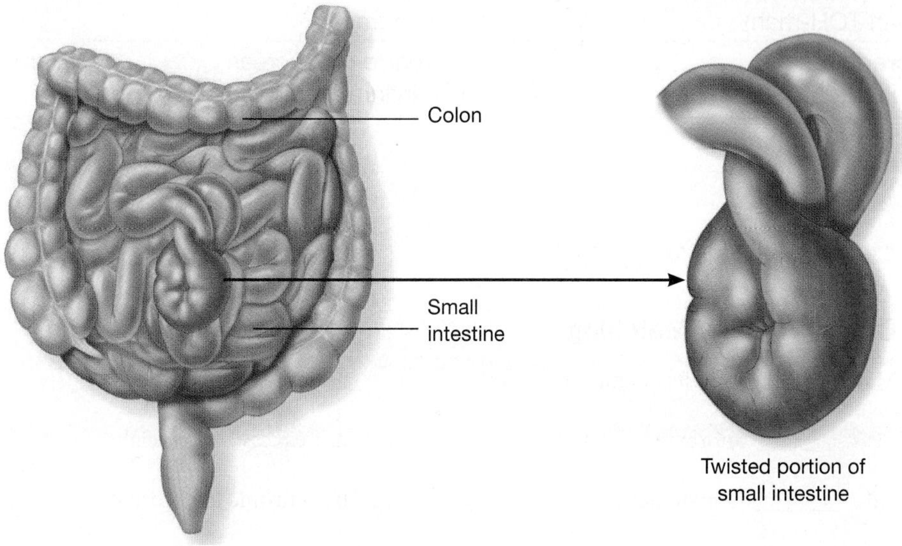

■ **Figure 8.15** Endoscopic view of a polyp in the colon. Note the mushroom-like shape, an enlarged top growing at the end of a stem. It is being removed by means of a wire loop slipped over the polyp and then tightened to cut it off. *(David M. Martin, M.D./Science Source)*

■ **Figure 8.16** Volvulus. A length of small intestine has twisted around itself, cutting off blood circulation to the twisted loop.

Pathology (continued)

Term	Word Parts	Definition
Accessory Organs		
cholecystitis (koh-lee-sis-TYE-tis)	cholecyst/o = gallbladder -itis = inflammation	Inflammation of the gallbladder; most commonly caused by gallstones in the gallbladder or common bile duct that block the flow of bile.
cholelithiasis (koh-lee-lih-THIGH-ah-sis)	chol/e = bile -lithiasis = condition of stones	Presence of gallstones; may or may not cause symptoms such as *cholecystalgia*.

■ Figure 8.17 A) Common sites for cholelithiasis. B) A gallbladder specimen with multiple gallstones.
(Biophoto Associates/Science Source)

Term	Word Parts	Definition
cirrhosis (sih-ROH-sis)	cirrh/o = yellow -osis = abnormal condition	Chronic disease of the liver associated with failure of the liver to function properly.
hepatitis (hep-ah-TYE-tis)	hepat/o = liver -itis = inflammation	Inflammation of the liver, usually due to a viral infection. Different viruses are transmitted by different routes, such as sexual contact or from exposure to blood or fecally contaminated water or food.
hepatoma (hep-ah-TOH-mah)	hepat/o = liver -oma = tumor	Liver tumor.
pancreatitis (pan-kree-ah-TYE-tis)	pancreat/o = pancreas -itis = inflammation	Inflammation of the pancreas.

Practice As You Go

C. Terminology Matching

Match each term to its definition.

1. ________ anorexia
2. ________ hematemesis
3. ________ pyrosis

a. excess body weight
b. chronic liver disease
c. heartburn

4. ________ obesity
5. ________ constipation
6. ________ melena
7. ________ ascites
8. ________ cirrhosis
9. ________ spastic colon
10. ________ polyposis
11. ________ volvulus
12. ________ hiatal hernia
13. ________ ulcerative colitis
14. ________ dysentery
15. ________ jaundice

d. small colon tumors
e. fluid accumulation in abdominal cavity
f. vomit blood
g. bowel twists on self
h. inflammatory bowel disease
i. loss of appetite
j. difficulty having BM
k. irritable bowel syndrome
l. black tarry stool
m. yellow skin color
n. bloody diarrhea
o. diaphragmatocele

Diagnostic Procedures

Term	Word Parts	Definition
Clinical Laboratory Tests		
alanine transaminase (ALT) (AL-ah-neen / trans-AM-in-nase)		Enzyme normally present in the blood. Blood levels are increased in persons with liver disease.
aspartate transaminase (AST) (ass-PAR-tate / trans-AM-in-nase)		Enzyme normally present in the blood. Blood levels are increased in persons with liver disease.
fecal occult blood test (FOBT) (uh-CULT)	-al = pertaining to	Laboratory test on the feces to determine if microscopic amounts of blood are present. Also called *hemoccult* or *stool guaiac*.
ova and parasites (O&P) (OH-vah / PAR-ah-sights)		Laboratory examination of feces with a microscope for the presence of parasites or their eggs.
serum bilirubin (SEE-rum / BILLY-rubin)		Blood test to determine the amount of the waste product bilirubin in the bloodstream. Elevated levels indicate liver disease.
stool culture		Laboratory test of feces to determine if any pathogenic bacteria are present.
Diagnostic Imaging		
bite-wing X-ray		X-ray taken with a part of the film holder held between the teeth and parallel to the teeth.
cholecystogram (koh-lee-SIS-toh-gram)	cholecyst/o = gallbladder -gram = record	X-ray image of the gallbladder.

Diagnostic Procedures (continued)

Term	Word Parts	Definition
intravenous cholecystography (in-trah-VEE-nus / koh-lee-sis-TOG-rah-fee)	intra- = within ven/o = vein -ous = pertaining to cholecyst/o = gallbladder -graphy = process of recording	Dye is administered intravenously to the patient allowing for X-ray visualization of the gallbladder and bile ducts.
lower gastrointestinal series (lower GI series)	gastr/o = stomach -al = pertaining to	X-ray image of the colon and rectum is taken after the administration of barium (Ba), a radiopaque dye, by enema. Also called a *barium enema* (BE).
■ **Figure 8.18** Color enhanced X-ray of the colon taken during a barium enema. *(CNRI/Science Photo Library/Science Source)*		
percutaneous transhepatic cholangiography (PTC) (per-kyoo-TAY-nee-us / trans-heh PAT-ik / koh-lan-jee-OG-rah-fee)	per- = through cutane/o = skin -ous = pertaining to trans- = across hepat/o = liver -ic = pertaining to cholangi/o = bile duct -graphy = process of recording	Procedure in which contrast medium is injected directly into the liver to visualize the bile ducts. Used to detect obstructions such as gallstones in the common bile duct.
upper gastrointestinal (UGI) **series**	gastr/o = stomach -al = pertaining to	Patient is administered a barium (Ba) contrast material orally and then X-rays are taken to visualize the esophagus, stomach, and duodenum. Also called a *barium swallow*.
Endoscopic Procedures		
colonoscope (koh-LON-oh-scope)	colon/o = colon -scope = instrument to view	Instrument used to view the colon.
colonoscopy (koh-lon-OSS-koh-pee)	colon/o = colon -scopy = process of viewing	Flexible fiberscope called a *colonoscope* is passed through the anus, rectum, and colon; used to examine the upper portion of the colon. Polyps and small growths can be removed during this procedure (see again Figure 8.15).

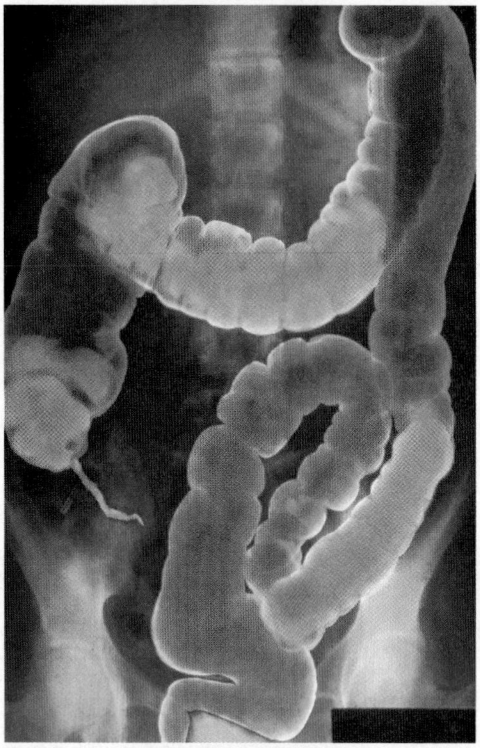

Diagnostic Procedures (continued)

Term	Word Parts	Definition
endoscopic retrograde cholangiopancreatography (ERCP) (en-doh-SKOP-ik / RET-roh-grayd / koh-lan-jee-oh-pan-kree-ah-TOG-rah-fee)	endo- = within -scopic = pertaining to visually examining retro- = backward cholangi/o = bile duct pancreat/o = pancreas -graphy = process of recording	Procedure using an endoscope to visually examine the hepatic duct, common bile duct, and pancreatic duct. First an endoscope is passed through the patient's mouth, esophagus, and stomach until it reaches the duodenum where the pancreatic and common bile ducts empty. Then a thin catheter is passed through the endoscope and into the ducts (in the retrograde direction). Contrast dye is then used to visualize these ducts on an X-ray.
esophagogastroduodenoscopy (EGD) (eh-soff-ah-go-gas-troh-duo-den-OSS-koh-pee)	esophag/o = esophagus gastr/o = stomach duoden/o = duodenum -scopy = process of viewing	Use of a flexible fiberoptic endoscope to visually examine the esophagus, stomach, and beginning of the duodenum.
gastroscope (GAS-troh-scope)	gastr/o = stomach -scope = instrument to view	Instrument used to view inside the stomach.
gastroscopy (gas-TROS-koh-pee)	gastr/o = stomach -scopy = process of viewing	Procedure in which a flexible *gastroscope* is passed through the mouth and down the esophagus in order to visualize inside the stomach. Used to diagnose peptic ulcers and gastric carcinoma.
laparoscope (LAP-ah-roh-scope)	lapar/o = abdomen -scope = instrument to view	Instrument used to view inside the abdomen.
laparoscopy (lap-ar-OSS-koh-pee)	lapar/o = abdomen -scopy = process of viewing	*Laparoscope* is passed into the abdominal wall through a small incision. The abdominal cavity is then visually examined for tumors and other conditions with this lighted instrument. Also called *peritoneoscopy*.
sigmoidoscope (sig-MOYD-oh-scope)	sigmoid/o = sigmoid colon -scope = instrument to view	Instrument used to view inside the sigmoid colon.
sigmoidoscopy (sig-moid-OSS-koh-pee)	sigmoid/o = sigmoid colon -scopy = process of viewing	Procedure using a flexible *sigmoidoscope* to visually examine the sigmoid colon. Commonly done to diagnose cancer and polyps.
Additional Diagnostic Procedures		
paracentesis (pair-ah-sin-TEE-sis)	-centesis = process of removing fluid	Insertion of a needle into the abdominal cavity to withdraw fluid. Tests to diagnose diseases may be conducted on the fluid.

Therapeutic Procedures

Term	Word Parts	Definition
Dental Procedures		
bridge		Dental appliance to replace missing teeth. It is attached to adjacent teeth for support.
crown		Artificial covering for a tooth that is created to replace the original enamel covering of the tooth.

Therapeutic Procedures (continued)

Term	Word Parts	Definition
denture (DEN-chur)	dent/o = tooth	Partial or complete set of artificial teeth that are set in plastic materials. Acts as a substitute for the natural teeth and related structures.
extraction	ex- = outward	Removing or "pulling" of teeth.
implant (IM-plant)		Prosthetic device placed in the jaw to which a tooth or denture may be anchored.
root canal	-al = pertaining to	Dental treatment involving the pulp cavity of the root of a tooth. Procedure is used to save a tooth that is badly infected or abscessed.
Medical Procedures		
gavage (guh-VAHZH)		Use of a nasogastric (NG) tube to place liquid nourishment directly into the stomach.
lavage (lah-VAHZH)		Use of a nasogastric (NG) tube to wash out the stomach, for example, after ingestion of dangerous substances.
nasogastric intubation (NG tube) (NAY-zo-gas-trik / in-two-BAY-shun)	nas/o = nose gastr/o = stomach -ic = pertaining to in- = inward	Procedure in which a flexible catheter is inserted into the nose and down the esophagus to the stomach. May be used for feeding or to suction out stomach fluids.
total parenteral nutrition (TPN) (pair-in-TARE-all)	-al = pertaining to	Providing 100% of a patient's nutrition intravenously. Used when a patient is unable to eat.
Surgical Procedures		
anastomosis (ah-nas-toh-MOH-sis)		To surgically create a connection between two organs or vessels. For example, joining together two cut ends of the intestines after a section is removed.
appendectomy (ap-en-DEK-toh-mee)	append/o = appendix -ectomy = surgical removal	Surgical removal of the appendix.
bariatric surgery (bear-ee-AT-rik)	bar/o = weight -iatric = pertaining to medical treatment	Group of surgical procedures such as stomach stapling and restrictive banding to reduce the size of the stomach. A treatment for morbid (extreme) obesity.
cholecystectomy (koh-lee-sis-TEK-toh-mee)	cholecyst/o = gallbladder -ectomy = surgical removal	Surgical removal of the gallbladder.
choledocholithotripsy (koh-led-oh-koh-LITH-oh-trip-see)	choledoch/o = common bile duct lith/o = stone -tripsy = surgical crushing	Crushing of a gallstone in the common bile duct.
colectomy (koh-LEK-toh-mee)	col/o = colon -ectomy = surgical removal	Surgical removal of the colon.

Therapeutic Procedures (continued)

Term	Word Parts	Definition
colostomy (koh-LOSS-toh-mee)	col/o = colon -ostomy = surgically create an opening	Surgical creation of an opening of some portion of the colon through the abdominal wall to the outside surface. Fecal material (stool) drains into a bag worn on the abdomen.

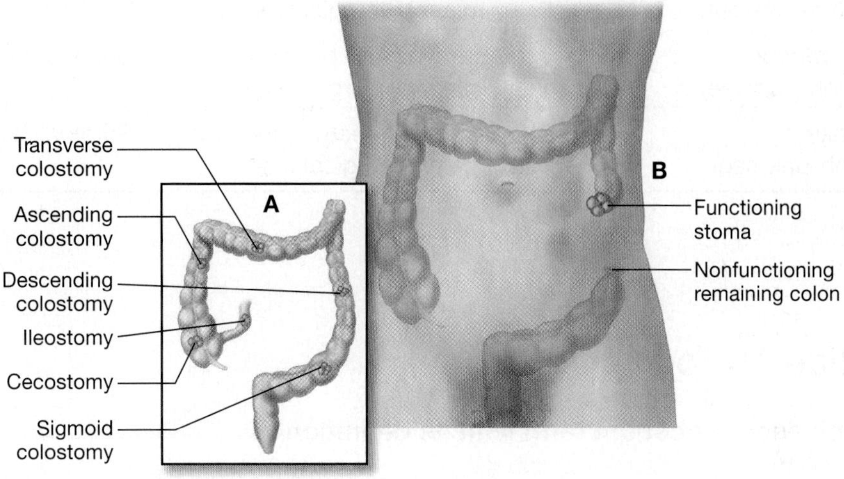

■ **Figure 8.19** A) The colon illustrating various ostomy sites. B) Colostomy in the descending colon, illustrating functioning stoma and nonfunctioning distal sigmoid colon and rectum.

Term	Word Parts	Definition
diverticulectomy (dye-ver-tik-yoo-LEK-toh-mee)	diverticul/o = pouch -ectomy = surgical removal	Surgical removal of a diverticulum.
exploratory laparotomy (ek-SPLOR-ah-tor-ee / lap-ah-ROT-oh-mee)	lapar/o = abdomen -otomy = cutting into	Abdominal operation for the purpose of examining the abdominal organs and tissues for signs of disease or other abnormalities.
fistulectomy (fis-tyoo-LEK-toh-mee)	-ectomy = surgical removal	Removal of an anal fistula.
gastrectomy (gas-TREK-toh-mee)	gastr/o = stomach -ectomy = surgical removal	Surgical removal of the stomach.
gastric stapling	gastr/o = stomach -ic = pertaining to	Procedure that closes off a large section of the stomach with rows of staples. Results in a much smaller stomach to assist very obese patients to lose weight.
gastrostomy (gas-TROSS-toh-mee)	gastr/o = stomach -ostomy = surgically create an opening	Surgical procedure to create an opening in the stomach.
hemorrhoidectomy (hem-oh-royd-EK-toh-mee)	-ectomy = surgical removal	Surgical removal of hemorrhoids from the anorectal area.
hernioplasty (her-nee-oh-PLAS-tee)	-plasty = surgical repair	Surgical repair of a hernia. Also called *herniorrhaphy*.
ileostomy (ill-ee-OSS-toh-mee)	ile/o = ileum -ostomy = surgically create an opening	Surgical creation of an opening in the ileum.
laparoscopic cholecystectomy (lap-ar-oh-SKOP-ik / koh-lee-sis-TEK-toh-mee)	lapar/o = abdomen -scopic = pertaining to visually examining cholecyst/o = gallbladder -ectomy = surgical removal	Surgical removal of the gallbladder through a very small abdominal incision with the assistance of a laparoscope.

Therapeutic Procedures (continued)

Term	Word Parts	Definition
laparotomy (lap-ah-ROT-oh-mee)	lapar/o = abdomen -otomy = cutting into	Surgical incision into the abdomen.
liver transplant		Transplant of a liver from a donor.
palatoplasty (pa-LOT-toh-plas-tee)	palat/o = palate -plasty = surgical repair	Surgical repair of the palate.
pharyngoplasty (fair-ING-oh-plas-tee)	pharyng/o = pharynx -plasty = surgical repair	Surgical repair of the throat.
proctopexy (PROK-toh-pek-see)	proct/o = rectum and anus -pexy = surgical fixation	Surgical fixation of the rectum and anus.

Practice As You Go

D. Match each procedure term with its definition

1. _______ serum bilirubin
2. _______ lavage
3. _______ bariatric surgery
4. _______ proctopexy
5. _______ lower GI series
6. _______ paracentesis
7. _______ fecal occult blood test
8. _______ laparoscopy

a. withdraws fluid from abdominal cavity
b. barium enema
c. visually examines abdominal cavity
d. stool guaiac
e. treatment for obesity
f. elevated levels indicate liver disease
g. to wash out the stomach
h. surgical fixation of rectum and anus

Pharmacology

Classification	Word Parts	Action	Examples
anorexiant (an-oh-REKS-ee-ant)	an- = without -orexia = appetite	Treats obesity by suppressing appetite.	phendimetrazine, Adipost, Obezine; phentermine, Zantryl, Adipex
antacid	anti- = against	Used to neutralize stomach acids.	calcium carbonate, Tums; aluminum hydroxide and magnesium hydroxide, Maalox, Mylanta
antidiarrheal (an-tee-dye-ah-REE-all)	anti- = against -al = pertaining to	Used to control diarrhea.	loperamide, Imodium; diphenoxylate and atropine, Lomotil; kaolin/pectin, Kaopectate

Pharmacology (continued)

Classification	Word Parts	Action	Examples
antiemetic (an-tye-ee-MEH-tik)	anti- = against -emetic = pertaining to vomiting	Treats nausea, vomiting, and motion sickness.	prochlorperazine, Compazine; promethazine, Phenergan
antivirals	anti- = against	Treat herpes simplex infection.	valacyclovir, Valtrex; famcyclovir, Famvir; acyclovir, Zovirax
H_2-receptor antagonist	anti- = against	Used to treat peptic ulcers and gastroesophageal reflux disease. When stimulated, H_2-receptors increase the production of stomach acid. Using an antagonist to block these receptors results in a low acid level in the stomach.	ranitidine, Zantac; cimetidine, Tagamet; famotidine, Pepcid
laxative Med Term Tip The term *laxative* comes from the Latin term meaning "to relax."		Treats constipation by stimulating a bowel movement.	senosides, Senokot; psyllium, Metamucil
proton pump inhibitors		Used to treat peptic ulcers and gastroesophageal reflux disease. Blocks the stomach's ability to secrete acid.	esomeprazole, Nexium; omeprazole, Prilosec

Abbreviations

ac	before meals	**HDV**	hepatitis D virus
ALT	alanine transaminase	**HEV**	hepatitis E virus
AST	aspartate transaminase	**HSV-1**	herpes simplex virus type 1
Ba	barium	**IBD**	inflammatory bowel disease
BE	barium enema	**IBS**	irritable bowel syndrome
BM	bowel movement	**IVC**	intravenous cholangiography
BS	bowel sounds	**n&v**	nausea and vomiting
CBD	common bile duct	**NG**	nasogastric (tube)
EGD	esophagogastroduodenoscopy	**NPO**	nothing by mouth
ERCP	endoscopic retrograde cholangiopancreatography	**O&P**	ova and parasites
FOBT	fecal occult blood test	**pc**	after meals
GB	gallbladder	**PO**	by mouth
GERD	gastroesophageal reflux disease	**pp**	postprandial
GI	gastrointestinal	**PTC**	percutaneous transhepatic cholangiography
HAV	hepatitis A virus	**PUD**	peptic ulcer disease
HBV	hepatitis B virus	**TPN**	total parenteral nutrition
HCl	hydrochloric acid	**UGI**	upper gastrointestinal series
HCV	hepatitis C virus		

Practice As You Go

E. What's the Abbreviation?

1. nasogastric ______________________________

2. gastrointestinal ______________________________

3. hepatitis B virus ______________________________

4. fecal occult blood test ______________________________

5. inflammatory bowel disease ______________________________

6. herpes simplex virus type 1 ______________________________

7. aspartate transaminase ______________________________

8. after meals ______________________________

9. peptic ulcer disease ______________________________

10. gastroesophageal reflux disease ______________________________

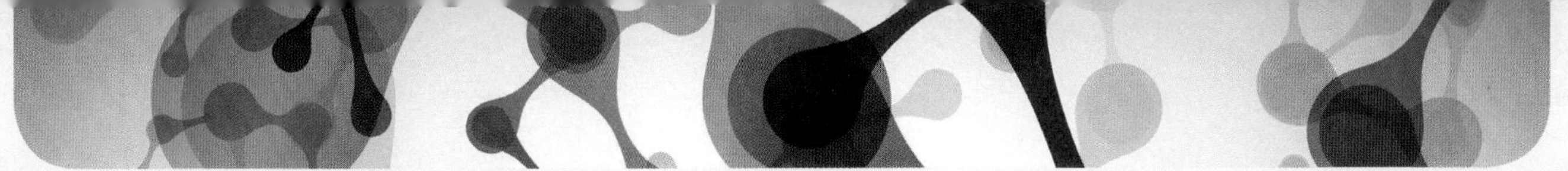

Chapter Review

Real-World Applications

Medical Record Analysis

This Gastroenterology Consultation Report contains 12 medical terms. Underline each term and write it in the list below the report. Then define each term.

Gastroenterology Consultation Report

Reason for Consultation:	Evaluation of recurrent epigastric pain with anemia and melena.
History of Present Illness:	Patient is a 56-year-old male. He reports a long history of mild dyspepsia characterized by burning epigastric pain, especially when his stomach is empty. This pain has been relieved by over-the-counter antacids. Approximately two weeks ago, the pain became significantly worse and he noted that his stool were dark and tarry.
Results of Physical Examination:	CBC indicates anemia, and a fecal occult blood test is positive for blood. A blood test for *Helicobacter pylori* is positive. Gastroscopy located an ulcer in the lining of the stomach. This ulcer is 1.5 cm in diameter and deep. There is evidence of active bleeding from the ulcer.
Assessment:	Peptic ulcer disease.
Recommendations:	A gastrectomy to remove the ulcerated portion of the stomach is indicated because the ulcer is already bleeding.

	Term	Definition
1.	______________	______________________________
2.	______________	______________________________
3.	______________	______________________________
4.	______________	______________________________
5.	______________	______________________________
6.	______________	______________________________
7.	______________	______________________________
8.	______________	______________________________
9.	______________	______________________________
10.	______________	______________________________
11.	______________	______________________________
12.	______________	______________________________

Chart Note Transcription

The chart note below contains 12 phrases that can be reworded with a medical term that you learned in this chapter. Each phrase is identified with an underline. Determine the medical term and write your answers in the space provided.

Pearson General Hospital Consultation Report

Task Edit View Time Scale Options Help Download Archive Date: 17 May 2015

Current Complaint:	Patient is a 74-year-old female seen by a physician who specializes in the treatment of the gastrointestinal tract **1** with complaints of severe lower abdominal pain and extreme difficulty with having a bowel movement. **2**
Past History:	Patient has a history of the presence of gallstones **3** requiring surgical removal of the gallbladder **4** 10 years ago and chronic acid backing up from the stomach into the esophagus. **5**
Signs and Symptoms:	The patient's abdomen is distended with fluid collecting in the abdominal cavity. **6** X-ray of the colon after inserting barium dye with an enema **7** revealed the presence of multiple small tumors growing on a stalk **8** throughout the colon. Visual examination of the colon by a scope inserted through the rectum **9** was performed, and biopsies taken for microscopic examination located a tumor.
Diagnosis:	Carcinoma of the section of colon between the descending colon and the rectum. **10**
Treatment:	Surgical removal of the colon **11** between the descending colon and the rectum with the surgical creation of an opening of the colon through the abdominal wall. **12**

1. ______________________________

2. ______________________________

3. ______________________________

4. ______________________________

5. ______________________________

6. ______________________________

7. ______________________________

8. ______________________________

9. ______________________________

10. ______________________________

11. ______________________________

12. ______________________________

Case Study

Below is a case study presentation of a patient with a condition discussed in this chapter. Read the case study and answer the questions below. Some questions will ask for information not included within this chapter. Use your text, a medical dictionary, or any other reference material you choose to answer these questions.

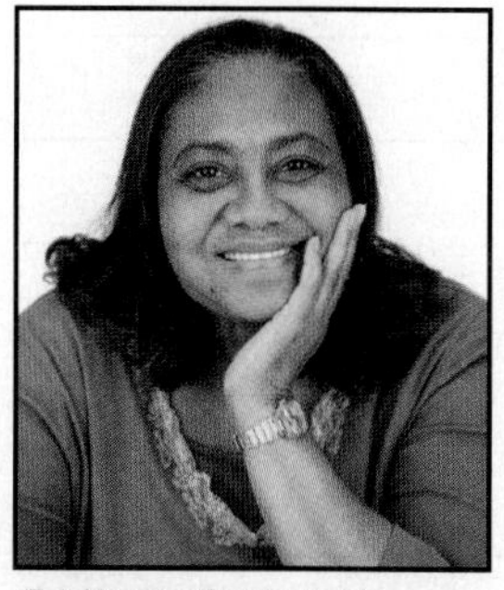
(Rob Marmion/Shutterstock)

A 60-year-old obese female has come into the ER due to severe RUQ pain for the past two hours. Patient also reports increasing nausea but denies emesis. Patient states she has been told she has cholelithiasis by her family physician following a milder episode of this pain two years ago. In addition to severe pain, patient displays a moderate degree of scleral jaundice. Abdominal ultrasound identified acute cholecystitis and a large number of gallstones. Because of the jaundice a PTC was performed and confirmed choledocholithiasis. Patient was sent to surgery for laparoscopic cholecystectomy to remove the gallbladder and all gallstones. She recovered without incident.

Questions

1. Define each of the patient's symptoms.

____

____

2. The patient has severe RUQ pain. What organs are located in the RUQ?

____

____

3. After reading the definition of jaundice, what is most likely causing this patient to have it?

____

____

4. Describe the diagnostic imaging procedures this patient received.

____

____

5. What is the difference between cholelithiasis and cholecystitis?

____

____

6. The patient's gallbladder was removed laparoscopically. What does that mean?

____

____

Practice Exercises

A. Word Building Practice

The combining form **gastr/o** refers to the stomach. Use it to write a term that means:

1. inflammation of the stomach ______
2. study of the stomach and small intestines ______
3. removal of the stomach ______
4. visual exam of the stomach ______
5. stomach pain ______
6. enlargement of the stomach ______
7. cutting into the stomach ______

The combining form **esophag/o** refers to the esophagus. Use it to write a term that means:

8. inflammation of the esophagus ______
9. visual examination of the esophagus ______
10. surgical repair of the esophagus ______
11. pertaining to the esophagus ______
12. stretched-out esophagus ______

The combining form **proct/o** refers to the rectum and anus. Use it to write a term that means:

13. surgical fixation of the rectum and anus ______
14. drooping of the rectum and anus ______
15. inflammation of the rectum and anus ______
16. specialist in the study of the rectum and anus ______

The combining form **cholecyst/o** refers to the gallbladder. Use it to write a term that means:

17. removal of the gallbladder ______
18. condition of having gallbladder stones ______
19. gallbladder stone surgical crushing ______
20. gallbladder inflammation ______

The combining form **lapar/o** refers to the abdomen. Use it to write a term that means:

21. instrument to view inside the abdomen ______
22. cutting into the abdomen ______
23. visual examination of the abdomen ______

The combining form **hepat/o** refers to the liver. Use it to write a term that means:

24. liver tumor ______
25. enlargement of the liver ______
26. pertaining to the liver ______
27. inflammation of the liver ______

The combining form **pancreat/o** refers to the pancreas. Use it to write a term that means:

28. inflammation of the pancreas ______
29. pertaining to the pancreas ______

The combining form **col/o** refers to the colon. Use it to write a term that means:

30. surgically create an opening in the colon ______
31. inflammation of the colon ______

B. Define the Combining Form

	Definition	Example from Chapter
1. **esophag/o**	______	______
2. **hepat/o**	______	______
3. **ile/o**	______	______
4. **proct/o**	______	______
5. **gloss/o**	______	______
6. **labi/o**	______	______
7. **jejun/o**	______	______
8. **sigmoid/o**	______	______
9. **rect/o**	______	______
10. **gingiv/o**	______	______
11. **cholecyst/o**	______	______
12. **duoden/o**	______	______
13. **an/o**	______	______
14. **enter/o**	______	______
15. **dent/o**	______	______

C. Suffix Practice

Use the following suffixes to create a medical term for the following definitions.

-orexia	**-phagia**	**-pepsia**
-emesis	**-lithiasis**	**-prandial**

1. after meals ______
2. condition of having gallstones ______
3. no appetite ______
4. difficulty swallowing ______
5. vomiting blood ______
6. slow digestion ______

D. What Does it Stand For?

1. BM ______
2. UGI ______
3. BE ______
4. BS ______
5. n & v ______
6. O & P ______
7. PO ______
8. CBD ______
9. NPO ______
10. pp ______

E. Define the Term

1. colonoscopy ______
2. bite wing X-ray ______
3. hematochezia ______
4. serum bilirubin ______
5. cachexia ______
6. lavage ______
7. hernioplasty ______
8. extraction ______
9. choledocholithotripsy ______
10. anastomosis ______

F. Fill in the Blank

colonoscopy	barium swallow	lower GI series
gastric stapling	colostomy	colectomy
total parenteral nutrition	choledocholithotripsy	liver biopsy
ileostomy	fecal occult blood test	intravenous cholecystography

1. Excising a small piece of hepatic tissue for microscopic examination is called a(n) ______________________.
2. When a surgeon performs a total or partial colectomy for cancer, she may have to create an opening on the surface of the skin for fecal matter to leave the body. This procedure is called a(n) ______________________.
3. Another name for an upper GI series is a(n) ______________________.
4. Mr. White has had a radiopaque material placed into his large bowel by means of an enema for the purpose of viewing his colon. This procedure is called a(n) ______________________.
5. A(n) ______________________ is the surgical removal of the colon.
6. Jessica has been on a red meat–free diet in preparation for a test of her feces for the presence of hidden blood. This test is called a(n) ______________________.
7. Dr. Mendez uses equipment to crush gallstones in the common bile duct. This procedure is called a(n) ____________.
8. Mrs. Alcazar required ______________________ because she could not eat following her intestinal surgery.
9. Mr. Bright had a(n) ______________________ to treat his morbid obesity.
10. Visualizing the gallbladder and bile ducts by injecting a dye into the patient's arm is called a(n) ____________.
11. Passing an instrument into the anus and rectum in order to see the colon is called a(n) ______________________.
12. Ms. Fayne suffers from Crohn's disease, which has necessitated the removal of much of her small intestine. She has had a surgical passage created for the external disposal of waste material from the ileum. This is called a(n) ____________.

G. Terminology Matching

Match each term to its definition.

1. ________ dentures	a. tooth decay
2. ________ cementum	b. prosthetic device used to anchor a tooth
3. ________ root canal	c. inflammation of the gums
4. ________ crown	d. full set of artificial teeth
5. ________ bridge	e. portion of the tooth covered by enamel
6. ________ implant	f. replacement for missing teeth
7. ________ gingivitis	g. anchors root in bony socket of jaw
8. ________ dental caries	h. surgery on the tooth pulp

H. Pharmacology Challenge

Fill in the classification for each drug description, then match the brand name.

	Drug Description	Classification	Brand Name
1.	________ Controls diarrhea	______________	a. Pepcid
2.	________ Blocks stomach's ability to secrete acid	______________	b. Obezine
3.	________ Treats motion sickness	______________	c. Metamucil
4.	________ Blocks acid-producing receptors	______________	d. Compazine
5.	________ Suppresses appetite	______________	e. Maalox
6.	________ Stimulates a bowel movement	______________	f. Imodium
7.	________ Neutralizes stomach acid	______________	g. Valtrex
8.	________ Treats herpes simplex infection	______________	h. Nexium

Labeling Exercise

Image A

Write the labels for this figure on the numbered lines provided.

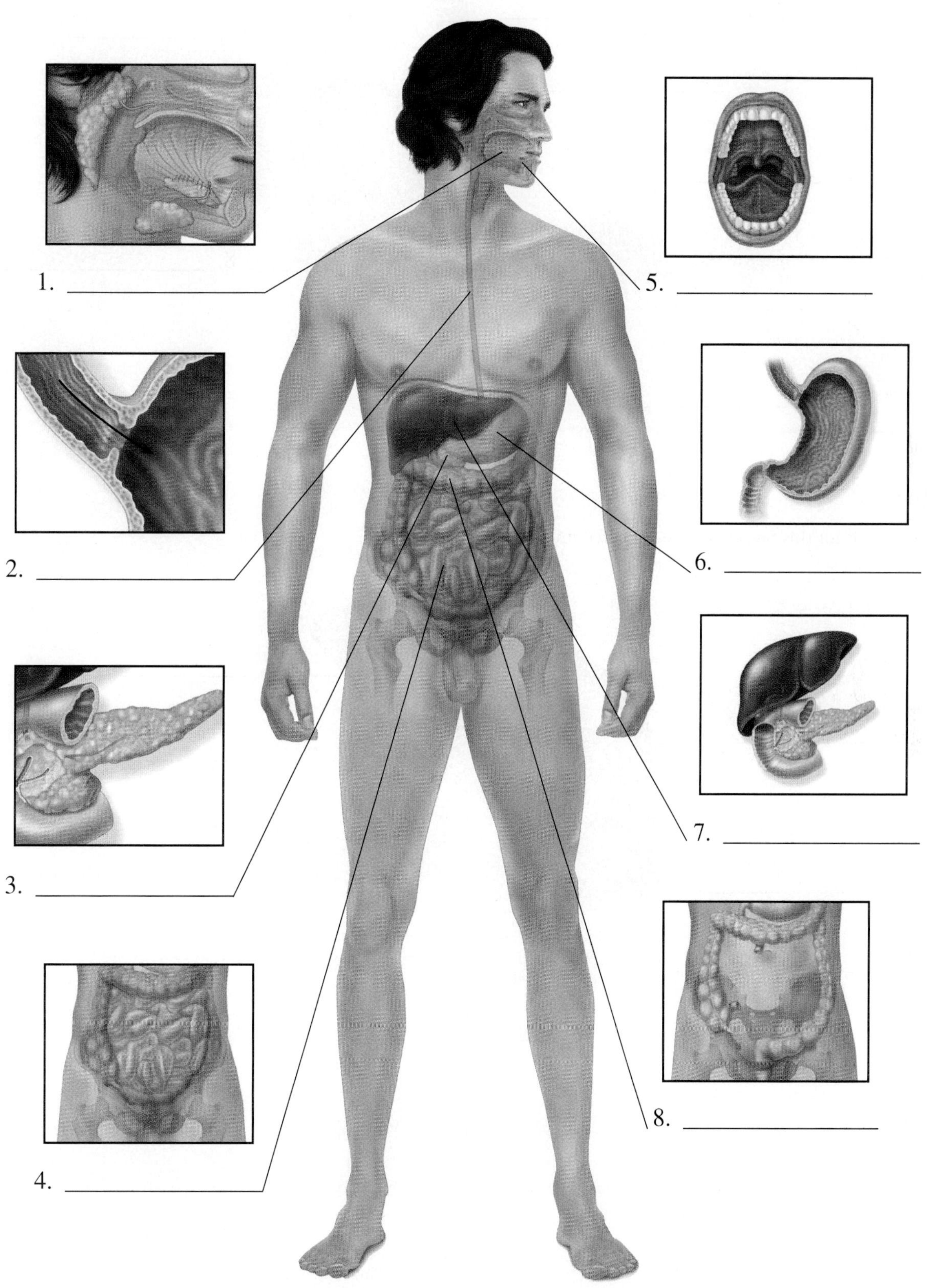

Image B

Write the labels for this figure on the numbered lines provided.

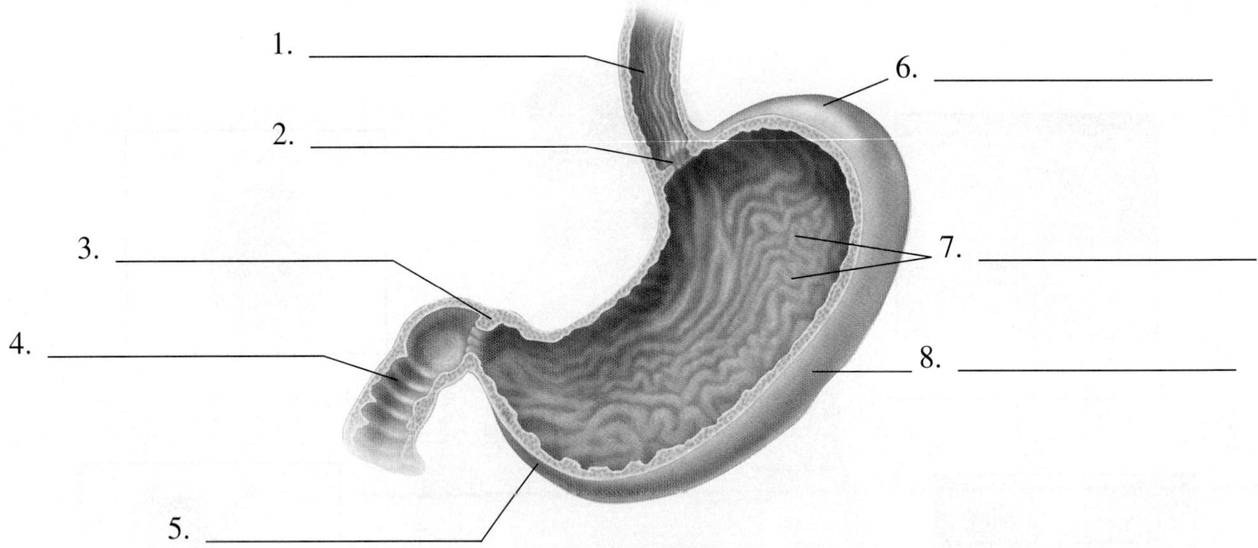

Image C

Write the labels for this figure on the numbered lines provided.

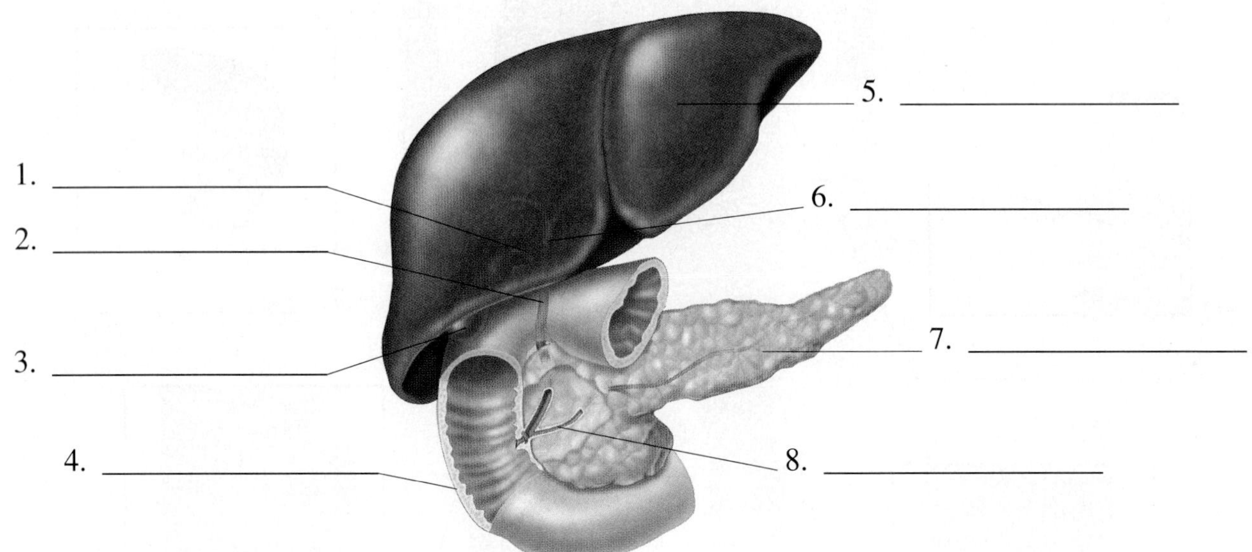

9

Urinary System

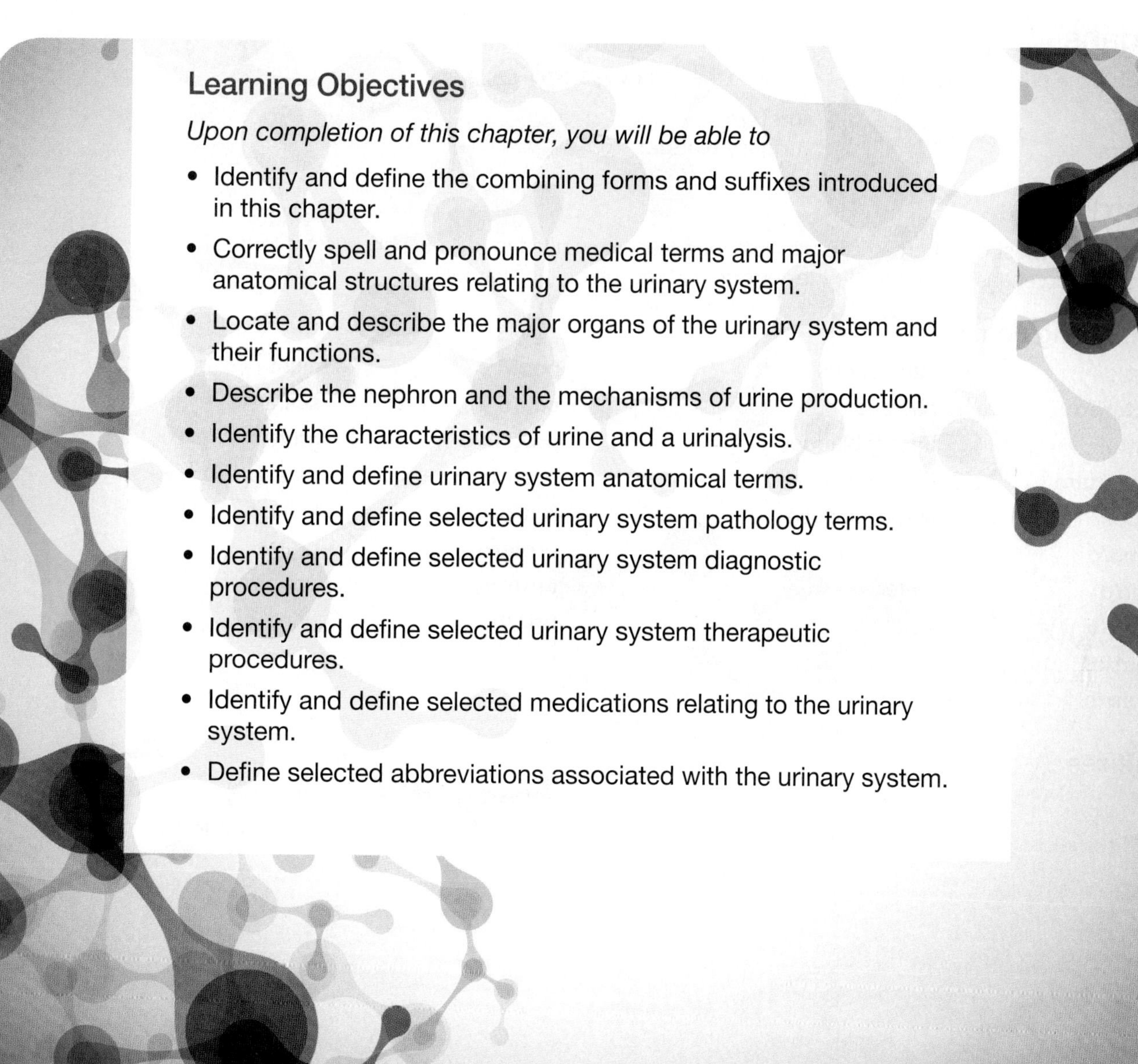

Learning Objectives

Upon completion of this chapter, you will be able to

- Identify and define the combining forms and suffixes introduced in this chapter.
- Correctly spell and pronounce medical terms and major anatomical structures relating to the urinary system.
- Locate and describe the major organs of the urinary system and their functions.
- Describe the nephron and the mechanisms of urine production.
- Identify the characteristics of urine and a urinalysis.
- Identify and define urinary system anatomical terms.
- Identify and define selected urinary system pathology terms.
- Identify and define selected urinary system diagnostic procedures.
- Identify and define selected urinary system therapeutic procedures.
- Identify and define selected medications relating to the urinary system.
- Define selected abbreviations associated with the urinary system.

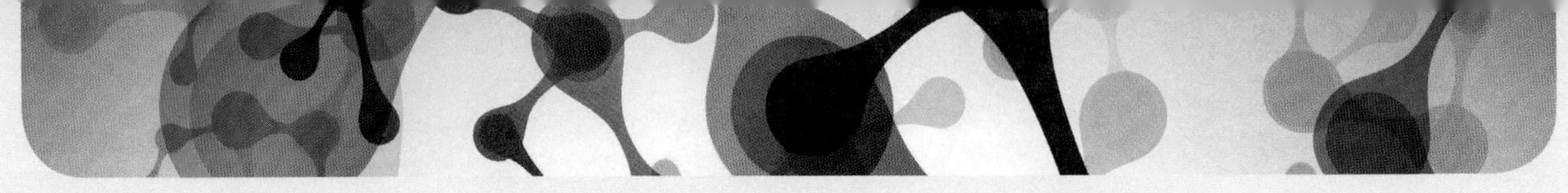

Urinary System at a Glance

Function

The urinary system is responsible for maintaining a stable internal environment for the body. In order to achieve this state, the urinary system removes waste products, adjusts water and electrolyte levels, and maintains the correct pH.

Organs

Here are the primary structures that comprise the urinary system:

kidneys
urethra
ureters
urinary bladder

Word Parts

Here are the most common word parts (with their meanings) used to build urinary system terms. For a more comprehensive list, refer to the Terminology section of this chapter.

Combining Forms

azot/o	nitrogenous waste
bacteri/o	bacteria
cyst/o	urinary bladder
glomerul/o	glomerulus
glycos/o	sugar, glucose
home/o	sameness
hydr/o	water
keton/o	ketones
meat/o	meatus
nephr/o	kidney
noct/i	night
olig/o	scanty
protein/o	protein
pyel/o	renal pelvis
ren/o	kidney
ureter/o	ureter
urethr/o	urethra
urin/o	urine
ur/o	urine

Suffixes

-lith	stone
-lysis	to destroy
-ptosis	drooping
-uria	urine condition

Urinary System Illustrated

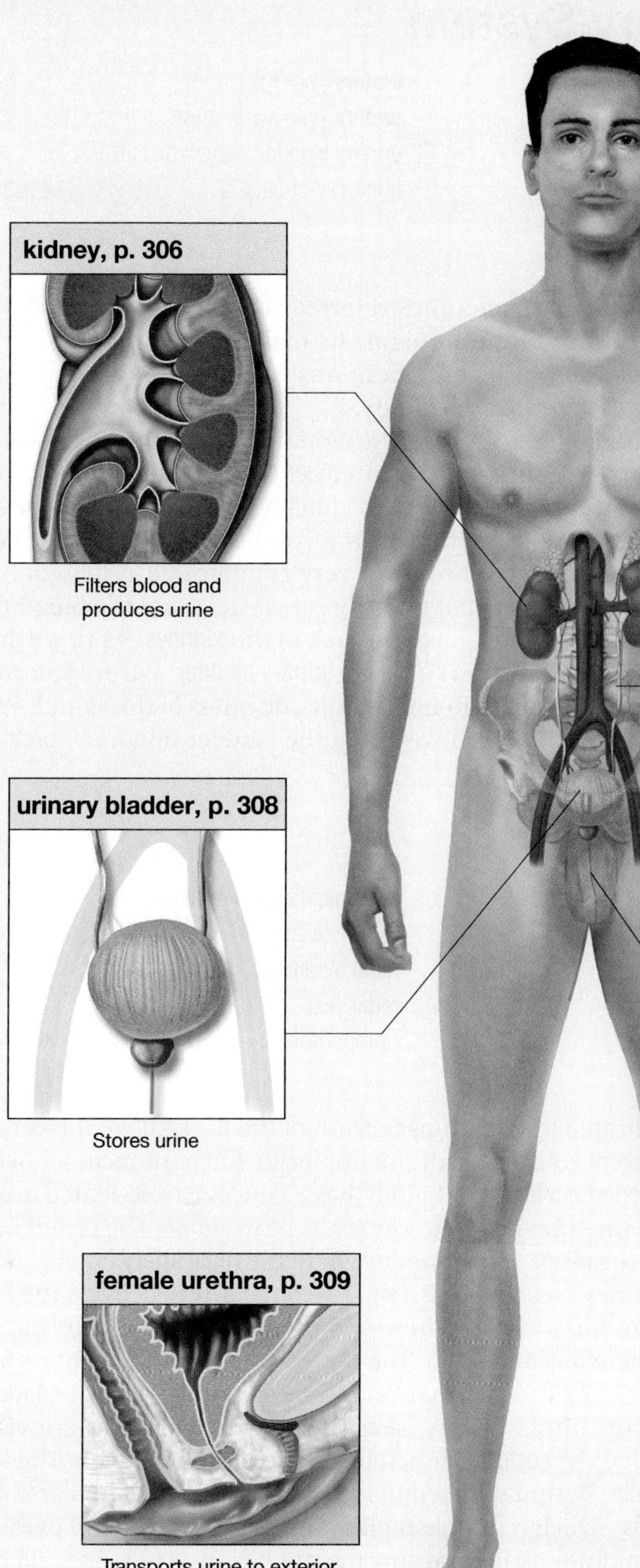

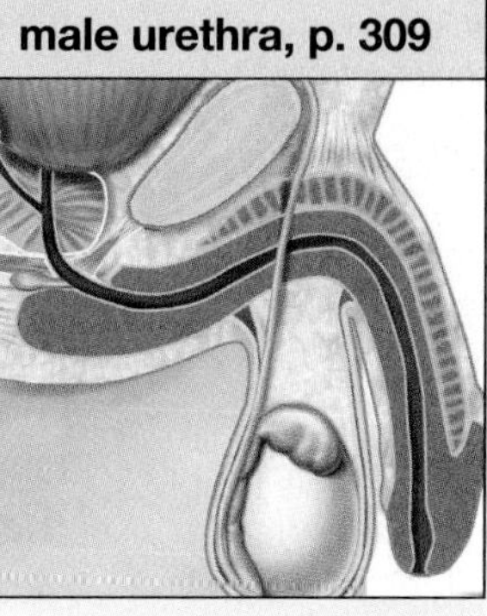

What's In A Name?
Look for these word parts:
genit/o = genitals
urin/o = urine
-ary = pertaining to

Anatomy and Physiology of the Urinary System

genitourinary system (jen-ih-toh-YOO-rih-nair-ee)
kidneys
nephrons (NEF-ronz)
uremia (yoo-REE-mee-ah)
ureters (YOO-reh-ters)
urethra (yoo-REE-thrah)
urinary bladder (YOO-rih-nair-ee)
urine (YOO-rin)

Think of the urinary system, sometimes referred to as the **genitourinary** (GU) **system**, as similar to a water filtration plant. Its main function is to filter and remove waste products from the blood. These waste materials result in the production and excretion of **urine** from the body.

Med Term Tip
The urinary system and the male reproductive system share some of the same organs, particularly the urethra. Hence, the term *genitourinary* (GU) is sometimes used to describe the urinary system. The reproductive system is discussed in Chapter 10.

The urinary system is one of the hardest working systems of the body. All the body's metabolic processes result in the production of waste products. These waste products are a natural part of life but quickly become toxic if they are allowed to build up in the blood, resulting in a condition called **uremia**. Waste products in the body are removed through a very complicated system of blood vessels and kidney tubules. The actual filtration of wastes from the blood takes place in millions of **nephrons**, which make up each of the **kidneys**. As urine drains from each kidney, the **ureters** transport it to the **urinary bladder**. We are constantly producing urine, and our bladders can hold about one quart of this liquid. When the urinary bladder empties, urine moves from the bladder down the **urethra** to the outside of the body.

What's In A Name?
Look for these word parts:
peritone/o = peritoneum
-al = pertaining to
retro- = behind

Med Term Tip
From the time of early man, there has been an interest in urine. Drawings on cave walls and hieroglyphics in Egyptian pyramids reveal interest in urine as a means of determining the physical state of the body. Some of the first doctors, called *pisse prophets*, believed that examining the urine would help treat a patient. Now urologists treat disorders of the urinary tract in both men and women, as well as disorders of the male reproductive tract.

Kidneys

calyx (KAY-liks)
cortex (KOR-teks)
hilum (HIGH-lum)
medulla (meh-DULL-ah)
renal artery
renal papilla (pah-PILL-ah)
renal pelvis
renal pyramids
renal vein
retroperitoneal (ret-roh-pair-ih-toh-NEE-al)

The two kidneys are located in the lumbar region of the back above the waist on either side of the vertebral column. They are not inside the peritoneal sac, a location referred to as **retroperitoneal**. Each kidney has a concave or indented area on the edge toward the center that gives the kidney its bean shape. The center of this concave area is called the **hilum**. The hilum is where the **renal artery** enters and the **renal vein** leaves the kidney (see Figure 9.1 ■). The renal artery delivers the blood that is full of waste products to the kidney and the renal vein returns the now cleansed blood to the general circulation. The ureters also leave the kidneys at the hilum. The ureters are narrow tubes that lead from the kidneys to the bladder.

When a surgeon cuts into a kidney, several structures or areas are visible. The outer portion, called the **cortex**, is much like a shell for the kidney. The inner area is called the **medulla**. Within the medulla are a dozen or so triangular-shaped areas, the **renal pyramids**, which resemble their namesake, the Egyptian pyramids. The tip of each pyramid points inward toward the hilum. At its tip, called the **renal papilla**, each pyramid opens into a **calyx** (plural is *calyces*), which is continuous with the **renal pelvis**. The calyces and ultimately the renal pelvis collect urine as it is formed. The ureter for each kidney arises from the renal pelvis (see Figure 9.2 ■).

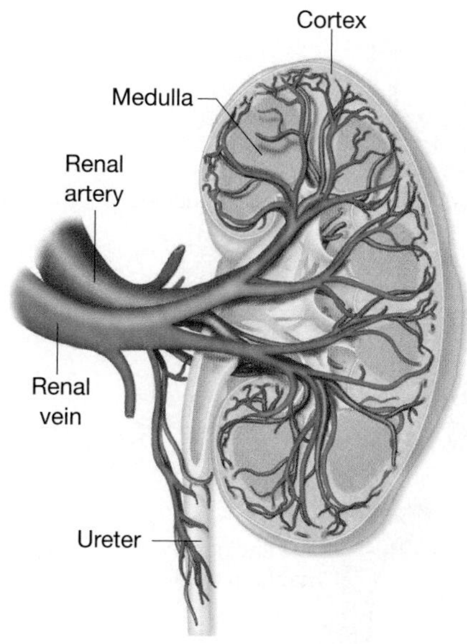

■ **Figure 9.1** Kidney structure. Longitudinal section showing the renal artery entering and the renal vein and ureter exiting at the hilum of the kidney.

■ **Figure 9.2** Longitudinal section of a kidney illustrating the internal structures.

Nephrons

afferent arteriole (AFF-er-ent)
Bowman's capsule
collecting tubule
distal convoluted tubule (DISS-tall / con-voh-LOOT-ed)
efferent arteriole (EF-er-ent)
glomerular capsule (glom-AIR-yoo-lar)
glomerulus (glom-AIR-yoo-lus)
loop of Henle
nephron (NEF-ron)
nephron loop
proximal convoluted tubule (PROK-sim-al / con-voh-LOOT-ed)
renal corpuscle (KOR-pus-ehl)
renal tubule

Med Term Tip

The kidney bean is so named because it resembles a kidney in shape. Each organ weighs four to six ounces, is two to three inches wide and approximately one inch thick, and is about the size of your fist. In most people the left kidney is slightly higher and larger than the right kidney. Functioning kidneys are necessary for life, but it is possible to live with only one functioning kidney.

The functional or working unit of the kidney is the **nephron**. There are more than one million of these microscopic structures in each human kidney. Each nephron consists of the **renal corpuscle** and the **renal tubule** (see Figure 9.3 ■). The renal corpuscle is the blood-filtering portion of the nephron. It has a double-walled cuplike structure called the **glomerular capsule** (also known as **Bowman's capsule**) that encases a ball of capillaries called the **glomerulus**. An **afferent arteriole** carries blood to the glomerulus, and an **efferent arteriole** carries blood away from the glomerulus.

Water and substances that were removed from the bloodstream in the renal corpuscle flow into the renal tubules to finish the urine production process. This continuous tubule is divided into four sections: the **proximal convoluted tubule**, followed by the narrow **nephron loop** (also known as the **loop of Henle**), then the **distal convoluted tubule**, and finally the **collecting tubule**.

What's In A Name?

Look for these word parts:
dist/o = away from
proxim/o = near to
-al = pertaining to

Med Term Tip

Afferent, meaning "moving toward," and *efferent*, meaning "moving away from," are terms used when discussing moving either toward or away from the central point in many systems. For example, there are afferent and efferent nerves in the nervous system.

Ureters

As urine drains out of the renal pelvis it enters the ureter, which carries it down to the urinary bladder (see Figure 9.4 ■). Ureters are very narrow tubes measuring less than ¼-inch wide and 10–12 inches long that extend from the renal pelvis to the urinary bladder. Mucous membrane lines the ureters just as it lines most passages that open to the external environment.

■ **Figure 9.3** The structure of a nephron, illustrating the nephron structure in relation to the circulatory system.

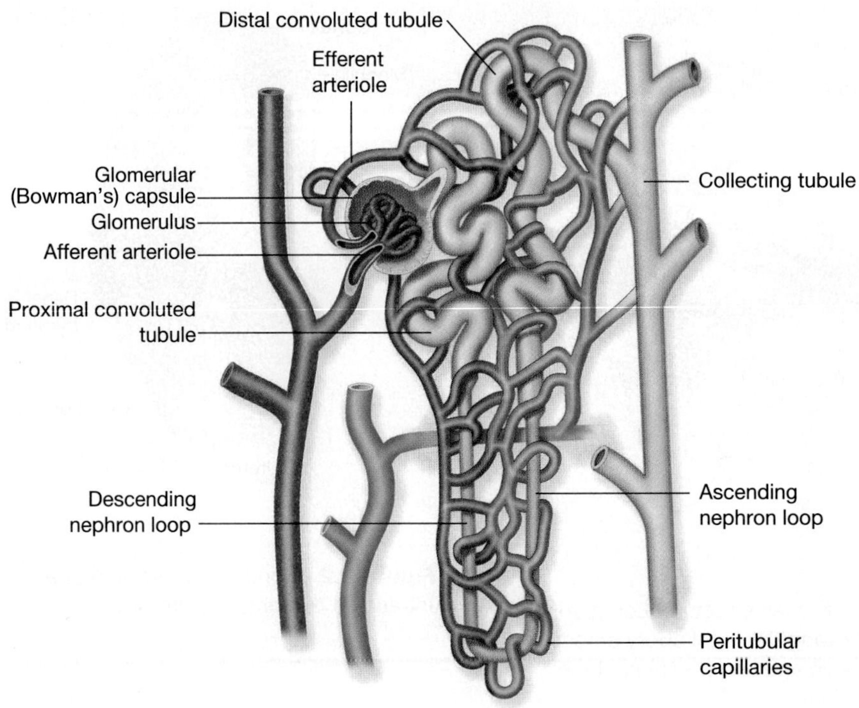

What's In A Name?

Look for these word parts:
ex- = outward
in- = inward
-al = pertaining to

Word Watch

The terms *ureter* and *urethra* are frequently confused. Remember that there are two ureters carrying urine from the kidneys into the bladder. There is only one urethra, and it carries urine from the bladder to the outside of the body.

Med Term Tip

Terms such as *micturition*, *voiding*, and *urination* all mean basically the same thing—the process of releasing urine from the body.

Urinary Bladder

external sphincter (SFINGK-ter)
internal sphincter
rugae (ROO-gay)
urination

The urinary bladder is an elastic muscular sac that lies in the base of the pelvis just behind the pubic symphysis (see Figure 9.5 ■). It is composed of three layers of smooth muscle tissue lined with mucous membrane containing **rugae** or folds that allow it to stretch. The bladder receives the urine directly from the ureters, stores it, and excretes it by **urination** through the urethra.

Generally, an adult bladder will hold 250 mL of urine. This amount then creates an urge to void or empty the bladder. Involuntary muscle action causes the bladder to contract and the **internal sphincter** to relax. The internal sphincter protects us from having our bladder empty at the wrong time. Voluntary action

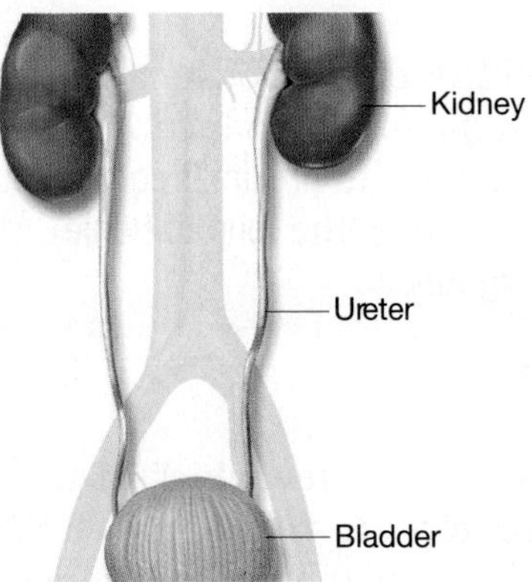

■ **Figure 9.4** The ureters extend from the kidneys to the urinary bladder.

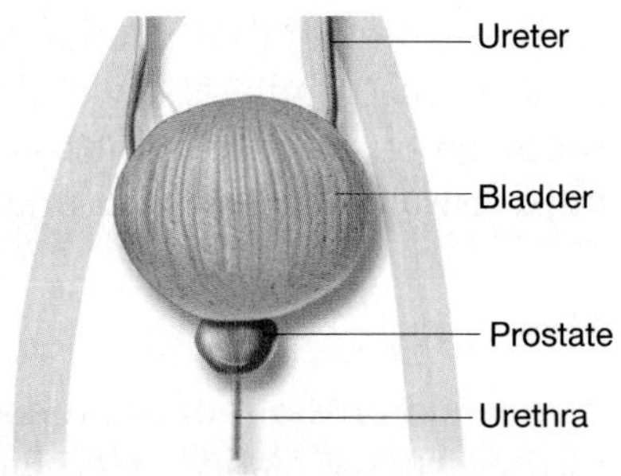

■ **Figure 9.5** The structure of the urinary bladder. (Note the prostate gland.)

controls the **external sphincter**, which opens on demand to allow the intentional emptying of the bladder. The act of controlling the emptying of urine is developed sometime after a child is two years of age.

Urethra

urinary meatus (mee-AY-tus)

The urethra is a tubular canal that carries the flow of urine from the bladder to the outside of the body (see Figure 9.6 ■). The external opening through which urine passes out of the body is called the **urinary meatus**. Mucous membrane also lines the urethra as it does other structures of the urinary system. This is one of the reasons that infection spreads up the urinary tract. The urethra is one to two inches long in the female and eight inches long in the male. In a woman it functions only as the outlet for urine and is in front of the vagina. In the male, however, it has two functions: an outlet for urine and the passageway for semen to leave the body.

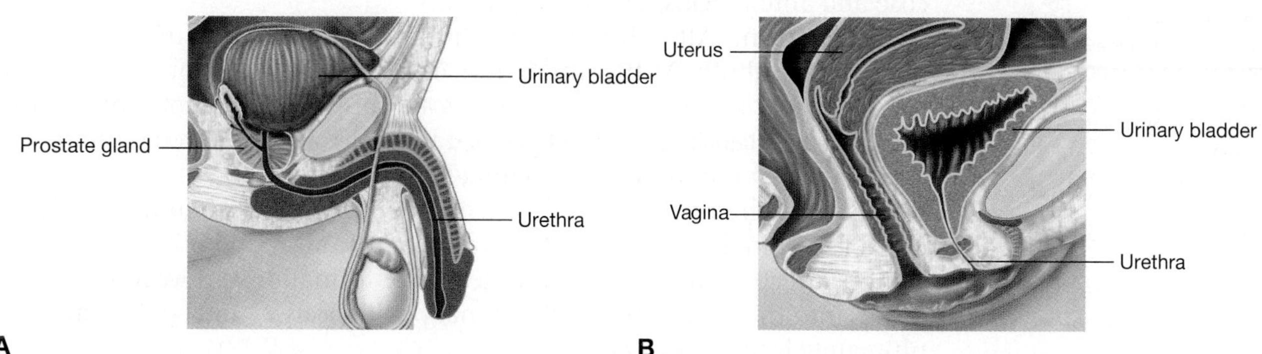

■ **Figure 9.6** A) The male urethra extends from the urinary bladder in the floor of the pelvis through the penis to the urinary meatus. B) The much shorter female urethra extends from the urinary bladder to the floor of the pelvis and exits just in front of the vaginal opening.

Role of Kidneys in Homeostasis

electrolytes (ee-LEK-troh-lites)   **homeostasis** (hoh-mee-oh-STAY-sis)

The kidneys are responsible for **homeostasis** or balance in the body. They continually adjust the chemical conditions in the body, allowing us to survive. Because of its interaction with the bloodstream and its ability to excrete substances from the body, the urinary system maintains the body's proper balance of water (H_2O) and chemicals. If the body is low on water, the kidneys conserve it, or in the opposite case, if there is excess water in the body, the kidneys excrete the excess. In addition to water, the kidneys regulate the level of **electrolytes**—small biologically important molecules such as sodium (Na^+), potassium (K^+), chloride (Cl^-), and bicarbonate (HCO_3^-). Finally, the kidneys play an important role in maintaining the correct pH range within the body, making sure we do not become too acidic or too alkaline. The kidneys accomplish these important tasks through the production of urine.

Med Term Tip

Mucous membranes will carry infections up the urinary tract from the urinary meatus and urethra into the bladder and eventually up the ureters and the kidneys if not stopped. It is never wise to ignore a simple bladder infection or what is called *cystitis*.

What's In A Name?

Look for these word parts:
home/o = sameness
-stasis = standing still

What's In A Name?

Look for these word parts:
-ar = pertaining to
peri- = around
re- = again

Med Term Tip

At any one time, about 20% of your blood is being filtered by your kidneys. In this way, all your blood is cleansed every few minutes.

Med Term Tip

The amount of water and other fluids processed by the kidneys each day is astonishing. Approximately 190 quarts of fluid are filtered out of the glomerular blood every day. Most of this fluid returns to the body through the reabsorption process. About 99% of the water that leaves the blood each day through the filtration process returns to the blood by proximal tubule reabsorption.

Stages of Urine Production

filtration
glomerular filtrate (glom-AIR-yoo-lar)
peritubular capillaries (pair-ih-TOO-byoo-lar)
reabsorption
secretion

As wastes and unnecessary substances are removed from the bloodstream by the nephrons, many desirable molecules are also removed initially. Waste products are eliminated from the body, but other substances such as water, electrolytes, and nutrients must be returned to the bloodstream. Urine, in its final form ready for elimination from the body, is the ultimate product of this entire process.

Urine production occurs in three stages: **filtration**, **reabsorption**, and **secretion**. Each of these steps is performed by a different section of the nephrons (see Figure 9.7 ■).

1. **Filtration.** The first stage is the filtering of particles, which occurs in the renal corpuscle. The pressure of blood flowing through the glomerulus forces material out of the bloodstream, through the wall of the glomerular capsule, and into the renal tubules. This fluid in the tubules is called the **glomerular filtrate** and consists of water, electrolytes, nutrients such as glucose and amino acids, wastes, and toxins.
2. **Reabsorption.** After filtration, the filtrate passes through the four sections of the tubule. As the filtrate moves along its twisted journey, most of the water and much of the electrolytes and nutrients are reabsorbed into the **peritubular capillaries**, a capillary bed that surrounds the renal tubules. They can then reenter the circulating blood.
3. **Secretion.** The final stage of urine production occurs when the special cells of the renal tubules secrete ammonia, uric acid, and other waste substances directly into the renal tubule. Urine formation is now finished; it passes into the collecting tubules, renal papilla, calyx, renal pelvis, and ultimately into the ureter.

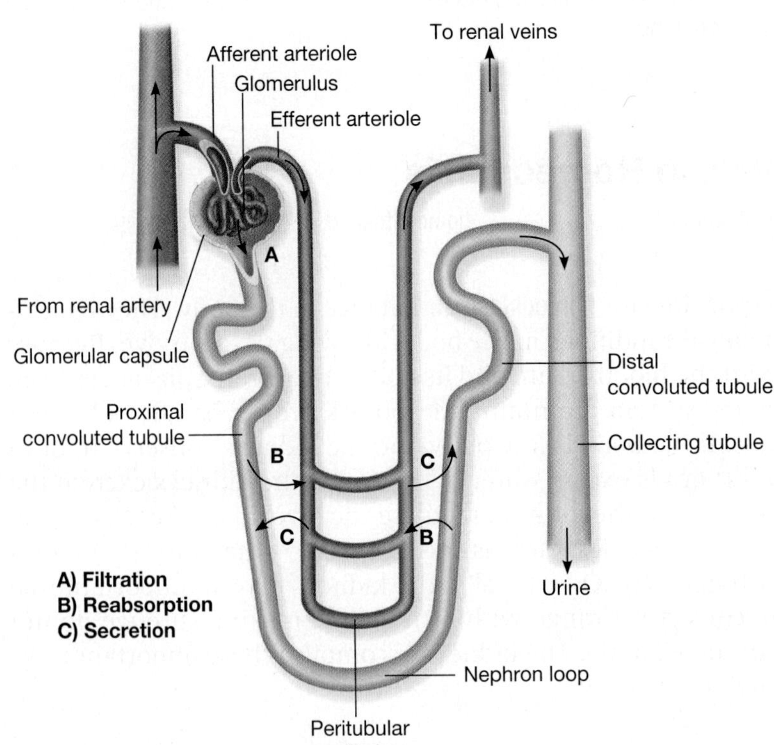

■ **Figure 9.7** The three stages of urine production: filtration, reabsorption, and secretion.

Urine

albumin (al-BEW-min)
nitrogenous wastes (nigh-TROJ-eh-nus)
specific gravity
urinalysis (yoo-rih-NAL-ih-sis)

Urine is normally straw-colored to clear, depending on how dilute it is. As it is being produced and collecting in the bladder, it is sterile. However, as it passes through the urethra to the outside, it may become contaminated by bacteria. Although it is 95% water, it also contains many dissolved substances, such as electrolytes, toxins, and **nitrogenous wastes**, the by-products of muscle metabolism. At times the urine also contains substances that should not be there, such as glucose, blood, or **albumin**, a protein that should remain in the blood. This is the reason for performing a **urinalysis**, a physical and chemical analysis of urine, which gives medical personnel important information regarding disease processes occurring in a patient. Normally, during a 24-hour period the output of urine will be 1,000–2,000 mL, depending on the amount of fluid consumed and the general health of the person. Normal urine is acidic because this is one way our bodies dispose of excess acids. **Specific gravity** indicates the amount of dissolved substances in urine. The specific gravity of pure water is 1.000. The specific gravity of urine varies from 1.001 to 1.030. Highly concentrated urine has a higher specific gravity, while the specific gravity of very dilute urine is close to that of water. See Table 9.1 ■ for the normal values for urine testing and Table 9.2 ■ for abnormal findings.

What's In A Name?

Look for these word parts:
urin/o = urine
-lysis = to destroy
-ous = pertaining to

Med Term Tip

The color, odor, volume, and sugar content of urine have been examined for centuries. Color charts for urine were developed by 1140, and "taste testing" was common in the late 17th century. By the 19th century, urinalysis was a routine part of a physical examination.

Table 9.1 Values for Urinalysis Testing

Element	Normal Findings
Color	Straw-colored, pale yellow to deep gold
Odor	Aromatic
Appearance	Clear
Specific gravity	1.001–1.030
pH	5.0–8.0
Protein	Negative to trace
Glucose	None
Ketones	None
Blood	Negative

Table 9.2 Abnormal Urinalysis Findings

Element	Implications
Color	Color varies depending on the patient's fluid intake and output or medication. Brown or black urine color indicates a serious disease process.
Odor	A fetid or foul odor may indicate infection, while a fruity odor may be found in diabetes mellitus, dehydration, or starvation. Other odors may be due to medication or foods.
Appearance	Cloudiness may mean that an infection is present.
Specific gravity	Concentrated urine has a higher specific gravity. Dilute urine, such as can be found with diabetes insipidus, acute tubular necrosis, or salt-restricted diets, has a lower specific gravity.
pH	A pH value below 7.0 (acidic) is common in urinary tract infections, metabolic or respiratory acidosis, diets high in fruits or vegetables, or administration of some drugs. A pH higher than 7.0 (basic or alkaline) is common in metabolic or respiratory alkalosis, fever, high-protein diets, and taking ascorbic acid.
Protein	Protein may indicate glomerulonephritis or preeclampsia in a pregnant woman.
Glucose	Small amounts of glucose may be present as the result of eating a high-carbohydrate meal, stress, pregnancy, and taking some medications, such as aspirin or corticosteroids. Higher levels may indicate poorly controlled diabetes, Cushing's syndrome, or infection.
Ketones	The presence of ketones may indicate poorly controlled diabetes, dehydration, starvation, or ingestion of large amounts of aspirin.
Blood	Blood may indicate glomerulonephritis, cancer of the urinary tract, some types of anemia, taking of some medications (such as blood thinners), arsenic poisoning, reactions to transfusion, trauma, burns, and convulsions.

Practice As You Go

A. Complete the Statement

1. The functional or working units of the kidneys are the ____________________.
2. The three stages of urine production are ____________________, ____________________, and ____________________.
3. Na^+, K^+, and Cl^- are collectively known as ____________________.
4. The term that describes the location of the kidneys is ____________________.
5. The glomerular capsule surrounds the ____________________.
6. The tip of each renal pyramid opens into a(n) ____________________.
7. There are ____________________ ureters and ____________________ urethra.
8. Urination can also be referred to as ____________________ or ____________________.

Terminology

Word Parts Used to Build Urinary System Terms

The following lists contain the combining forms, suffixes, and prefixes used to build terms in the remaining sections of this chapter.

Combining Forms

azot/o	nitrogenous waste
bacteri/o	bacteria
bi/o	life
carcin/o	cancer
corpor/o	body
cyst/o	bladder, pouch
glomerul/o	glomerulus
glycos/o	sugar
hem/o	blood
hemat/o	blood

hydr/o	water
keton/o	ketones
lith/o	stone
meat/o	meatus
necr/o	death
nephr/o	kidney
neur/o	nerve
noct/i	night
olig/o	scanty
peritone/o	peritoneum

protein/o	protein
py/o	pus
pyel/o	renal pelvis
ren/o	kidney
ur/o	urine
ureter/o	ureter
urethr/o	urethra
urin/o	urine
ven/o	vein

Suffixes

-al	pertaining to
-algia	pain
-ar	pertaining to
-ary	pertaining to

-cele	protrusion
-eal	pertaining to
-ectasis	dilated
-ectomy	surgical removal

-emia	blood condition
-genic	producing
-gram	record

Suffixes (continued)

-graphy	process of recording
-ic	pertaining to
-itis	inflammation
-lith	stone
-lithiasis	condition of stones
-logy	study of
-lysis	to destroy (to break down)
-malacia	abnormal softening
-megaly	enlarged
-meter	instrument to measure

-oma	tumor
-ory	pertaining to
-osis	abnormal condition
-ostomy	surgically create an opening
-otomy	cutting into
-ous	pertaining to
-pathy	disease
-pexy	surgical fixation
-plasty	surgical repair
-ptosis	drooping
-rrhagia	abnormal flow condition

-sclerosis	hardening
-scope	instrument to visually examine
-scopy	process of visually examining
-stenosis	narrowing
-tic	pertaining to
-tripsy	surgical crushing
-uria	urine condition

Prefixes

an-	without
anti-	against
dys-	painful, difficult

extra-	outside of
intra-	within
poly-	many

retro-	backward

Adjective Forms of Anatomical Terms

Term	Word Parts	Definition
cystic (SIS-tik)	cyst/o = bladder -ic = pertaining to	Pertaining to the bladder.
glomerular (glom-AIR-yoo-lar)	glomerul/o = glomerulus -ar = pertaining to	Pertaining to a glomerulus.
meatal (mee-AY-tal)	meat/o = meatus -al = pertaining to	Pertaining to the meatus.
pyelitic (pye-eh-LIT-ik)	pyel/o = renal pelvis -tic = pertaining to	Pertaining to the renal pelvis.
renal (REE-nal)	ren/o = kidney -al = pertaining to	Pertaining to the kidney.
ureteral (yoo-REE-ter-all)	ureter/o = ureter -al = pertaining to **Word Watch** Be particularly careful when using the three very similar combining forms: *uter/o* meaning "uterus," *ureter/o* meaning "ureter," and *urethr/o* meaning "urethra."	Pertaining to the ureter.
urethral (yoo-REE-thral)	urethr/o = urethra -al = pertaining to	Pertaining to the urethra.
urinary (yoo-rih-NAIR-ee)	urin/o = urine -ary = pertaining to	Pertaining to urine.

Practice As You Go

B. Give the adjective form for each anatomical structure

1. The ureter ______________________
2. The kidney ______________________
3. A glomerulus ______________________
4. Urine ______________________
5. The urethra ______________________

Pathology

Term	Word Parts	Definition
Medical Specialties		
nephrology (neh-FROL-oh-jee)	nephr/o = kidney -logy = study of	Branch of medicine involved in diagnosis and treatment of diseases and disorders of the kidney. Physician is a *nephrologist.*
urology (yoo-RAL-oh-jee)	ur/o = urine -logy = study of	Branch of medicine involved in diagnosis and treatment of diseases and disorders of the urinary system (and male reproductive system). Physician is a *urologist.*
Signs and Symptoms		
anuria (an-YOO-ree-ah)	an- = without -uria = urine condition	Complete suppression of urine formed by the kidneys and a complete lack of urine excretion.
azotemia (a-zo-TEE-mee-ah)	azot/o = nitrogenous waste -emia = blood condition	Accumulation of nitrogenous waste in the bloodstream. Occurs when the kidney fails to filter these wastes from the blood.
bacteriuria (back-teer-ree-YOO-ree-ah)	bacteri/o = bacteria -uria = urine condition	Presence of bacteria in the urine.
calculus (KAL-kew-lus) ■ **Figure 9.8** Photograph of sectioned kidney specimen illustrating extensive renal calculi. *(Science Source)*		Stone formed within an organ by an accumulation of mineral salts. Found in the kidney, renal pelvis, ureters, bladder, or urethra. Plural is *calculi*.

Pathology (continued)

Term	Word Parts	Definition
cystalgia (sis-TAL-jee-ah)	cyst/o = bladder -algia = pain **Word Watch** Be careful using the combining forms *cyst/o* meaning "bladder" and *cyt/o* meaning "cell."	Urinary bladder pain.
cystolith (SIS-toh-lith)	cyst/o = bladder -lith = stone	Bladder stone.
cystorrhagia (sis-toh-RAH-jee-ah)	cyst/o = bladder -rrhagia = abnormal flow condition	Profuse bleeding from the urinary bladder.
diuresis (dye-yoo-REE-sis)		Increased formation and excretion of urine.
dysuria (dis-YOO-ree-ah)	dys- = painful, difficult -uria = urine condition	Difficult or painful urination.
enuresis (en-yoo-REE-sis)		Involuntary discharge of urine after the age by which bladder control should have been established. This usually occurs by the age of five. *Nocturnal enuresis* refers to bed-wetting at night.
frequency		Greater-than-normal occurrence in the urge to urinate, without an increase in the total daily volume of urine. Frequency is an indication of inflammation of the bladder or urethra.
glycosuria (glye-kohs-YOO-ree-ah)	glycos/o = sugar -uria = urine condition	Presence of sugar in the urine.
hematuria (hee-mah-TOO-ree-ah)	hemat/o = blood -uria = urine condition	Presence of blood in the urine.
hesitancy		Decrease in the force of the urine stream, often with difficulty initiating the flow. It is often a symptom of a blockage along the urethra, such as an enlarged prostate gland.
ketonuria (key-tone-YOO-ree-ah)	keton/o = ketones -uria = urine condition	Presence of ketones in the urine. This occurs when the body burns fat instead of glucose for energy, such as in uncontrolled diabetes mellitus.
nephrolith (NEF-roh-lith)	nephr/o = kidney -lith = stone	Kidney stone.
nephromalacia (nef-roh-mah-LAY-she-ah)	nephr/o = kidney -malacia = abnormal softening	Kidney is abnormally soft.
nephromegaly (nef-roh-MEG-ah-lee)	nephr/o = kidney -megaly = enlarged	Kidney is enlarged.
nephrosclerosis (nef-roh-skleh-ROH-sis)	nephr/o = kidney -sclerosis = hardening	Kidney tissue has become hardened.
nocturia (nok-TOO-ree-ah)	noct/i = night -uria = urine condition	Having to urinate frequently during the night.

Pathology (continued)

Term	Word Parts	Definition
oliguria (ol-ig-YOO-ree-ah)	olig/o = scanty -uria = urine condition	Producing too little urine.
polyuria (pol-ee-YOO-ree-ah)	poly- = many -uria = urine condition	Producing an unusually large volume of urine.
proteinuria (pro-teen-YOO-ree-ah)	protein/o = protein -uria = urine condition	Presence of protein in the urine.
pyuria (pye-YOO-ree-ah)	py/o = pus -uria = urine condition	Presence of pus in the urine.
renal colic (KOL-ik)	ren/o = kidney -al = pertaining to -ic = pertaining to	Pain caused by a kidney stone. Can be an excruciating pain and generally requires medical treatment.
stricture (STRIK-chur)		Narrowing of a passageway in the urinary system.
uremia (yoo-REE-mee-ah)	ur/o = urine -emia = blood condition	Accumulation of waste products (especially nitrogenous wastes) in the bloodstream. Associated with renal failure.
ureterectasis (yoo-ree-ter-EK-tah-sis)	ureter/o = ureter -ectasis = dilated	Ureter is stretched out or dilated.
ureterolith (yoo-REE-teh-roh-lith)	ureter/o = ureter -lith = stone	Stone in the ureter.
ureterostenosis (yoo-ree-ter-oh-sten-OH-sis)	ureter/o = ureter -stenosis = narrowing	Ureter has become narrow.
urethralgia (yoo-ree-THRAL-jee-ah)	urethr/o = urethra -algia = pain	Urethral pain.
urethrorrhagia (yoo-ree-throh-RAH-jee-ah)	urethr/o = urethra -rrhagia = abnormal flow condition	Profuse bleeding from the urethra.
urethrostenosis (yoo-ree-throh-steh-NOH-sis)	urethr/o = urethra -stenosis = narrowing	Urethra has become narrow.
urgency (ER-jen-see)		Feeling the need to urinate immediately.
urinary incontinence (in-CON-tin-ens)	urin/o = urine -ary = pertaining to	Involuntary release of urine. In some patients an indwelling catheter is inserted into the bladder for continuous urine drainage.

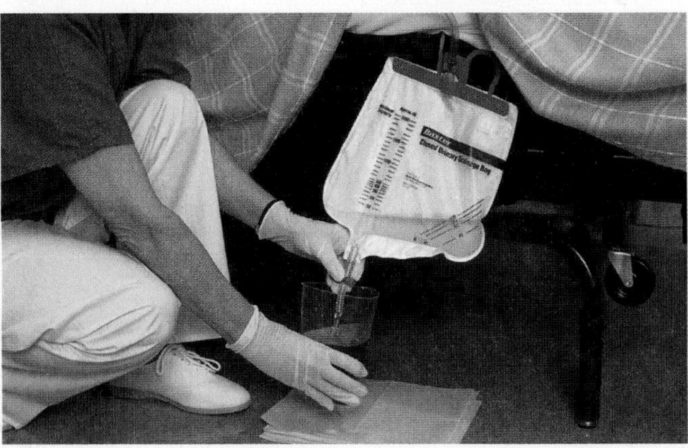

■ **Figure 9.9** Healthcare worker draining urine from a bladder catheter bag. *(Michal Heron, Pearson Education)*

Pathology (continued)

Term	Word Parts	Definition
urinary retention	**urin/o** = urine -**ary** = pertaining to	Inability to fully empty the bladder, often indicates a blockage in the urethra.
Kidney		
acute tubular necrosis (ATN) (ne-KROH-sis)	-**ar** = pertaining to **necr/o** = death -**osis** = abnormal condition	Damage to the renal tubules due to presence of toxins in the urine or to ischemia. Results in oliguria.
diabetic nephropathy (ne-FROH-path-ee)	-**ic** = pertaining to **nephr/o** = kidney -**pathy** = disease	Accumulation of damage to the glomerulus capillaries due to the chronic high blood sugars of diabetes mellitus.
glomerulonephritis (gloh-mair-yoo-loh-neh-FRYE-tis)	**glomerul/o** = glomerulus **nephr/o** = kidney -**itis** = inflammation	Inflammation of the kidney (primarily of the glomerulus). Since the glomerular membrane is inflamed, it becomes more permeable and will allow protein and blood cells to enter the filtrate. Results in protein in the urine (proteinuria) and hematuria.
hydronephrosis (high-droh-neh-FROH-sis)	**hydr/o** = water **nephr/o** = kidney -**osis** = abnormal condition	Distention of the renal pelvis due to urine collecting in the kidney; often a result of the obstruction of a ureter.
nephritis (neh-FRYE-tis)	**nephr/o** = kidney -**itis** = inflammation	Kidney inflammation.
nephrolithiasis (nef-roh-lith-EYE-a-sis)	**nephr/o** = kidney -**lithiasis** = condition of stones	Presence of calculi in the kidney. Usually begins with the solidification of salts present in the urine.
nephroma (neh-FROH-ma)	**nephr/o** = kidney -**oma** = tumor	Kidney tumor.
nephropathy (neh-FROP-ah-thee)	**nephr/o** = kidney -**pathy** = disease	General term describing the presence of kidney disease.
nephroptosis (nef-rop-TOH-sis)	**nephr/o** = kidney -**ptosis** = drooping	Downward displacement of the kidney out of its normal location; commonly called a *floating kidney.*
nephrotic syndrome (NS)	**nephr/o** = kidney -**tic** = pertaining to	Damage to the glomerulus resulting in protein appearing in the urine, proteinuria, and the corresponding decrease in protein in the bloodstream. Also called *nephrosis.*
polycystic kidneys (POL-ee-sis-tik)	**poly-** = many **cyst/o** = pouch -**tic** = pertaining to	Formation of multiple cysts within the kidney tissue. Results in the destruction of normal kidney tissue and uremia.

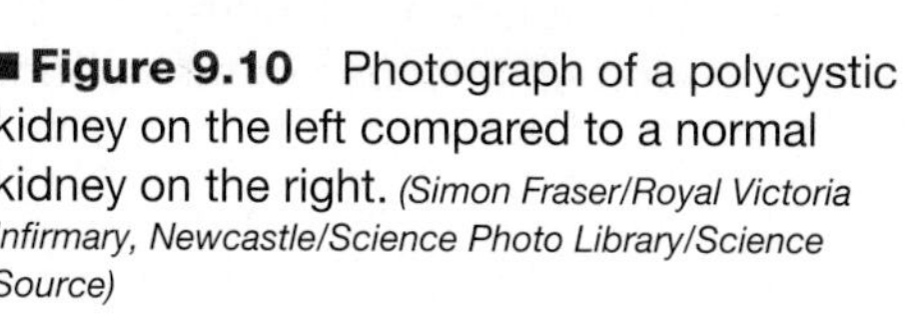

■ **Figure 9.10** Photograph of a polycystic kidney on the left compared to a normal kidney on the right. *(Simon Fraser/Royal Victoria Infirmary, Newcastle/Science Photo Library/Science Source)*

Pathology (continued)

Term	Word Parts	Definition
pyelitis (pye-eh-LYE-tis)	pyel/o = renal pelvis -itis = inflammation	Renal pelvis inflammation.
pyelonephritis (pye-eh-loh-neh-FRYE-tis)	pyel/o = renal pelvis nephr/o = kidney -itis = inflammation	Inflammation of the renal pelvis and the kidney. One of the most common types of kidney disease; may be the result of a lower urinary tract infection that moved up to the kidney by way of the ureters. Large quantities of white blood cells and bacteria in the urine are possible. Blood (hematuria) may even be present in the urine in this condition. Can occur with any untreated or persistent case of cystitis.
renal cell carcinoma	ren/o = kidney -al = pertaining to carcin/o = cancer -oma = tumor	Cancerous tumor that arises from kidney tubule cells.
renal failure	ren/o = kidney -al = pertaining to	Inability of the kidneys to filter wastes from the blood resulting in uremia. May be acute or chronic. Major reason for a patient being placed on dialysis.
Wilms' tumor (VILMZ)		Malignant kidney tumor found most often in children.
Urinary Bladder		
bladder cancer		Cancerous tumor that arises from the cells lining the bladder; major sign is hematuria.
bladder neck obstruction (BNO)		Blockage of the bladder outlet. Often caused by an enlarged prostate gland in males.
cystitis (sis-TYE-tis)	cyst/o = bladder -itis = inflammation	Urinary bladder inflammation.
cystocele (SIS-toh-seel)	cyst/o = bladder -cele = protrusion	Protrusion (or herniation) of the urinary bladder into the wall of the vagina.
interstitial cystitis (in-ter-STISH-al / sis-TYE-tis)	-al = pertaining to cyst/o = bladder -itis = inflammation	Disease of unknown cause in which there is inflammation and irritation of the bladder. Most commonly seen in middle-aged women.
neurogenic bladder (noo-roh-JEN-ik)	neur/o = nerve -genic = producing	Loss of nervous control that leads to retention; may be caused by spinal cord injury or multiple sclerosis.
urinary tract infection (UTI)	urin/o = urine -ary = pertaining to	Infection, usually from bacteria, of any organ of the urinary system. Most often begins with cystitis and may ascend into the ureters and kidneys. Most common in women because of their shorter urethra.

Practice As You Go

C. Terminology Matching

Match each term to its definition.

1. ________ Wilms' tumor	a. kidney stones
2. ________ azotemia	b. feeling the need to urinate immediately
3. ________ urinary retention	c. childhood malignant kidney tumor
4. ________ nephroptosis	d. swelling of the kidney due to urine collecting in the renal pelvis
5. ________ nocturia	e. involuntary release of urine
6. ________ incontinence	f. frequent urination at night
7. ________ hydronephrosis	g. excess nitrogenous waste in bloodstream
8. ________ urgency	h. inability to fully empty bladder
9. ________ nephrolithiasis	i. a floating kidney
10. ________ polycystic kidney disease	j. multiple cysts in the kidneys

Diagnostic Procedures

Term	Word Parts	Definition
Clinical Laboratory Tests		
blood urea nitrogen (BUN) (yoo-REE-ah / NIGH-troh-jen)		Blood test to measure kidney function by the level of nitrogenous waste (urea) that is in the blood.
clean catch specimen (CC)		Urine sample obtained after cleaning off the urinary opening and catching or collecting a urine sample in midstream (halfway through the urination process) to minimize contamination from the genitalia.
creatinine clearance (kree-AT-tih-neen)		Test of kidney function. Creatinine is a waste product cleared from the bloodstream by the kidneys. For this test, urine is collected for 24 hours, and the amount of creatinine in the urine is compared to the amount of creatinine that remains in the bloodstream.
urinalysis (U/A, UA) (yoo-rih-NAL-ih-sis)	urin/o = urine -lysis = to destroy (to break down)	Laboratory test consisting of the physical, chemical, and microscopic examination of urine.
urine culture and sensitivity (C&S)		Laboratory test of urine for bacterial infection. Attempt to grow bacteria on a culture medium in order to identify it and determine which antibiotics it is sensitive to.
urinometer (yoo-rin-OH-meter)	urin/o = urine -meter = instrument to measure	Instrument to measure the specific gravity of urine; part of a urinalysis.

Diagnostic Procedures (continued)

Term	Word Parts	Definition
Diagnostic Imaging		
cystogram (SIS-toh-gram)	**cyst/o** = bladder **-gram** = record	X-ray record of the urinary bladder.
cystography (sis-TOG-rah-fee)	**cyst/o** = bladder **-graphy** = process of recording	Process of instilling a contrast material or dye into the bladder by catheter to visualize the urinary bladder on X-ray.
excretory urography (EU) (EKS-kreh-tor-ee / yoo-ROG-rah-fee)	**-ory** = pertaining to **ur/o** = urine **-graphy** = process of recording	Injecting dye into the bloodstream and then taking an X-ray to trace the action of the kidney as it excretes the dye.
intravenous pyelography (IVP) (in-trah-VEE-nus / pye-eh-LOG-rah-fee)	**intra-** = within **ven/o** = vein **-ous** = pertaining to **pyel/o** = renal pelvis **-graphy** = process of recording	Diagnostic X-ray procedure in which a dye is injected into a vein and then X-rays are taken to visualize the renal pelvis as the dye is removed by the kidneys.
kidneys, ureters, bladder (KUB)		X-ray taken of the abdomen demonstrating the kidneys, ureters, and bladder without using any contrast dye. Also called a *flat-plate abdomen.*
nephrogram (NEH-fro-gram)	**nephr/o** = kidney **-gram** = record	X-ray record of the kidney.
pyelogram (PYE-eh-loh-gram)	**pyel/o** = renal pelvis **-gram** = record	X-ray record of the renal pelvis.
retrograde pyelography (RP) (RET-roh-grayd/ pye-eh-LOG-rah-fee) ■ **Figure 9.11** Color enhanced retrograde pyelogram X-ray. Radiopaque dye outlines urinary bladder, ureters, and renal pelvis. *(Clinique Ste. Catherine/CNRI/ Science Photo Library/Science Source)*	**retro-** = backward **pyel/o** = renal pelvis **-graphy** = process of recording	Diagnostic X-ray procedure in which dye is inserted through the urethra to outline the bladder, ureters, and renal pelvis.
voiding cystourethrography (VCUG) (sis-toh-yoo-ree-THROG-rah-fee)	**cyst/o** = bladder **urethr/o** = urethra **-graphy** = process of recording	X-ray taken to visualize the urethra while the patient is voiding after a contrast dye has been placed in the bladder.

Diagnostic Procedures (continued)

Term	Word Parts	Definition
Endoscopic Procedure		
cystoscope (SIS-toh-scope)	cyst/o = bladder -scope = instrument to visually examine	Instrument used to visually examine the inside of the urinary bladder.
cystoscopy (cysto) (sis-TOSS-koh-pee)	cyst/o = bladder -scopy = process of visually examining	Visual examination of the urinary bladder using an instrument called a *cystoscope.*
urethroscope (yoo-REE-throh-scope)	urethr/o = urethra -scope = instrument to visually examine	Instrument to visually examine the inside of the urethra.

Therapeutic Procedures

Term	Word Parts	Definition
Medical Treatments		
catheter (KATH-eh-ter)		Flexible tube inserted into the body for the purpose of moving fluids into or out of the body. Most commonly used to refer to a tube threaded through the urethra into the bladder to withdraw urine (see again Figure 9.9).
catheterization (cath) (kath-eh-ter-ih-ZAY-shun)		Insertion of a tube through the urethra and into the urinary bladder for the purpose of withdrawing urine or inserting dye.
extracorporeal shockwave lithotripsy (ESWL) (eks-trah-cor-POR-ee-al / shockwave / LITH-oh-trip-see)	extra- = outside of corpor/o = body -eal = pertaining to lith/o = stone -tripsy = surgical crushing	Use of ultrasound waves to break up stones. Process does not require invasive surgery.

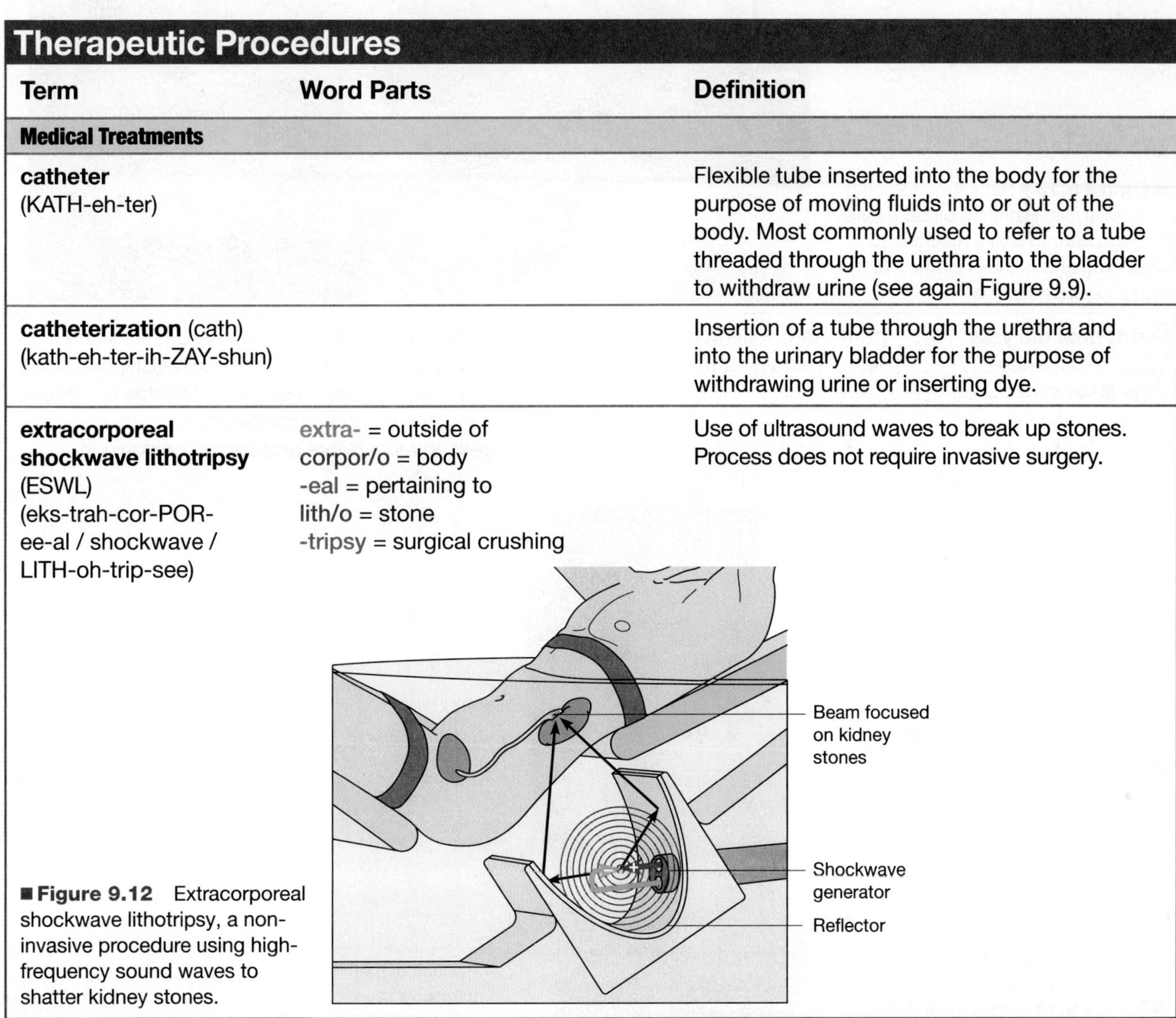

■ **Figure 9.12** Extracorporeal shockwave lithotripsy, a non-invasive procedure using high-frequency sound waves to shatter kidney stones.

Therapeutic Procedures (continued)

Term	Word Parts	Definition
hemodialysis (HD) (hee-moh-dye-AL-ih-sis)	hem/o = blood	Use of an artificial kidney machine that filters the blood of a person to remove waste products. Use of this technique in patients who have defective kidneys is lifesaving.

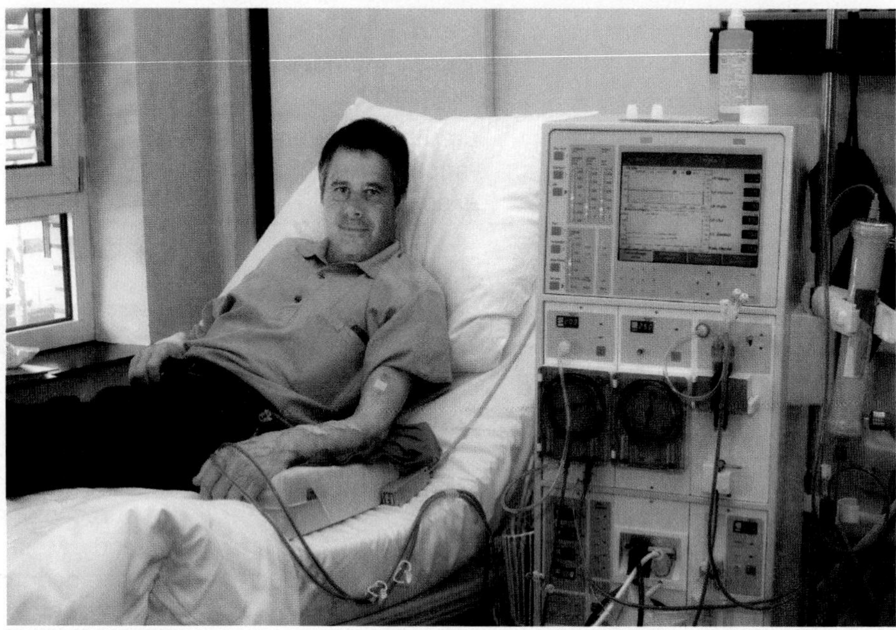

■ **Figure 9.13** Patient undergoing hemodialysis. Patient's blood passes through hemodialysis machine for cleansing and is then returned to the body. *(gopixa/Shutterstock)*

Term	Word Parts	Definition
peritoneal dialysis (pair-ih-TOH-nee-al / dye-AL-ih-sis)	peritone/o = peritoneum -eal = pertaining to	Removal of toxic waste substances from the body by placing warm chemically balanced solutions into the peritoneal cavity. Wastes are filtered out of the blood across the peritoneum. Used in treating renal failure and certain poisonings.

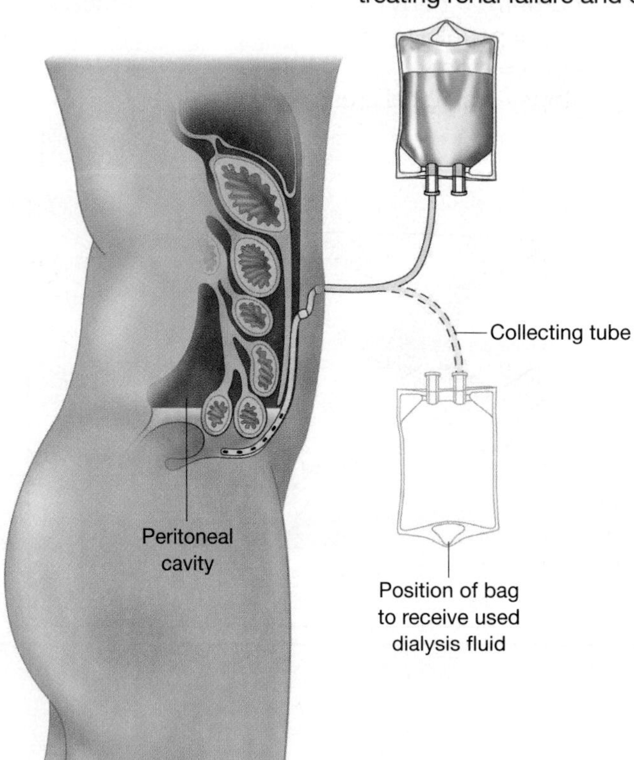

■ **Figure 9.14** Peritoneal dialysis. Chemically balanced solution is placed into the abdominal cavity to draw impurities out of the bloodstream. It is removed after several hours.

Therapeutic Procedures (continued)

Term	Word Parts	Definition
Surgical Treatments		
cystectomy (sis-TEK-toh-mee)	cyst/o = bladder -ectomy = surgical removal	Surgical removal of the urinary bladder.
cystopexy (SIS-toh-pek-see)	cyst/o = bladder -pexy = surgical fixation	Surgical fixation of the urinary bladder. Performed to correct a cystocele.
cystoplasty (SIS-toh-plas-tee)	cyst/o = bladder -plasty = surgical repair	To repair a defect in the urinary bladder by surgical means.
cystostomy (sis-TOSS-toh-mee)	cyst/o = bladder -ostomy = surgically create an opening	To surgically create an opening into the urinary bladder through the abdominal wall.
cystotomy (sis-TOT-oh-mee)	cyst/o = bladder -otomy = cutting into	To cut into the urinary bladder.
lithotomy (lith-OT-oh-mee)	lith/o = stone -otomy = cutting into	To cut into an organ for the purpose of removing a stone.
lithotripsy (LITH-oh-trip-see)	lith/o = stone -tripsy = surgical crushing	Destroying or crushing stones in the bladder or urethra.
meatotomy (mee-ah-TOT-oh-mee)	meat/o = meatus -otomy = cutting into	To cut into the meatus in order to enlarge the opening of the urethra.
nephrectomy (ne-FREK-toh-mee)	nephr/o = kidney -ectomy = surgical removal	Surgical removal of a kidney.
nephrolithotomy (nef-roh-lith-OT-oh-mee)	nephr/o = kidney lith/o = stone -otomy = cutting into	To cut into the kidney in order to remove stones.
nephropexy (NEF-roh-pek-see)	nephr/o = kidney -pexy = surgical fixation	Surgical fixation of a kidney; to anchor it in its normal anatomical position.
nephrostomy (neh-FROS-toh-mee)	nephr/o = kidney -ostomy = surgically create an opening	To surgically create an opening into the kidney through the abdominal wall.
nephrotomy (neh-FROT-oh-mee)	nephr/o = kidney -otomy = cutting into	To cut into the kidney.
pyeloplasty (PIE-ah-loh-plas-tee)	pyel/o = renal pelvis -plasty = surgical repair	To repair the renal pelvis by surgical means.
renal transplant	ren/o = kidney -al = pertaining to	Surgical placement of a donor kidney.

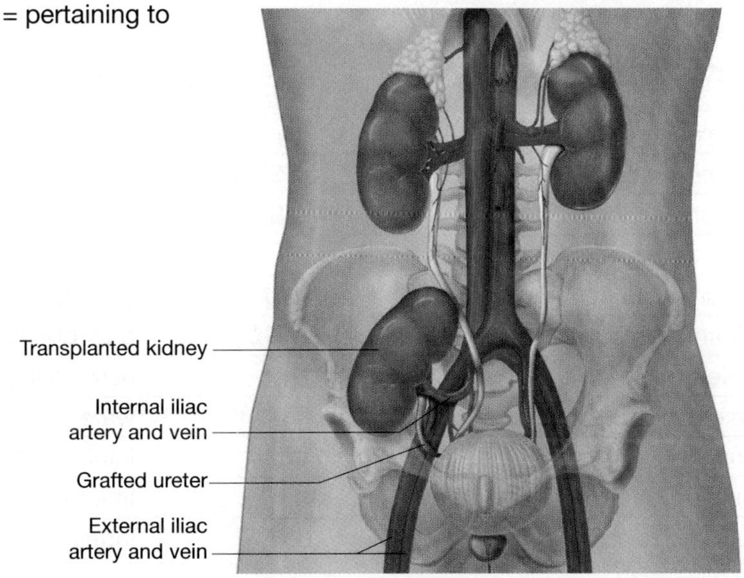

■ **Figure 9.15** Figure illustrates location utilized for implantation of donor kidney.

Practice As You Go

D. Match each procedure term with its definition

1. ________ clean catch specimen
2. ________ hemodialysis
3. ________ pyeloplasty
4. ________ urinometer
5. ________ lithotripsy
6. ________ cystoscopy
7. ________ catheter
8. ________ kidneys, ureters, bladder

a. measures specific gravity
b. abdominal X-ray
c. visual examination of the bladder
d. a flexible tube inserted into the body
e. removes waste products from blood
f. method of obtaining urine sample
g. crushing of a stone
h. surgical repair of the renal pelvis

Pharmacology

Classification	Word Parts	Action	Examples
antibiotic	anti- = against bi/o = life -tic = pertaining to	Used to treat bacterial infections of the urinary tract.	ciprofloxacin, Cipro; nitrofurantoin, Macrobid
antispasmodic (an-tye-spaz-MAH-dik)	anti- = against -ic = pertaining to	Used to prevent or reduce bladder muscle spasms.	oxybutynin, Ditropan; neostigmine, Prostigmine
diuretic (dye-yoo-REH-tik)	-tic = pertaining to	Increases the volume of urine produced by the kidneys. Useful in the treatment of edema, kidney failure, heart failure, and hypertension.	furosemide, Lasix; spironolactone, Aldactone

Abbreviations

AGN	acute glomerulonephritis	**cysto**	cystoscopy
ARF	acute renal failure	**ESRD**	end-stage renal disease
ATN	acute tubular necrosis	**ESWL**	extracorporeal shockwave lithotripsy
BNO	bladder neck obstruction	**EU**	excretory urography
BUN	blood urea nitrogen	**GU**	genitourinary
CAPD	continuous ambulatory peritoneal dialysis	**HCO_3^-**	bicarbonate
cath	catheterization	**HD**	hemodialysis
CC	clean catch urine specimen	**H_2O**	water
Cl^-	chloride	**I&O**	intake and output
CRF	chronic renal failure	**IPD**	intermittent peritoneal dialysis
C&S	culture and sensitivity	**IVP**	intravenous pyelogram

Abbreviations (continued)

K^+	potassium	**RP**	retrograde pyelogram
KUB	kidneys, ureters, bladder	**SG, sp. gr.**	specific gravity
mL	milliliter	**U/A, UA**	urinalysis
Na^+	sodium	**UC**	urine culture
NS	nephrotic syndrome	**UTI**	urinary tract infection
pH	acidity or alkalinity of urine	**VCUG**	voiding cystourethrography

Practice As You Go

E. What Does it Stand For?

1. KUB ______
2. cath ______
3. cysto ______
4. GU ______
5. ESWL ______
6. UTI ______
7. UC ______
8. RP ______
9. ARF ______
10. BUN ______
11. CRF ______
12. H_2O ______

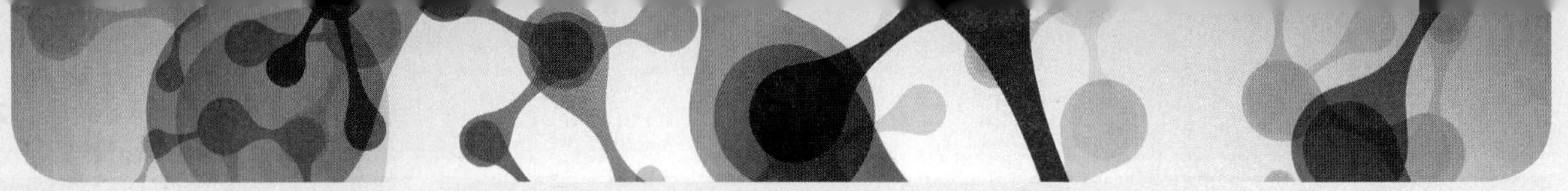

Chapter Review

Real-World Applications

Medical Record Analysis

This Discharge Summary contains 13 medical terms. Underline each term and write it in the list below the report. Then define each term.

Discharge Summary

Admitting Diagnosis:	Severe right side pain and hematuria.
Final Diagnosis:	Pyelonephritis right kidney, complicated by chronic cystitis.
History of Present Illness:	Patient has long history of frequent bladder infections, but denies any recent lower pelvic pain or dysuria. Earlier today he had rapid onset of severe right side pain and is unable to stand fully erect. His temperature was 101°F, and his skin was sweaty and flushed. He was admitted from the ER for further testing and diagnosis.
Summary of Hospital Course:	Clean catch urinalysis revealed gross hematuria and pyuria, but no albuminuria. A culture and sensitivity was ordered to identify the pathogen and an antibiotic was started. Cystoscopy showed evidence of chronic cystitis, bladder irritation, and a bladder neck obstruction. The obstruction appears to be congenital and the probable cause of the chronic cystitis. The patient was catheterized to ensure complete emptying of the bladder, and fluids were encouraged. Patient responded well to the antibiotic therapy and fluids, and his symptoms improved.
Discharge Plans:	Patient was discharged home after three days in the hospital. He was switched to an oral antibiotic for the pyelonephritis and chronic cystitis. A repeat urinalysis is scheduled for next week. After all inflammation is corrected, will repeat cystoscopy to reevaluate bladder neck obstruction.

	Term	Definition
1.	______________	______________________________
2.	______________	______________________________
3.	______________	______________________________
4.	______________	______________________________
5.	______________	______________________________
6.	______________	______________________________
7.	______________	______________________________
8.	______________	______________________________
9.	______________	______________________________
10.	______________	______________________________
11.	______________	______________________________
12.	______________	______________________________
13.	______________	______________________________

Chart Note Transcription

The chart note below contains 11 phrases that can be reworded with a medical term that you learned in this chapter. Each phrase is identified with an underline. Determine the medical term and write your answers in the space provided.

Pearson General Hospital Consultation Report

Task Edit View Time Scale Options Help Download Archive Date: 17 May 2015

Current Complaint:	A 36-year-old male was seen by the specialist in the treatment of diseases of the urinary system **1** because of right flank pain and blood in the urine. **2**
Past History:	Patient has a history of bladder infection; **3** denies experiencing any symptoms for two years.
Signs and Symptoms:	A technique used to obtain an uncontaminated urine sample **4** obtained for laboratory analysis of the urine **5** revealed blood in the urine, but no pus in the urine. **6** A kidney X-ray made after inserting dye into the bladder **7** was normal on the left, but dye was seen filling the right tube between the kidney and bladder **8** only halfway to the kidney.
Diagnosis:	Stone in the tube between the kidney and the bladder **9** on the right.
Treatment:	Patient underwent the use of ultrasound waves to break up stones. **10** Pieces of dissolved kidney stones **11** were flushed out, after which symptoms resolved.

1. ______________________________

2. ______________________________

3. ______________________________

4. ______________________________

5. ______________________________

6. ______________________________

7. ______________________________

8. ______________________________

9. ______________________________

10. ______________________________

11. ______________________________

Case Study

Below is a case study presentation of a patient with a condition discussed in this chapter. Read the case study and answer the questions below. Some questions will ask for information not included within this chapter. Use your text, a medical dictionary, or any other reference material you choose to answer these questions.

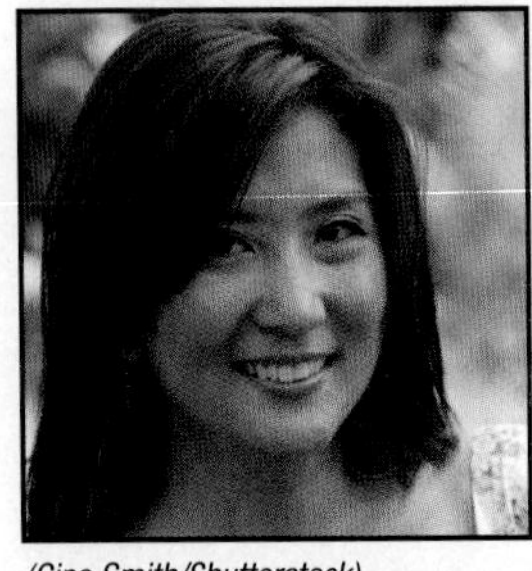

(Gina Smith/Shutterstock)

A 32-year-old female is seen in the urologist's office because of a fever, chills, and generalized fatigue. She also reported urgency, frequency, dysuria, and hematuria. In addition, she noticed that her urine was cloudy with a fishy odor. The physician ordered the following tests: a clean catch specimen for a U/A, a urine C&S, and a KUB. The U/A revealed pyuria, bacteriuria, and a slightly acidic pH. A common type of bacteria was grown in the culture. X-rays reveal acute pyelonephritis resulting from cystitis, which has spread up to the kidney from the bladder. The patient was placed on an antibiotic and encouraged to "push fluids" by drinking two liters of water a day.

Questions

1. This patient has two urinary system infections in different locations; name them. Which one caused the other and how?

____

____

2. List and define each of the patient's presenting symptoms in your own words.

____

____

3. What diagnostic tests did the urologist order? Describe them in your own words.

____

____

4. Explain the results of each diagnostic test in your own words.

____

____

5. What were the physician's treatment instructions for this patient? Explain the purpose of each treatment.

____

____

6. Describe the normal appearance of urine.

____

____

Practice Exercises

A. Word Building Practice

The combining form **nephr/o** refers to the kidney. Use it to write a term that means:

1. surgical fixation of the kidney ____________
2. X-ray record of the kidney ____________
3. condition of kidney stones ____________
4. removal of a kidney ____________
5. inflammation of the kidney ____________
6. kidney disease ____________
7. hardening of the kidney ____________

The combining form **cyst/o** refers to the urinary bladder. Use it to write a term that means:

8. inflammation of the bladder ____________
9. abnormal flow condition from the bladder ____________
10. surgical repair of the bladder ____________
11. instrument to view inside the bladder ____________
12. bladder pain ____________

The combining form **pyel/o** refers to the renal pelvis. Use it to write a term that means:

13. surgical repair of the renal pelvis ____________
14. inflammation of the renal pelvis ____________
15. X-ray record of the renal pelvis ____________

The combining form **ureter/o** refers to one or both of the ureters. Use it to write a term that means:

16. a ureteral stone ____________
17. ureter dilation ____________
18. ureter narrowing ____________

The combining form **urethr/o** refers to the urethra. Use it to write a term that means:

19. urethra inflammation ____________
20. instrument to view inside the urethra ____________

B. Define the Combining Form

	Definition	Example from Chapter
1. **ur/o**	____________	____________
2. **meat/o**	____________	____________

	Definition	Example from Chapter
3. **cyst/o**	______	______
4. **ren/o**	______	______
5. **pyel/o**	______	______
6. **glycos/o**	______	______
7. **noct/i**	______	______
8. **olig/o**	______	______
9. **ureter/o**	______	______
10. **glomerul/o**	______	______

C. Pharmacology Challenge

Fill in the classification for each drug description, then match the brand name.

	Drug Description	Classification	Brand Name
1.	______ Reduces bladder muscle spasms	______	a. Lasix
2.	______ Treats bacterial infections	______	b. Ditropan
3.	______ Increases volume of urine produced	______	c. Cipro

D. Define the Term

1. micturition ______
2. diuretic ______
3. renal colic ______
4. catheterization ______
5. pyelitis ______
6. glomerulonephritis ______
7. lithotomy ______
8. enuresis ______
9. meatotomy ______
10. diabetic nephropathy ______
11. urinalysis ______
12. hesitancy ______

E. Name That Term

1. absence of urine ______
2. blood in the urine ______
3. kidney stone ______
4. crushing a stone ______
5. inflammation of the urethra ______
6. pus in the urine ______
7. bacteria in the urine ______
8. painful urination ______
9. ketones in the urine ______
10. protein in the urine ______
11. (too) much urine ______

F. What's the Abbreviation?

1. potassium ______
2. sodium ______
3. urinalysis ______
4. blood urea nitrogen ______
5. specific gravity ______
6. intravenous pyelogram ______
7. bladder neck obstruction ______
8. intake and output ______
9. acute tubular necrosis ______
10. end-stage renal disease ______

G. Define the Suffix

	Definition	Example from Chapter
1. **-ptosis**	______	______
2. **-uria**	______	______
3. **-lith**	______	______
4. **-tripsy**	______	______
5. **-lithiasis**	______	______

H. Fill in the Blank

renal transplant	ureterectomy	intravenous pyelogram (IVP)
cystostomy	pyelolithectomy	nephropexy
renal biopsy	cystoscopy	urinary tract infection

1. Juan suffered from chronic renal failure. His sister, Maria, donated one of her normal kidneys to him, and he had a(n)____________________.
2. Anesha's floating kidney needed surgical fixation. Her physician performed a surgical procedure known as ____________________.
3. Kenya's physician stated that she had a general infection that he referred to as a UTI. The full name for this infection is ____________________.
4. Surgeons operated on Robert to remove calculi from his renal pelvis. The name of this surgery is ____________________.
5. Charles had to have a small piece of his kidney tissue removed so that the physician could perform a microscopic evaluation. This procedure is called a(n) ____________________.
6. Naomi had to have one of her ureters removed due to a stricture. This procedure is called ____________________.
7. The physician had to create a temporary opening between Eric's bladder and his abdominal wall. This procedure is called ____________________.
8. Sally's bladder was visually examined using a special instrument. This procedure is called a(n) ____________________.
9. The doctors believe that Jacob has a tumor of the right kidney. They are going to do a test called a(n) ____________________ that requires them to inject a radiopaque contrast medium intravenously so that they can see the kidney on X-ray.

Labeling Exercise

Image A

Write the labels for this figure on the numbered lines provided.

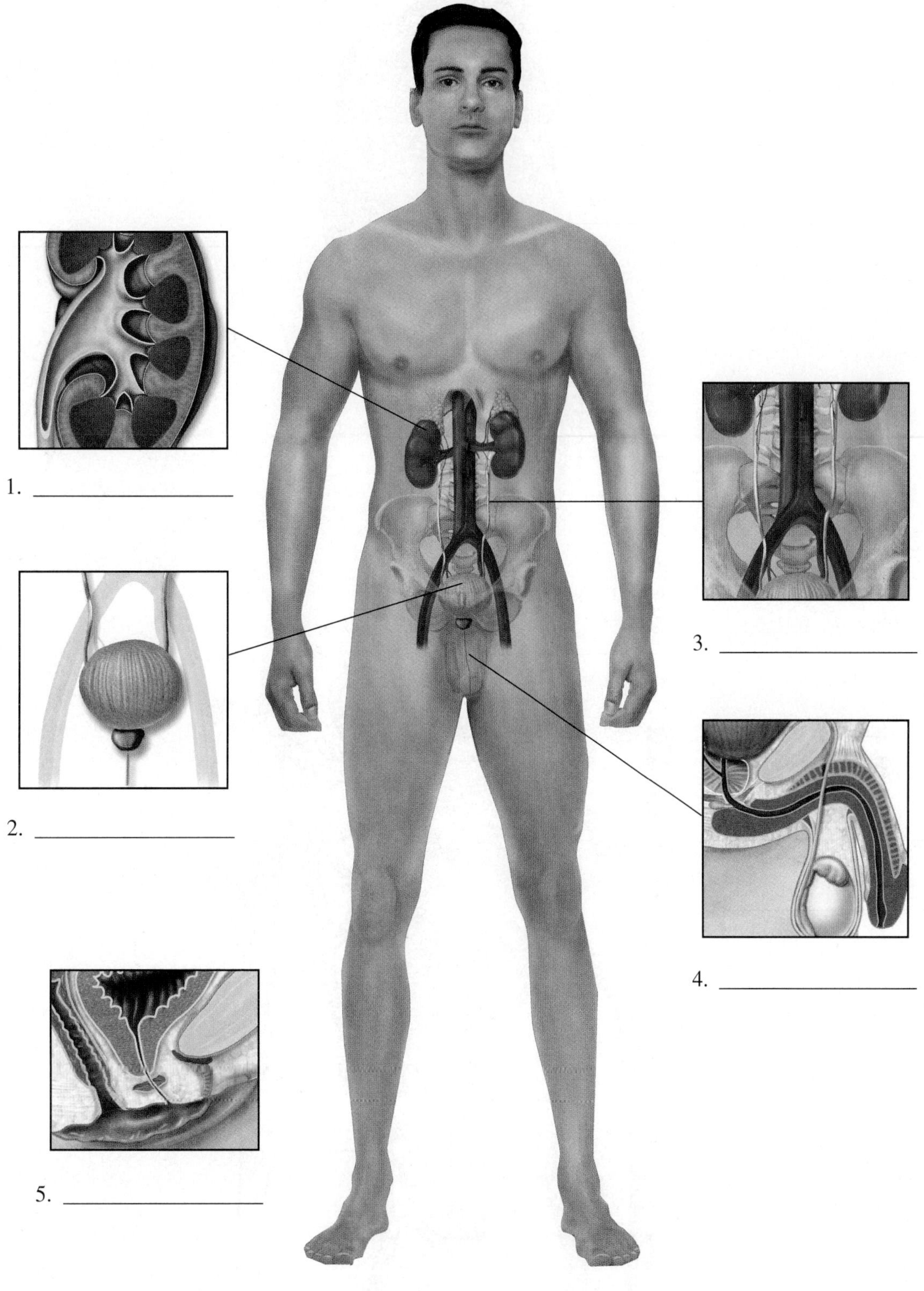

Image B

Write the labels for this figure on the numbered lines provided.

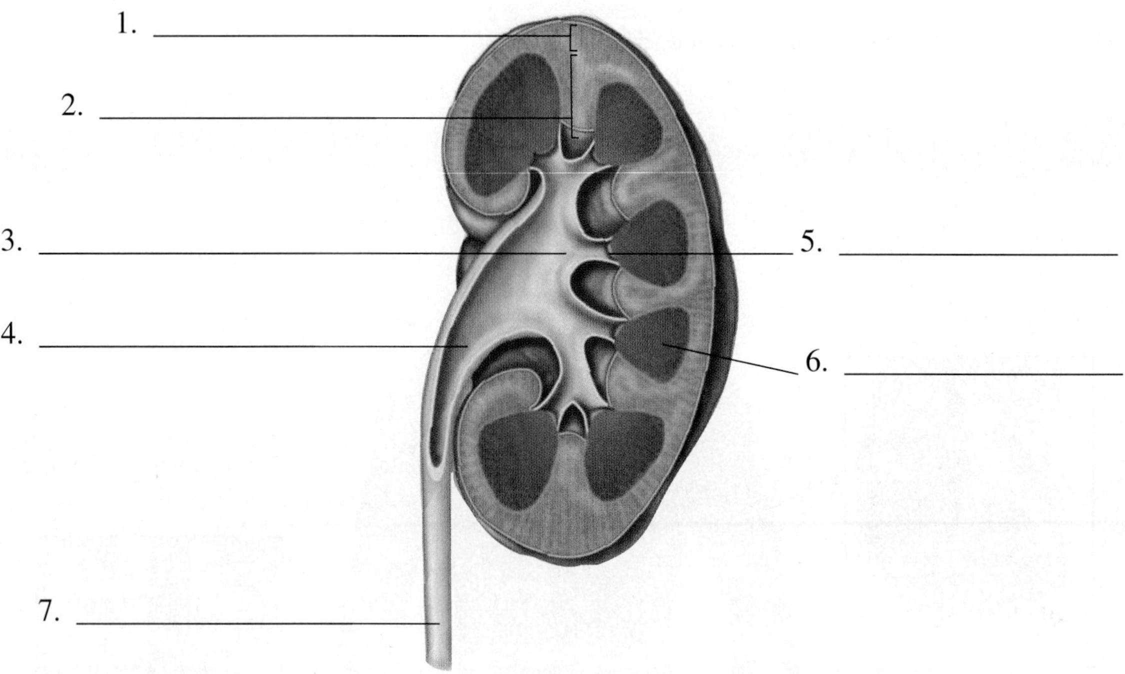

Image C

Write the labels for this figure on the numbered lines provided.

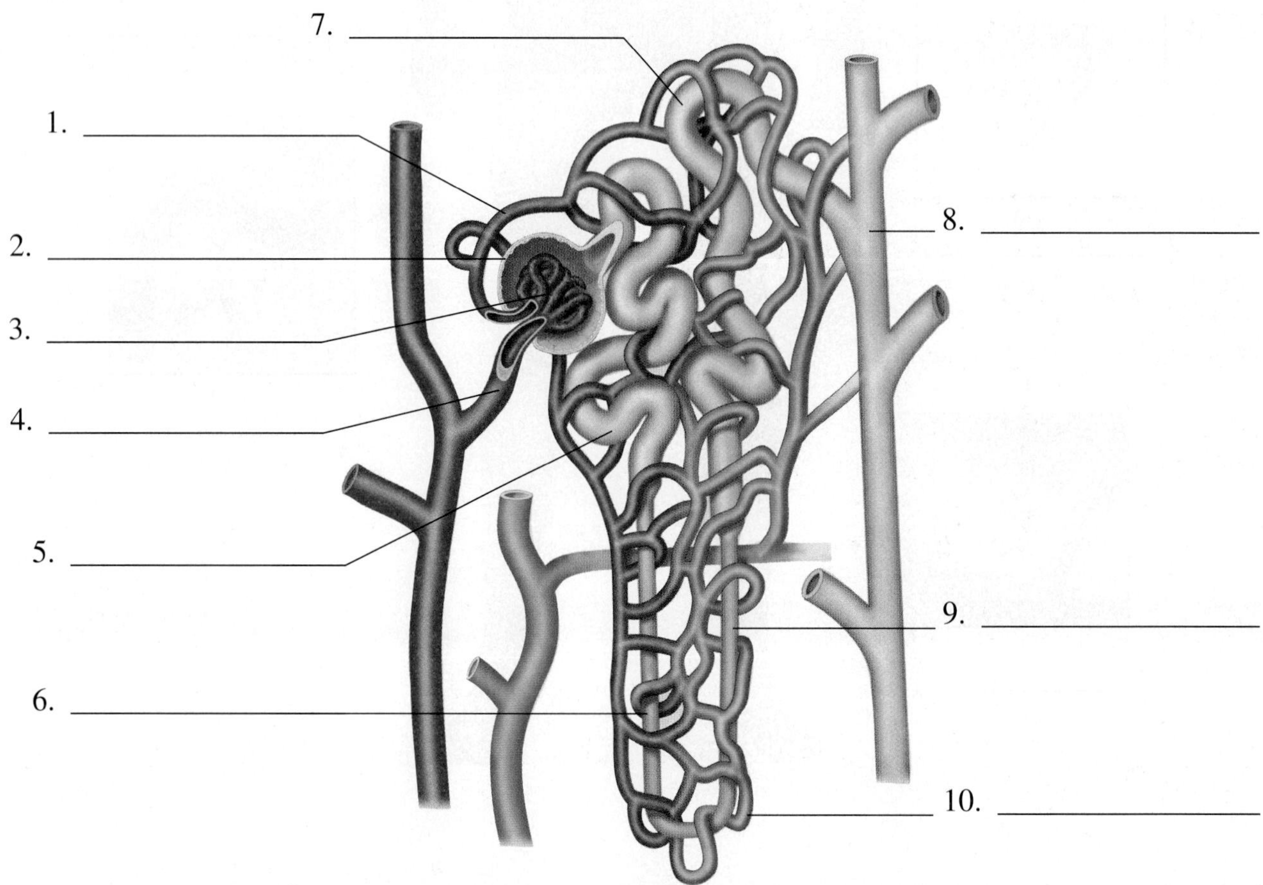

10

Reproductive System

Learning Objectives

Upon completion of this chapter, you will be able to

- Identify and define the combining forms, suffixes, and prefixes introduced in this chapter.
- Correctly spell and pronounce medical terms and major anatomical structures relating to the reproductive systems.
- Locate and describe the major organs of the reproductive systems and their functions.
- Use medical terms to describe circumstances relating to pregnancy.
- Identify and define reproductive system anatomical terms.
- Identify and define selected reproductive system pathology terms.
- Identify the symptoms and origin of sexually transmitted diseases.
- Identify and define selected reproductive system diagnostic procedures.
- Identify and define selected reproductive system therapeutic procedures.
- Identify and define selected medications relating to the reproductive systems.
- Define selected abbreviations associated with the reproductive systems.

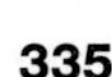

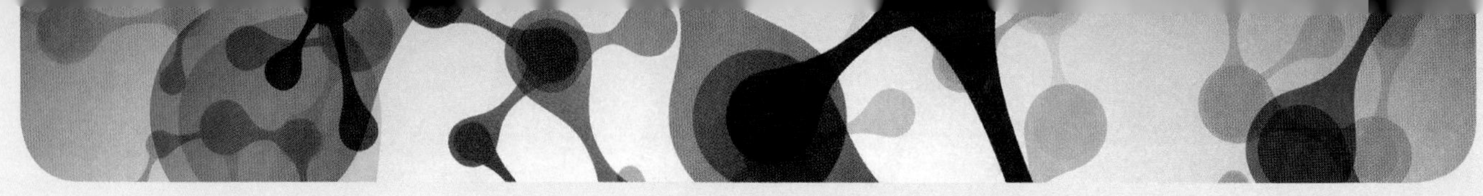

Section I: Female Reproductive System at a Glance

Function

The female reproductive system produces ova (the female reproductive cells), provides a location for fertilization and growth of a baby, and secretes female sex hormones. In addition, the breasts produce milk to nourish the newborn.

Organs

Here are the primary structures that comprise the female reproductive system:

breasts
uterine tubes
ovaries
uterus
vagina
vulva

Word Parts

Here are the most common word parts (with their meanings) used to build female reproductive system terms. For a more comprehensive list, refer to the Terminology section of this chapter.

Combining Forms

amni/o	amnion
cervic/o	neck, cervix
chori/o	chorion
colp/o	vagina
culd/o	cul-de-sac
dilat/o	to widen
embry/o	embryo
episi/o	vulva
estr/o	female
fet/o	fetus
gynec/o	woman, female
hymen/o	hymen
hyster/o	uterus
lact/o	milk
mamm/o	breast
mast/o	breast
men/o	menses, menstruation
metr/o	uterus
nat/o	birth
o/o	egg
oophor/o	ovary
ov/o, ov/i	ovum
ovari/o	ovary
perine/o	perineum
radic/o	root
salping/o	uterine (fallopian) tubes
tox/o	poison
uter/o	uterus
vagin/o	vagina
vulv/o	vulva

Suffixes

-arche	beginning
-cyesis	state of pregnancy
-genesis	produces
-gravida	pregnancy
-oid	resembling
-para	to bear (offspring)
-partum	childbirth
-salpinx	uterine tube
-tocia	labor, childbirth

Prefixes

ante-	before, in front of
contra-	against
primi-	first

Female Reproductive System Illustrated

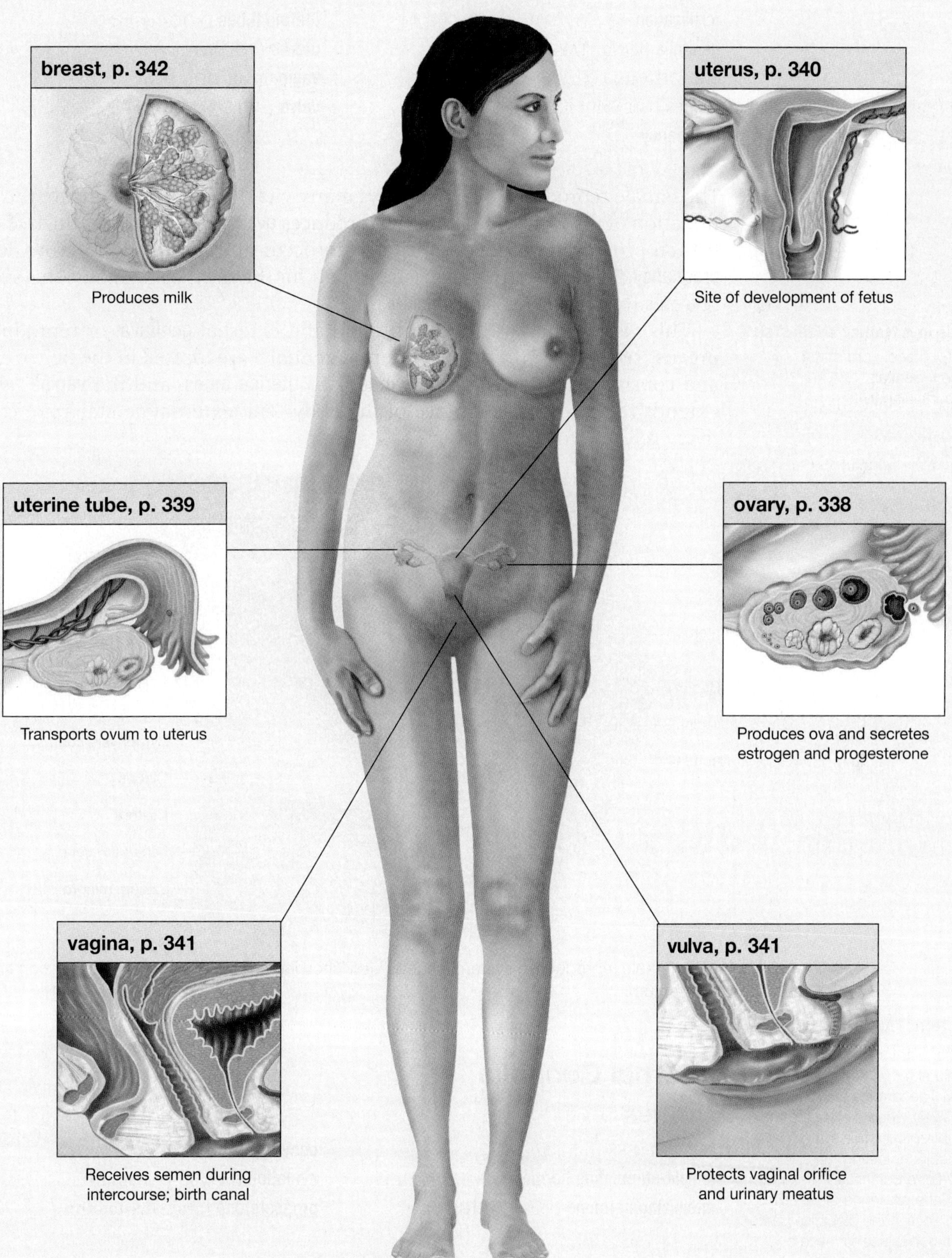

Anatomy and Physiology of the Female Reproductive System

breasts
fertilization
genitalia (jen-ih-TAY-lee-ah)
ova (OH-vah)
ovaries (OH-vah-reez)
pregnancy
sex hormones
uterine tubes (YOO-ter-in)
uterus (YOO-ter-us)
vagina (vah-JIGH-nah)
vulva (VULL-vah)

The female reproductive system plays many vital functions that ensure the continuation of the human race. First, it produces **ova**, the female reproductive cells. It then provides a place for **fertilization** to occur and for a baby to grow during **pregnancy**. The **breasts** provide nourishment for the newborn. Finally, this system secretes the female **sex hormones**.

What's In A Name?
Look for these word parts:
genit/o = genitals
-al = pertaining to

This system consists of both internal and external **genitalia**, or reproductive organs (see Figure 10.1 ■). The internal genitalia are located in the pelvic cavity and consist of the **uterus**, two **ovaries**, two **uterine tubes**, and the **vagina**, which extends to the external surface of the body. The external genitalia are collectively referred to as the **vulva**.

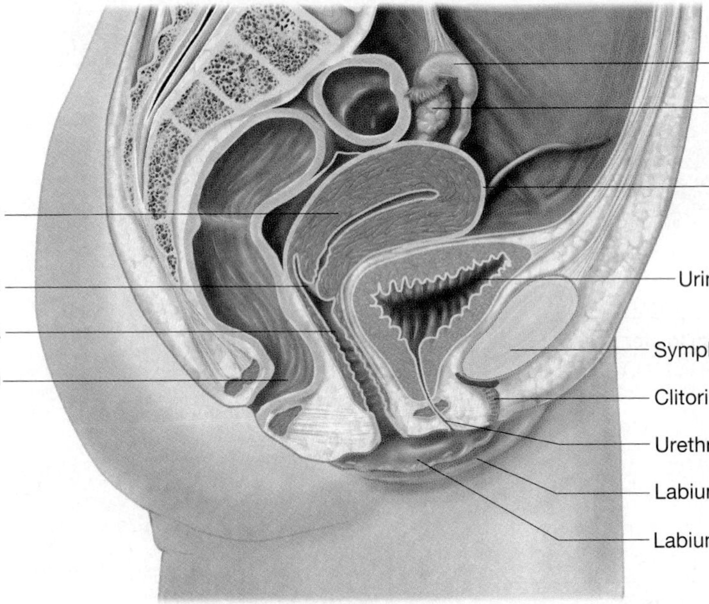

■ **Figure 10.1** The female reproductive system, sagittal view showing organs of the system in relation to the urinary bladder and rectum.

Med Term Tip
The singular for egg is *ovum*. The plural term for many eggs is *ova*. The term *ova* is not used exclusively when discussing the human reproductive system. For instance, testing the stool for ova and parasites is used to detect the presence of parasites or their ova in the digestive tract, a common cause for severe diarrhea. Ova are produced in the ovary by a process called *oogenesis* (*o/o* = egg and *-genesis* = produce).

Internal Genitalia

Ovaries

estrogen (ESS-troh-jen)
follicle-stimulating hormone (FOLL-ih-kl)
luteinizing hormone (loo-teh-NIGH-zing)
oocyte (oh-oh-site)
ovulation (ov-yoo-LAY-shun)
progesterone (proh-JES-ter-ohn)

There are two ovaries, one located on each side of the uterus within the pelvic cavity (see again Figure 10.1). These are small almond-shaped glands that produce ova (singular is *ovum*) and the female sex hormones (see Figure 10.2 ■).

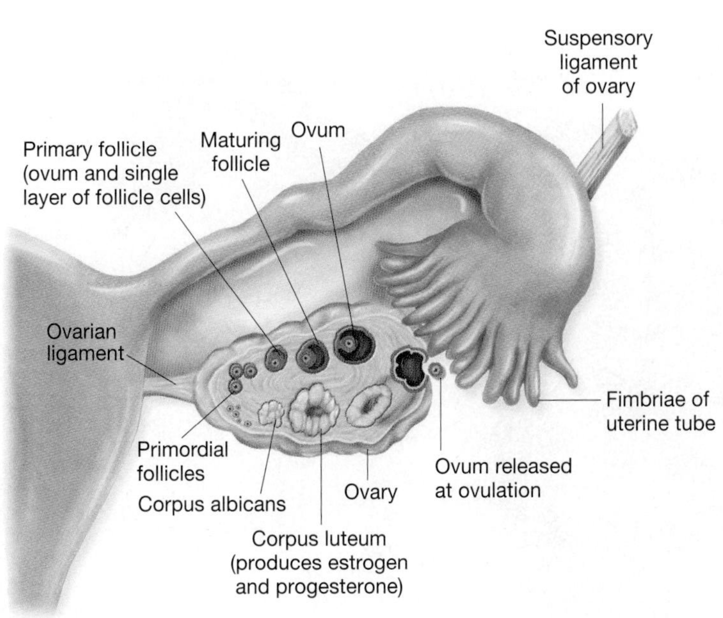

■ **Figure 10.2** Structure of the ovary and fallopian (uterine) tube. Figure illustrates stages of ovum development and the relationship of the ovary to the uterine tube.

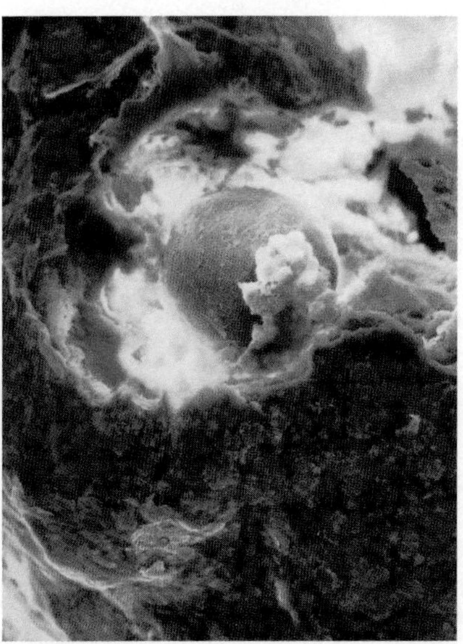

■ **Figure 10.3** Color-enhanced scanning electron micrograph showing an ovum (pink) released by the ovary at ovulation surrounded by follicle (white) tissue. The external surface of the ovary is brown in this photo.
(P.M. Motta and J. Van Blekrom/Science Photo Library/ Science Source)

In humans approximately every 28 days hormones from the anterior pituitary, **follicle-stimulating hormone** (FSH) and **luteinizing hormone** (LH), stimulate maturation of ovum and trigger **ovulation**, the process by which one ovary releases an ovum (or **oocyte**) (see Figure 10.3 ■). The principal female sex hormones produced by the ovaries, **estrogen** and **progesterone**, stimulate the lining of the uterus to be prepared to receive a fertilized ovum. These hormones are also responsible for the female secondary sexual characteristics.

What's In A Name?
Look for these word parts:
estr/o = female
o/o = egg
ov/o = ovum
-cyte = cell
-gen = that which produces
pro- = before

Uterine Tubes

conception (con-SEP-shun)
fallopian tubes (fah-LOH-pee-an)
fimbriae (FIM-bree-ay)
oviducts (OH-vih-ducts)

The uterine tubes, also called the **fallopian tubes** or **oviducts**, are approximately 5½ inches long and run from the area around each ovary to either side of the upper portion of the uterus (see Figure 10.4 ■ and Figure 10.5 ■). As they near the

What's In A Name?
Look for these word parts:
ov/i = ovum

Med Term Tip
When the fertilized egg adheres or implants to the uterine tube instead of moving into the uterus, a condition called *tubal pregnancy* exists. There is not enough room in the uterine tube for the fetus to grow normally. Implantation of the fertilized egg in any location other than the uterus is called an *ectopic pregnancy. Ectopic* is a general term meaning "in the wrong place."

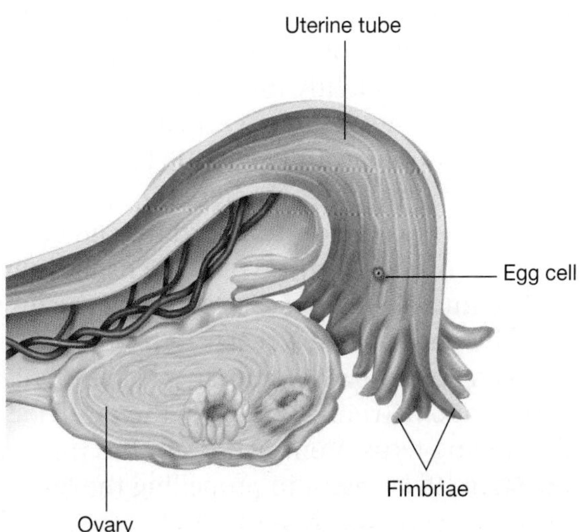

■ **Figure 10.4** Uterine (fallopian) tube, showing released ovum within the uterine tube.

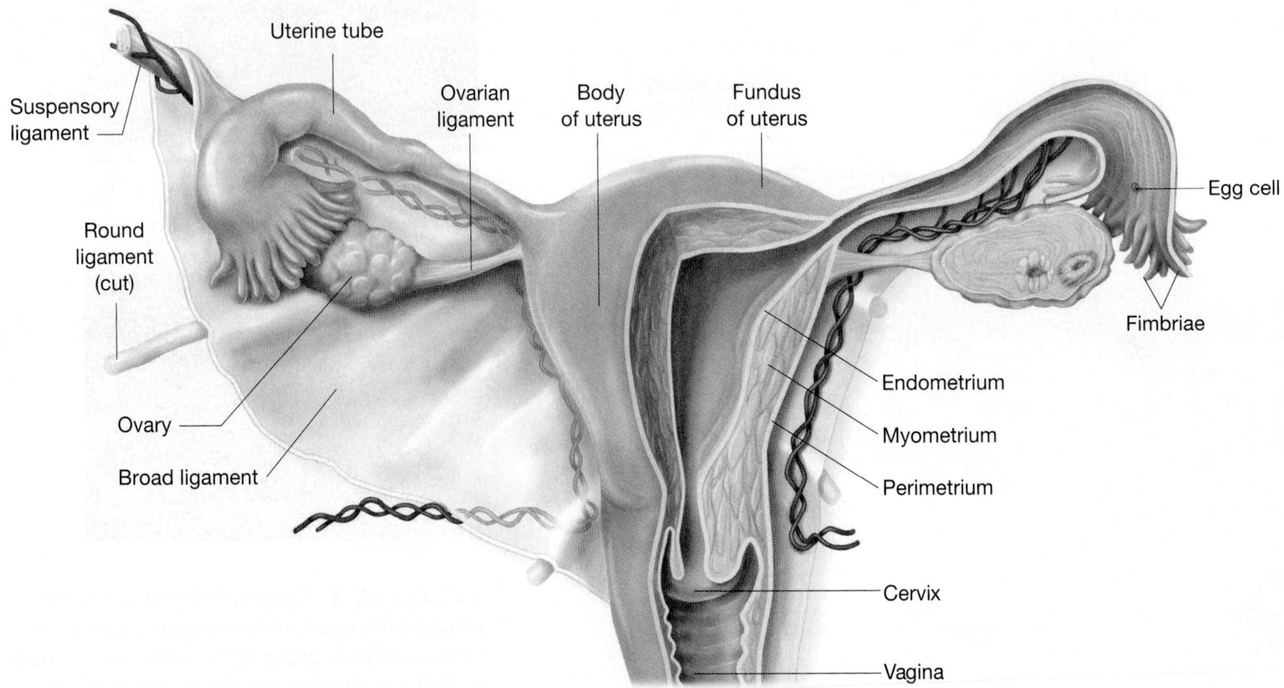

■ **Figure 10.5** The uterus. Cutaway view shows regions of the uterus and cervix and its relationship to the uterine (fallopian) tubes and vagina.

ovaries, the unattached ends of these two tubes expand into finger-like projections called **fimbriae**. The fimbriae catch an ovum after ovulation and direct it into the uterine tube. The uterine tube can then propel the ovum from the ovary to the uterus so that it can implant. The meeting of the egg and sperm, called fertilization or **conception**, normally takes place within the upper one-half of the uterine tubes.

What's In A Name?

Look for these word parts:
flex/o = to bend
men/o = menses
metr/o = uterus
my/o = muscle
-al = pertaining to
-arche = beginning
-ion = action
ante- = in front of
endo- = inner
peri- = around

Uterus

anteflexion (an-tee-FLEK-shun)
cervix (SER-viks)
corpus (KOR-pus)
endometrium (en-doh-MEE-tre-um)
fundus (FUN-dus)
menarche (men-AR-kee)
menopause (MEN-oh-pawz)
menstrual period (MEN-stroo-all)
menstruation (men-stroo-AY-shun)
myometrium (my-oh-MEE-tre-um)
perimetrium (pear-ee-MEE-tre-um)
puberty (PEW-ber-tee)

The uterus is a hollow, pear-shaped organ that contains a thick muscular wall, a mucous membrane lining, and a rich supply of blood (see again Figure 10.5). It lies in the center of the pelvic cavity between the bladder and the rectum. It is normally bent slightly forward, which is called **anteflexion**, and is held in position by strong fibrous ligaments anchored in the outer layer of the uterus, called the **perimetrium** (see again Figure 10.1). The uterus has three sections: the **fundus** or upper portion, between where the uterine tubes connect to the uterus; **corpus** or body, which is the central portion; and **cervix** (Cx), or lower portion, also called the neck of the uterus, which opens into the vagina.

Med Term Tip

During pregnancy, the height of the fundus is an important measurement for estimating the stage of pregnancy and the size of the fetus. Following birth, massaging the fundus with pressure applied in a circular pattern stimulates the uterine muscle to contract to help stop bleeding. Patients may be more familiar with a common term for uterus, *womb*. However, the correct medical term is *uterus*.

The inner layer, or **endometrium**, of the uterine wall contains a rich blood supply. The endometrium reacts to hormonal changes every month that prepare it to receive a fertilized ovum. In a normal pregnancy the fertilized ovum implants in the endometrium, which can then provide nourishment and protection for the developing fetus. Contractions of the thick muscular walls of the uterus, called the **myometrium**, assist in propelling the fetus through the birth canal at delivery.

If a pregnancy is not established, most of the endometrium is sloughed off, resulting in **menstruation** or the **menstrual period**. During a pregnancy, the lining of the uterus does not leave the body but remains to nourish the fetus. A girl's first menstrual period occurs during **puberty** (the sequence of events by which a child becomes a young adult capable of reproduction) and is called **menarche**. In the United States, the average age for menarche is 12½ years. The ending of menstrual activity and childbearing years is called **menopause**. This generally occurs between the ages of 40 and 55.

Word Watch
Be careful using the combining forms *uter/o* meaning "uterus" and *ureter/o* meaning "ureter."

Vagina

Bartholin's glands (BAR-toh-linz)
hymen (HIGH-men)
vaginal orifice (VAJ-ih-nal / OR-ih-fis)

The vagina is a muscular tube lined with mucous membrane that extends from the cervix of the uterus to the outside of the body (see Figure 10.6 ■). The vagina allows for the passage of the menstrual flow. In addition, during intercourse, it receives the male's penis and semen, which is the fluid containing sperm. The vagina also serves as the birth canal through which the baby passes during a normal vaginal birth.

The **hymen** is a thin membranous tissue that partially covers the external vaginal opening or **vaginal orifice**. This membrane may be broken by the use of tampons, during physical activity, or during sexual intercourse. A pair of glands (called **Bartholin's glands**) are located on either side of the vaginal orifice and secrete mucus for lubrication during intercourse.

Vulva

clitoris (KLIT-oh-ris)
erectile tissue (ee-REK-tile)
labia majora (LAY-bee-ah / mah-JOR-ah)
labia minora (LAY-bee-ah / min-NOR-ah)
perineum (pair-ih-NEE-um)
urinary meatus (YOO-rih-nair-ee / mee-AY-tus)

Word Watch
Be careful using the combining forms *colp/o* meaning "vagina" and *culd/o* meaning "cul-de-sac (rectouterine pouch)."

The vulva is a general term that refers to the group of structures that make up the female external genitalia. The **labia majora** and **labia minora** are folds of skin that serve as protection for the genitalia, the vaginal orifice, and the **urinary meatus** (see Figure 10.7 ■). Since the urinary tract and the reproductive organs are located in proximity to one another and each contains mucous membranes that can transport infection, there is a danger of infection entering the urinary tract. The **clitoris** is a small organ containing sensitive **erectile tissue** that is aroused during sexual stimulation and corresponds to the glans penis in the male. The region between the vaginal orifice and the anus is referred to as the **perineum**.

What's In A Name?
Look for these word parts:
labi/o = lip
urin/o = urine
-ary = pertaining to

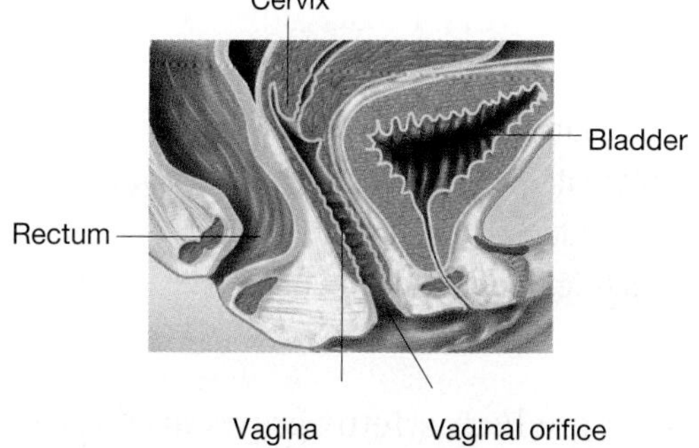

■ **Figure 10.6** The vagina, sagittal section showing the location of the vagina and its relationship to the cervix, uterus, rectum, and bladder.

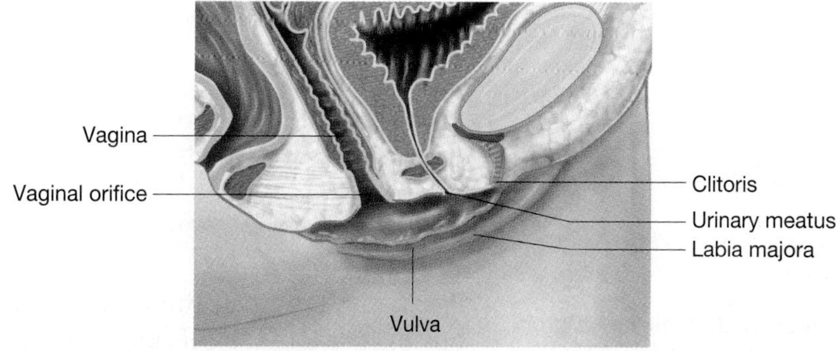

■ **Figure 10.7** The vulva, sagittal section illustrating how the labia major and labia minora cover and protect the vaginal orifice, clitoris, and urinary meatus.

Breast

areola (ah-REE-oh-la)
lactation (lak-TAY-shun)
lactiferous ducts (lak-TIF-er-us)
lactiferous glands (lak-TIF-er-us)
mammary glands (MAM-ah-ree)
nipple
nurse

What's In A Name?
Look for these word parts:
lact/o = milk

The breasts, or **mammary glands**, play a vital role in the reproductive process because they produce milk, a process called **lactation**, to nourish the newborn. The size of the breasts, which varies greatly from woman to woman, has no bearing on the ability to **nurse** or feed a baby. Milk is produced by the **lactiferous glands** and is carried to the **nipple** by the **lactiferous ducts** (see Figure 10.8 ■). The **areola** is the pigmented area around the nipple. As long as the breast is stimulated by the nursing infant, the breast will continue to secrete milk.

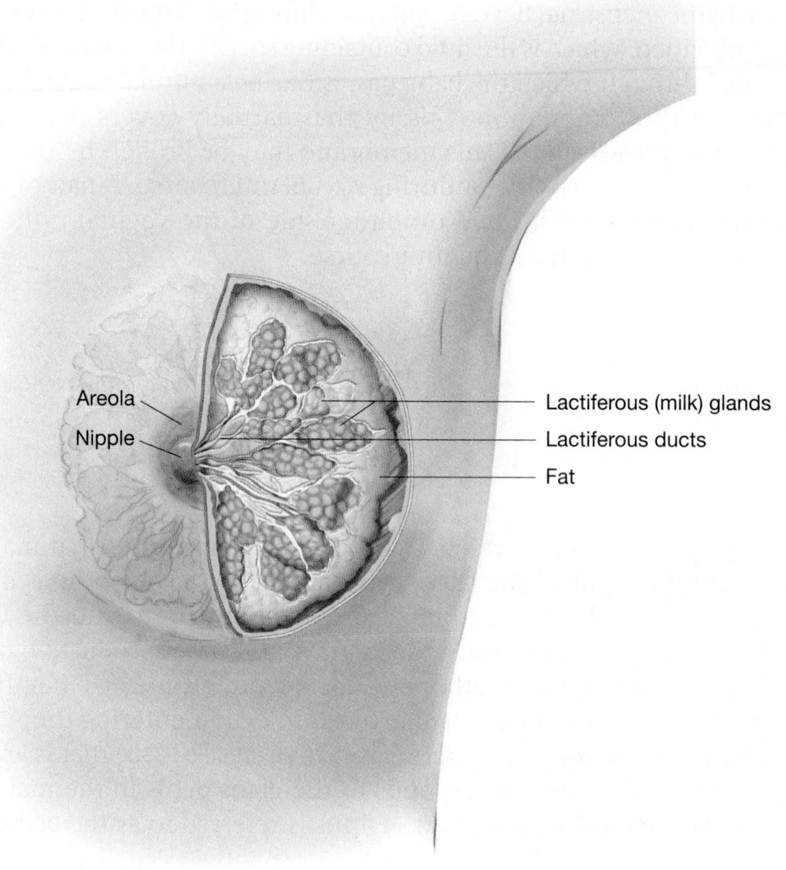

■ **Figure 10.8** The breast, cutaway view showing both internal and external features.

Pregnancy

amnion (AM-nee-on)
amniotic fluid (am-nee-OT-ik)
chorion (KOR-ree-on)
embryo (EM-bree-oh)
fetus (FEE-tus)
gestation (jess-TAY-shun)
placenta (plah-SEN-tah)
premature
umbilical cord (um-BILL-ih-kal)

What's In A Name?
Look for these word parts:
-al = pertaining to
pre- = before

Pregnancy refers to the period of time during which a fetus grows and develops in its mother's uterus (see Figure 10.9 ■). The normal length of time for a pregnancy (**gestation**) is 40 weeks. If a baby is born before completing at least 37 weeks of gestation, it is considered **premature**.

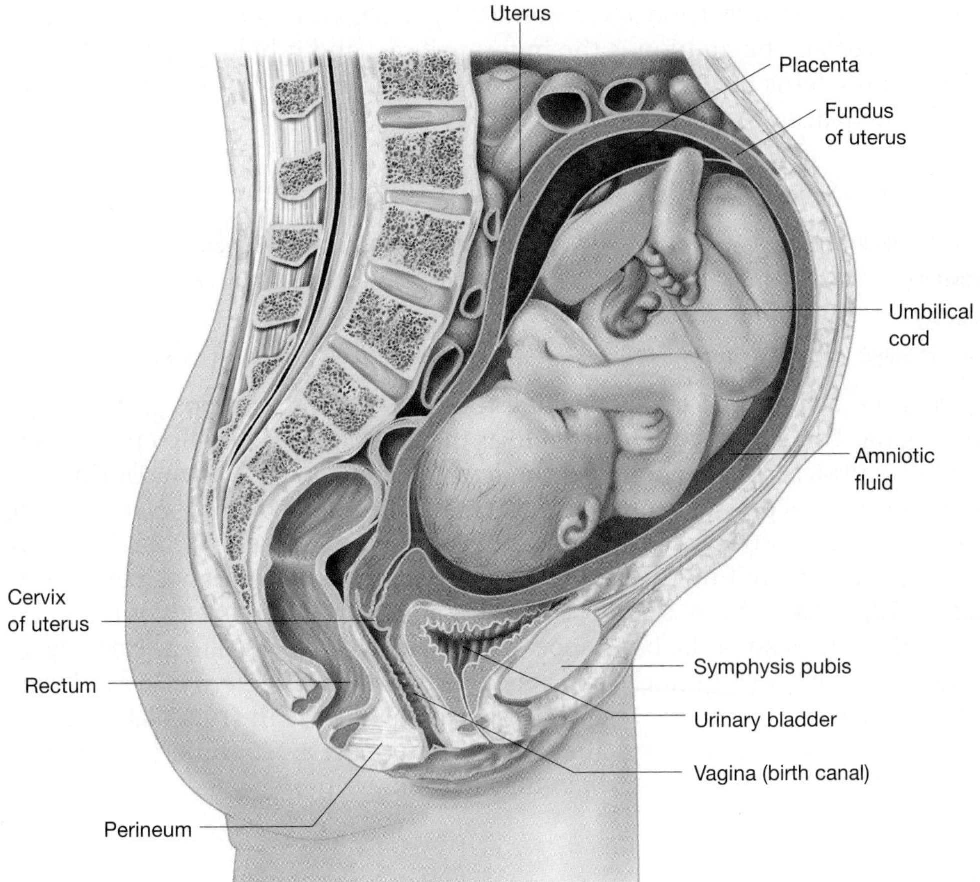

■ **Figure 10.9** A full-term pregnancy. Image illustrates position of the fetus and the structures associated with pregnancy.

During pregnancy the female body undergoes many changes. In fact, all of the body systems become involved in the development of a healthy infant. From the time the fertilized egg implants in the uterus until approximately the end of the eighth week, the infant is referred to as an **embryo** (see Figure 10.10■). During this period all the major organs and body systems are formed. Following the embryo stage and lasting until birth, the infant is called a **fetus** (see Figure 10.11■). During this time, the longest period of gestation, the organs mature and begin to function.

The fetus receives nourishment from its mother by way of the **placenta**, which is a spongy, blood-filled organ that forms in the uterus next to the fetus. The placenta is commonly referred to as the afterbirth because it is delivered through the birth canal after the birth of a baby. The fetus is attached to the placenta by

Med Term Tip

During the embryo stage of gestation, the organs and organ systems of the body are formed. Therefore, this is a very common time for *congenital anomalies*, or birth defects, to occur. This may happen before the woman is even aware of being pregnant.

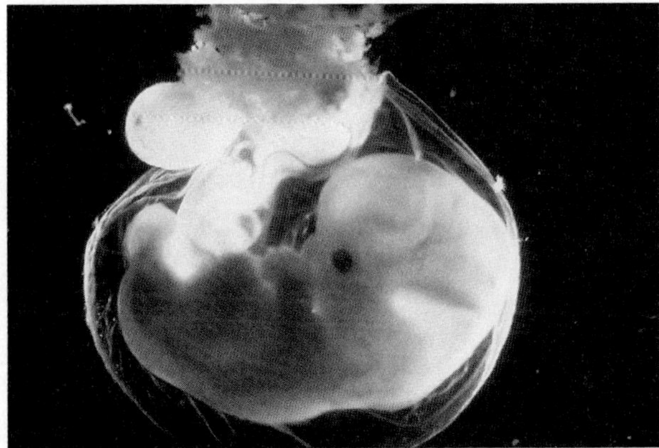

■ **Figure 10.10** Photograph illustrating the development of an embryo. *(Science Source)*

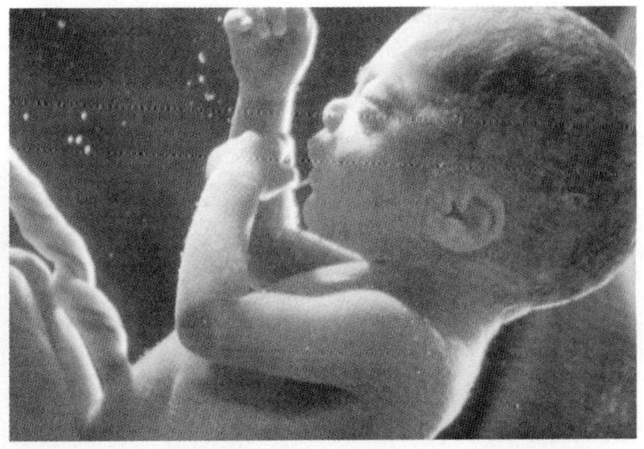

■ **Figure 10.11** Photograph illustrating the development of a fetus. *(Petit Format/Science Source)*

Med Term Tip

The term *placenta* comes from the Latin word meaning "a flat cake." This refers to the appearance of the placenta, which is a solid mass, flattened along the inner wall of the uterus.

way of the **umbilical cord** and is surrounded by two membranous sacs, the **amnion** and the **chorion**. The amnion is the innermost sac, and it holds the **amniotic fluid** in which the fetus floats. The chorion is an outer, protective sac and also forms part of the placenta.

Labor and Delivery

breech presentation
crowning
delivery
dilation stage (dye-LAY-shun)
effacement (eh-FACE-ment)
expulsion stage (ex-PULL-shun)
labor
placental stage (plah-SEN-tal)

What's In A Name?

Look for these word parts:
dilat/o = to widen
-al = pertaining to
ex- = outward

Labor is the actual process of expelling the fetus from the uterus and through the vagina. The first stage is referred to as the **dilation stage**, in which the uterine muscle contracts strongly to expel the fetus (see Figure 10.12A ■). During this process the fetus presses on the cervix and causes it to dilate or expand. As the cervix dilates, it also becomes thinner, referred to as **effacement**. When the cervix is completely dilated to 10 centimeters, the second stage of labor begins (see Figure 10.12B ■). This is the **expulsion stage** and ends with **delivery** of the baby. Generally, the head of the baby appears first, which is referred to as **crowning**. In some cases the baby's buttocks will appear first, and this is referred to as a **breech presentation** (see Figure 10.13 ■). The last stage of labor is the **placental stage** (see Figure 10.12C ■). Immediately after childbirth, the uterus continues to contract, causing the placenta to be expelled through the vagina.

A

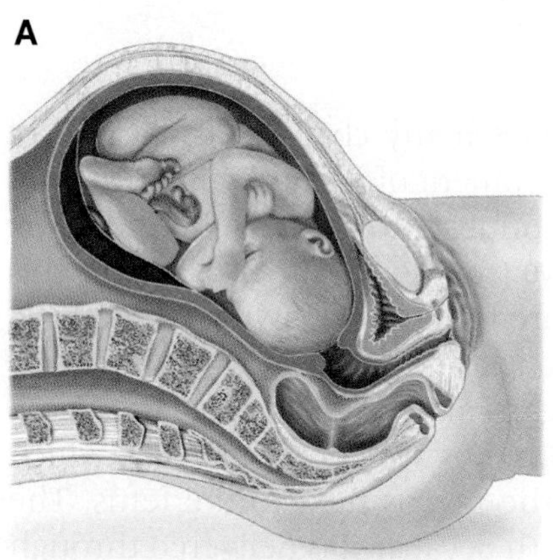

DILATION STAGE:
Uterine contractions dilate cervix

B

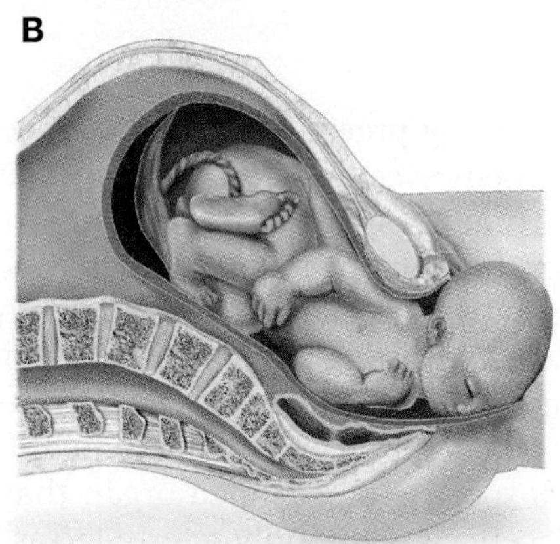

EXPULSION STAGE:
Birth of baby or expulsion

C

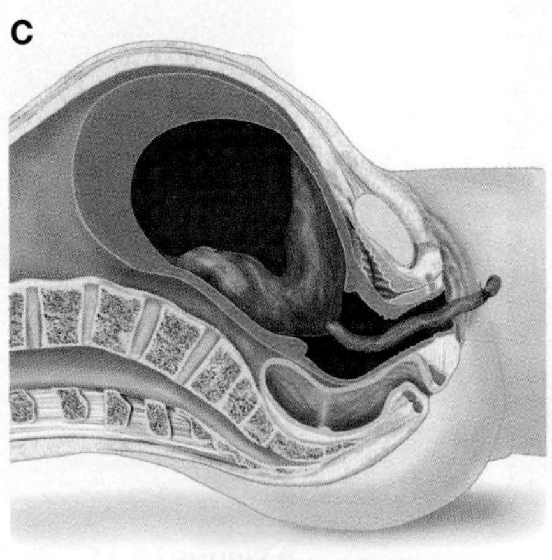

PLACENTAL STAGE:
Delivery of placenta

■ **Figure 10.12** The stages of labor and delivery. A) During the dilation stage the cervix thins and dilates to 10 cm. B) During the expulsion stage the infant is delivered. C) During the placental stage the placenta is delivered.

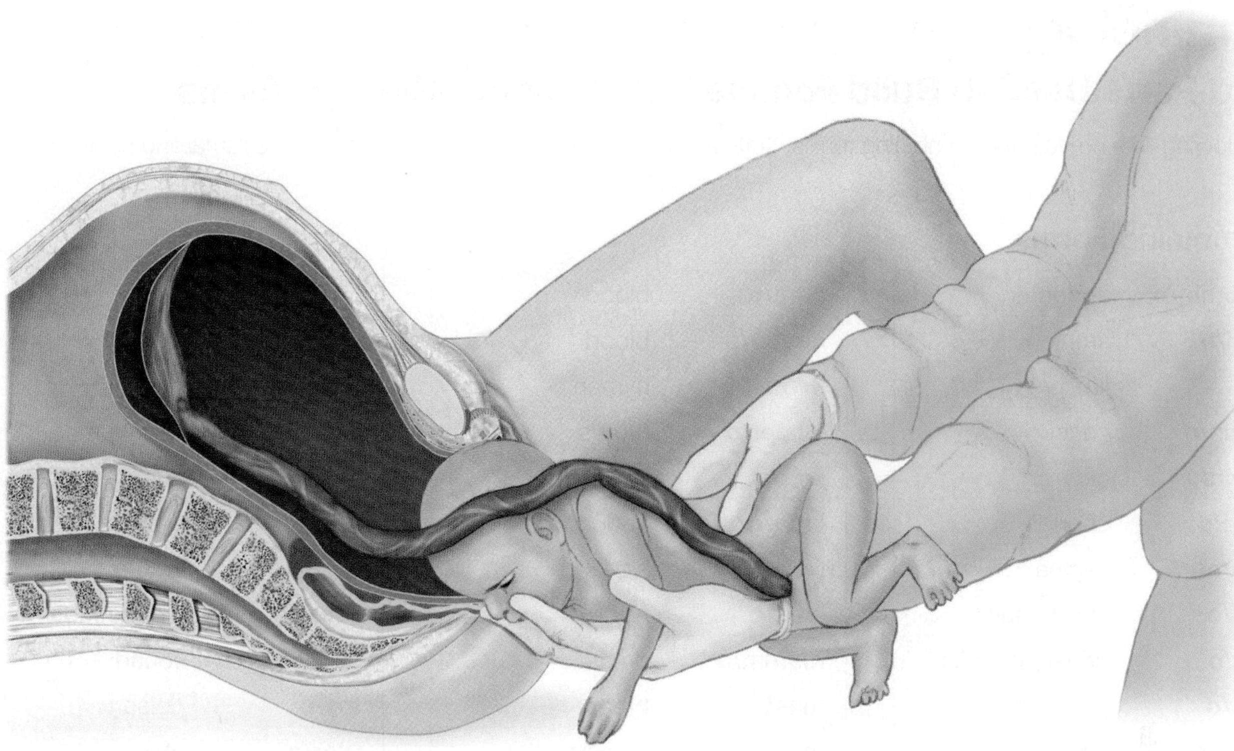

■ **Figure 10.13** A breech birth. This image illustrates a newborn that has been delivered buttocks first.

Practice As You Go

A. Complete the Statement

1. The tubes that extend from the outer edges of the uterus and assist in transporting the ova and sperm are called ____________________.
2. The time required for the development of a fetus is called ____________________.
3. The three stages of labor and delivery are the ____________________ stage, the ____________________ stage, and the ____________________ stage.
4. The cessation of menstruation is called ____________________.
5. The female sex cell is a(n) ____________________.
6. The inner lining of the uterus is called the ____________________.
7. The organ in which the developing fetus resides is called the ____________________.

Terminology

Word Parts Used to Build Female Reproductive System Terms

The following lists contain the combining forms, suffixes, and prefixes used to build terms in the remaining sections of this chapter.

Combining Forms

abdomin/o	abdomen
amni/o	amnion
bi/o	life
carcin/o	cancer
cervic/o	cervix
chori/o	chorion
colp/o	vagina
culd/o	cul-de-sac
cyst/o	urinary bladder
dilat/o	to widen
embry/o	embryo
episi/o	vulva
fet/o	fetus
fibr/o	fibers
gynec/o	woman

hem/o	blood
hemat/o	blood
hymen/o	hymen
hyster/o	uterus
lact/o	milk
lapar/o	abdomen
later/o	side
leuk/o	white
mamm/o	breast
mast/o	breast
men/o	menstruation
metr/o	uterus
nat/o	birth
olig/o	scanty
oophor/o	ovary

or/o	mouth
ovari/o	ovary
pelv/o	pelvis
perine/o	perineum
py/o	pus
radic/o	root
rect/o	rectum
salping/o	uterine tube
son/o	sound
tox/o	poison
uter/o	uterus
vagin/o	vagina
vulv/o	vulva

Suffixes

-al	pertaining to
-algia	pain
-an	pertaining to
-ar	pertaining to
-ary	pertaining to
-cele	protrusion
-centesis	puncture to withdraw fluid
-cyesis	pregnancy
-ectomy	surgical removal
-gram	record
-graphy	process of recording
-gravida	pregnancy
-ia	condition

-iasis	abnormal condition
-ic	pertaining to
-ine	pertaining to
-itis	inflammation
-logy	study of
-lytic	destruction
-nic	pertaining to
-oid	resembling
-oma	tumor
-opsy	view of
-osis	abnormal condition
-otomy	cutting into
-para	to bear

-partum	childbirth
-pexy	surgical fixation
-plasty	surgical repair
-rrhagia	abnormal flow condition
-rrhaphy	suture
-rrhea	discharge
-rrhexis	rupture
-salpinx	uterine tube
-scope	instrument for viewing
-scopy	process of viewing
-tic	pertaining to
-tocia	labor and childbirth

Prefixes

a-	without
ante-	before
bi-	two
contra-	against
dys-	painful
endo-	inner, within

in-	not
intra-	within
multi-	many
neo-	new
nulli-	none
peri-	around

post-	after
pre-	before
primi-	first
pseudo-	false
ultra-	beyond

Adjective Forms of Anatomical Terms

Term	Word Parts	Definition
amniotic (am-nee-OT-ik)	amni/o = amnion -tic = pertaining to	Pertaining to the amnion.
cervical (SER-vih-kal)	cervic/o = cervix -al = pertaining to	Pertaining to the cervix.
chorionic (koh-ree-ON-ik)	chori/o = chorion -nic = pertaining to	Pertaining to the chorion.
embryonic (em-bree-ON-ik)	embry/o = embryo -nic = pertaining to	Pertaining to the embryo.
endometrial (en-doh-MEE-tree-al)	endo- = inner metr/o = uterus -al = pertaining to	Pertaining to the inner lining of the uterus.
fetal (FEE-tal)	fet/o = fetus -al = pertaining to	Pertaining to the fetus.
lactic (LAK-tik)	lact/o = milk -ic = pertaining to	Pertaining to milk.
mammary (MAM-mah-ree)	mamm/o = breast -ary = pertaining to	Pertaining to the breast.
ovarian (oh-VAIR-ee-an)	ovari/o = ovary -an = pertaining to	Pertaining to the ovary.
perineal (per-ih-NEE-al)	perine/o = perineum -al = pertaining to	Pertaining to the perineum.
uterine (YOO-ter-in)	uter/o = uterus -ine = pertaining to	Pertaining to the uterus.
vaginal (VAJ-ih-nal)	vagin/o = vagina -al = pertaining to	Pertaining to the vagina.
vulvar (VUL-var)	vulv/o = vulva -ar = pertaining to	Pertaining to the vulva.

Practice As You Go

B. Give the adjective form for each anatomical structure

1. The embryo ______
2. The fetus ______
3. The uterus ______
4. An ovary ______
5. A breast ______
6. The vagina ______

Pregnancy Terms

Term	Word Parts	Definition
antepartum (an-tee-PAR-tum)	ante- = before -partum = childbirth	Period of time before birth.
colostrum (kuh-LOS-trum)		Thin fluid first secreted by the breast after delivery. It does not contain much protein, but is rich in antibodies.
fraternal twins	-al = pertaining to	Twins that develop from two different ova fertilized by two different sperm. Although twins, these siblings do not have identical DNA.
identical twins	-al = pertaining to	Twins that develop from the splitting of one fertilized ovum. These siblings have identical DNA.
meconium (meh-KOH-nee-um)		First bowel movement of a newborn. It is greenish-black in color and consists of mucus and bile.
multigravida (mull-tih-GRAV-ih-dah)	multi- = many -gravida = pregnancy	A woman who has been pregnant two or more times.
multipara (mull-TIP-ah-rah)	multi- = many -para = to bear	A woman who has given birth to a live infant two or more times.
neonate (NEE-oh-nayt)	neo- = new nat/o = birth	Term for a newborn baby.
nulligravida (null-ih-GRAV-ih-dah)	nulli- = none -gravida = pregnancy	A woman who has not been pregnant.
nullipara (null-IP-ah-rah)	nulli- = none -para = to bear	A woman who has not given birth to a live infant.
postpartum (post-PAR-tum)	post- = after -partum = childbirth	Period of time shortly after birth.
primigravida (GI, grav I) (pry-mih-GRAV-ih-dah)	primi- = first -gravida = pregnancy	A woman who is pregnant for the first time.
primipara (PI, para I) (pry-MIP-ah-rah)	primi- = first -para = to bear	A woman who has given birth to a live infant once.

Pathology (continued)

Term	Word Parts	Definition
hysterorrhexis (hiss-ter-oh-REK-sis)	hyster/o = uterus -rrhexis = rupture	Rupture of the uterus; may occur during labor.
menometrorrhagia (men-oh-mee-troh-RAY-jee-ah)	men/o = menstruation metr/o = uterus -rrhagia = abnormal flow condition	Excessive bleeding during the menstrual period and at intervals between menstrual periods.
premenstrual syndrome (PMS) (pre-MEN-stroo-al / SIN-drohm)	pre- = before men/o = menstruation -al = pertaining to	Symptoms that develop just prior to the onset of a menstrual period, which can include irritability, headache, tender breasts, and anxiety.
prolapsed uterus (pro-LAPS'D / YOO-ter-us)		Fallen uterus that can cause the cervix to protrude through the vaginal opening. Generally caused by weakened muscles from vaginal delivery or as the result of pelvic tumors pressing down.
Vagina		
candidiasis (kan-dih-DYE-ah-sis) Med Term Tip The term *candida* comes from a Latin term meaning "dazzling white." Candida is the scientific name for yeast and refers to the very white discharge that is the hallmark of a yeast infection.	-iasis = abnormal condition	Yeast infection of the skin and mucous membranes that can result in white plaques on the tongue and vagina.
cystocele (SIS-toh-seel)	cyst/o = urinary bladder -cele = protrusion	Hernia or outpouching of the bladder that protrudes into the vagina. This may cause urinary frequency and urgency.
rectocele (REK-toh-seel)	rect/o = rectum -cele = protrusion	Protrusion or herniation of the rectum into the vagina.
toxic shock syndrome (TSS)	tox/o = poison -ic = pertaining to	Rare and sometimes fatal staphylococcus infection that generally occurs in menstruating women. Initial infection of the vagina is associated with prolonged wearing of a super-absorbent tampon.
vaginitis (vaj-ih-NIGH-tis)	vagin/o = vagina -itis = inflammation	Inflammation of the vagina.
Pelvic Cavity		
endometriosis (en-doh-mee-tree-OH-sis)	endo- = within metr/o = uterus -osis = abnormal condition	Abnormal condition of endometrium tissue appearing throughout the pelvis or on the abdominal wall. This tissue is normally found within the uterus.
pelvic inflammatory disease (PID) (PELL-vik / in-FLAM-mah-toh-ree)	pelv/o = pelvis -ic = pertaining to	Chronic or acute infection, usually bacterial, that has ascended through the female reproductive organs and out into the pelvic cavity. May result in scarring that interferes with fertility.
perimetritis (pair-ih-meh-TRY-tis)	peri- = around metr/o = uterus -itis = inflammation	Inflammation in the pelvic cavity around the outside of the uterus.

Pathology (continued)

Term	Word Parts	Definition
Breast		
breast cancer		Malignant tumor of the breast. Usually forms in the milk-producing gland tissue or the lining of the milk ducts.

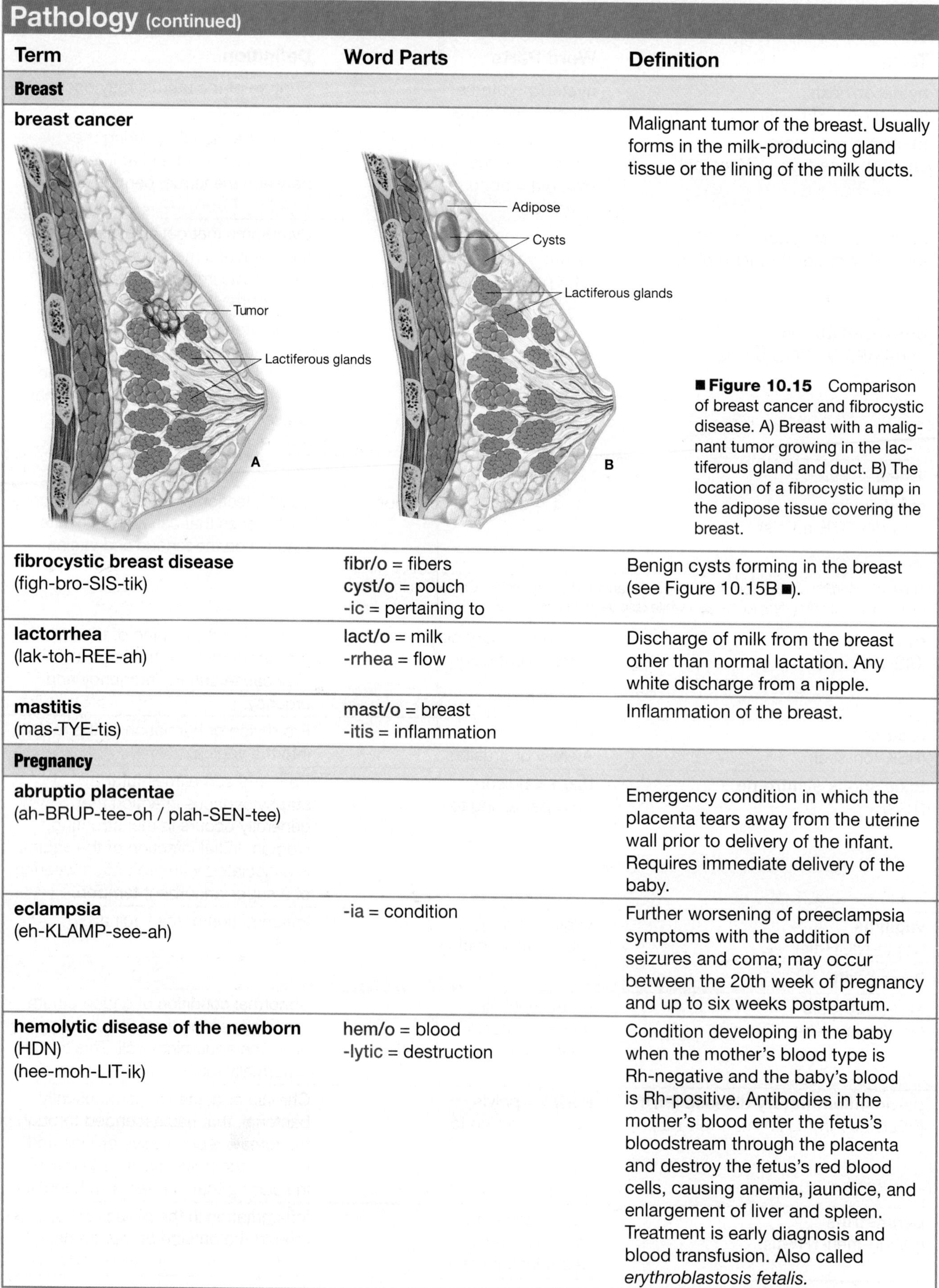

■ **Figure 10.15** Comparison of breast cancer and fibrocystic disease. A) Breast with a malignant tumor growing in the lactiferous gland and duct. B) The location of a fibrocystic lump in the adipose tissue covering the breast.

Term	Word Parts	Definition
fibrocystic breast disease (figh-bro-SIS-tik)	fibr/o = fibers cyst/o = pouch -ic = pertaining to	Benign cysts forming in the breast (see Figure 10.15B ■).
lactorrhea (lak-toh-REE-ah)	lact/o = milk -rrhea = flow	Discharge of milk from the breast other than normal lactation. Any white discharge from a nipple.
mastitis (mas-TYE-tis)	mast/o = breast -itis = inflammation	Inflammation of the breast.
Pregnancy		
abruptio placentae (ah-BRUP-tee-oh / plah-SEN-tee)		Emergency condition in which the placenta tears away from the uterine wall prior to delivery of the infant. Requires immediate delivery of the baby.
eclampsia (eh-KLAMP-see-ah)	-ia = condition	Further worsening of preeclampsia symptoms with the addition of seizures and coma; may occur between the 20th week of pregnancy and up to six weeks postpartum.
hemolytic disease of the newborn (HDN) (hee-moh-LIT-ik)	hem/o = blood -lytic = destruction	Condition developing in the baby when the mother's blood type is Rh-negative and the baby's blood is Rh-positive. Antibodies in the mother's blood enter the fetus's bloodstream through the placenta and destroy the fetus's red blood cells, causing anemia, jaundice, and enlargement of liver and spleen. Treatment is early diagnosis and blood transfusion. Also called *erythroblastosis fetalis.*

Pathology (continued)

Term	Word Parts	Definition
infertility	in- = not	Inability to produce children. Generally defined as no pregnancy after properly timed intercourse for one year.
placenta previa (plah-SEN-tah / PREE-vee-ah)		A placenta that is implanted in the lower portion of the uterus and, in turn, blocks the birth canal.
preeclampsia (pre-eh-KLAMP-see-ah)	pre- = before	Metabolic disease of pregnancy. If untreated, it may progress to eclampsia. Symptoms include hypertension, headaches, albumin in the urine, and edema. May occur between the 20th week of pregnancy and up to six weeks postpartum. Also called *toxemia* or *pregnancy-induced hypertension* (PIH).
prolapsed umbilical cord (pro-LAPSD / um-BILL-ih-kal)		When the umbilical cord of the baby is expelled first during delivery and is squeezed between the baby's head and the vaginal wall. This presents an emergency situation since the baby's circulation is compromised.
pseudocyesis (soo-doh-sigh-EE-sis)	pseudo- = false -cyesis = pregnancy	Condition in which the body reacts as if there is a pregnancy (especially hormonal changes), but there is no pregnancy.
salpingocyesis (sal-ping-goh-sigh-EE-sis)	salping/o = uterine tube -cyesis = pregnancy	Pregnancy that occurs in the uterine tube instead of in the uterus.
spontaneous abortion		Unplanned loss of a pregnancy due to the death of the embryo or fetus before the time it is viable, commonly referred to as a *miscarriage*.
stillbirth		Birth in which a viable-aged fetus dies shortly before or at the time of delivery.

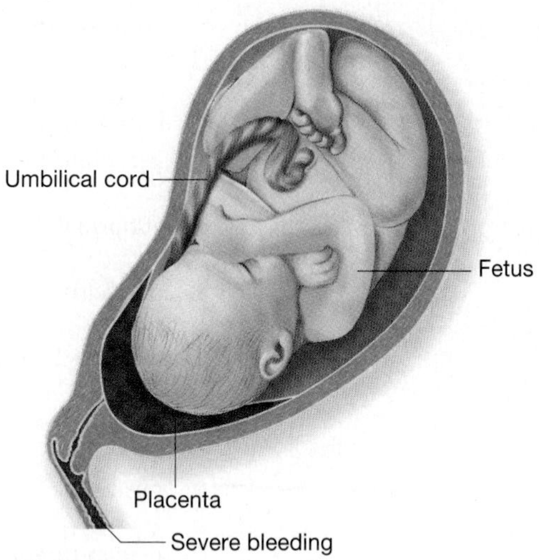

Umbilical cord
Fetus
Placenta
Severe bleeding

■ **Figure 10.16** Placenta previa, longitudinal section showing the placenta growing over the opening into the cervix.

Med Term Tip

The term *abortion* (AB) has different meanings for medical professionals and the general population. The general population equates the term *abortion* specifically with the planned termination of a pregnancy. However, to the medical community, *abortion* is a broader medical term meaning that a pregnancy has ended before a fetus is *viable*, meaning before it can live on its own.

Practice As You Go

C. Terminology Matching

Match each term to its definition.

1. ________ hemolytic disease of the newborn
2. ________ dysmenorrhea
3. ________ breech presentation
4. ________ abruptio placentae
5. ________ eclampsia
6. ________ pyosalpinx
7. ________ fibroid
8. ________ candidiasis
9. ________ lactorrhea
10. ________ neonate

a. seizures and coma during pregnancy
b. erythroblastosis fetalis
c. detached placenta
d. yeast infection
e. abnormal discharge from breast
f. newborn
g. buttocks first to appear in birth canal
h. painful menstruation
i. pus in the uterine tube
j. benign tumor

Diagnostic Procedures

Term	Word Parts	Definition
Clinical Laboratory Tests		
Pap (Papanicolaou) **smear** (pap-ah-NIK-oh-low)		Test for the early detection of cancer of the cervix named after the developer of the test, George Papanicolaou, a Greek physician. A scraping of cells is removed from the cervix for examination under a microscope.
pregnancy test (PREG-nan-see)		Chemical test that can determine a pregnancy during the first few weeks. Can be performed in a physician's office or with a home-testing kit.
Diagnostic Imaging		
hysterosalpingography (HSG) (hiss-ter-oh-sal-pin-GOG-rah-fee)	hyster/o = uterus salping/o = uterine tube -graphy = process of recording	Taking of an X-ray after injecting radiopaque material into the uterus and uterine tubes.
mammogram (MAM-moh-gram)	mamm/o = breast -gram = record	X-ray record of the breast.
mammography (mam-OG-rah-fee)	mamm/o = breast -graphy = process of recording	X-ray to diagnose breast disease, especially breast cancer.

Diagnostic Procedures (continued)

Term	Word Parts	Definition
pelvic ultrasonography (PELL-vik / ull-trah-son-OG-rah-fee)	pelv/o = pelvis -ic = pertaining to ultra- = beyond son/o = sound -graphy = process of recording	Use of high-frequency sound waves to produce an image or photograph of an organ, such as the uterus, ovaries, or fetus.
Endoscopic Procedures		
colposcope (KOL-poh-scope)	colp/o = vagina -scope = instrument for viewing	Instrument used to view inside the vagina.
colposcopy (kol-POS-koh-pee)	colp/o = vagina -scopy = process of viewing	Examination of vagina using an instrument called a *colposcope.*
culdoscopy (kul-DOS-koh-pee)	culd/o = cul-de-sac -scopy = process of viewing	Examination of the female pelvic cavity, particularly behind the uterus, by introducing an endoscope through the wall of the vagina.
laparoscope (LAP-ah-row-scope)	lapar/o = abdomen -scope = instrument for viewing	Instrument used to view inside the abdomen.
laparoscopy (lap-ar-OS-koh-pee)	lapar/o = abdomen -scopy = process of viewing	Examination of the peritoneal cavity using an instrument called a *laparoscope.* The instrument is passed through a small incision made by the surgeon into the abdominopelvic cavity.

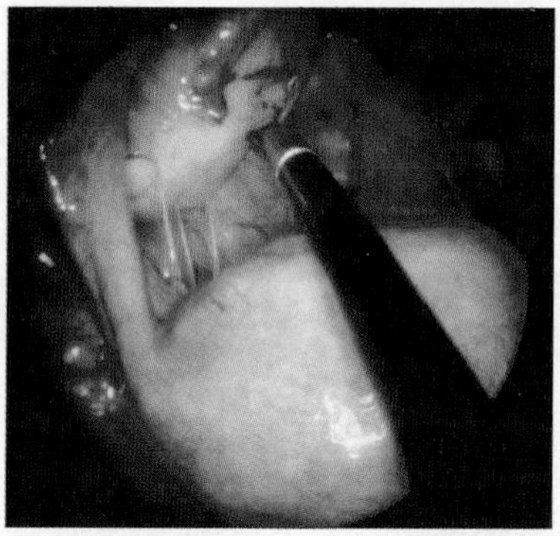

■ **Figure 10.17** Photograph taken during a laparoscopic procedure. The fundus of the uterus is visible below the probe, the ovary is at the tip of the probe, and the uterine tube extends along the left side of the photo. *(Southern Illinois University/Photo Researchers, Inc.)*

Term	Word Parts	Definition
Obstetrical Diagnostic Procedures		
amniocentesis (am-nee-oh-sen-TEE-sis)	amni/o = amnion -centesis = puncture to withdraw fluid	Puncturing of the amniotic sac using a needle and syringe for the purpose of withdrawing amniotic fluid for testing. Can assist in determining fetal maturity, development, and genetic disorders.
Apgar score (AP-gar)		Evaluation of a neonate's adjustment to the outside world. Observes color, heart rate, muscle tone, respiratory rate, and response to stimulus at one minute and five minutes after birth.
chorionic villus sampling (CVS) (kor-ree-ON-ik / vill-us)	chori/o = chorion -nic = pertaining to	Removal of a small piece of the chorion for genetic analysis. May be done at an earlier stage of pregnancy than amniocentesis.

Diagnostic Procedures (continued)

Term	Word Parts	Definition
fetal monitoring (FEE-tal)	fet/o = fetus -al = pertaining to	Using electronic equipment placed on the mother's abdomen or the fetus' scalp to check the fetal heart rate (FHR) (also called fetal heart tone [FHT]) during labor. The normal heart rate of the fetus is rapid, ranging from 120 to 160 beats per minute. A drop in the fetal heart rate indicates the fetus is in distress.
Additional Diagnostic Procedures		
cervical biopsy (SER-vih-kal / BYE-op-see)	cervic/o = cervix -al = pertaining to bi/o = life -opsy = view of	Taking a sample of tissue from the cervix to test for the presence of cancer cells.
endometrial biopsy (EMB) (en-doh-MEE-tre-al BYE-op-see)	endo- = inner metr/o = uterus -al = pertaining to bi/o = life -opsy = view of	Taking a sample of tissue from the lining of the uterus to test for abnormalities.
pelvic examination (PELL-vik)	pelv/o = pelvis -ic = pertaining to	Physical examination of the vagina and adjacent organs performed by a physician placing the fingers of one hand into the vagina. An instrument called a *speculum* is used to open the vagina.

■ **Figure 10.18** A speculum used to hold the vagina open in order to visualize the cervix. *(Patrick Watson, Pearson Education)*

Therapeutic Procedures

Term	Word Parts	Definition
Medical Procedures		
barrier contraception (kon-trah-SEP-shun)	contra- = against	Prevention of a pregnancy using a device to prevent sperm from meeting an ovum. Examples include condoms, diaphragms, and cervical caps.
hormonal contraception	-al = pertaining to contra- = against	Use of hormones to block ovulation and prevent conception. May be in the form of a pill, a patch, an implant under the skin, or an injection.
intrauterine device (IUD) (in-trah-YOO-ter-in)	intra- = within uter/o = uterus -ine = pertaining to	Device inserted into the uterus by a physician for the purpose of contraception (see Figure 10.19 ■).

Therapeutic Procedures (continued)

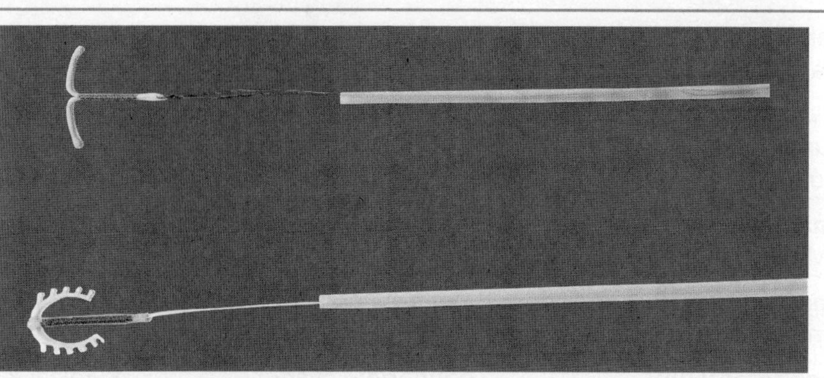

■ **Figure 10.19** Photograph illustrating the shape of two different Intrauterine devices (IDUs). The intrauterine portion is approximately 1-1/4 inches long. The thin thread attached to the end of the device extends through the cervix into the vagina. This allows a woman to check that the IUD remains properly in place. *(Jules Selmes and Debi Treloar/Dorling Kindersley Media Library)*

Term	Word Parts	Definition
Surgical Procedures		
amniotomy (am-nee-OT-oh-mee)	amni/o = amnion -otomy = cutting into	Surgically cutting open the amnion; commonly referred to as "breaking the water."
cervicectomy (ser-vih-SEK-toh-mee)	cervic/o = cervix -ectomy = surgical removal	Surgical removal of the cervix.
cesarean section (CS, C-section) (see-SAYR-ee-an)		Surgical delivery of a baby through an incision into the abdominal and uterine walls. Legend has it that the Roman emperor, Julius Caesar, was the first person born by this method.
conization (kon-ih-ZAY-shun)		Surgical removal of a core of cervical tissue. Also refers to partial removal of the cervix.
dilation and curettage (D & C) (dye-LAY-shun / koo-reh-TAZH)	dilat/o = to widen	Surgical procedure in which the opening of the cervix is dilated and the uterus is scraped or suctioned of its lining or tissue. Often performed after a spontaneous abortion and to stop excessive bleeding from other causes.
elective abortion		Legal termination of a pregnancy for nonmedical reasons.
episiorrhaphy (eh-peez-ee-OR-ah-fee)	episi/o = vulva -rrhaphy = suture	To suture the perineum; postpartum procedure to repair an episiotomy or any tearing of the perineum that occurred during birth. Note that the combining form *episi/o* is used even though the perineum is not part of the vulva.
episiotomy (eh-peez-ee-OT-oh-mee)	episi/o = vulva -otomy = cutting into	Surgical incision of the perineum to facilitate the delivery process. Can prevent an irregular tearing of tissue during birth. Note that the combining form *episi/o* is used even though the perineum is not part of the vulva.
hymenectomy (high-men-EK-toh-mee)	hymen/o = hymen -ectomy = surgical removal	Surgical removal of the hymen.
hysterectomy (hiss-ter-EK-toh-mee)	hyster/o = uterus -ectomy = surgical removal	Surgical removal of the uterus.
hysteropexy (HISS-ter-oh-pek-see)	hyster/o = uterus -pexy = surgical fixation	To surgically anchor the uterus to its proper location in the pelvic cavity; a treatment for a prolapsed uterus.

Therapeutic Procedures (continued)

Term	Word Parts	Definition
laparotomy (lap-ah-ROT-oh-mee)	lapar/o = abdomen -otomy = cutting into	To cut open the abdomen; performed in order to complete other surgical procedures inside the abdomen or performed during a C-section.
lumpectomy (lump-EK-toh-mee)	-ectomy = surgical removal	Removal of only a breast tumor and the tissue immediately surrounding it.
mammoplasty (MAM-moh-plas-tee)	mamm/o = breast -plasty = surgical repair	Surgical repair or reconstruction of the breast.
mastectomy (mass-TEK-toh-mee)	mast/o = breast -ectomy = surgical removal	Surgical removal of the breast.
oophorectomy (oh-off-oh-REK-toh-mee)	oophor/o = ovary -ectomy = surgical removal	Surgical removal of the ovary.
radical mastectomy (mast-EK-toh-mee)	radic/o = root -al = pertaining to mast/o = breast -ectomy = surgical removal	Surgical removal of the breast tissue plus chest muscles and axillary lymph nodes.
salpingectomy (sal-ping-JECK-toh-mee)	salping/o = uterine tube -ectomy = surgical removal	Surgical removal of the uterine tube.
simple mastectomy (mast-EK-toh-mee)	mast/o = breast -ectomy = surgical removal	Surgical removal of only breast tissue; all underlying tissue is left intact.
therapeutic abortion		Termination of a pregnancy for the health of the mother or another medical reason.
total abdominal hysterectomy—bilateral salpingo-oophorectomy (TAH-BSO) (hiss-ter-EK-toh-me / sal-ping-goh / oh-oh-foe-REK-toh-mee)	abdomin/o = abdomen -al = pertaining to hyster/o = uterus -ectomy = surgical removal bi- = two later/o = side -al = pertaining to salping/o = uterine tube oophor/o = ovary -ectomy = surgical removal	Removal of the entire uterus, cervix, both ovaries, and both uterine tubes.
tubal ligation (TOO-bal / lye-GAY-shun)	-al = pertaining to	Surgical tying-off of the uterine tubes to prevent conception from taking place. Results in sterilization of the female.
vaginal hysterectomy (VAJ-ih-nal / hiss-ter-EK-toh-me)	vagin/o = vagina -al = pertaining to hyster/o = uterus -ectomy = surgical removal	Removal of the uterus through the vagina rather than through an abdominal incision.

Practice As You Go

D. Terminology Matching

Match each term to its definition.

1. ________ Pap smear
2. ________ intrauterine device
3. ________ colposcopy
4. ________ Apgar
5. ________ chorionic villus sampling
6. ________ lumpectomy
7. ________ episiotomy
8. ________ tubal ligation

a. measures newborn's adjustment to outside world
b. widens birth canal; facilitates delivery
c. removes only tumor and tissue around it
d. visually examines vagina
e. test for cervical cancer
f. sterilization procedure
g. birth control method
h. obtains cells for genetic testing

Pharmacology

Classification	Word Parts	Action	Examples
abortifacient (ah-bore-tih-FAY-shee-ent)		Terminates a pregnancy.	mifepristone, Mifeprex; dinoprostone, Prostin E2
fertility drug		Triggers ovulation. Also called *ovulation stimulant.*	clomiphene, Clomid; follitropin alfa, Gonal-F
hormone replacement therapy (HRT)		Replaces hormones missing from menopause or lost ovaries, which can result in the lack of estrogen production. Replacing this hormone may prevent some of the consequences of menopause, especially in younger women who have surgically lost their ovaries.	conjugated estrogens, Cenestin, Premarin
oral contraceptive pills (OCPs) (kon-trah-SEP-tive)	or/o = mouth -al = pertaining to contra- = against	Form of birth control that uses low doses of female hormones to prevent conception by blocking ovulation.	desogestrel/ethinyl estradiol, Ortho-Cept; ethinyl estradiol/ norgestrel, Lo/Ovral
oxytocin (ox-ee-TOH-sin)		A natural hormone that begins or improves uterine contractions during labor and delivery.	oxytocin, Pitocin, Syntocinon

Abbreviations

AB	abortion	**HPV**	human papilloma virus
AI	artificial insemination	**HRT**	hormone replacement therapy
BSE	breast self-examination	**HSG**	hysterosalpingography
CS, C-section	cesarean section	**IUD**	intrauterine device
CVS	chorionic villus sampling	**IVF**	*in vitro* fertilization
Cx	cervix	**LBW**	low birth weight
D & C	dilation and curettage	**LH**	luteinizing hormone
EDC	estimated date of confinement	**LMP**	last menstrual period
EMB	endometrial biopsy	**NB**	newborn
ERT	estrogen replacement therapy	**OB**	obstetrics
FEKG	fetal electrocardiogram	**OCPs**	oral contraceptive pills
FHR	fetal heart rate	**Pap**	Papanicolaou test
FHT	fetal heart tone	**PI, para I**	first delivery
FSH	follicle-stimulating hormone	**PID**	pelvic inflammatory disease
FTND	full-term normal delivery	**PIH**	pregnancy-induced hypertension
GI, grav I	first pregnancy	**PMS**	premenstrual syndrome
GYN, gyn	gynecology	**TAH-BSO**	total abdominal hysterectomy–bilateral salpingo-oophorectomy
HCG, hCG	human chorionic gonadotropin	**TSS**	toxic shock syndrome
HDN	hemolytic disease of the newborn	**UC**	uterine contractions

Practice As You Go

E. What's the Abbreviation?

1. first pregnancy ______
2. artificial insemination ______
3. uterine contractions ______
4. full-term normal delivery ______
5. intrauterine device ______
6. dilation and curettage ______
7. hormone replacement therapy ______
8. gynecology ______
9. abortion ______
10. oral contraceptive pills ______

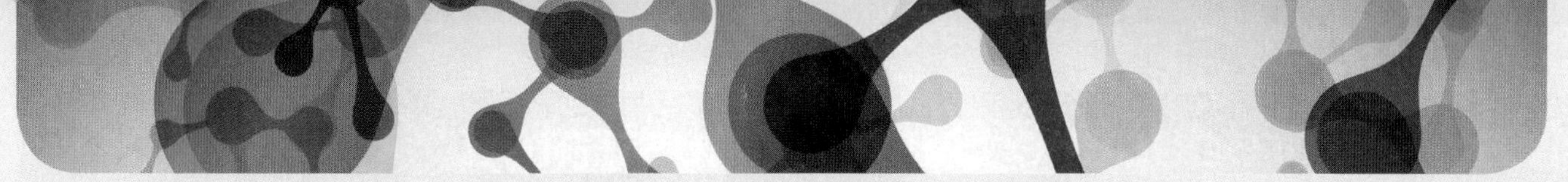

Section II: Male Reproductive System at a Glance

Function

Similar to the female reproductive system, the male reproductive system is responsible for producing sperm, the male reproductive cell, secreting the male sex hormones, and delivering sperm to the female reproductive tract.

Organs

Here are the primary structures that comprise the male reproductive system:

bulbourethral glands
epididymis
penis
prostate gland
seminal vesicles
testes
vas deferens

Word Parts

Here are the most common word parts (with their meanings) used to build male reproductive system terms. For a more comprehensive list, refer to the Terminology section of this chapter.

Combining Forms

andr/o	male
balan/o	glans penis
crypt/o	hidden
epididym/o	epididymis
orch/o	testes
orchi/o	testes
orchid/o	testes
pen/o	penis
prostat/o	prostate
spermat/o	sperm
testicul/o	testes
vas/o	vas deferens
vesicul/o	seminal vesicle

Suffixes

-cide	to kill
-plasia	formation of cells
-spermia	condition of sperm

Male Reproductive System Illustrated

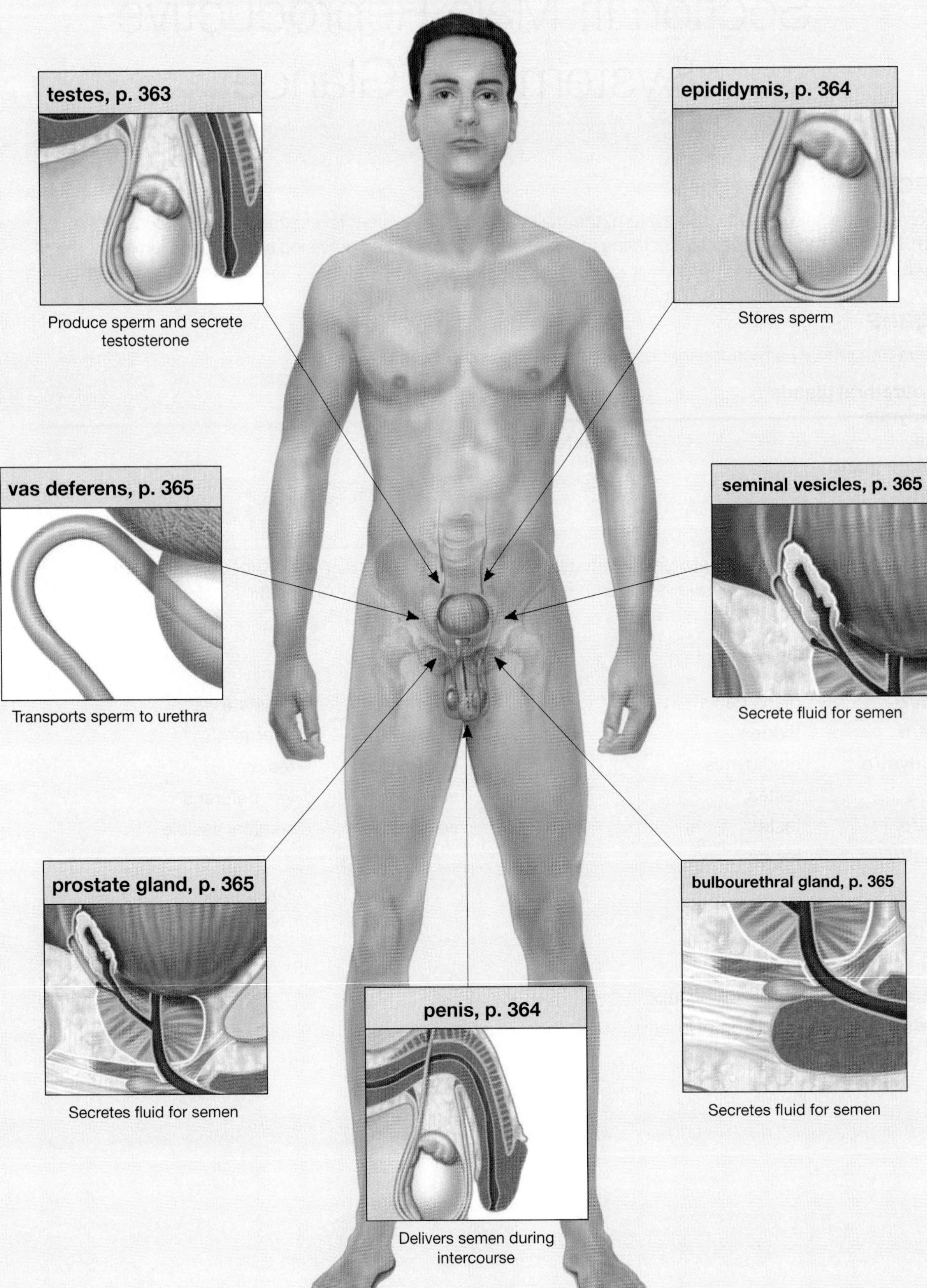

Anatomy and Physiology of the Male Reproductive System

bulbourethral glands (buhl-boh-yoo-REE-thral)
epididymis (ep-ih-DID-ih-mis)
genitourinary system (jen-ih-toh-YOO-rih-nair-ee)
penis (PEE-nis)
prostate gland (PROSS-tayt)
semen (SEE-men)
seminal vesicles (SEM-ih-nal / VESS-ih-kls)
sex hormones
sperm
testes (TESS-teez)
vas deferens (VAS / DEF-er-enz)

The male reproductive system has two main functions. The first is to produce **sperm**, the male reproductive cell; the second is to secrete the male **sex hormones**. In the male, the major organs of reproduction are located outside the body: the **penis**, and the two **testes**, each with an **epididymis** (see Figure 10.20 ■). The penis contains the urethra, which carries both urine and **semen** to the outside of the body. For this reason, this system is sometimes referred to as the **genitourinary system** (GU).

The internal organs of reproduction include two **seminal vesicles**, two **vas deferens**, the **prostate gland**, and two **bulbourethral glands**.

What's In A Name?
Look for these word parts:
genit/o = genitals
urethr/o = urethra
urin/o = urine
-al = pertaining to
-ary = pertaining to

External Organs of Reproduction

Testes

androgen (AN-droh-jen)
perineum
scrotum (SKROH-tum)
seminiferous tubules (sem-ih-NIF-er-us / TOO-byools)
spermatogenesis (sper-mat-oh-JEN-eh-sis)
testicles (test-IH-kles)
testosterone (tess-TAHS-ter-own)

What's In A Name?
Look for these word parts:
andr/o = male
spermat/o = sperm
-gen = that which produces
-genesis = produces
-ous = pertaining to

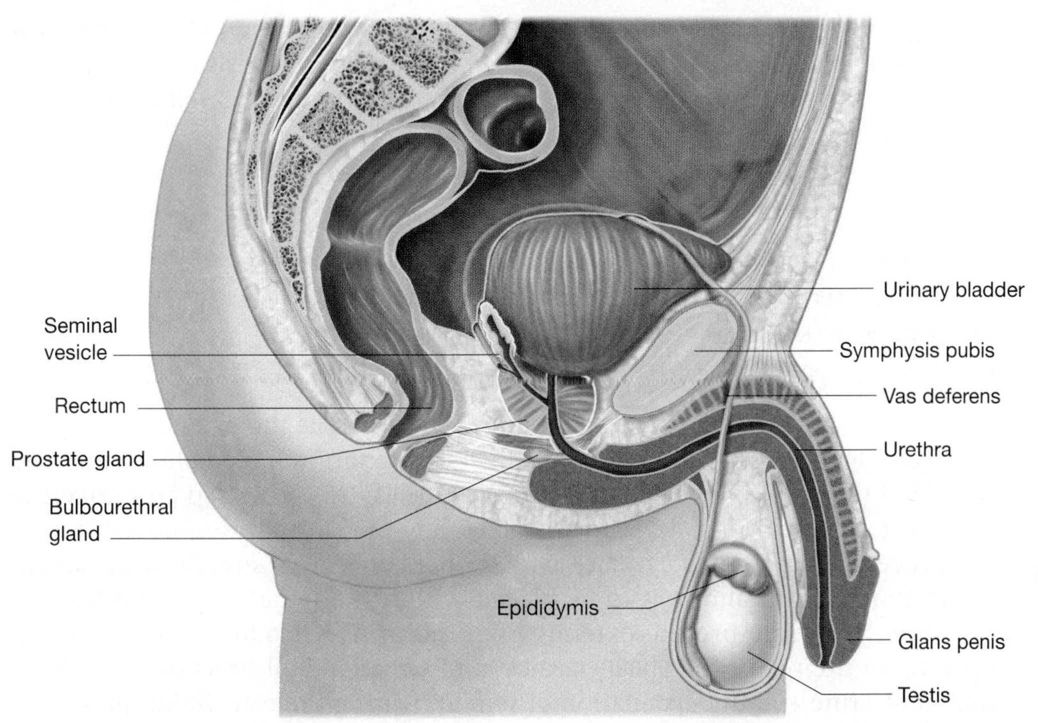

■ **Figure 10.20** The male reproductive system, sagittal section showing the organs of the system and their relation to the urinary bladder and rectum.

Med Term Tip

Spermatozoon and its plural form, *spermatozoa*, are other terms that mean "sperm." You have no doubt realized that there can be several terms with the same meaning in medical terminology. You must continue to remain flexible when working with these terms in your career. In some cases, one term will be more commonly used, depending on the type of medical specialty or even what part of the country you are in.

The testes (singular is *testis*) or **testicles** are oval in shape and are responsible for the production of sperm (see again Figure 10.20). This process, called **spermatogenesis**, takes place within the **seminiferous tubules** that make up the insides of the testes (see Figure 10.21 ■). The testes must be maintained at the proper temperature for the sperm to survive. This lower temperature level is achieved by the placement of the testes suspended in the **scrotum**, a sac outside the body. The **perineum** of the male is similar to that in the female and is the area between the scrotum and the anus. The chief **androgen** (male sex hormone) is **testosterone**, which is responsible for the development of the male reproductive organs, sperm, and secondary sex characteristics, and is also produced by the testes.

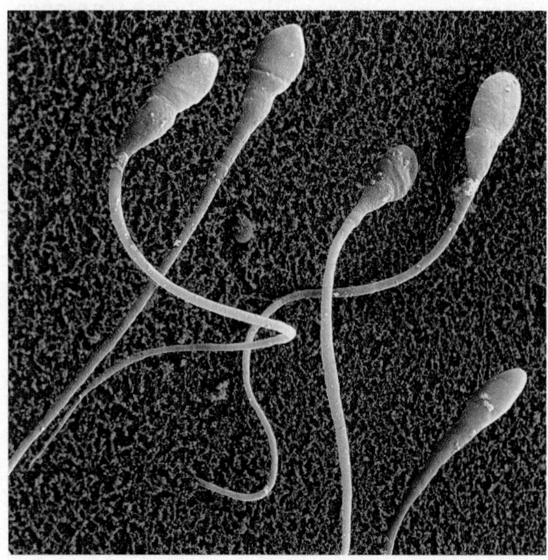

■ **Figure 10.21** Electron-micrograph of human sperm.
(Juergen Berger, Max-Planck Institute/Science Photo Library/Science Source)

Epididymis

Each epididymis is a coiled tubule that lies on top of the testes within the scrotum (see again Figure 10.20). This elongated structure serves as the location for sperm maturation and storage until they are ready to be released into the vas deferens.

Penis

What's In A Name?

Look for these word parts:
urin/o = urine
-ary = pertaining to
-ile = pertaining to
circum- = around

circumcision (ser-kum-SIH-zhun)
ejaculation (ee-jak-yoo-LAY-shun)
erectile tissue (ee-REK-tile)
glans penis (GLANS / PEE-nis)
prepuce (PREE-pyoos)
sphincter (SFINGK-ter)
urinary meatus (YOO-rih-nair-ee / me-AY-tus)

The penis is the male sex organ containing **erectile tissue** that is encased in skin (see again Figure 10.20). This organ delivers semen into the female vagina. The soft tip of the penis is referred to as the **glans penis**. It is protected by a covering called the **prepuce** or foreskin. It is this covering of skin that is removed during the procedure known as **circumcision**. The penis becomes erect during sexual stimulation, which allows it to be placed within the female for the **ejaculation** of semen. The male urethra extends from the urinary bladder to the external opening in the penis, the **urinary meatus**, and serves a dual function: the elimination of urine and the ejaculation of semen. During the ejaculation process, a **sphincter** closes to keep urine from escaping.

Med Term Tip

During sexual intercourse, which is also referred to as *coitus*, the male can eject up to 100 million sperm cells. The adult male produces nearly 200 million sperm daily.

Internal Organs of Reproduction

Vas Deferens

spermatic cord (sper-MAT-ik)

Each vas deferens carries sperm from the epididymis up into the pelvic cavity. They travel up in front of the urinary bladder, over the top, and then back down the posterior side of the bladder to empty into the urethra (see again Figure 10.20). They, along with nerves, arteries, veins, and lymphatic vessels running between the pelvic cavity and the testes, form the **spermatic cord.**

Seminal Vesicles

The two seminal vesicles are small glands located at the base of the urinary bladder (see again Figure 10.20). These vesicles are connected to the vas deferens just before it empties into the urethra. The seminal vesicles secrete a glucose-rich fluid that nourishes the sperm. This liquid, along with the sperm and secretions from other male reproductive glands, constitutes semen, the fluid that is eventually ejaculated during sexual intercourse.

Prostate Gland

The single prostate gland is located just below the urinary bladder (see again Figure 10.20). It surrounds the urethra and when enlarged can cause difficulty in urination. The prostate is important for the reproductive process since it secretes an alkaline fluid that assists in keeping the sperm alive by neutralizing the pH of the urethra and vagina.

Bulbourethral Glands

Cowper's glands (KOW-perz)

The bulbourethral glands, also known as **Cowper's glands**, are two small glands located on either side of the urethra just below the prostate (see again Figure 10.20). They produce a mucuslike lubricating fluid that joins with semen to become a part of the ejaculate.

Practice As You Go

F. Complete the Statement

1. The male reproductive system is a combination of the __________________ and __________________ systems.
2. The male's external organs of reproduction consist of the __________________, __________________, and __________________.
3. Another term for the prepuce is the __________________.
4. The organs responsible for developing the sperm cells are the __________________.
5. The glands of lubrication and fluid production at each side of the male urethra are the __________________.
6. The male sex hormone is __________________.
7. The area between the scrotum and the anus is called the __________________.

Terminology

Word Parts Used to Build Male Reproductive System Terms

The following lists contain the combining forms, suffixes, and prefixes used to build terms in the remaining sections of this chapter.

Combining Forms

andr/o	male
balan/o	glans penis
carcin/o	cancer
crypt/o	hidden
epididym/o	epididymis
genit/o	genital
hydr/o	water
immun/o	protection

olig/o	scanty
orch/o	testes
orchi/o	testes
orchid/o	testes
pen/o	penis
prostat/o	prostate gland
rect/o	rectum

spermat/o	sperm
testicul/o	testicle
ur/o	urine
urethr/o	urethra
varic/o	dilated vein
vas/o	vas deferens
vesicul/o	seminal vesicle

Suffixes

-al	pertaining to
-ar	pertaining to
-cele	protrusion
-cide	to kill
-ectomy	surgical removal
-gen	that which produces
-iasis	abnormal condition
-ic	pertaining to

-ile	pertaining to
-ism	state of
-itis	inflammation
-logy	study of
-lysis	to destroy
-oid	resembling
-oma	tumor
-osis	abnormal condition

-ostomy	surgically create an opening
-otomy	cutting into
-pexy	surgical fixation
-plasia	formation of cells
-plasty	surgical repair
-rrhea	discharge
-spermia	sperm condition

Prefixes

a-	without
an-	without
anti-	against

dys-	abnormal
epi-	above
hyper-	excessive

hypo-	below
trans-	across

Adjective Forms of Anatomical Terms

Term	Word Parts	Definition
balanic (buh-LAN-ik)	balan/o = glans penis -ic = pertaining to	Pertaining to the glans penis.
epididymal (ep-ih-DID-ih-mal)	epididym/o = epididymis -al = pertaining to	Pertaining to the epididymis.
penile (PEE-nile)	pen/o = penis -ile = pertaining to	Pertaining to the penis.
prostatic (pross-TAT-ik)	prostat/o = prostate gland -ic = pertaining to	Pertaining to the prostate gland.

Adjective Forms of Anatomical Terms (continued)

Term	Word Parts	Definition
spermatic (sper-MAT-ik)	spermat/o = sperm -ic = pertaining to	Pertaining to sperm.
testicular (tes-TIK-yoo-lar)	testicul/o = testes -ar = pertaining to	Pertaining to the testes.
vasal (VAY-sal)	vas/o = vas deferens -al = pertaining to	Pertaining to the vas deferens.
vesicular (veh-SIC-yoo-lar)	vesicul/o = seminal vesicle -ar = pertaining to **Word Watch** Be careful using the combining forms *vesic/o* meaning "bladder" and *vesicul/o* meaning "seminal vesicle."	Pertaining to the seminal vesicle.

Practice As You Go

G. Give the adjective form for each anatomical structure

1. A testis ______
2. Sperm ______
3. A seminal vesicle ______
4. The penis ______
5. The prostate gland ______

Pathology

Term	Word Parts	Definition
Medical Specialties		
urology (yoo-RAL-oh-jee)	ur/o = urine -logy = study of	Branch of medicine involved in diagnosis and treatment of diseases and disorders of the urinary system and male reproductive system. Physician is a *urologist.*
Signs and Symptoms		
aspermia (ah-SPER-mee-ah)	a- = without -spermia = sperm condition	Condition of having no sperm.
balanorrhea (bah-lah-noh-REE-ah)	balan/o = glans penis -rrhea = discharge	Discharge from the glans penis.
oligospermia (ol-ih-goh-SPER-mee-ah)	olig/o = scanty -spermia = sperm condition	Condition of having too few sperm, making the chances of fertilization very low.
spermatolysis (sper-mah-TOL-ih-sis)	spermat/o = sperm -lysis = to destroy	Term that refers to anything that destroys sperm.

Pathology (continued)

Term	Word Parts	Definition
Testes		
anorchism (an-OR-kizm)	an- = without orch/o = testes -ism = state of	The absence of testes; may be congenital or as the result of an accident or surgery.
cryptorchidism (kript-OR-kid-izm)	crypt/o = hidden orchid/o = testes -ism = state of	Failure of the testes to descend into the scrotal sac before birth. Usually, the testes will descend before birth. A surgical procedure called *orchidopexy* may be required to bring the testes down into the scrotum permanently. Failure of the testes to descend could result in sterility in the male or an increased risk of testicular cancer.
hydrocele (HIGH-droh-seel)	hydr/o = water -cele = protrusion	Accumulation of fluid around the testes or along the spermatic cord. Common in infants.
orchitis (or-KIGH-tis)	orch/o = testes -itis = inflammation	Inflammation of one or both testes.
sterility		Inability to father children due to a problem with spermatogenesis.
testicular carcinoma (kar-sih-NOH-mah)	testicul/o = testicle -ar = pertaining to carcin/o = cancer -oma = tumor	Cancer of one or both testicles; most common cancer in men under age 40.
testicular torsion	testicul/o = testicle -ar = pertaining to	Twisting of the spermatic cord.
varicocele (VAIR-ih-koh-seel)	varic/o = dilated vein -cele = protrusion	Enlargement of the veins of the spermatic cord that commonly occurs on the left side of adolescent males.
Epididymis		
epididymitis (ep-ih-did-ih-MYE-tis)	epididym/o = epididymis -itis = inflammation	Inflammation of the epididymis.
Prostate Gland		
benign prostatic hyperplasia (BPH) (bee-NINE / pross-TAT-ik / high-per-PLAY-zhee-ah)	prostat/o = prostate gland -ic = pertaining to hyper- = excessive -plasia = formation of cells	Noncancerous enlargement of the prostate gland commonly seen in males over age 50. Formerly called *benign prostatic hypertrophy.*
prostate cancer (PROSS-tayt)		Slow-growing cancer that affects a large number of males after age 50. The prostate-specific antigen (PSA) test is used to assist in early detection of this disease.
prostatitis (pross-tah-TYE-tis)	prostat/o = prostate gland -itis = inflammation	Inflammation of the prostate gland.
Penis		
balanitis (bal-ah-NYE-tis)	balan/o = glans penis -itis = inflammation	Inflammation of the glans penis.

Pathology (continued)

Term	Word Parts	Definition
epispadias (ep-ih-SPAY-dee-as)	epi- = above	Congenital opening of the urethra on the dorsal surface of the penis.
erectile dysfunction (ED) (ee-REK-tile)	-ile = pertaining to dys- = abnormal, difficult	Inability to engage in sexual intercourse due to inability to maintain an erection. Also called *impotence.*
hypospadias (high-poh-SPAY-dee-as)	hypo- = below	Congenital opening of the male urethra on the underside of the penis.
phimosis (fih-MOH-sis)	-osis = abnormal condition	Narrowing of the foreskin over the glans penis resulting in difficulty with hygiene. This condition can lead to infection or difficulty with urination. The condition is treated with circumcision, the surgical removal of the foreskin.
priapism (pri-ah-pizm)	-ism = state of	A persistent and painful erection due to pathological causes, not sexual arousal.
Sexually Transmitted Diseases		
chancroid (SHANG-kroyd)	-oid = resembling	Highly infectious nonsyphilitic venereal ulcer.
■ **Figure 10.22** Photograph showing a chancroid on the glans penis. *(Joe Miller/Centers for Disease Control and Prevention [CDC])*	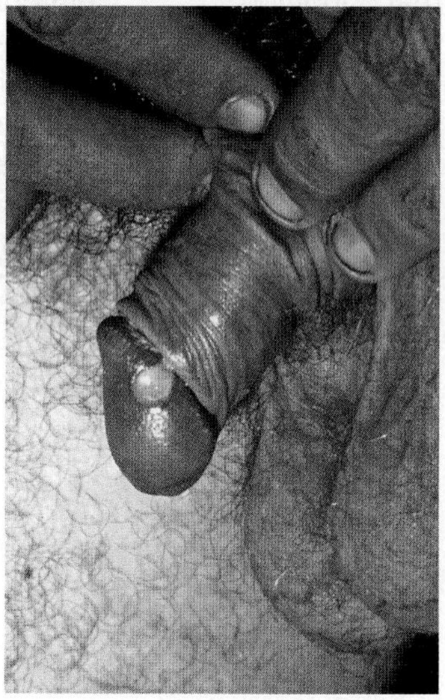	
chlamydia (klah-MID-ee-ah)		Bacterial infection causing genital inflammation in males and females. Can lead to pelvic inflammatory disease in females and eventual infertility.
genital herpes (JEN-ih-tal / HER-peez)	genit/o = genital -al = pertaining to	Spreading skin disease that can appear like a blister or vesicle on the genital region of males and females; may spread to other areas of the body. Caused by a sexually transmitted virus.

Pathology (continued)

Term	Word Parts	Definition
genital warts (JEN-ih-tal)	genit/o = genital -al = pertaining to	Growth of warts on the genitalia of both males and females that can lead to cancer of the cervix in females. Caused by the sexual transmission of the human papilloma virus (HPV).
gonorrhea (GC) (gon-oh-REE-ah)	-rrhea = discharge	Sexually transmitted bacterial infection of the mucous membranes of either sex. Can be passed on to an infant during the birth process.
human immunodeficiency virus (HIV)	immun/o = protection	Sexually transmitted virus that attacks the immune system.
sexually transmitted disease (STD)		Disease usually acquired as the result of sexual intercourse. Also called *sexually transmitted infections* (STI). Formerly referred to as *venereal disease* (VD).
syphilis (SIF-ih-lis)		Infectious, chronic, bacterial venereal disease that can involve any organ. May exist for years without symptoms, but is fatal if untreated. Treated with the antibiotic penicillin.
trichomoniasis (trik-oh-moh-NYE-ah-sis)	-iasis = abnormal condition	Genitourinary infection caused by a single-cell protist that is usually without symptoms (asymptomatic) in both males and females. In women the disease can produce itching and/or burning, a foul-smelling discharge, and result in vaginitis.

Practice As You Go

H. Terminology Matching

Match each term to its definition.

1. ________ aspermia
2. ________ phimosis
3. ________ balanitis
4. ________ chancroid
5. ________ varicocele
6. ________ oligospermia

a. inflammation of glans penis
b. having no sperm
c. venereal ulcer
d. having too few sperm
e. narrowing of foreskin
f. enlarged spermatic cord veins

Diagnostic Procedures

Term	Word Parts	Definition
Clinical Laboratory Tests		
prostate-specific antigen (PSA) (PROSS-tayt-specific / AN-tih-jen)	anti- = against -gen = that which produces	Blood test to screen for prostate cancer. Elevated blood levels of PSA are associated with prostate cancer.
semen analysis (SEE-men / ah-NAL-ih-sis)		Procedure used when performing a fertility workup to determine if the male is able to produce sperm. Semen is collected by the patient after abstaining from sexual intercourse for a period of three to five days. The sperm in the semen are analyzed for number, swimming strength, and shape. Also used to determine if a vasectomy has been successful. After a period of six weeks, no further sperm should be present in a sample from the patient.
Additional Diagnostic Procedures		
digital rectal exam (DRE) (DIJ-ih-tal / REK-tal)	rect/o = rectum -al = pertaining to	Manual examination for an enlarged prostate gland performed by palpating (feeling) the prostate gland through the wall of the rectum.

Therapeutic Procedures

Term	Word Parts	Definition
Surgical Procedures		
balanoplasty (BAL-ah-noh-plas-tee)	balan/o = glans penis -plasty = surgical repair	Surgical repair of the glans penis.
castration (kass-TRAY-shun)		Removal of the testicles in the male or the ovaries in the female.
circumcision (ser-kum-SIH-zhun)		Surgical removal of the prepuce, or foreskin, of the penis. Generally performed on the newborn male at the request of the parents. The primary reason is for ease of hygiene. Circumcision is also a ritual practice in some religions.
epididymectomy (ep-ih-did-ih-MEK-toh-mee)	epididym/o = epididymis -ectomy = surgical removal	Surgical removal of the epididymis.
orchidectomy (or-kid-EK-toh-mee)	orchid/o = testes -ectomy = surgical removal	Surgical removal of one or both testes.
orchidopexy (OR-kid-oh-peck-see)	orchid/o = testes -pexy = surgical fixation	Surgical fixation to move undescended testes into the scrotum and to attach them to prevent retraction. Used to treat cryptorchidism.
orchiectomy (or-kee-EK-toh-mee)	orchi/o = testes -ectomy = surgical removal	Surgical removal of one or both testes.
orchiotomy (or-kee-OT-oh-mee)	orchi/o = testes -otomy = cutting into	To cut into the testes.
orchioplasty (OR-kee-oh-plas-tee)	orchi/o = testes -plasty = surgical repair	Surgical repair of the testes.

Therapeutic Procedures (continued)

Term	Word Parts	Definition
prostatectomy (pross-tah-TEK-toh-mee)	prostat/o = prostate gland -ectomy = surgical removal	Surgical removal of the prostate gland.
sterilization (ster-ih-lih-ZAY-shun)		Process of rendering a male or female sterile or unable to conceive children.
transurethral resection of the prostate (TUR, TURP) (trans-yoo-REE-thrall / REE-sek-shun / PROSS-tayt)	trans- = across urethr/o = urethra -al = pertaining to	Surgical removal of the part of the prostate gland that is blocking urine flow by inserting a device through the urethra and removing prostate tissue.
vasectomy (vas-EK-toh-mee)	vas/o = vas deferens -ectomy = surgical removal	Removal of a segment or all of the vas deferens to prevent sperm from leaving the male body. Used for contraception purposes.

Med Term Tip

The vas deferens is the tubing that is severed during a procedure called a *vasectomy*. A vasectomy results in the sterilization of the male since the sperm are no longer able to travel into the urethra and out of the penis during sexual intercourse. The surgical procedure to reverse a vasectomy is a *vasovasostomy*. A new opening is created in order to reconnect one section of the vas deferens to another section of the vas deferens, thereby reestablishing an open tube for sperm to travel through.

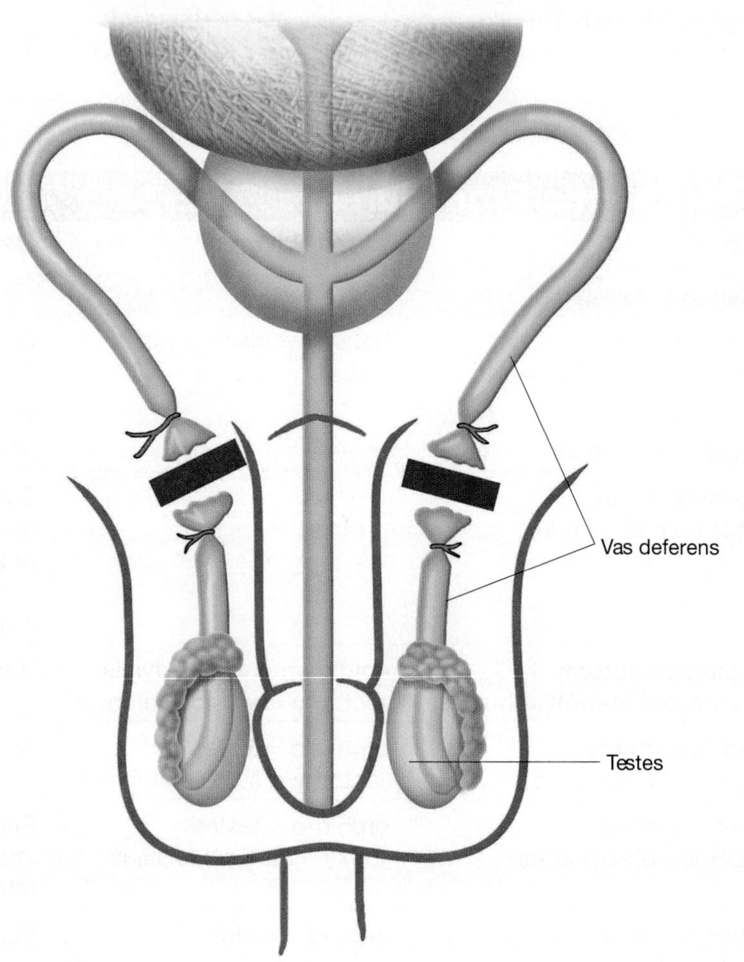

■ **Figure 10.23** A vasectomy, showing how each vas deferens is tied off in two places and then a section is removed from the middle. This prevents sperm from traveling through the vas deferens during ejaculation.

Term	Word Parts	Definition
vasovasostomy (vas-oh-vay-ZOS-toh-mee)	vas/o = vas deferens -ostomy = surgically create an opening	Surgical procedure to reconnect the vas deferens to reverse a vasectomy.

Practice As You Go

I. Terminology Matching

Match each term to its definition.

1. ________ digital rectal exam
2. ________ circumcision
3. ________ vasectomy
4. ________ orchidopexy
5. ________ semen analysis

a. removes prepuce
b. surgical fixation of testis
c. examination for enlarged prostate
d. sterilization procedure
e. part of a fertility workup

Pharmacology

Classification	Word Parts	Action	Examples
androgen therapy (AN-droh-jen)	andr/o = male -gen = that which produces	Replaces male hormones to treat patients who produce insufficient hormone naturally.	testosterone cypionate, Andronate, depAndro
antiprostatic agents (an-tye-pross-TAT-ik)	anti- = against prostat/o = prostate gland -ic = pertaining to	Treat early cases of benign prostatic hyperplasia. May prevent surgery for mild cases.	finasteride, Proscar; dutasteride, Avodart
erectile dysfunction agents (ee-REK-tile)	-ile = pertaining to dys- = abnormal	Temporarily produce an erection in patients with erectile dysfunction.	sildenafil citrate, Viagra; tadalafil, Cialis
spermatocide (SPER-mah-toh-side)	spermat/o = sperm -cide = to kill	Destroys sperm. One form of birth control is the use of spermatolytic creams.	octoxynol 9, Semicid, Ortho-Gynol

Abbreviations

BPH	benign prostatic hyperplasia	**SPP**	suprapubic prostatectomy
DRE	digital rectal exam	**STD**	sexually transmitted disease
ED	erectile dysfunction	**STI**	sexually transmitted infection
GC	gonorrhea	**TUR**	transurethral resection
GU	genitourinary	**TURP**	transurethral resection of the prostate
PSA	prostate-specific antigen	**VD**	venereal disease
RPR	rapid plasma reagin (test for syphilis)		

Practice As You Go

J. What's the Abbreviation?

1. erectile dysfunction ______________________________

2. gonorrhea ______________________________

3. digital rectal exam ______________________________

4. transurethral resection of the prostate ______________________________

5. sexually transmitted infection ______________________________

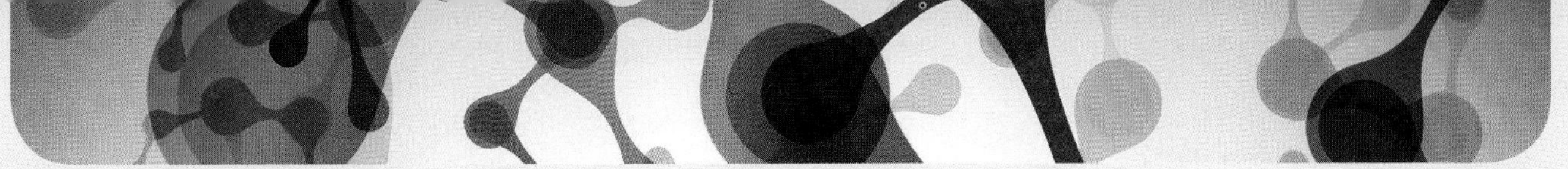

Chapter Review

Real-World Applications

Medical Record Analysis

This High-Risk Obstetrics Consultation Report contains 12 medical terms. Underline each term and write it in the list below the report. Then define each term.

High-Risk Obstetrics Consultation Report

Reason for Consultation:	High-risk pregnancy with late-term bleeding
History of Present Illness:	Patient is 23 years old. She is currently estimated to be at 175 days' gestation. Amniocentesis at 20 weeks shows a normally developing male fetus. She noticed a moderate degree of bleeding this morning but denies any cramping or pelvic pain. She immediately saw her obstetrician who referred her for high-risk evaluation.
Past Medical History:	This patient is multigravida but nullipara with three early miscarriages without obvious cause.
Results of Physical Examination:	Patient appears well nourished and abdominal girth appears consistent with length of gestation. Pelvic ultrasound indicates placenta previa with placenta almost completely overlying cervix. However, there is no evidence of abruptio placentae at this time. Fetal size estimate is consistent with 25 weeks' gestation. The fetal heartbeat is strong with a rate of 130 beats/minute.
Recommendations:	Fetus appears to be developing well and in no distress at this time. The placenta appears to be well attached on ultrasound, but the bleeding is cause for concern. With the extremely low position of the placenta, this patient is at very high risk for abruptio placentae. She will require C-section at onset of labor.

	Term	Definition
1.	______________	______________________________
2.	______________	______________________________
3.	______________	______________________________
4.	______________	______________________________
5.	______________	______________________________
6.	______________	______________________________
7.	______________	______________________________
8.	______________	______________________________
9.	______________	______________________________
10.	______________	______________________________
11.	______________	______________________________
12.	______________	______________________________

Chart Note Transcription

The chart note below contains 10 phrases that can be reworded with a medical term that you learned in this chapter. Each phrase is identified with an underline. Determine the medical term and write your answers in the space provided.

Pearson General Hospital Consultation Report

Task Edit View Time Scale Options Help Download Archive Date: 17 May 2015

Current Complaint:	Patient is a 77-year-old male seen by the urologist with complaints of nocturia and difficulty with the release of semen from the urethra. **1**
Past History:	Medical history revealed that the patient had failure of the testes to descend into the scrotum **2** at birth, which was repaired by surgical fixation of the testes. **3** He had also undergone elective sterilization by removal of a segment of the vas deferens **4** at the age of 41.
Signs and Symptoms:	Patient states he first noted these symptoms about five years ago. They have become increasingly severe and now he is not able to sleep without waking to urinate up to 20 times a night. He has difficulty with release of semen. **5** Palpation of the prostate gland through the rectum **6** revealed multiple round, firm nodules in prostate gland. A needle biopsy was negative for slow-growing cancer that frequently affects males over age 50 **7** and a blood test for prostate cancer **8** was normal.
Diagnosis:	Noncancerous enlargement of the prostate gland. **9**
Treatment:	Patient was scheduled for a surgical removal of prostate tissue through the urethra. **10**

1. ______________________________
2. ______________________________
3. ______________________________
4. ______________________________
5. ______________________________
6. ______________________________
7. ______________________________
8. ______________________________
9. ______________________________
10. ______________________________

Case Study

Below is a case study presentation of a patient with a condition covered by this chapter. Read the case study and answer the questions below. Some questions will ask for information not included within this chapter. Use your text,a medical dictionary, or any other reference material you choose to answer these questions.

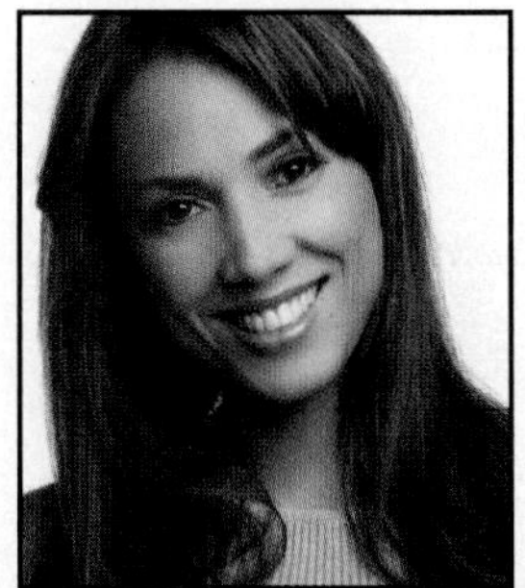
(Jason Stitt/Shutterstock)

A 22-year-old female has come into the gynecologist's office complaining of fever, malaise, dysuria, and vaginal leukorrhea. Upon examination the physician observes fluid-filled vesicles on her cervix, vulva, and perineum. Several have ruptured into ulcers with marked erythema and edema. Palpation revealed painful and enlarged inguinal lymph nodes. She also has an extragenital lesion on her mouth.
Her diagnosis is genital herpes.

Questions

1. What pathological condition does this patient have? Look this condition up in a reference source and include a short description of it.

____

____

2. List and define each of the patient's presenting symptoms in your own words.

____

____

3. Describe the results of the physician's examination in your own words.

____

____

4. Explain what extragenital lesion means.

____

____

5. Explain what palpation means.

____

____

6. What is the potential effect of having this virus present in open genital lesions on the patient's future pregnancy and childbirth?

____

____

Practice Exercises

A. What Does it Stand For?

1. SPP ______
2. TUR ______
3. GU ______
4. BPH ______
5. PSA ______
6. Cx ______
7. LMP ______
8. FHR ______
9. PID ______
10. GYN ______
11. CS ______
12. NB ______
13. PMS ______
14. TSS ______
15. LBW ______

B. Define the Term

1. spermatogenesis ______
2. hydrocele ______
3. transurethral resection of the prostate (TURP) ______
4. sterility ______
5. orchiectomy ______
6. vasectomy ______
7. castration ______
8. gestation ______
9. meconium ______
10. nulligravida ______
11. dystocia ______
12. metrorrhea ______

13. fibroid tumor ______

14. fibrocystic disease ______

15. placenta previa ______

C. Word Building Practice

The combining form **colp/o** refers to the vagina. Use it to write a term that means:

1. visual examination of the vagina ______
2. instrument used to examine the vagina ______

The combining form **cervic/o** refers to the cervix. Use it to write a term that means:

3. removal of the cervix ______
4. inflammation of the cervix ______

The combining form **hyster/o** also refers to the uterus. Use it to write a term that means:

5. surgical fixation of the uterus ______
6. removal of the uterus ______
7. rupture of the uterus ______

The combining form **oophor/o** refers to the ovaries. Use it to write a term that means:

8. inflammation of an ovary ______
9. removal of an ovary ______

The combining form **mamm/o** refers to the breasts. Use it to write a term that means:

10. record of breast ______
11. surgical repair of breast ______

The combining form **amni/o** refers to the amnion. Use it to write a term that means:

12. cutting into amnion ______
13. flow from amnion ______

The combining form **prostat/o** refers to the prostate. Use this to write a term that means:

14. removal of prostate ______
15. inflammation of the prostate ______

The combining form **orchi/o** refers to the testes. Use this to write a term that means:

16. removal of the testes ______
17. surgical repair of the testes ______
18. incision into the testes ______

The suffix **-spermia** refers to a sperm condition. Use this to write a term that means:

19. condition of being without sperm ______________________________

20. condition of having too few (scanty) sperm ______________________________

The combining form **spermat/o** refers to sperm. Use this to write a term that means:

21. sperm forming ______________________________

22. to destroy sperm ______________________________

D. Define the Combining Form

	Definition	Example from Chapter
1. **metr/o**	______________	______________
2. **hyster/o**	______________	______________
3. **gynec/o**	______________	______________
4. **episi/o**	______________	______________
5. **oophor/o**	______________	______________
6. **ovari/o**	______________	______________
7. **salping/o**	______________	______________
8. **men/o**	______________	______________
9. **vagin/o**	______________	______________
10. **mast/o**	______________	______________
11. **spermat/o**	______________	______________
12. **orchi/o**	______________	______________
13. **andr/o**	______________	______________
14. **pen/o**	______________	______________
15. **prostat/o**	______________	______________

E. Define the Suffix

	Definition	Example from Chapter
1. -tocia	__________	__________
2. -gravida	__________	__________
3. -arche	__________	__________
4. -cyesis	__________	__________
5. -partum	__________	__________
6. -para	__________	__________
7. -salpinx	__________	__________
8. -spermia	__________	__________

F. Fill in the Blank

premenstrual syndrome	stillbirth	conization	laparoscopy
D & C	puberty	endometriosis	eclampsia
fibroid tumor	cesarean section		

1. Kesha had a core of tissue from her cervix removed for testing. This is called ____________________.
2. Joan delivered a baby that had died while still in the uterus. She had a(n) ____________________.
3. Ashley has just started her first menstrual cycle. She is said to have entered ____________________.
4. Kimberly is experiencing tender breasts, headaches, and some irritability just prior to her monthly menstrual cycle. This may be ____________________.
5. Ana has been scheduled for an examination in which her physician will use an instrument to observe her abdominal cavity to rule out the diagnosis of severe endometriosis. The physician will insert the instrument through a small incision. This procedure is called a(n) ____________________.
6. Lenora is scheduled to have a hysterectomy as a result of a long history of large benign growths in her uterus that have caused pain and bleeding. Lenora has a(n) ____________________.
7. Tiffany's physician has recommended that she have a uterine scraping to stop excessive bleeding after a miscarriage. She will be scheduled for a(n) ____________________.
8. Stacey is having frequent prenatal checkups to prevent the serious condition of pregnancy called ____________________.
9. Marion has experienced painful menstrual periods as a result of the lining of her uterus being displaced into her pelvic cavity. This is called ____________________.
10. Because her cervix was not dilating, Shataundra was informed that she will probably require a(n) ____________________ for her baby's delivery.

G. Terminology Matching

Match each term to its definition.

1. _______ gonorrhea	a. also called STD
2. _______ genital herpes	b. caused by parasitic microorganism
3. _______ human immunodeficiency virus	c. treated with penicillin
4. _______ syphilis	d. caused by human papilloma virus
5. _______ venereal disease	e. can pass to infant during birth
6. _______ genital warts	f. genitourinary infection
7. _______ chancroid	g. venereal ulcer
8. _______ chlamydia	h. attacks the immune system
9. _______ trichomoniasis	i. skin disease with vesicles

H. Pharmacology Challenge

Fill in the classification for each drug description, then match the brand name.

Drug Description	Classification	Brand Name
1. _______ replacement male hormone	_______________	a. Pitocin
2. _______ improves uterine contractions	_______________	b. Avodart
3. _______ treats early BPH	_______________	c. Clomid
4. _______ blocks ovulation	_______________	d. Semicid
5. _______ kills sperm	_______________	e. Mifeprex
6. _______ produces an erection	_______________	f. Andronate
7. _______ replaces estrogen	_______________	g. Ortho-Cept
8. _______ terminates a pregnancy	_______________	h. Viagra
9. _______ triggers ovulation	_______________	i. Premarin

MyMedicalTerminologyLab™

MyMedicalTerminologyLab is a premium online homework management system that includes a host of features to help you study. Registered users will find:

- Learning activities and homework assignments
- Fun games and activities built within a virtual hospital
- Powerful tools that track and analyze your results—allowing you to create a personalized learning experience
- Videos, flashcards, and audio pronunciations to help enrich your progress
- Streaming lesson presentations and self-paced learning modules
- A space where you and your instructors can view and manage your assignments

Labeling Exercise

Image A

Write the labels for this figure on the numbered lines provided.

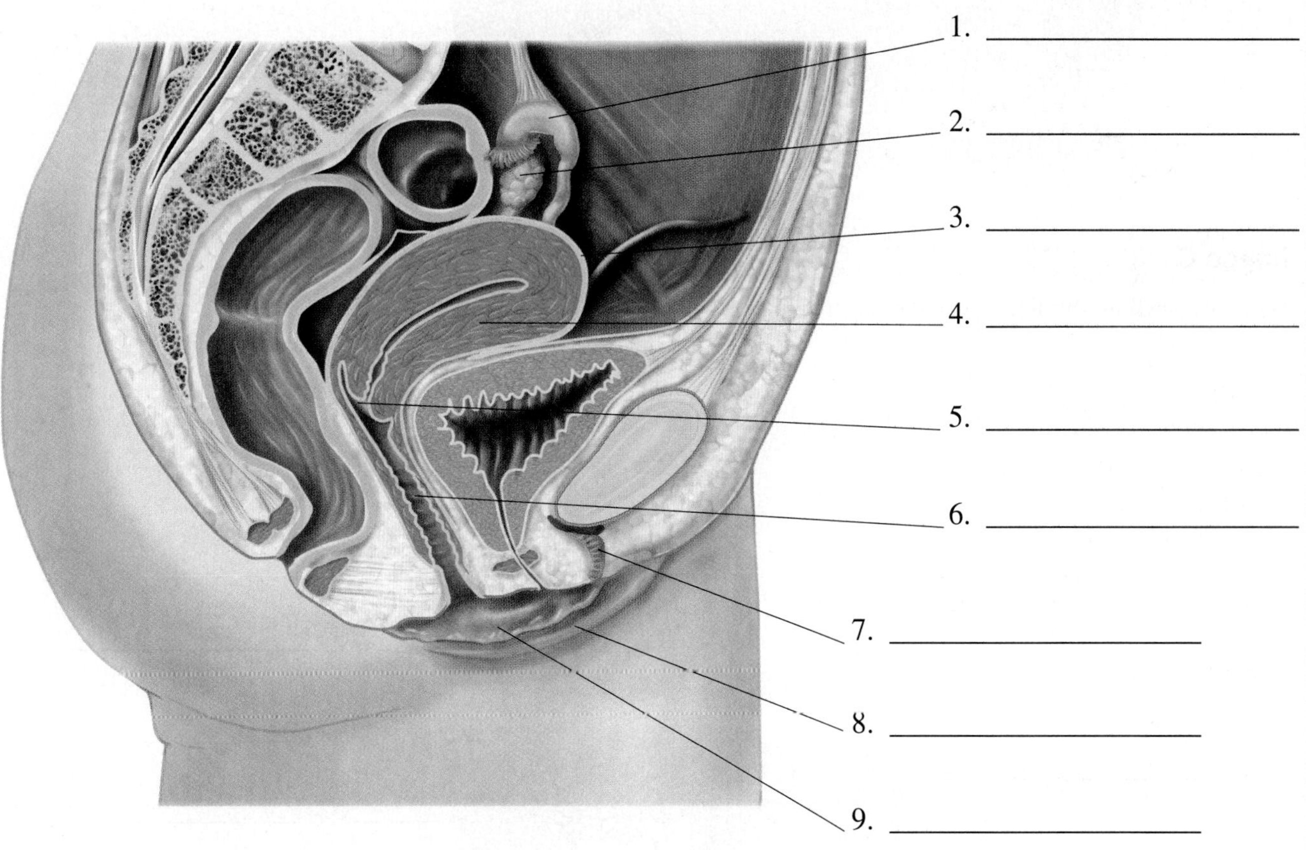

Image B

Write the labels for this figure on the numbered lines provided.

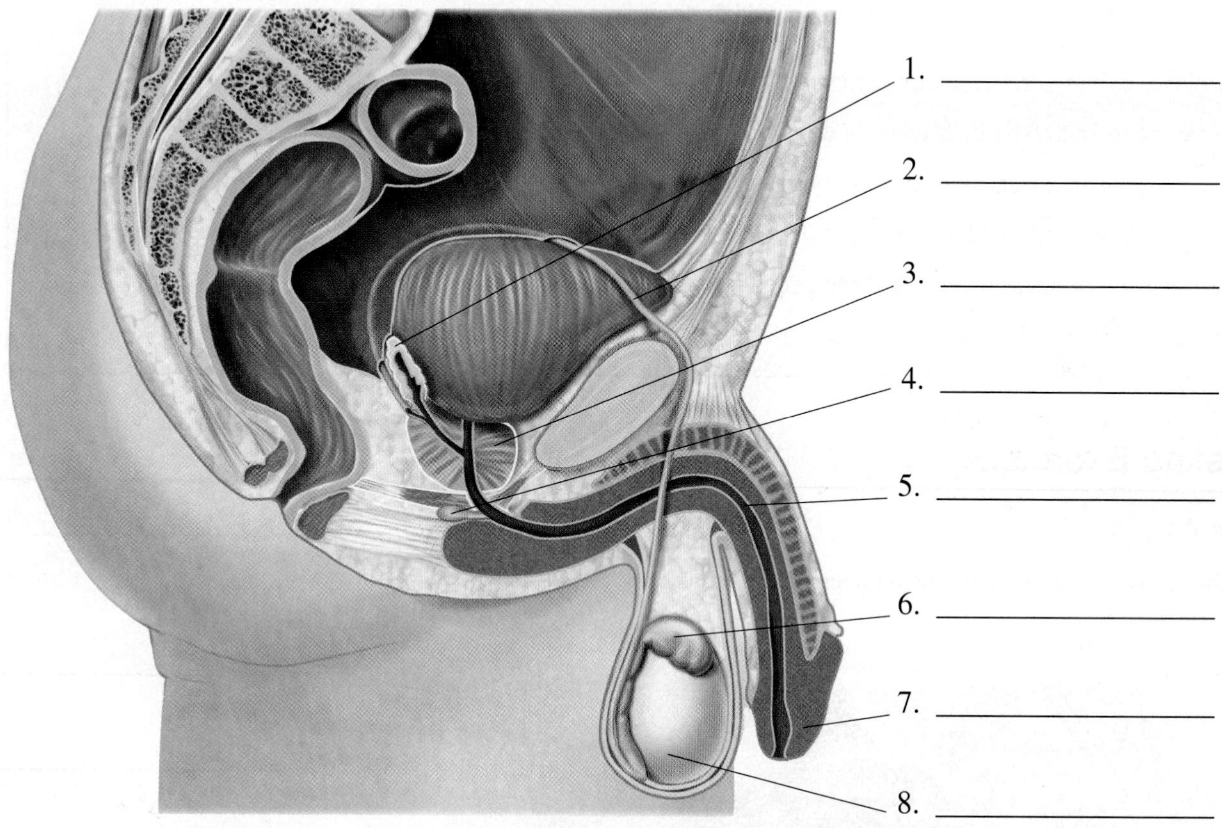

Image C

Write the labels for this figure on the numbered lines provided.

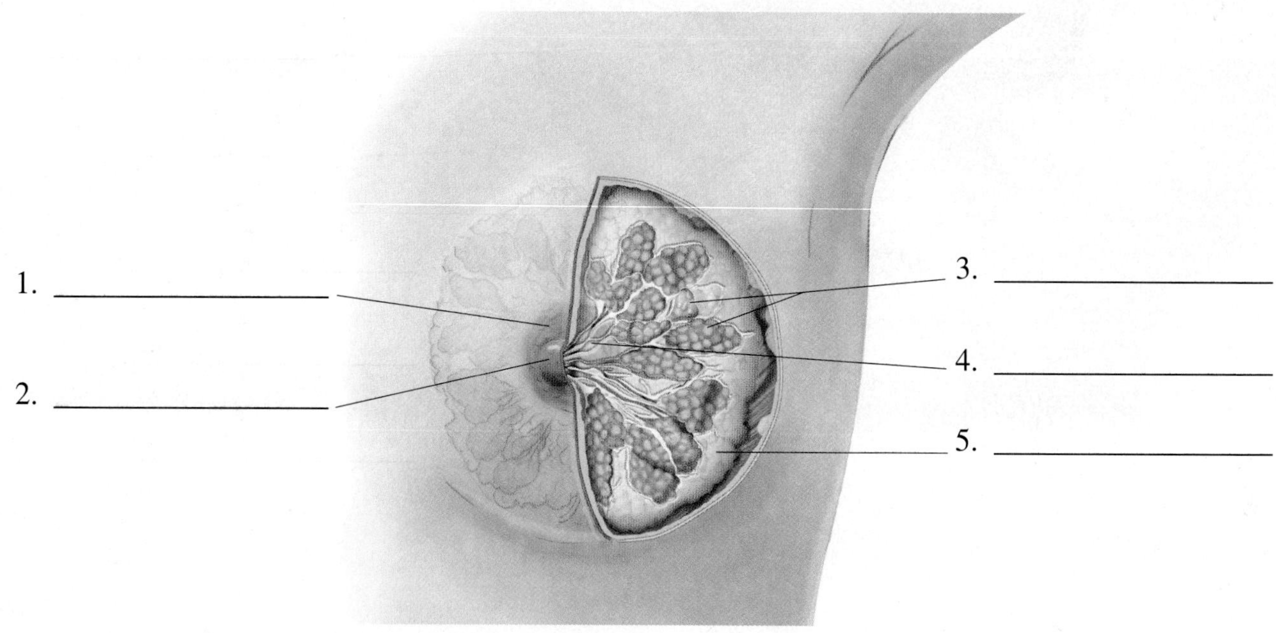

11

Endocrine System

Learning Objectives

Upon completion of this chapter, you will be able to

- Identify and define the combining forms and suffixes introduced in this chapter.
- Correctly spell and pronounce medical terms and major anatomical structures relating to the endocrine system.
- Locate and describe the major organs of the endocrine system and their functions.
- List the major hormones secreted by each endocrine gland and describe their functions.
- Identify and define endocrine system anatomical terms.
- Identify and define selected endocrine system pathology terms.
- Identify and define selected endocrine system diagnostic procedures.
- Identify and define selected endocrine system therapeutic procedures.
- Identify and define selected medications relating to the endocrine system.
- Define selected abbreviations associated with the endocrine system.

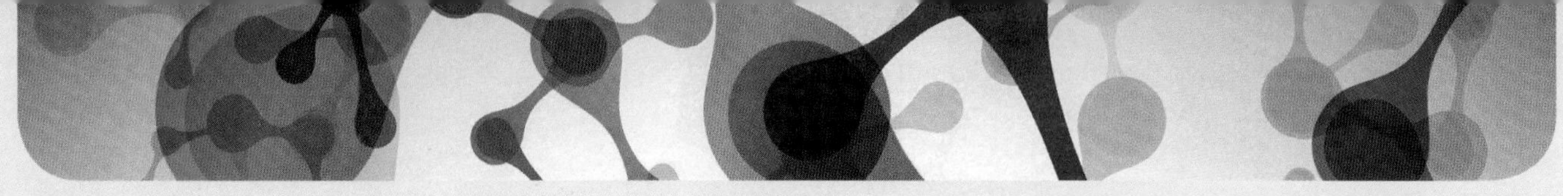

Endocrine System at a Glance

Function

Endocrine glands secrete hormones that regulate many body activities such as metabolic rate, water and mineral balance, immune system reactions, and sexual functioning.

Organs

Here are the primary structures that comprise the endocrine system:

adrenal glands
ovaries
pancreas (islets of Langerhans)
parathyroid glands
pineal gland
pituitary gland
testes
thymus gland
thyroid gland

Word Parts

Here are the most common word parts used to build endocrine system terms. For a more comprehensive list, refer to the Terminology section of this chapter.

Combining Forms

acr/o	extremities
aden/o	gland
adren/o	adrenal glands
adrenal/o	adrenal glands
andr/o	male
calc/o	calcium
crin/o	to secrete
estr/o	female
gluc/o	glucose
glyc/o	sugar
gonad/o	sex glands
iod/o	iodine
kal/i	potassium
ket/o	ketones
mineral/o	minerals, electrolytes
natr/o	sodium
ovari/o	ovary
pancreat/o	pancreas
parathyroid/o	parathyroid gland
pineal/o	pineal gland
pituitar/o	pituitary gland
radi/o	radiation
somat/o	body
testicul/o	testes
thym/o	thymus gland
thyr/o	thyroid gland
thyroid/o	thyroid gland
toxic/o	poison

Suffixes

-dipsia	thirst
-emic	pertaining to a blood condition
-pressin	to press down
-tropic	pertaining to stimulating
-tropin	to stimulate

Endocrine System Illustrated

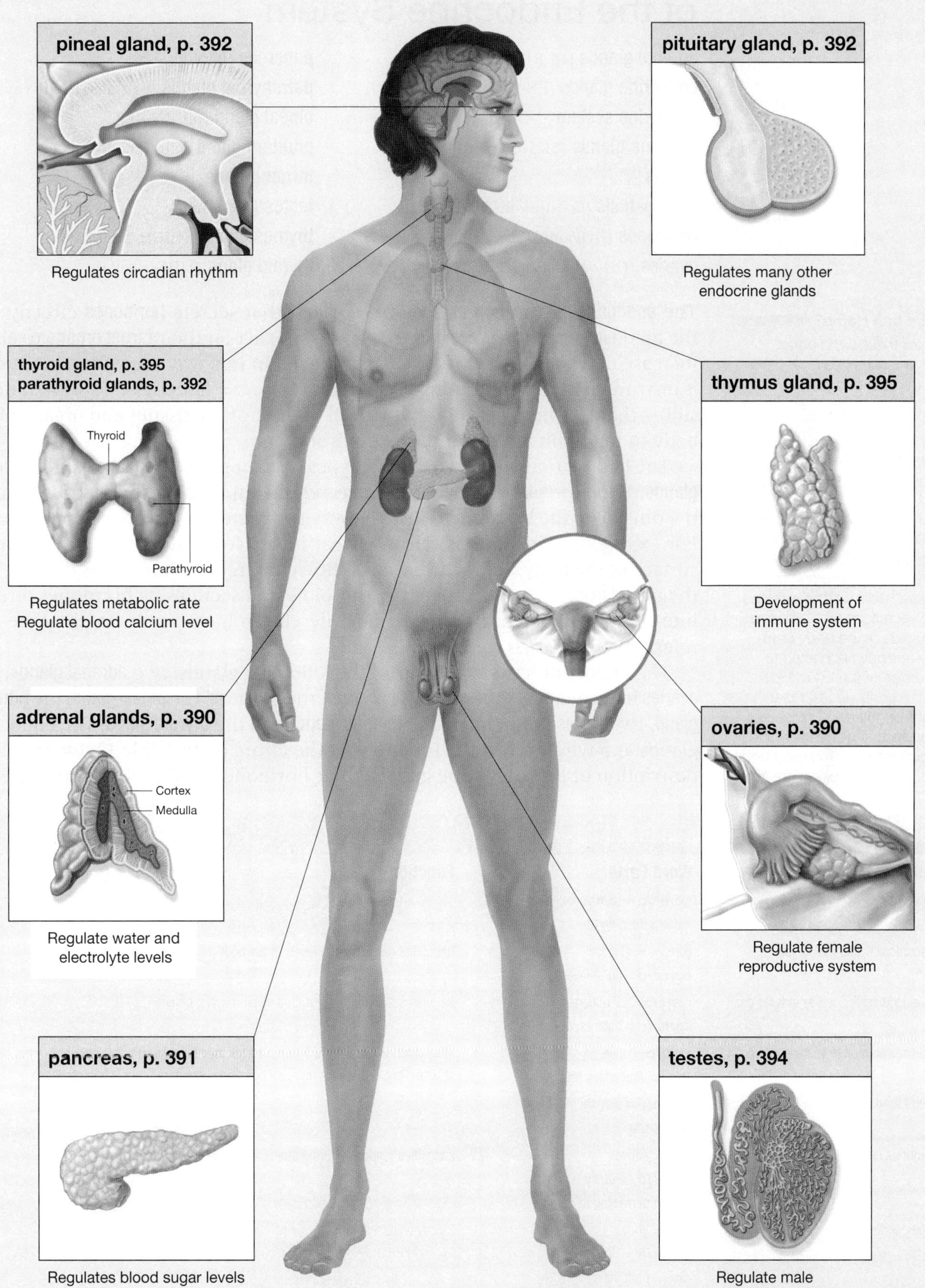

pineal gland, p. 392
Regulates circadian rhythm
pituitary gland, p. 392
Regulates many other endocrine glands
thyroid gland, p. 395
parathyroid glands, p. 392
Thyroid
Parathyroid
Regulates metabolic rate
Regulate blood calcium level
thymus gland, p. 395
Development of immune system
adrenal glands, p. 390
Cortex
Medulla
Regulate water and electrolyte levels
ovaries, p. 390
Regulate female reproductive system
pancreas, p. 391
Regulates blood sugar levels
testes, p. 394
Regulate male reproductive system

Anatomy and Physiology of the Endocrine System

adrenal glands (ad-REE-nal)
endocrine glands (EN-doh-krin)
endocrine system
exocrine glands (EKS-oh-krin)
glands
homeostasis (hoe-me-oh-STAY-sis)
hormones (HOR-mohnz)
ovaries (OH-vah-reez)
pancreas (PAN-kree-ass)
parathyroid glands (pair-ah-THIGH-royd)
pineal gland (pih-NEAL)
pituitary gland (pih-TOO-ih-tair-ee)
target organs
testes (TESS-teez)
thymus gland (THIGH-mus)
thyroid gland (THIGH-royd)

What's In A Name?
Look for these word parts:
home/o = sameness
-stasis = standing still

Med Term Tip
The terms *endocrine* and *exocrine* were constructed to reflect the function of each type of gland. As glands, they both secrete, indicated by the combining form *crin/o*. The prefix *exo-*, meaning "external" or "outward," tells us that exocrine gland secretions are carried to the outside of the body or to a passageway connected to the outside of the body. However, the prefix *endo-*, meaning "within" or "internal," indicates that endocrine gland secretions are carried to other internal body structures by the bloodstream.

The **endocrine system** is a collection of **glands** that secrete **hormones** directly into the bloodstream. Hormones are chemicals that act on their **target organs** to either increase or decrease the target's activity level. In this way the endocrine system is instrumental in maintaining **homeostasis** (*home/o* = sameness; *-stasis* = standing still)—that is, adjusting the activity level of most of the tissues and organs of the body to maintain a stable internal environment.

The body actually has two distinct types of glands: **exocrine glands** and **endocrine glands**. Exocrine glands release their secretions into a duct that carries them to the outside of the body or to a passageway connected to the outside of the body. For example, sweat glands release sweat into a sweat duct that travels to the surface of the body. Endocrine glands, however, release hormones directly into the bloodstream. For example, the thyroid gland secretes its hormones directly into the bloodstream. Because endocrine glands have no ducts, they are also referred to as *ductless glands*.

The endocrine system consists of the following glands: two **adrenal glands**, two **ovaries** in the female, four **parathyroid glands**, the **pancreas**, the **pineal gland**, the **pituitary gland**, two **testes** in the male, the **thymus gland**, and the **thyroid gland**. The endocrine glands as a whole affect the functions of the entire body. Table 11.1 ■ presents a description of the endocrine glands, their hormones, and their functions.

Table 11.1 Endocrine Glands and Their Hormones

Gland and Hormone	Word Parts	Function
Adrenal cortex	adren/o = adrenal gland -al = pertaining to	
Glucocorticoids such as cortisol	gluc/o = glucose cortic/o = outer layer	Regulates carbohydrate levels in the body.
Mineralocorticoids such as aldosterone	mineral/o = minerals, electrolytes cortic/o = outer layer	Regulates electrolytes and fluid volume in the body.
Steroid sex hormones such as androgen	andr/o = male -gen = that which produces	Male sex hormones from adrenal cortex may be converted to estrogens in the bloodstream. Responsible for reproduction and secondary sexual characteristics.
Adrenal medulla	adren/o = adrenal gland -al = pertaining to	
Epinephrine (adrenaline)	epi- = above nephr/o = kidney -ine = pertaining to	Intensifies response during stress; "fight-or-flight" response.
Norepinephrine	epi- = above nephr/o = kidney -ine = pertaining to	Chiefly a vasoconstrictor.

Table 11.1 Endocrine Glands and Their Hormones (continued)

Gland and Hormone	Word Parts	Function
Ovaries		
Estrogen	estr/o = female -gen = that which produces	Stimulates development of secondary sex characteristics in females; regulates menstrual cycle.
Progesterone	pro- = before estr/o = female	Prepares for conditions of pregnancy.
Pancreas		
Glucagon		Stimulates liver to release glucose into the blood.
Insulin		Regulates and promotes entry of glucose into cells.
Parathyroid glands	para- = beside	
Parathyroid hormone (PTH)	para- = beside	Stimulates bone breakdown; regulates calcium level in the blood.
Pineal gland	pineal/o = pineal gland -al = pertaining to	
Melatonin		Regulates circadian rhythm.
Pituitary anterior lobe	-ary = pertaining to anter/o = front -ior = pertaining to	
Adrenocorticotropic hormone (ACTH)	adren/o = adrenal gland cortic/o = outer layer -tropic = pertaining to stimulating	Regulates secretion of some adrenal cortex hormones.
Gonadotropins	gonad/o = gonads -tropin = to stimulate	Consists of two hormones, follicle-stimulating hormone and luteinizing hormone.
Follicle-stimulating hormone (FSH)		Stimulates growth of eggs in female and sperm in males.
Luteinizing hormone (LH)		Regulates function of male and female gonads and plays a role in releasing ova in females.
Growth hormone (GH)		Stimulates growth of the body.
Melanocyte-stimulating hormone (MSH)	melan/o = black -cyte = cell	Stimulates pigment in skin.
Prolactin	pro- = before lact/o = milk	Stimulates milk production.
Thyroid-stimulating hormone (TSH)		Regulates function of thyroid gland.
Pituitary posterior lobe	-ary = pertaining to poster/o = back -ior = pertaining to	
Antidiuretic hormone (ADH)	anti- = against -tic = pertaining to	Stimulates reabsorption of water by the kidneys.
Oxytocin		Stimulates uterine contractions and releases milk into ducts.
Testes		
Testosterone		Promotes sperm production and development of secondary sex characteristics in males.
Thymus		
Thymosin	thym/o = thymus gland	Promotes development of cells in immune system.
Thyroid gland		
Calcitonin (CT)		Stimulates deposition of calcium into bone.
Thyroxine (T_4)	thyr/o = thyroid gland -ine = pertaining to	Stimulates metabolism in cells.
Triiodothyronine (T_3)	tri- = three iod/o = iodine thyr/o = thyroid gland -ine = pertaining to	Stimulates metabolism in cells.

Adrenal Glands

adrenal cortex (KOR-tex)
adrenal medulla (meh-DOOL-lah)
adrenaline (ah-DREN-ah-lin)
aldosterone (al-DOSS-ter-ohn)
androgens (AN-druh-jenz)
corticosteroids (kor-tih-koh-STAIR-oydz)
cortisol (KOR-tih-sal)
epinephrine (ep-ih-NEF-rin)
estrogen (ESS-troh-jen)
glucocorticoids (gloo-koh-KOR-tih-koydz)
mineralocorticoids (min-er-al-oh-KOR-tih-koydz)
norepinephrine (nor-ep-ih-NEF-rin)
progesterone (proh-JESS-ter-ohn)
steroid sex hormones (STAIR-oyd)

What's In A Name?

Look for these word parts:
adrenal/o = adrenal gland
-ine = pertaining to

Med Term Tip

The term *adrenal* contains the word part ren/o, meaning "kidney." Likewise, the term *epinephrine* contains another word part meaning "kidney," nephr/o. But neither the adrenal gland nor epinephrine have anything to do with the kidney. Both received their names because the adrenal glands sit on top of the kidney, but have no connection to it.

Med Term Tip

The term *cortex* is frequently used in anatomy to indicate the outer layer of an organ such as the adrenal gland or the kidney. The term *cortex* means "bark," as in the bark of a tree. The term *medulla* means "marrow." Because marrow is found in the inner cavity of bones, the term came to stand for the middle of an organ.

The two adrenal glands are located above each of the kidneys (see Figure 11.1 ■). Each gland is composed of two sections: **adrenal cortex** and **adrenal medulla.**

The outer adrenal cortex manufactures several different families of hormones: **mineralocorticoids**, **glucocorticoids**, and **steroid sex hormones** (see again Table 11.1). However, because they are all produced by the cortex, they are collectively referred to as **corticosteroids**. The mineralocorticoid hormone, **aldosterone**, regulates sodium (Na^+) and potassium (K^+) levels in the body. The glucocorticoid hormone, **cortisol**, regulates carbohydrates in the body. The adrenal cortex of both men and women secretes steroid sex hormones, **androgens** (which may be converted to **estrogen** once released into the bloodstream). These hormones regulate secondary sexual characteristics. All hormones secreted by the adrenal cortex are steroid hormones.

The inner adrenal medulla is responsible for secreting the hormones **epinephrine**, also called **adrenaline**, and **norepinephrine**. These hormones are critical during emergency situations because they increase blood pressure, heart rate, and respiration levels. This helps the body perform better during emergencies or otherwise stressful times.

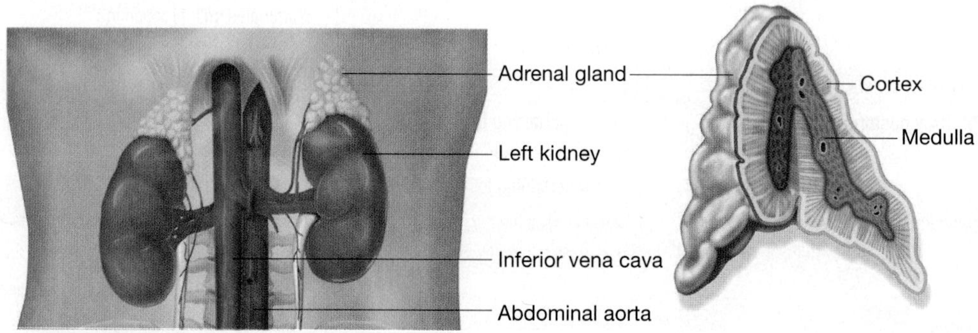

■ **Figure 11.1** The adrenal glands. These glands sit on top of each kidney. Each adrenal is subdivided into an outer cortex and an inner medulla. Each region secretes different hormones.

Ovaries

estrogen
gametes (GAM-eats)
gonads (GOH-nadz)
menstrual cycle (MEN-stroo-al)
ova
progesterone

What's In A Name?

Look for these word parts:
men/o = menses, menstruation
-al = pertaining to

The two ovaries are located in the lower abdominopelvic cavity of the female (see Figure 11.2 ■). They are the female **gonads**. Gonads are organs that produce **gametes** or the reproductive sex cells. In the case of females, the gametes are the **ova**. Of importance to the endocrine system, the ovaries produce the female sex hormones, **estrogen** and **progesterone** (see again Table 11.1). Estrogen is responsible for the appearance of the female sexual characteristics and regulation of the **menstrual cycle.** Progesterone helps to maintain a suitable uterine environment for pregnancy.

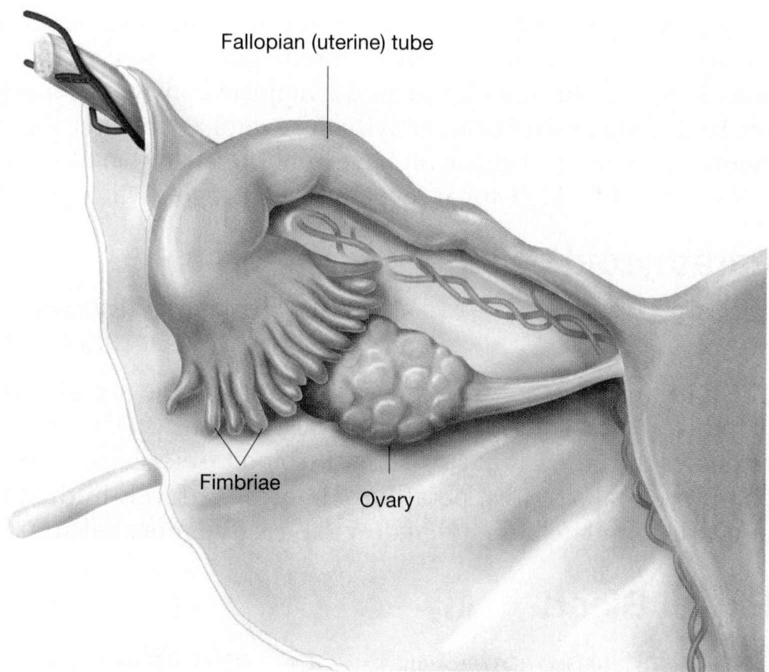

■ **Figure 11.2**
The ovaries. In addition to producing ova, the ovaries secrete the female sex hormones, estrogen and progesterone.

Pancreas

glucagon (GLOO-koh-gon)
insulin (IN-suh-lin)
islets of Langerhans (EYE-lets / of / LAHNG-er-hahnz)
pancreatic islets (pan-kree-AT-ik / EYE-lets)

The pancreas is located along the lower curvature of the stomach (see Figure 11.3A ■). It is the only organ in the body that has both endocrine and exocrine functions. The exocrine portion of the pancreas releases digestive enzymes through a duct into the duodenum of the small intestine. The endocrine sections of the pancreas are the **pancreatic islets** or **islets of Langerhans** (see Figure 11.3B ■). The islets cells produce two different hormones: **insulin** and **glucagon** (see again Table 11.1). Insulin, produced by beta (β) islet cells, stimulates the cells of the body to take in glucose from the bloodstream, lowering the body's blood sugar level. This occurs after a meal has been eaten and the carbohydrates are absorbed into the bloodstream. In this way the cells obtain the glucose they need for cellular respiration.

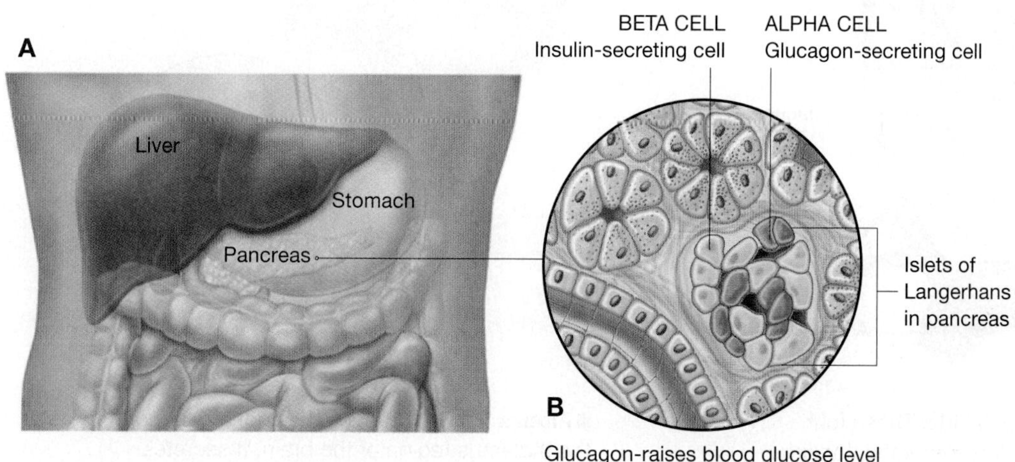

■ **Figure 11.3**
The pancreas. This organ sits just below the stomach and is both an exocrine and an endocrine gland. The endocrine regions of the pancreas are called the islets of Langerhans and they secrete insulin and glucagon.

Another set of islet cells, the alpha (α) cells, secrete a different hormone, glucagon, which stimulates the liver to release glucose, thereby raising the blood glucose level. Glucagon is released when the body needs more sugar, such as at the beginning of strenuous activity or several hours after the last meal has been digested. Insulin and glucagon have opposite effects on blood sugar level. Insulin will reduce the blood sugar level, while glucagon will increase it.

Parathyroid Glands

calcium

parathyroid hormone (pair-ah-THIGH-royd / HOR-mohn)

Med Term Tip

A calcium deficiency in the system can result in a condition called *tetany*, or muscle excitability and tremors. If the parathyroid glands are removed during thyroid surgery, calcium replacement in the body is often necessary.

The four tiny parathyroid glands are located on the dorsal surface of the thyroid gland (see Figure 11.4■). The **parathyroid hormone** (PTH) secreted by these glands regulates the amount of **calcium** in the blood (see again Table 11.1). If blood calcium levels fall too low, parathyroid hormone levels in the blood are increased and will stimulate bone breakdown to release more calcium into the blood.

Pineal Gland

circadian rhythm (seer-KAY-dee-an)

melatonin (mel-ah-TOH-nin)

thalamus (THALL-mus)

Med Term Tip

The pineal gland is an example of an organ named for its shape. *Pineal* means "shaped like a pine cone."

The pineal gland is a small pine cone-shaped gland that is part of the **thalamus** region of the brain (see Figure 11.5■). The pineal gland secretes **melatonin**, a hormone not well understood, but that plays a role in regulating the body's **circadian rhythm** (see again Table 11.1). This is the 24-hour clock that governs our periods of wakefulness and sleepiness.

Pituitary Gland

adrenocorticotropic hormone (ah-dree-noh-kor-tih-koh-TROH-pik)

anterior lobe

antidiuretic hormone (an-tye-dye-yoo-RET-ik)

follicle-stimulating hormone (FOLL-ih-kl / STIM-yoo-lay-ting)

gonadotropins (go-nad-oh-TROH-pins)

growth hormone

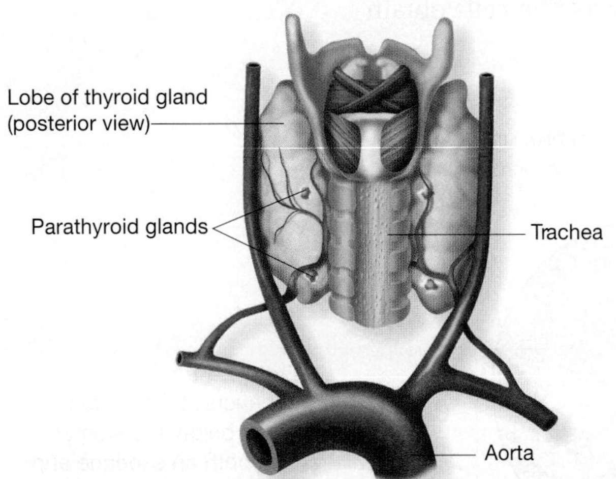

■ **Figure 11.4** The parathyroid glands. These four glands are located on the posterior side of the thyroid gland. They secrete parathyroid hormone.

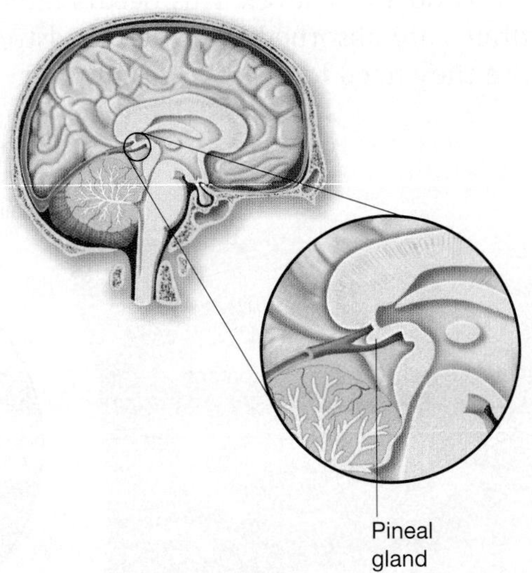

■ **Figure 11.5** The pineal gland is a part of the thalamus region of the brain. It secretes melatonin.

luteinizing hormone (LOO-tee-in-eye-zing)
melanocyte-stimulating hormone
oxytocin (ok-see-TOH-sin)
posterior lobe
hypothalamus (high-poh-THAL-ah-mus)
prolactin (proh-LAK-tin)
somatotropin (so-mat-oh-TROH-pin)
thyroid-stimulating hormone

The pituitary gland is located underneath the brain (see Figure 11.6 ■). The small marble-shaped gland is divided into an **anterior lobe** and a **posterior lobe**. Both lobes are controlled by the **hypothalamus**, a region of the brain active in regulating automatic body responses.

The anterior pituitary secretes several different hormones (see again Table 11.1 and Figure 11.7 ■). **Growth hormone** (GH), also called **somatotropin**, promotes growth of the body by stimulating cells to rapidly increase in size and divide. **Thyroid-stimulating hormone** (TSH) regulates the function of the thyroid gland. **Adrenocorticotropic hormone** (ACTH) regulates the function of the adrenal cortex. **Prolactin** (PRL) stimulates milk production in the breast following pregnancy and birth. **Follicle-stimulating hormone** (FSH) and **luteinizing hormone** (LH) both exert their influence on the male and female gonads. Therefore, these two hormones together are referred to as the **gonadotropins**. Follicle-stimulating hormone is responsible for the development of ova in ovaries and sperm in testes. It also stimulates the ovary to secrete estrogen. Luteinizing hormone stimulates secretion of sex hormones in both males and females and plays a role in releasing ova in females. **Melanocyte-stimulating hormone** (MSH) stimulates melanocytes to produce more melanin, thereby darkening the skin.

The posterior pituitary secretes two hormones, **antidiuretic hormone** (ADH) and **oxytocin** (see again Table 11.1). Antidiuretic hormone promotes water reabsorption by the kidney tubules. Oxytocin stimulates uterine contractions during labor and delivery, and after birth the release of milk from the mammary glands.

What's In A Name?

Look for these word parts:
somat/o = body
-tropin = to stimulate
hypo- = below

Med Term Tip

The pituitary gland is sometimes referred to as the "master gland" because several of its secretions regulate other endocrine glands.

Med Term Tip

Many people use the term *diabetes* to refer to diabetes mellitus (DM). But there is another type of diabetes, called *diabetes insipidus* (DI), that is a result of the inadequate secretion of the antidiuretic hormone (ADH) from the pituitary gland.

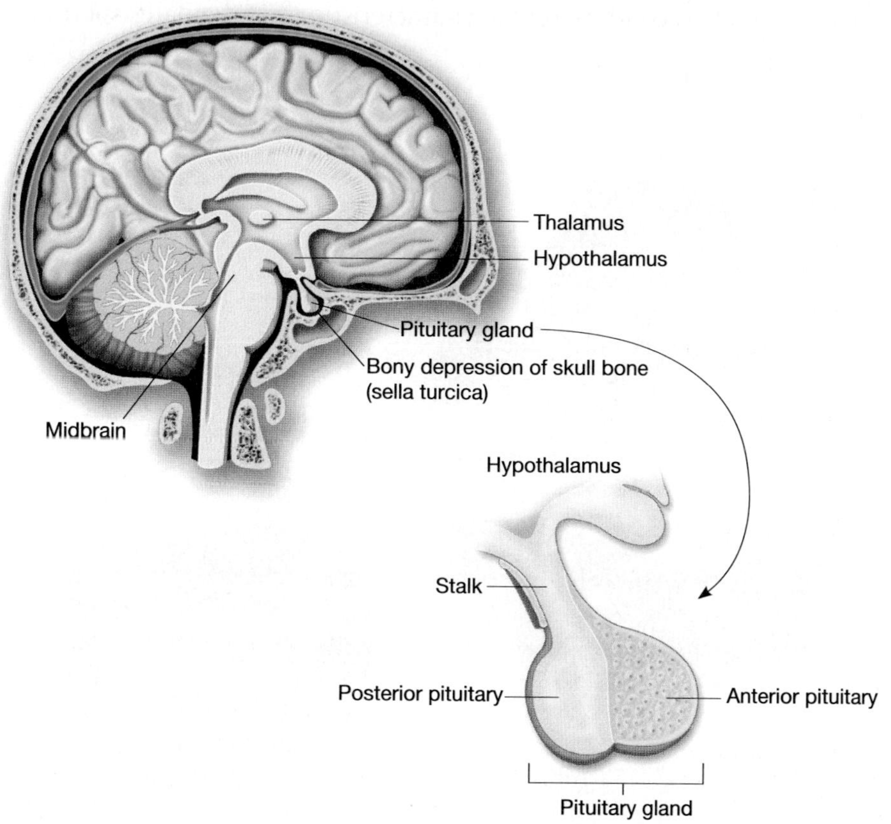

■ **Figure 11.6** The pituitary gland lies just underneath the brain. It is subdivided into anterior and posterior lobes. Each lobe secretes different hormones.

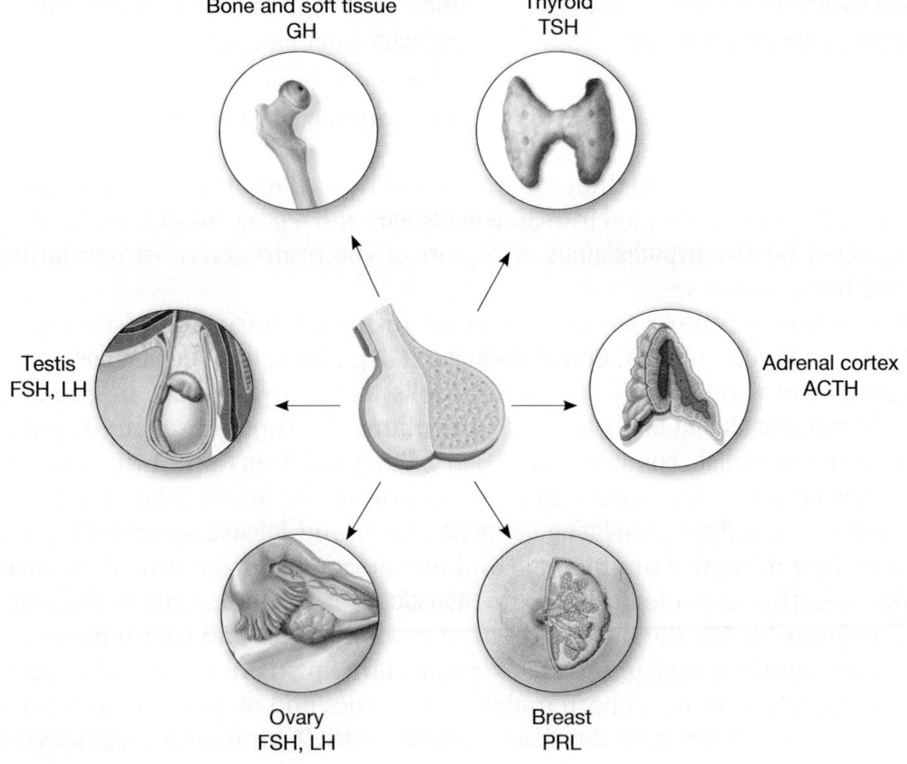

■ **Figure 11.7** The anterior pituitary is sometimes called the master gland because it secretes many hormones that regulate other glands. This figure illustrates the different hormones and target tissues for the anterior pituitary.

Testes

sperm **testosterone** (tess-TAHS-ter-own)

The testes are two oval glands located in the scrotal sac of the male (see Figure 11.8■). They are the male gonads, which produce the male gametes, **sperm**, and the male sex hormone, **testosterone** (see again Table 11.1). Testosterone produces the male secondary sexual characteristics and regulates sperm production.

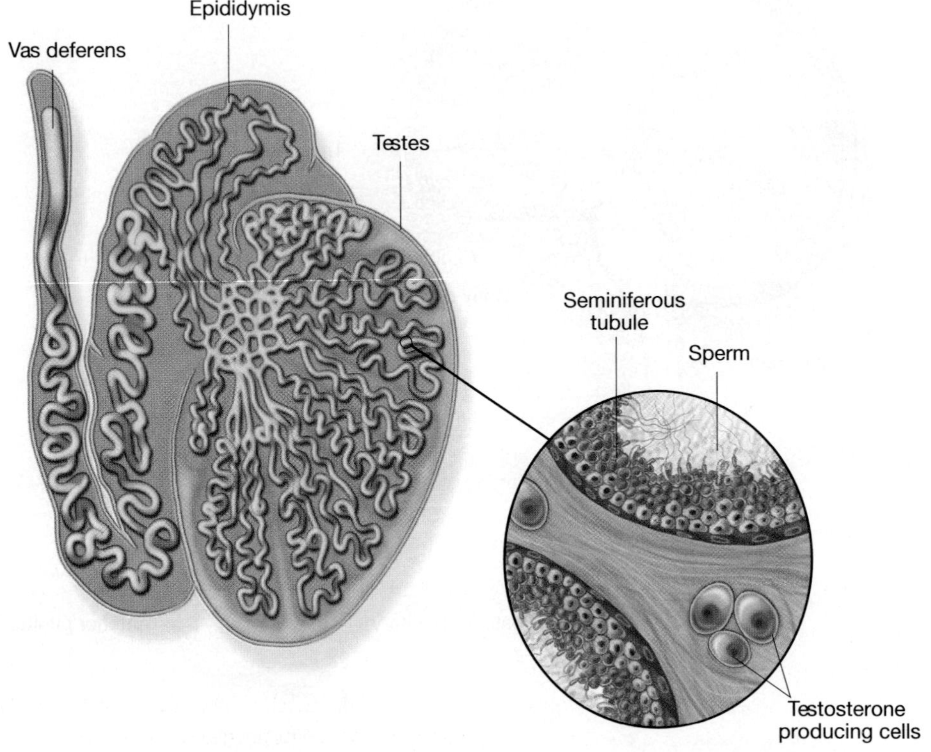

■ **Figure 11.8** The testes. In addition to producing sperm, the testes secrete the male sex hormones, primarily testosterone.

Thymus Gland

T cells **thymosin** (thigh-MOH-sin)

In addition to its role as part of the immune system, the thymus is also one of the endocrine glands because it secretes the hormone **thymosin** (see again Table 11.1). Thymosin, like the rest of the thymus gland, is important for proper development of the immune system. The thymus gland is located in the mediastinal cavity anterior and superior to the heart (see Figure 11.9 ■). The thymus is present at birth and grows to its largest size during puberty. At puberty it begins to shrink and eventually is replaced with connective and adipose tissue.

The most important function of the thymus is the development of the immune system in the newborn. It is essential to the growth and development of thymic lymphocytes or **T cells**, which are critical for the body's immune system.

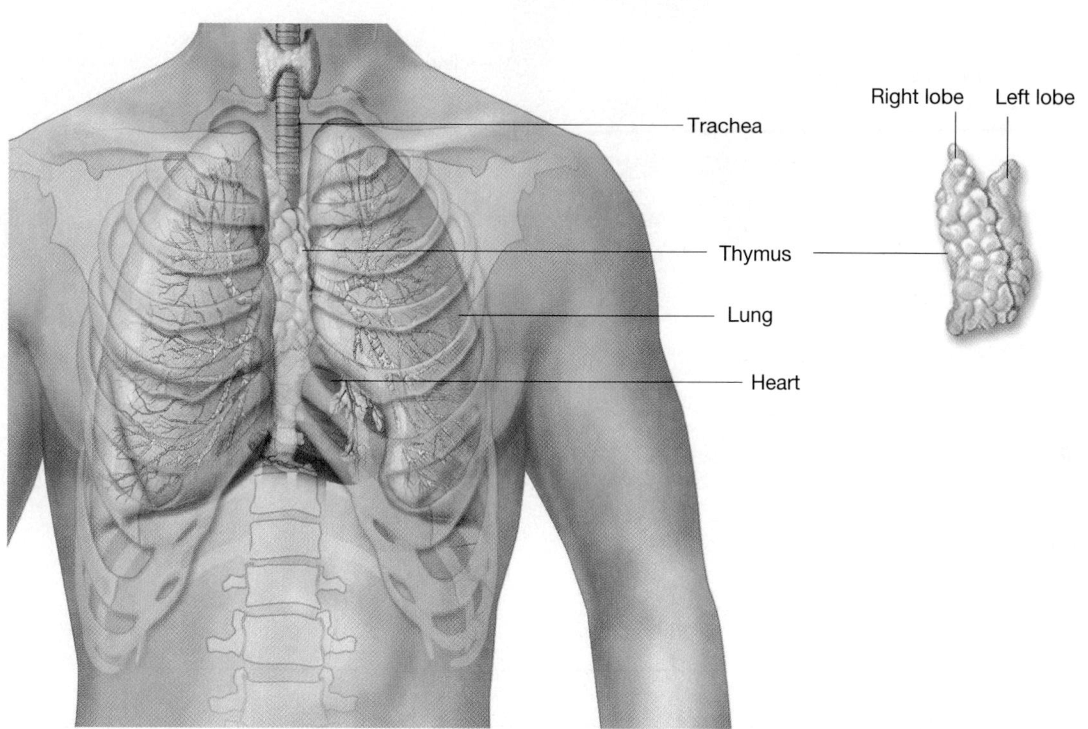

■ **Figure 11.9** The thymus gland. This gland lies in the mediastinum of the thoracic cavity, just above the heart. It secretes thymosin.

Thyroid Gland

basal metabolic rate
calcitonin (kal-sih-TOH-nin)
iodine (EYE-oh-dine)
thyroxine (thigh-ROKS-in)
triiodothyronine (try-eye-oh-doh-THIGH-roh-neen)

The thyroid gland, which resembles a butterfly in shape, has right and left lobes (see Figure 11.10 ■). It is located on either side of the trachea and larynx. The thyroid cartilage, or Adam's apple, is located just above the thyroid gland. This gland produces the hormones **thyroxine** (T_4) and **triiodothyronine** (T_3) (see again Table 11.1). These hormones are produced in the thyroid gland from the mineral

What's In A Name?
Look for these word parts:
bas/o = base
-al = pertaining to
-ic = pertaining to

Med Term Tip

Iodine is found in many foods, including vegetables and seafood. It is also present in iodized salt, which is one of the best sources of iodine for people living in the Goiter Belt, composed of states located away from saltwater. A lack of iodine in the diet can lead to thyroid disorders, including *goiter.*

iodine. Thyroxine and triiodothyronine help to regulate the production of energy and heat in the body to adjust the body's metabolic rate. The minimum rate of metabolism necessary to support the function of the body at rest is called the **basal metabolic rate** (BMR).

The thyroid gland also secretes **calcitonin** (CT) in response to hypercalcemia (too high blood calcium level). Its action is the opposite of parathyroid hormone and stimulates the increased deposition of calcium into bone, thereby lowering blood levels of calcium.

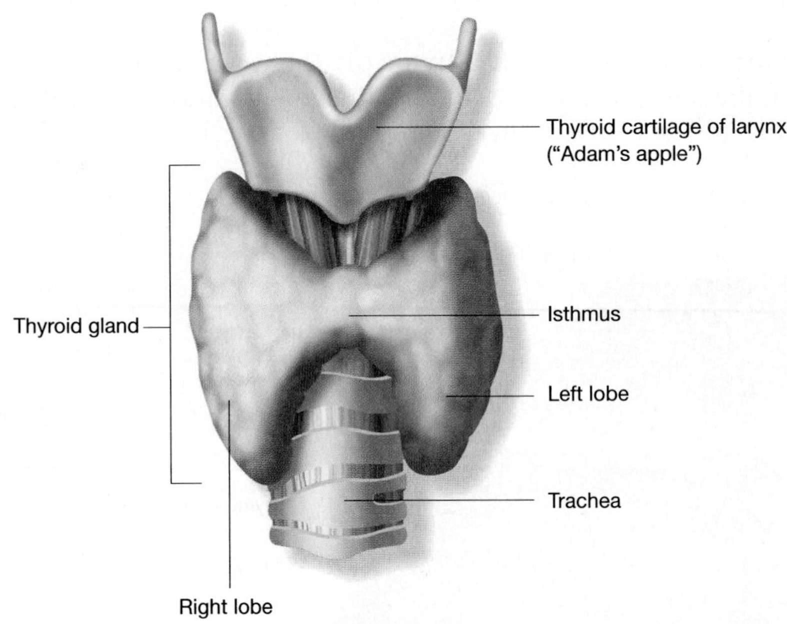

■ Figure 11.10 The thyroid gland is subdivided into two lobes, one on each side of the trachea.

Practice As You Go

A. Complete the Statement

1. The study of the endocrine system is called ______.
2. The master endocrine gland is the ______.
3. ______ is a general term for the sexual organs that produce gametes.
4. The term for the hormones produced by the outer layer of the adrenal cortex is ______.
5. The hormone produced by the testes is ______.
6. The two hormones produced by the ovaries are ______ and ______.
7. An inadequate supply of the hormone ______ causes diabetes insipidus.
8. The endocrine gland associated with the immune system is the ______.

Terminology

Word Parts Used to Build Endocrine System Terms

The following lists contain the combining forms, suffixes, and prefixes used to build terms in the remaining sections of this chapter.

Combining Forms

acr/o	extremities
aden/o	gland
adren/o	adrenal gland
adrenal/o	adrenal gland
calc/o	calcium
carcin/o	cancer
chem/o	drug
cortic/o	outer layer
crin/o	to secrete
cyt/o	cell
glyc/o	sugar
glycos/o	sugar
gynec/o	female

immun/o	protection
kal/i	potassium
ket/o	ketones
lapar/o	abdomen
lob/o	lobe
mast/o	breast
natr/o	sodium
neur/o	nerve
ophthalm/o	eye
or/o	mouth
ovari/o	ovary
pancreat/o	pancreas

parathyroid/o	parathyroid gland
pineal/o	pineal gland
pituitar/o	pituitary gland
radi/o	radiation
retin/o (see Chapter 13)	retina
testicul/o	testes
thym/o	thymus gland
thyr/o	thyroid gland
thyroid/o	thyroid gland
toxic/o	poison
vas/o	vessel

Suffixes

-al	pertaining to
-an	pertaining to
-ar	pertaining to
-ary	pertaining to
-dipsia	thirst
-ectomy	surgical removal
-edema	swelling
-emia	blood condition
-emic	pertaining to a blood condition

-graphy	process of recording
-ia	condition
-ic	pertaining to
-ism	state of
-itis	inflammation
-logy	study of
-megaly	enlarged
-meter	instrument to measure
-oma	tumor

-osis	abnormal condition
-pathy	disease
-prandial	pertaining to a meal
-pressin	to press down
-scopic	pertaining to visually examining
-tic	pertaining to
-uria	urine condition

Prefixes

anti-	against
endo-	within
ex-	outward

hyper-	excessive
hypo-	insufficient
pan-	all

poly-	many
post-	after

Adjective Forms of Anatomical Terms

Term	Word Parts	Definition
adrenal (ah-DREE-nall)	adren/o = adrenal gland -al = pertaining to	Pertaining to the adrenal glands.
ovarian (oh-VAIR-ee-an)	ovari/o = ovary -an = pertaining to	Pertaining to the ovary.
pancreatic (pan-kree-AT-ik)	pancreat/o = pancreas -ic = pertaining to	Pertaining to the pancreas.
parathyroidal (pair-ah-THIGH-roy-dal)	parathyroid/o = parathyroid gland -al = pertaining to	Pertaining to the parathyroid gland.
pineal (pih-NEAL)	pineal/o = pineal gland -al = pertaining to	Pertaining to the pineal gland.
pituitary (pih-TOO-ih-tair-ee)	pituitar/o = pituitary gland -ary = pertaining to	Pertaining to the pituitary gland.
testicular (tes-TIK-yoo-lar)	testicul/o = testes -ar = pertaining to	Pertaining to the testes.
thymic (THIGH-mik)	thym/o = thymus gland -ic = pertaining to	Pertaining to the thymus gland.
thyroidal (thigh-ROYD-all)	thyroid/o = thyroid gland -al = pertaining to	Pertaining to the thyroid gland.

Practice As You Go

B. Give the adjective form for each anatomical structure

1. The thymus gland ______________________
2. The pancreas ______________________
3. The thyroid gland ______________________
4. An ovary ______________________
5. A testis ______________________

Pathology

Term	Word Parts	Definition
Medical Specialties		
endocrinology (en-doh-krin-ALL-oh-jee)	endo- = within crin/o = to secrete -logy = study of	Branch of medicine involving diagnosis and treatment of conditions and diseases of endocrine glands. Physician is an *endocrinologist.*
Signs and Symptoms		
adrenomegaly (ad-ree-noh-MEG-ah-lee)	adren/o = adrenal gland -megaly = enlarged	Having one or both adrenal glands enlarged.

Pathology (continued)

Term	Word Parts	Definition
adrenopathy (ad-ren-OP-ah-thee)	adren/o = adrenal gland -pathy = disease	General term for adrenal gland disease.
edema (eh-DEE-mah)	**Word Watch** Watch how the term edema is used in this condition. It may also appear as the suffix -edema.	Condition in which the body tissues contain excessive amounts of fluid.
endocrinopathy (en-doh-krin-OP-ah-thee)	endo- = within crin/o = to secrete -pathy = disease	General term for diseases of the endocrine system.
exophthalmos (eks-off-THAL-mohs)	ex- = outward ophthalm/o = eye	Condition in which the eyeballs protrude, such as in Graves' disease. This is generally caused by an overproduction of thyroid hormone.
Figure 11.11 A photograph of a woman with exophthalmos. This condition is associated with hypersecretion of the thyroid gland. *(Petit Format/ Science Source)*		
glycosuria (glye-kohs-YOO-ree-ah)	glycos/o = sugar -uria = urine condition	Having a high level of sugar excreted in the urine.
gynecomastia (gigh-neh-koh-MAST-ee-ah)	gynec/o = female mast/o = breast -ia = condition	Development of breast tissue in males. May be a symptom of adrenal feminization.
hirsutism (HER-soot-izm)	-ism = state of	Condition of having an excessive amount of hair. Term generally used to describe females who have the adult male pattern of hair growth. Can be the result of a hormonal imbalance.
hypercalcemia (high-per-kal-SEE-mee-ah)	hyper- = excessive calc/o = calcium -emia = blood condition	Condition of having a high level of calcium in the blood; associated with hypersecretion of parathyroid hormone.
hyperglycemia (high-per-glye-SEE-mee-ah)	hyper- = excessive glyc/o = sugar -emia = blood condition	Condition of having a high level of sugar in the blood; associated with diabetes mellitus.
hyperkalemia (high-per-kal-EE-mee-ah)	hyper- = excessive kal/i = potassium -emia = blood condition	The condition of having a high level of potassium in the blood.
hypersecretion	hyper- = excessive	Excessive hormone production by an endocrine gland.
hypocalcemia (high-poh-kal-SEE-mee-ah)	hypo- = insufficient calc/o = calcium -emia = blood condition	The condition of having a low level of calcium in the blood; associated with hyposecretion of parathyroid hormone. Hypocalcemia may result in tetany.
hypoglycemia (high-poh-glye-SEE-mee-ah)	hypo- = insufficient glyc/o = sugar -emia = blood condition	Condition of having a low level of sugar in the blood.

Pathology (continued)

Term	Word Parts	Definition
hyponatremia (high-poh-nah-TREE-mee-ah)	hypo- = insufficient natr/o = sodium -emia = blood condition	Condition of having a low level of sodium in the blood.
hyposecretion	hypo- = insufficient	Deficient hormone production by an endocrine gland.
obesity (oh-BEE-sih-tee)		Having an abnormal amount of fat in the body.
polydipsia (pall-ee-DIP-see-ah)	poly- = many -dipsia = thirst	Excessive feeling of thirst.
polyuria (pall-ee-YOO-ree-ah)	poly- = many -uria = urine condition	Condition of producing an excessive amount of urine.
syndrome (SIN-drohm)		Group of symptoms and signs that, when combined, present a clinical picture of a disease or condition.
thyromegaly (thigh-roh-MEG-ah-lee)	thyr/o = thyroid gland -megaly = enlarged	Having an enlarged thyroid gland.
Adrenal Glands		
Addison's disease (AD-ih-sons)		Disease named for British physician Thomas Addison; results from a deficiency in adrenocortical hormones. There may be an increased pigmentation of the skin, generalized weakness, and weight loss.
adrenal feminization (ad-REE-nal / fem-ih-nigh-ZAY-shun)	adren/o = adrenal gland -al = pertaining to	Development of female secondary sexual characteristics (such as breasts) in a male. Often as a result of increased estrogen secretion by the adrenal cortex.
adrenal virilism (ad-REE-nal / VIR-ill-izm)	adren/o = adrenal gland -al = pertaining to -ism = state of	Development of male secondary sexual characteristics (such as deeper voice and facial hair) in a female. Often as a result of increased androgen secretion by the adrenal cortex.
adrenalitis (ad-ree-nal-EYE-tis)	adrenal/o = adrenal gland -itis = inflammation	Inflammation of one or both adrenal glands.
Cushing's syndrome (CUSH-ings / SIN-drohm)		Set of symptoms caused by excessive levels of cortisol due to high doses of corticosteroid drugs and adrenal tumors. The syndrome may present symptoms of weakness, edema, excess hair growth, skin discoloration, and osteoporosis.
pheochromocytoma (fee-oh-kroh-moh-sigh-TOH-ma)	cyt/o = cell -oma = tumor	Usually benign tumor of the adrenal medulla that secretes epinephrine. Symptoms include anxiety, heart palpitations, dyspnea, profuse sweating, headache, and nausea.

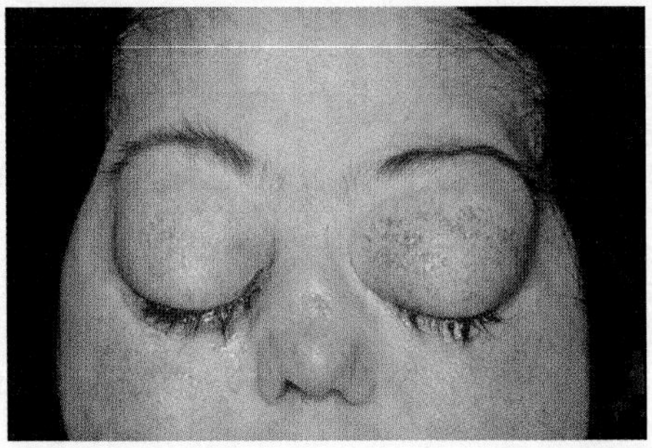

■ **Figure 11.12** Cushing's syndrome. A photograph of a woman with the characteristic facial features of Cushing's syndrome. *(Biophoto Photo Associates/ Science Scource)*

Pathology (continued)

Term	Word Parts	Definition
Pancreas		
diabetes mellitus (DM) (dye-ah-BEE-teez / MELL-ih-tus)		Chronic disorder of carbohydrate metabolism resulting in hyperglycemia and glycosuria. There are two distinct forms of diabetes mellitus: *insulin-dependent diabetes mellitus* (IDDM) or *type 1*, and *non-insulin-dependent diabetes mellitus* (NIDDM) or *type 2.*
diabetic retinopathy (dye-ah-BET-ik / ret-in-OP-ah-thee)	-tic = pertaining to retin/o = retina -pathy = disease	Secondary complication of diabetes that affects the blood vessels of the retina, resulting in visual changes and even blindness.
insulin-dependent diabetes mellitus (IDDM) (dye-ah-BEE-teez / MELL-ih-tus)		Also called *type 1 diabetes mellitus.* It develops early in life when the pancreas stops insulin production. Patient must take daily insulin injections.
insulinoma (in-sue-lin-OH-mah)	-oma = tumor	Tumor of the islets of Langerhans cells of the pancreas that secretes an excessive amount of insulin.
ketoacidosis (KEE-toh-ass-ih-DOH-sis)	ket/o = ketones -osis = abnormal condition	Acidosis due to an excess of acidic ketone bodies (waste products). A serious condition requiring immediate treatment that can result in death for the diabetic patient if not reversed. Also called *diabetic acidosis.*
non-insulin-dependent diabetes mellitus (NIDDM) (dye-ah-BEE-teez / MELL-ih-tus)		Also called *type 2 diabetes mellitus.* It typically develops later in life. The pancreas produces normal to high levels of insulin, but the cells fail to respond to it. Patients may take oral hypoglycemics to improve insulin function, or may eventually have to take insulin.
peripheral neuropathy (per-IF-eh-rall / noo-ROP-ah-thee)	-al = pertaining to neur/o = nerve -pathy = disease	Damage to the nerves in the lower legs and hands as a result of diabetes mellitus. Symptoms include either extreme sensitivity or numbness and tingling.
Parathyroid Glands		
hyperparathyroidism (HIGH-per-pair-ah-THIGH-royd-izm)	hyper- = excessive parathyroid/o = parathyroid gland -ism = state of	Hypersecretion of parathyroid hormone; may result in hypercalcemia and Recklinghausen disease.
hypoparathyroidism (HIGH-poh-pair-ah-THIGH-royd-izm)	hypo- = insufficient parathyroid/o = parathyroid gland -ism = state of	Hyposecretion of parathyroid hormone; may result in hypocalcemia and tetany.
Recklinghausen disease (REK-ling-how-zen)		Excessive production of parathyroid hormone resulting in degeneration of the bones.
tetany (TET-ah-nee)		Nerve irritability and painful muscle cramps resulting from hypocalcemia. Hypoparathyroidism is one cause of tetany.

Pathology (continued)

Term	Word Parts	Definition
Pituitary Gland		
acromegaly (ak-roh-MEG-ah-lee)	acr/o = extremities -megaly = enlarged	Chronic disease of adults that results in an elongation and enlargement of the bones of the head and extremities. There can also be mood changes. Due to an excessive amount of growth hormone in an adult.
■ **Figure 11.13** Skull X-ray (lateral view) of person with acromegaly showing abnormally enlarged mandible. *(Zephyr/Science Source)*		
diabetes insipidus (DI) (dye-ah-BEE-teez / in-SIP-ih-dus)		Disorder caused by the inadequate secretion of antidiuretic hormone by the posterior lobe of the pituitary gland. There may be polyuria and polydipsia.
dwarfism (DWARF-izm)	-ism = state of	Condition of being abnormally short in height. It may be the result of a hereditary condition or a lack of growth hormone.
gigantism (JYE-gan-tizm)	-ism = state of	Excessive development of the body due to the overproduction of the growth hormone by the pituitary gland in a child or teenager. The opposite of *dwarfism*.
hyperpituitarism (HIGH-per-pih-TOO-ih-tuh-rizm)	hyper- = excessive pituitar/o = pituitary gland -ism = state of	Hypersecretion of one or more pituitary gland hormones.
hypopituitarism (HIGH-poh-pih-TOO-ih-tuh-rizm)	hypo- = insufficient pituitar/o = pituitary gland -ism = state of	Hyposecretion of one or more pituitary gland hormones.
panhypopituitarism (pan-high-poh-pih-TOO-ih-tuh-rizm)	pan- = all hypo- = insufficient pituitar/o = pituitary gland -ism = state of	Deficiency in all the hormones secreted by the pituitary gland. Often recognized because of problems with the glands regulated by the pituitary—adrenal cortex, thyroid, ovaries, and testes.

Pathology (continued)

Term	Word Parts	Definition
Thymus Gland		
thymitis (thigh-MY-tis)	thym/o = thymus gland -itis = inflammation	Inflammation of the thymus gland.
thymoma (thigh-MOH-mah)	thym/o = thymus gland -oma = tumor	A tumor in the thymus gland.
Thyroid Gland		
congenital hypothyroidism (high-poh-THIGH-royd-izm)	hypo- = below thyroid/o = thyroid gland -ism = state of	Congenital condition in which a lack of thyroid hormones may result in arrested physical and mental development. Formerly called *cretinism*.
goiter (GOY-ter) ■ **Figure 11.14** Goiter. A photograph of a male with an extreme goiter or enlarged thyroid gland. *(Eugene Gordon, Pearson Education)*		Enlargement of the thyroid gland.
Graves' disease		Condition named for Irish physician Robert Graves that results in overactivity of the thyroid gland and can cause a crisis situation. Symptoms include exophthalmos and goiter. A type of *hyperthyroidism.*
Hashimoto's thyroiditis (hash-ee-MOH-tohz / thigh-roy-DYE-tis)	thyroid/o = thyroid gland -itis = inflammation	Chronic autoimmune form of thyroiditis; results in hyposecretion of thyroid hormones.
hyperthyroidism (high-per-THIGH-royd-izm)	hyper- = excessive thyroid/o = thyroid gland -ism = state of	Hypersecretion of thyroid gland hormones.
hypothyroidism (high-poh-THIGH-royd-izm)	hypo- = insufficient thyroid/o = thyroid gland -ism = state of	Hyposecretion of thyroid gland hormones.
myxedema (miks-eh-DEE-mah)	-edema = swelling	Condition resulting from a hyposecretion of the thyroid gland in an adult. Symptoms can include swollen facial features, edematous skin, anemia, slow speech, drowsiness, and mental lethargy.

Pathology (continued)

Term	Word Parts	Definition
thyrotoxicosis (thigh-roh-toks-ih-KOH-sis)	thyr/o = thyroid gland toxic/o = poison -osis = abnormal condition	Condition resulting from marked overproduction of the thyroid gland. Symptoms include rapid heart action, tremors, enlarged thyroid gland, exophthalmos, and weight loss.
All Glands		
adenocarcinoma (ad-eh-no-car-sih-NO-mah)	aden/o = gland carcin/o = cancer -oma = tumor	Cancerous tumor in a gland that is capable of producing the hormones secreted by that gland. One cause of hypersecretion pathologies.

Practice As You Go

C. Terminology Matching

Match each term to its definition.

1. ________ Cushing's disease	a. enlarged thyroid
2. ________ goiter	b. overactive adrenal cortex
3. ________ acromegaly	c. hyperthyroidism
4. ________ gigantism	d. underactive adrenal cortex
5. ________ myxedema	e. enlarged bones of head and extremities
6. ________ diabetes mellitus	f. may cause polyuria and polydipsia
7. ________ diabetes insipidus	g. an autoimmune disease
8. ________ Hashimoto's thyroiditis	h. excessive growth hormone in a child
9. ________ Graves' disease	i. disorder of carbohydrate metabolism
10. ________ Addison's disease	j. insufficient thyroid hormone in an adult

Diagnostic Procedures

Term	Word Parts	Definition
Clinical Laboratory Tests		
blood serum test		Blood test to measure the level of substances such as calcium, electrolytes, testosterone, insulin, and glucose. Used to assist in determining the function of various endocrine glands.
fasting blood sugar (FBS)		Blood test to measure the amount of sugar circulating throughout the body after a 12-hour fast.

Diagnostic Procedures (continued)

Term	Word Parts	Definition
glucose tolerance test (GTT) (GLOO-kohs)		Test to determine the blood sugar level. A measured dose of glucose is given to a patient either orally or intravenously. Blood samples are then drawn at certain intervals to determine the ability of the patient to use glucose. Used for diabetic patients to determine their insulin response to glucose.
protein-bound iodine test (PBI)		Blood test to measure the concentration of thyroxine (T_4) circulating in the bloodstream. The iodine becomes bound to the protein in the blood and can be measured. Useful in establishing thyroid function.
radioimmunoassay (RIA) (ray-dee-oh-im-yoo-noh-ASS-ay)	**radi/o** = ray **immun/o** = protection	Blood test that uses radioactively tagged hormones and antibodies to measure the quantity of hormone in the plasma.
thyroid function test (TFT) (THIGH-royd)		Blood test used to measure the levels of thyroxine, triiodothyronine, and thyroid-stimulating hormone in the bloodstream to assist in determining thyroid function.
total calcium		Blood test to measure the total amount of calcium to assist in detecting parathyroid and bone disorders.
two-hour postprandial glucose tolerance test (post-PRAN-dee-al)	**post-** = after **-prandial** = pertaining to a meal	Blood test to assist in evaluating glucose metabolism. The patient eats a high-carbohydrate diet and then fasts overnight before the test. Then the blood sample is taken two hours after a meal.
Diagnostic Imaging		
thyroid echography (THIGH-royd / eh-KOG-rah-fee)	**-graphy** = process of recording	Ultrasound examination of the thyroid that can assist in distinguishing a thyroid nodule from a cyst.
thyroid scan (THIGH-royd)		Test in which radioactive iodine is administered that localizes in the thyroid gland. The gland can then be visualized with a scanning device to detect pathology such as tumors.

Therapeutic Procedures

Term	Word Parts	Definition
Medical Procedures		
chemical thyroidectomy (thigh-royd-EK-toh-mee)	**chem/o** = drug **-al** = pertaining to **thyroid/o** = thyroid gland **-ectomy** = surgical removal	Large dose of radioactive iodine (RAI) is given in order to kill thyroid gland cells without having to actually do surgery.
glucometer (glue-COM-eh-ter)	**gluc/o** = glucose **-meter** = instrument to measure	Device designed for a diabetic to use at home to measure the level of glucose in the bloodstream.
hormone replacement therapy (HRT)		Artificial replacement of hormones in patients with hyposecretion disorders. May be oral pills, injections, or adhesive skin patches.

Therapeutic Procedures (continued)

Term	Word Parts	Definition
Surgical Procedures		
adrenalectomy (ad-ree-nal-EK-toh-mee)	adrenal/o = adrenal gland -ectomy = surgical removal	Surgical removal of one or both adrenal glands.
laparoscopic adrenalectomy (lap-row-SKOP-ik / ad-ree-nal-EK-toh-mee)	lapar/o = abdomen -scopic = pertaining to visually examining adren/o = adrenal gland -ectomy = surgical removal	Removal of the adrenal gland through a small incision in the abdomen and using endoscopic instruments.
lobectomy (lobe-EK-toh-mee)	lob/o = lobe -ectomy = surgical removal	Removal of a lobe from an organ. In this case, one lobe of the thyroid gland.
parathyroidectomy (pair-ah-thigh-royd-EK-toh-mee)	parathyroid/o = parathyroid gland -ectomy = surgical removal	Surgical removal of one or more of the parathyroid glands.
pinealectomy (PIN-ee-ah-LEK-toh-mee)	pineal/o = pineal gland -ectomy = surgical removal	Surgical removal of the pineal gland.
thymectomy (thigh-MEK-toh-mee)	thym/o = thymus gland -ectomy = surgical removal	Surgical removal of the thymus gland.
thyroidectomy (thigh-royd-EK-toh-mee)	thyroid/o = thyroid gland -ectomy = surgical removal	Surgical removal of the thyroid gland.

Practice As You Go

D. Terminology Matching

Match the term to its definition.

1. ________ protein-bound iodine test
2. ________ fasting blood sugar
3. ________ radioimmunoassay
4. ________ thyroid scan
5. ________ two-hour postprandial glucose tolerance test
6. ________ glucose tolerance test
7. ________ glucometer
8. ________ chemical thyroidectomy

a. measures levels of hormones in the blood
b. determines glucose metabolism after patient receives a measured dose of glucose
c. test of glucose metabolism two hours after eating a meal
d. measures blood sugar level after 12-hour fast
e. measures T_4 concentration in the blood
f. uses radioactive iodine
g. used instead of a surgical procedure
h. instrument to measure blood glucose

Pharmacology

Classification	Word Parts	Action	Examples
antithyroid agents	anti- = against	Block production of thyroid hormones in patients with hypersecretion disorders.	methimazole, Tapazole; propylthiouracil
corticosteroids (kor-tih-koh-STAIR-oydz)	cortic/o = outer layer	Although the function of these hormones in the body is to regulate carbohydrate metabolism, they also have a strong anti-inflammatory action. Therefore they are used to treat severe chronic inflammatory diseases such as rheumatoid arthritis. Long-term use has adverse side effects such as osteoporosis and the symptoms of Cushing's disease. Also used to treat adrenal cortex hyposecretion disorders such as Addison's disease.	prednisone, Deltasone
human growth hormone therapy		Hormone replacement therapy with human growth hormone in order to stimulate skeletal growth. Used to treat children with abnormally short stature.	somatropin, Genotropin; somatrem, Protropin
insulin (IN-suh-lin)		Replaces insulin for type 1 diabetics or treats severe type 2 diabetics.	human insulin, Humulin L
oral hypoglycemic agents (high-poh-glye-SEE-mik)	or/o = mouth -al = pertaining to hypo- = insufficient glyc/o = sugar -emic = relating to a blood condition	Taken by mouth to cause a decrease in blood sugar; not used for insulin-dependent patients.	metformin, Glucophage; glipizide, Glucotrol
thyroid replacement hormone		Hormone replacement therapy for patients with hypothyroidism or who have had a thyroidectomy.	levothyroxine, Levo-T; liothyronine, Cytomel
vasopressin (vaz-oh-PRESS-in)	vas/o = vessel -pressin = to press down	Controls diabetes insipidus and promotes reabsorption of water in the kidney tubules.	desmopressin acetate, Desmopressin; conivaptan, Vaprisol

Abbreviations

α	alpha	**LH**	luteinizing hormone
ACTH	adrenocorticotropic hormone	**MSH**	melanocyte-stimulating hormone
ADH	antidiuretic hormone	**Na^+**	sodium
β	beta	**NIDDM**	non-insulin-dependent diabetes mellitus
BMR	basal metabolic rate	**NPH**	neutral protamine Hagedorn (insulin)
CT	calcitonin	**PBI**	protein-bound iodine
DI	diabetes insipidus	**PRL**	prolactin
DM	diabetes mellitus	**PTH**	parathyroid hormone
FBS	fasting blood sugar	**RAI**	radioactive iodine
FSH	follicle-stimulating hormone	**RIA**	radioimmunoassay
GH	growth hormone	**T_3**	triiodothyronine
GTT	glucose tolerance test	**T_4**	thyroxine
HRT	hormone replacement therapy	**TFT**	thyroid function test
IDDM	insulin-dependent diabetes mellitus	**TSH**	thyroid-stimulating hormone
K^+	potassium		

Practice As You Go

E. What's the Abbreviation?

1. non-insulin-dependent diabetes mellitus ____________________
2. insulin-dependent diabetes mellitus ____________________
3. adrenocorticotropic hormone ____________________
4. parathyroid hormone ____________________
5. triiodothyronine ____________________
6. thyroid-stimulating hormone ____________________
7. fasting blood sugar ____________________
8. prolactin ____________________

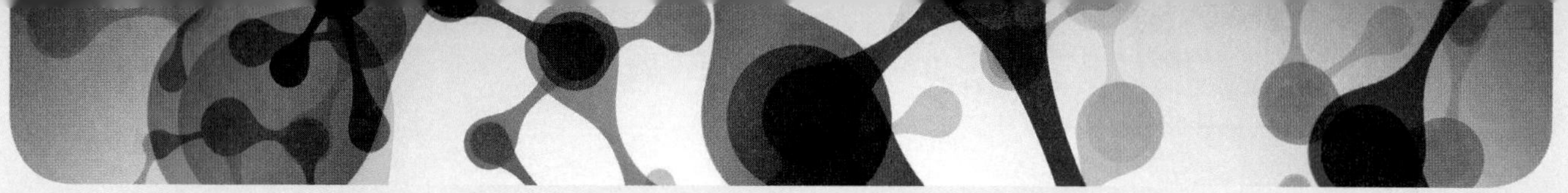

Chapter Review

Real-World Applications

Medical Record Analysis

This Discharge Summary below contains 10 medical terms. Underline each term and write it in the list below the report. Then define each term.

Discharge Summary

Admitting Diagnosis:	Hyperglycemia, ketoacidosis, glycosuria
Final Diagnosis:	New-onset type 1 diabetes mellitus
History of Present Illness:	A 12-year-old female patient presented to her physician's office with a two-month history of weight loss, fatigue, polyuria, and polydipsia. Her family history is significant for a grandfather, mother, and older brother with type 1 diabetes mellitus. The pediatrician found hyperglycemia with a fasting blood sugar and glycosuria with a urine dipstick. She is being admitted at this time for management of new-onset diabetes mellitus.
Summary of Hospital Course:	At the time of admission, the FBS was 300 mg/100 mL and she was in ketoacidosis. She rapidly improved after receiving insulin; her blood glucose level normalized. The next day a glucose tolerance test confirmed the diagnosis of diabetes mellitus. The patient was started on insulin injections. Patient and family were instructed on diabetes mellitus, insulin, diet, exercise, and long-term complications.
Discharge Plans:	Patient was discharged to home with her parents. Her parents are to check her blood glucose levels twice daily and call the office for insulin dosage. She is to return to the office in two weeks.

	Term	Definition
1.	______________	______________________________
2.	______________	______________________________
3.	______________	______________________________
4.	______________	______________________________
5.	______________	______________________________
6.	______________	______________________________
7.	______________	______________________________
8.	______________	______________________________
9.	______________	______________________________
10.	______________	______________________________

Chart Note Transcription

The chart note below contains 11 phrases that can be reworded with a medical term that you learned in this chapter. Each phrase is identified with an underline. Determine the medical term and write your answers in the space provided.

Pearson General Hospital Consultation Report

Task Edit View Time Scale Options Help Download Archive Date: 17 May 2015

Current Complaint: A 56-year-old female was referred to the specialist in the treatment of diseases of the endocrine glands **1** for evaluation of weakness, edema, an abnormal amount of fat in the body, **2** and an excessive amount of hair for a female. **3**

Past History: Patient reports she has been overweight most of her life in spite of a healthy diet and regular exercise. She was diagnosed with osteoporosis after incurring a pathological rib fracture following a coughing attack.

Signs and Symptoms: Patient has moderate edema in bilateral feet and lower legs as well as a puffy face and an upper lip moustache. She is 100 lbs. over normal body weight for her age and height. She moves slowly and appears generally lethargic. A test to measure the hormone levels in the blood plasma **4** reports increased steroid hormone that regulates carbohydrates in the body. **5** A CT scan demonstrates a gland tumor **6** in the right outer layer of the adrenal gland. **7**

Diagnosis: A group of symptoms associated with hypersecretion of the adrenal cortex **8** secondary to a gland tumor **9** in the right outer layer of the adrenal gland. **10**

Treatment: Surgical removal of the right adrenal gland. **11**

1. ______________________________
2. ______________________________
3. ______________________________
4. ______________________________
5. ______________________________
6. ______________________________
7. ______________________________
8. ______________________________
9. ______________________________
10. ______________________________
11. ______________________________

Case Study

Below is a case study presentation of a patient with a condition covered in this chapter. Read the case study and answer the questions below. Some questions will ask for information not included within this chapter. Use your text, a medical dictionary, or any other reference material you choose to answer these questions.

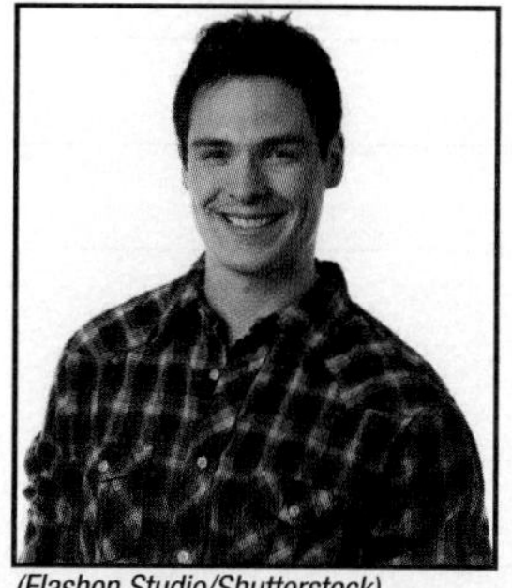

(Flashon Studio/Shutterstock)

A 22-year-old college student was admitted to the emergency room after his friends called an ambulance when he passed out in a bar. He had become confused, developed slurred speech, and had difficulty walking after having only consumed one beer. In the ER he was noted to have diaphoresis, rapid respirations and pulse, and was disoriented. Upon examination, needle marks were found on his abdomen and outer thighs. The physician ordered blood serum tests that revealed hyperglycemia and ketoacidosis. Unknown to his friends, this young man has had diabetes mellitus since early childhood. The patient quickly recovered following an insulin injection.

Questions

1. What pathological condition has this patient had since childhood? Look this condition up in a reference source and include a short description of it.

____

____

2. List and define each symptom noted in the ER in your own words.

____

____

3. What diagnostic test was performed? Describe it in your own words.

____

____

4. Explain the results of the test.

____

____

5. What specific type of diabetes does this young man probably have? Justify your answer.

____

____

6. Describe the other type of diabetes mellitus that this young man did not have.

____

____

Practice Exercises

A. Word Building Practice

The combining form **thyroid/o** refers to the thyroid. Use it to write a term that means:

1. removal of the thyroid ____________
2. pertaining to the thyroid ____________
3. state of excessive thyroid ____________

The combining form **pancreat/o** refers to the pancreas. Use it to write a term that means:

4. pertaining to the pancreas ____________
5. inflammation of the pancreas ____________
6. removal of the pancreas ____________
7. cutting into the pancreas ____________

The combining form **adren/o** refers to the adrenal glands. Use it to write a term that means:

8. pertaining to the adrenal glands ____________
9. enlargement of an adrenal gland ____________
10. adrenal gland disease ____________

The combining form **thym/o** refers to the thymus gland. Use it to write a term that means:

11. tumor of the thymus gland ____________
12. removal of the thymus gland ____________
13. pertaining to the thymus gland ____________
14. inflammation of the thymus gland ____________

B. Define the Combining Form

	Definition	Example from Chapter
1. **natr/o**	____________	____________
2. **estr/o**	____________	____________
3. **pineal/o**	____________	____________
4. **pituitar/o**	____________	____________
5. **kal/i**	____________	____________
6. **calc/o**	____________	____________
7. **parathyroid/o**	____________	____________
8. **acr/o**	____________	____________
9. **glyc/o**	____________	____________
10. **gonad/o**	____________	____________

C. What Does it Stand For?

1. PBI ______
2. K^+ ______
3. T_4 ______
4. GTT ______
5. DM ______
6. BMR ______
7. Na^+ ______
8. ADH ______

D. Suffix Practice

Use the following suffixes to create medical terms for the following definitions.

-pressin	**-uria**	**-tropin**
-dipsia	**-emia**	**-prandial**

1. the presence of sugar or glucose in the urine ______
2. to press down a vessel ______
3. excessive urination ______
4. condition of excessive calcium in the blood ______
5. excessive thirst ______
6. to stimulate the gonads ______
7. after a meal ______

E. Define the Term

1. corticosteroid ______
2. hirsutism ______
3. tetany ______
4. diabetic retinopathy ______
5. hyperglycemia ______
6. hypoglycemia ______
7. adrenaline ______
8. insulin ______
9. thyrotoxicosis ______
10. hypersecretion ______

F. Fill in the Blank

insulinoma	ketoacidosis	pheochromocytoma
gynecomastia	panhypopituitarism	Hashimoto's thyroiditis

1. The doctor found that Marsha's high level of insulin and hypoglycemia was caused by a(n) ______________________.
2. Kevin developed ______________________ as a result of his diabetes mellitus and required emergency treatment.
3. It was determined that Karen had ______________________ when doctors realized she had problems with her thyroid gland, adrenal cortex, and ovaries.
4. Luke's high epinephrine level was caused by a(n) ______________________.
5. When it was determined that Carl's thyroiditis was an autoimmune condition, it became obvious that he had ________.
6. Excessive sex hormones caused Jack to develop ______________________.

G. Pharmacology Challenge

Fill in the classification for each drug description, then match the brand name.

	Drug Description	Classification	Brand Name
1.	________ strong anti-inflammatory	______________	a. genotropin
2.	________ stimulates skeletal growth	______________	b. Desmopressin
3.	________ treats type 1 diabetes mellitus	______________	c. Tapazole
4.	________ blocks production of thyroid hormone	______________	d. Glucophage
5.	________ treats type 1 diabetes mellitus	______________	e. Deltasone
6.	________ controls diabetes insipidus	______________	f. Humulin

Labeling Exercise

Image A

Write the labels for this figure on the numbered lines provided.

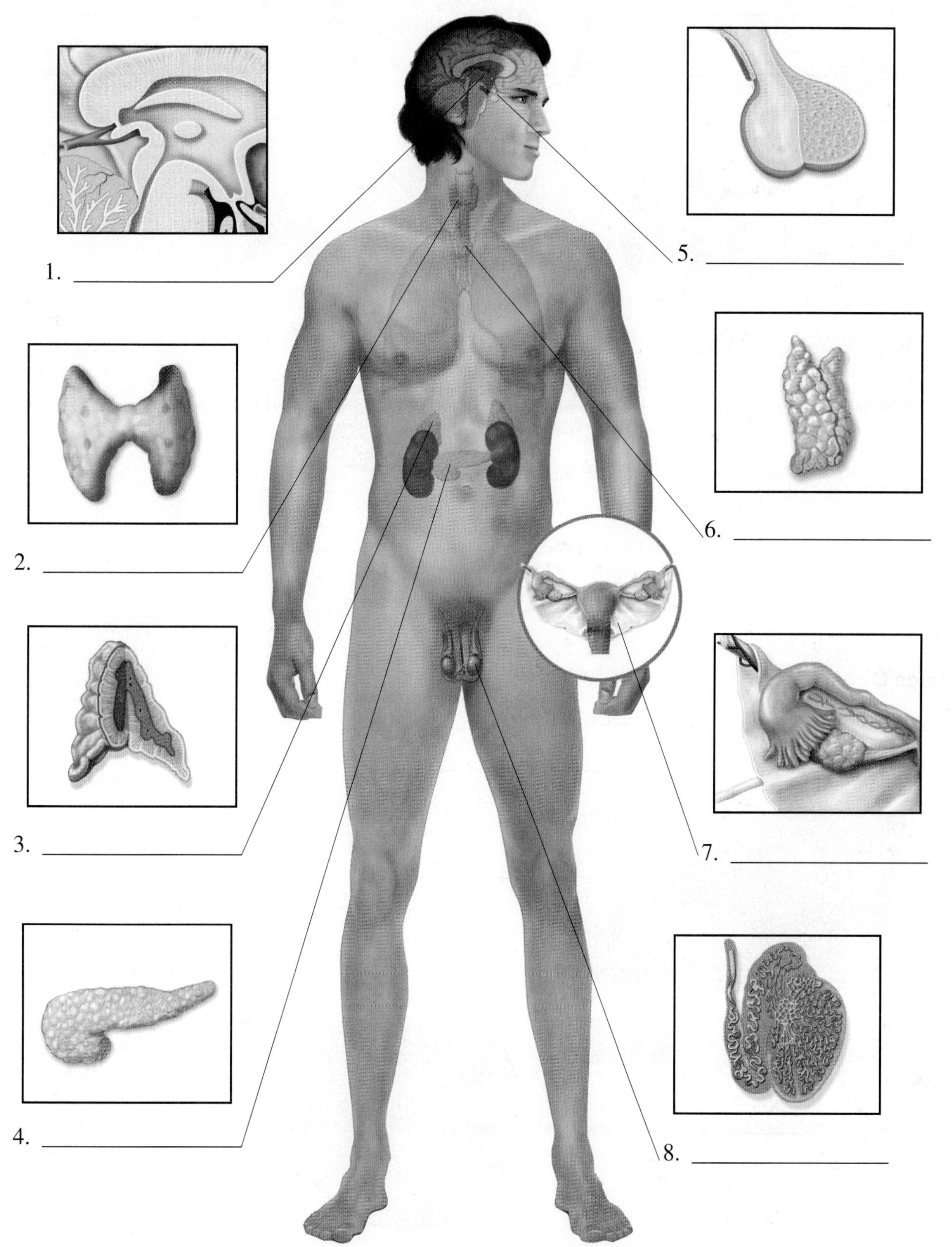

Image B

Write the labels for this figure on the numbered lines provided.

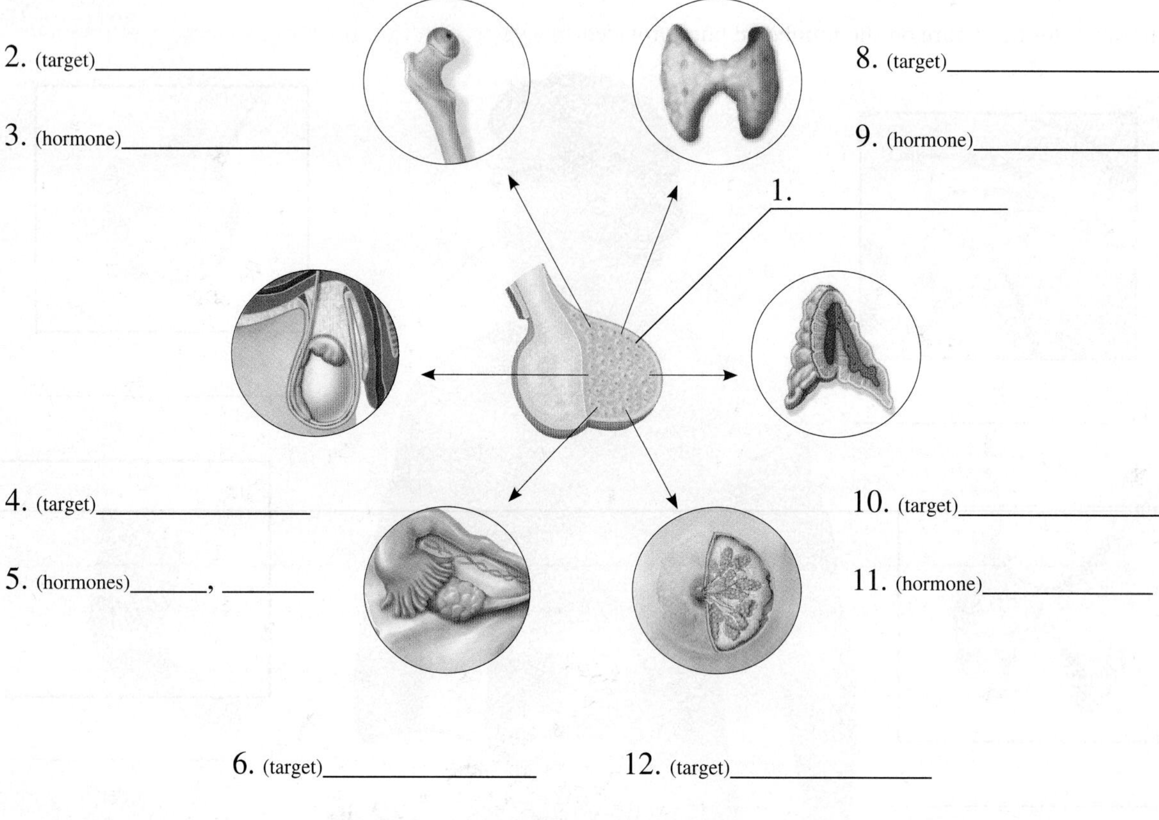

Image C

Write the labels for this figure on the numbered lines provided.

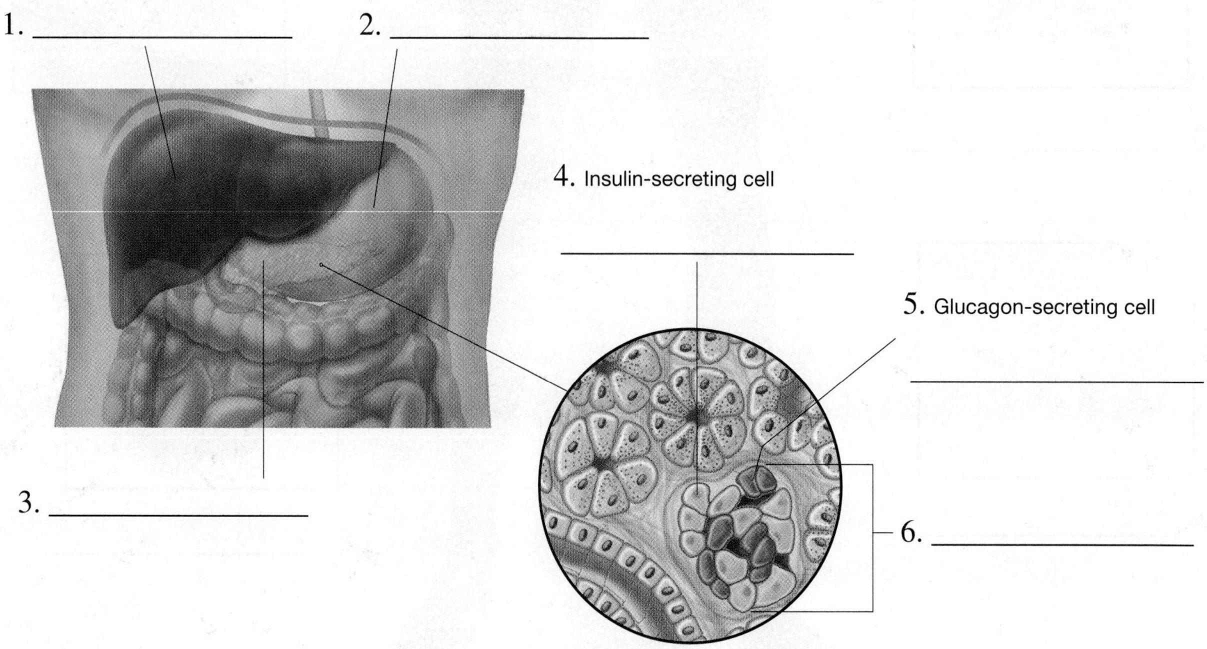

12

Nervous System

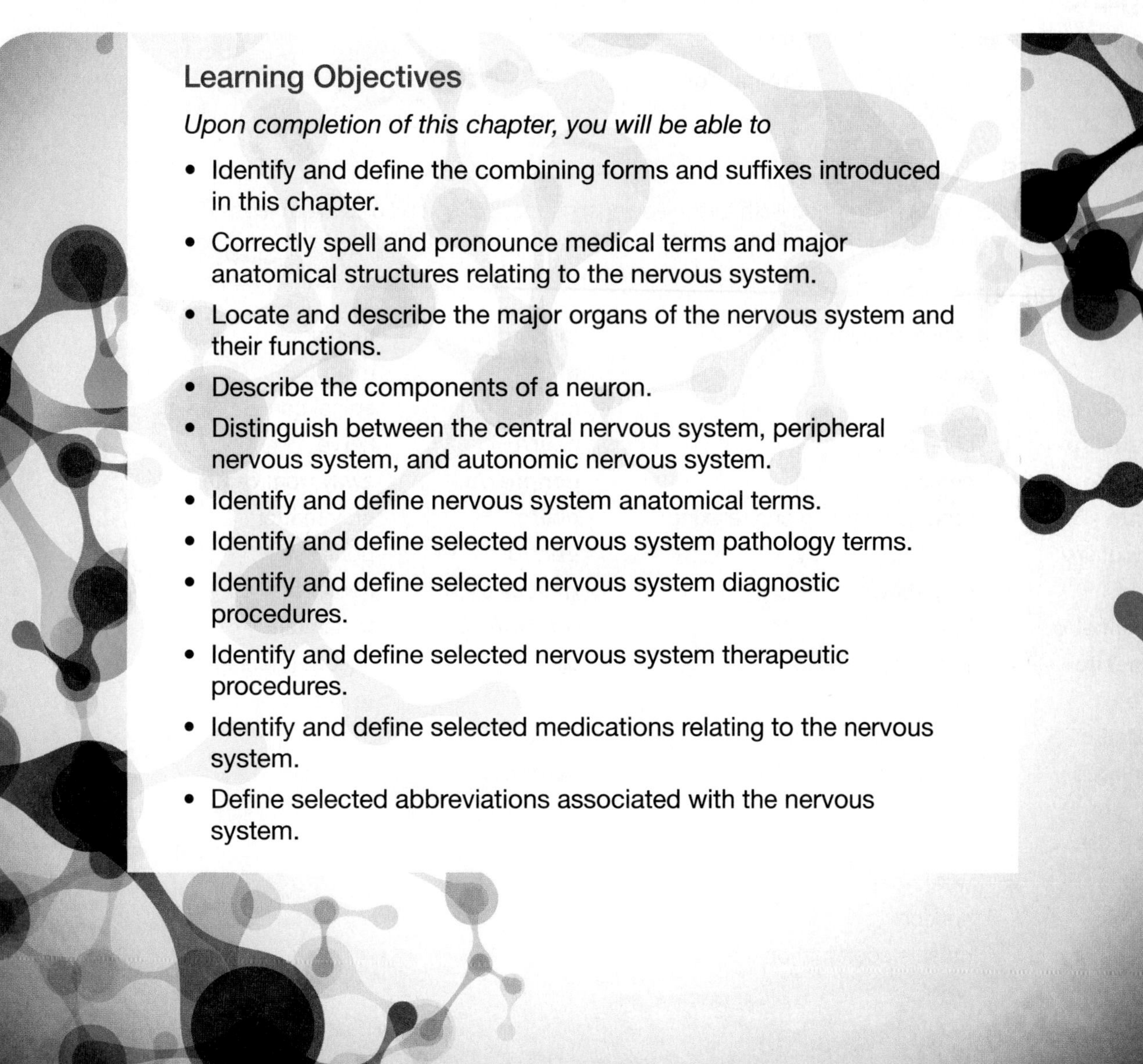

Learning Objectives

Upon completion of this chapter, you will be able to

- Identify and define the combining forms and suffixes introduced in this chapter.
- Correctly spell and pronounce medical terms and major anatomical structures relating to the nervous system.
- Locate and describe the major organs of the nervous system and their functions.
- Describe the components of a neuron.
- Distinguish between the central nervous system, peripheral nervous system, and autonomic nervous system.
- Identify and define nervous system anatomical terms.
- Identify and define selected nervous system pathology terms.
- Identify and define selected nervous system diagnostic procedures.
- Identify and define selected nervous system therapeutic procedures.
- Identify and define selected medications relating to the nervous system.
- Define selected abbreviations associated with the nervous system.

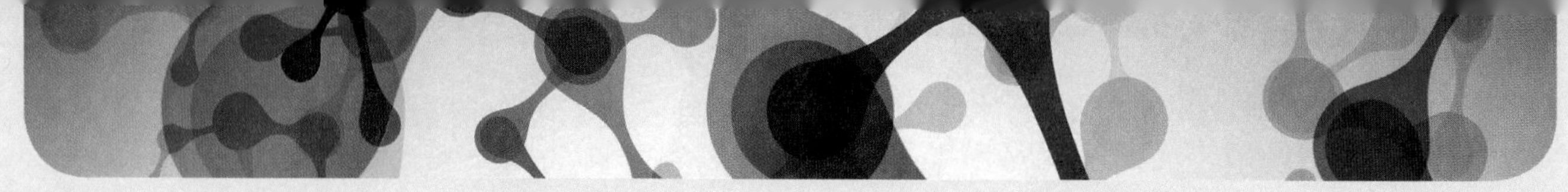

Nervous System at a Glance

Function

The nervous system coordinates and controls body function. It receives sensory input, makes decisions, and then orders body responses.

Organs

Here are the primary structures that comprise the nervous system:

brain
nerves
spinal cord

Word Parts

Here are the most common word parts (with their meanings) used to build nervous system terms. For a more comprehensive list, refer to the Terminology section of this chapter.

Combining Forms

alges/o	sense of pain
astr/o	star
centr/o	center
cerebell/o	cerebellum
cerebr/o	cerebrum
clon/o	rapid contracting and relaxing
concuss/o	to shake violently
dur/o	dura mater
encephal/o	brain
esthesi/o	sensation, feeling
gli/o	glue
medull/o	medulla oblongata
mening/o	meninges
meningi/o	meninges
ment/o	mind
myel/o	spinal cord
neur/o	nerve
peripher/o	away from center
poli/o	gray matter
pont/o	pons
radicul/o	nerve root
thalam/o	thalamus
thec/o	sheath (meninges)
tom/o	to cut
ton/o	tone
ventricul/o	ventricle

Suffixes

-paresis	weakness
-phasia	speech
-taxia	muscle coordination

Nervous System Illustrated

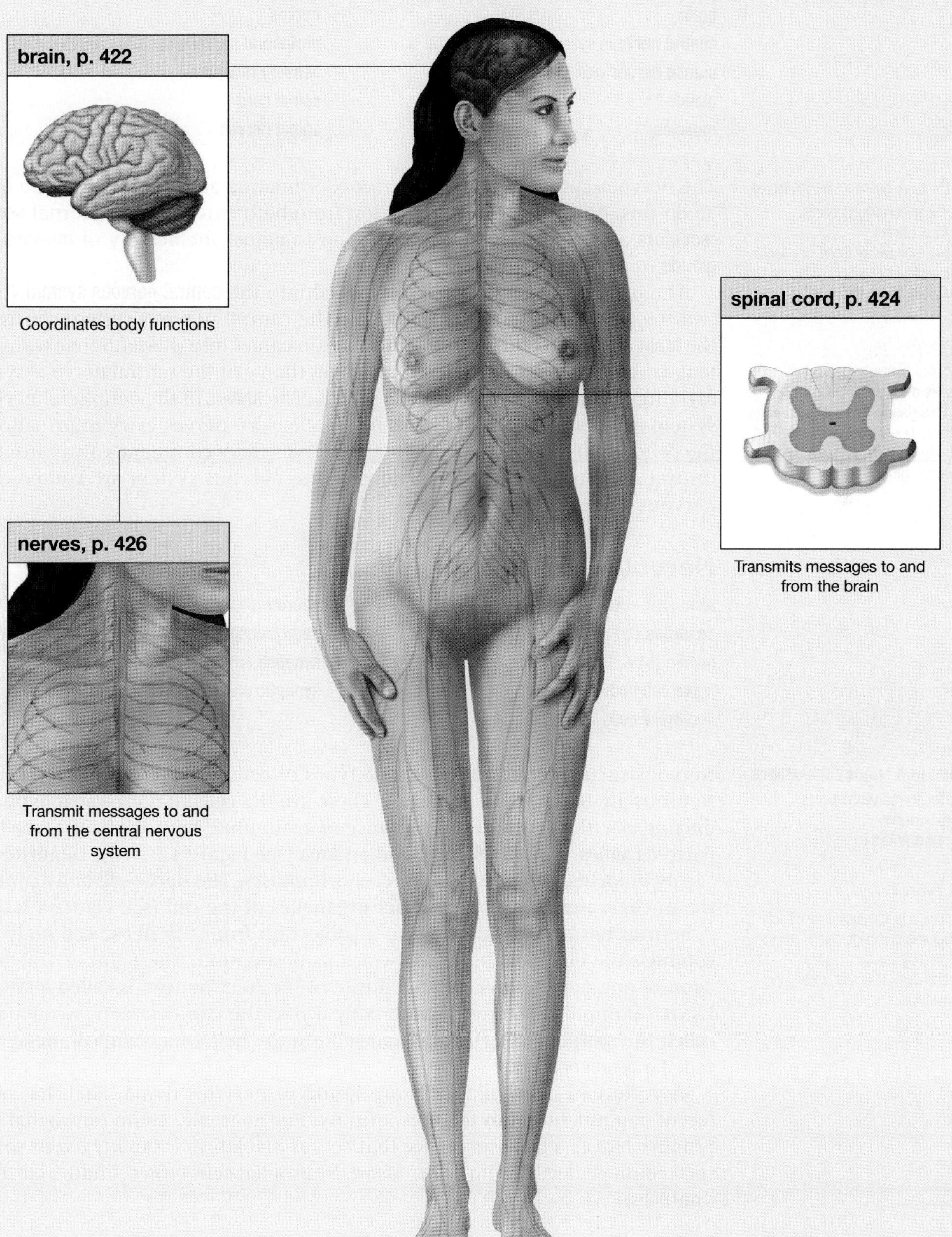

Anatomy and Physiology of the Nervous System

brain
central nervous system
cranial nerves (KRAY-nee-al)
glands
muscles
nerves
peripheral nervous system (per-IF-er-al)
sensory receptors
spinal cord
spinal nerves

What's In A Name?
Look for these word parts:
centr/o = center
peripher/o = away from center
-al = pertaining to
-ory = pertaining to

Med Term Tip
Neuroglial tissue received its name as a result of its function. This tissue holds neurons together. Therefore, it was called *neuroglial*, a term literally meaning "nerve glue."

The nervous system is responsible for coordinating all the activity of the body. To do this, it first receives information from both external and internal **sensory receptors** and then uses that information to adjust the activity of **muscles** and **glands** to match the needs of the body.

The nervous system can be subdivided into the **central nervous system** (CNS) and the **peripheral nervous system** (PNS). The central nervous system consists of the **brain** and **spinal cord**. Sensory information comes into the central nervous system, where it is processed. Motor messages then exit the central nervous system carrying commands to muscles and glands. The **nerves** of the peripheral nervous system are **cranial nerves** and **spinal nerves**. Sensory nerves carry information to the central nervous system, and motor nerves carry commands away from the central nervous system. All portions of the nervous system are composed of nervous tissue.

Nervous Tissue

axon (AK-son)
dendrites (DEN-drights)
myelin (MY-eh-lin)
nerve cell body
neuroglial cells (noo-ROH-glee-all)
neuron (NOO-ron)
neurotransmitter (noo-roh-TRANS-mit-ter)
synapse (sih-NAPSE)
synaptic cleft (sih-NAP-tik)

What's In A Name?
Look for these word parts:
neur/o = nerve
-tic = pertaining to

Med Term Tip
A synapse is the point at which two nerves contact each other. The term *synapse* comes from the Greek word meaning "connection."

Nervous tissue consists of two basic types of cells: **neurons** and **neuroglial cells**. Neurons are individual nerve cells. These are the cells that are capable of conducting electrical impulses in response to a stimulus. Neurons have three basic parts: **dendrites**, a **nerve cell body**, and an **axon** (see Figure 12.1A ■). Dendrites are highly branched projections that receive impulses. The nerve cell body contains the nucleus and many of the other organelles of the cell (see Figure 12.1B ■). A neuron has only a single axon, a projection from the nerve cell body that conducts the electrical impulse toward its destination. The point at which the axon of one neuron meets the dendrite of the next neuron is called a **synapse**. Electrical impulses cannot pass directly across the gap between two neurons, called the **synaptic cleft**. They instead require the help of a chemical messenger, called a **neurotransmitter**.

A variety of neuroglial cells are found in nervous tissue. Each has a different support function for the neurons. For example, some neuroglial cells produce **myelin**, a fatty substance that acts as insulation for many axons so that they conduct electrical impulses faster. Neuroglial cells *do not* conduct electrical impulses.

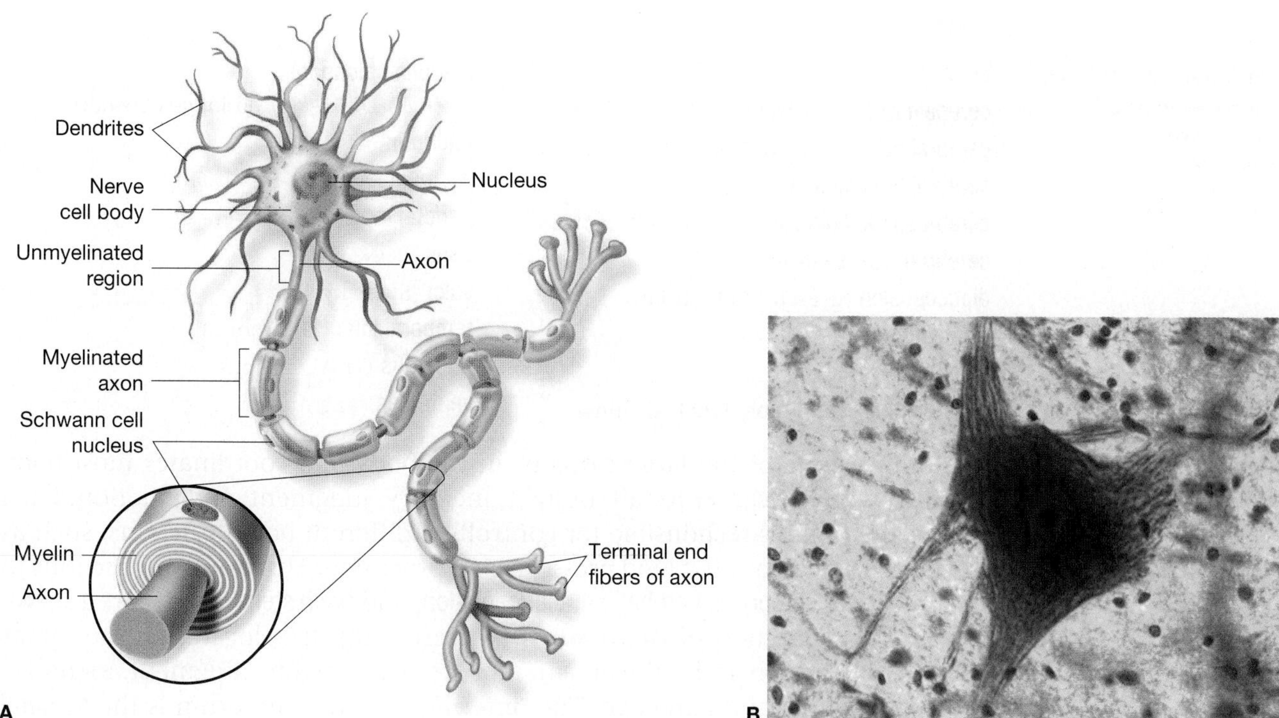

■ **Figure 12.1** A) The structure of a neuron, showing the dendrites, nerve cell body, and axon. B) Photomicrograph of typical neuron showing the nerve cell body, nucleus, and dendrites. *(Christopher Meade/Shutterstock)*

Central Nervous System

gray matter
meninges (men-IN-jeez)
myelinated (MY-eh-lih-nayt-ed)
tract
white matter

Because the central nervous system is a combination of the brain and spinal cord, it is able to receive impulses from all over the body, process this information, and then respond with an action. This system consists of both **gray matter** and **white matter.** Gray matter is comprised of unsheathed or uncovered cell bodies and dendrites. White matter is **myelinated** nerve fibers (see Figure 12.2■). The myelin sheath makes the nervous tissue appear white. Bundles of nerve fibers interconnecting different parts of the central nervous system are called **tracts.** The central nervous system is encased and protected by three membranes known as the **meninges.**

Med Term Tip

Myelin is a lipid and a very white molecule. This is why myelinated neurons are called *white matter*.

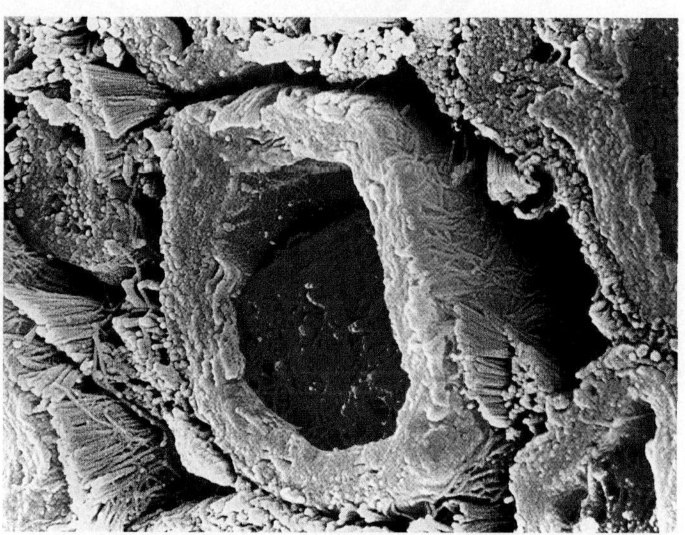

■ **Figure** 12.2 Electronmicrograph illustrating an axon (red) wrapped in its myelin sheath (blue). *(Quest/Science Photo Library/Science Source)*

Brain

What's In A Name?

Look for these word parts:
encephal/o = brain
-al = pertaining to
hypo- = below

brain stem
cerebellum (ser-eh-BELL-um)
cerebral cortex (seh-REE-bral / KOR-teks)
cerebral hemisphere
cerebrospinal fluid (ser-eh-broh-SPY-nal)
cerebrum (SER-eh-brum)
diencephalon (dye-en-SEFF-ah-lon)
frontal lobe
gyri (JYE-rye)
hypothalamus (high-poh-THAL-ah-mus)
medulla oblongata (meh-DULL-ah / ob-long-GAH-tah)
midbrain
occipital lobe (ock-SIP-ih-tal)
parietal lobe (pah-RYE-eh-tal)
pons (PONZ)
sulci (SULL-kye)
temporal lobe (TEM-por-al)
thalamus (THAL-ah-mus)
ventricles (VEN-trik-lz)

The brain is one of the largest organs in the body and coordinates most body activities. It is the center for all thought, memory, judgment, and emotion. Each part of the brain is responsible for controlling different body functions, such as temperature regulation, blood pressure, and breathing. There are four sections to the brain: the **cerebrum**, **cerebellum**, **diencephalon**, and **brain stem** (see Figure 12.3 ■).

The largest section of the brain is the cerebrum. It is located in the upper portion of the brain and is the area that processes thoughts, judgment, memory, problem solving, and language. The outer layer of the cerebrum is the **cerebral**

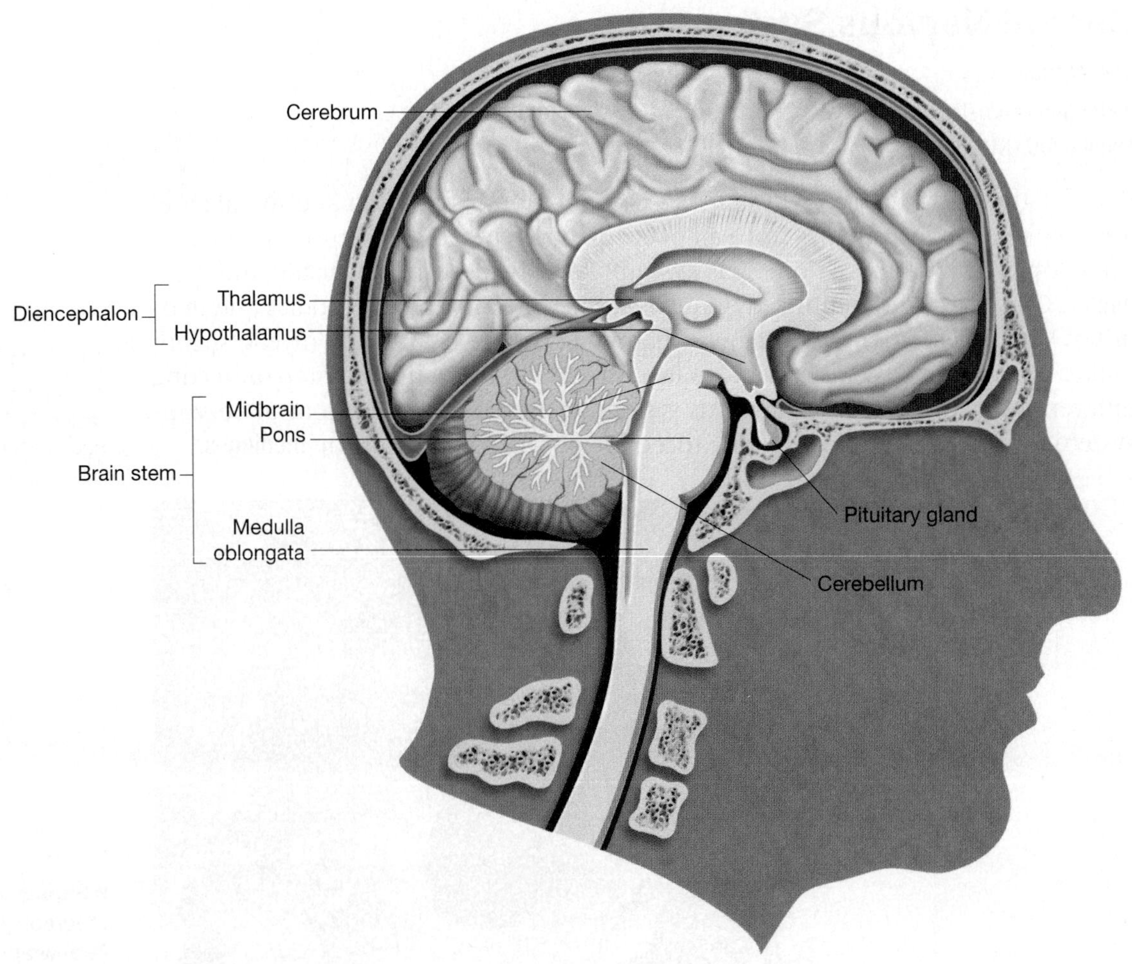

■ **Figure 12.3** The regions of the brain.

cortex, which is composed of folds of gray matter. The elevated portions of the cerebrum, or convolutions, are called **gyri** and are separated by fissures, or valleys, called **sulci**. The cerebrum is subdivided into left and right halves called **cerebral hemispheres**. Each hemisphere has four lobes. The lobes and their locations and functions are as follows (see Figure 12.4 ■):

1. **Frontal lobe:** Most anterior portion of the cerebrum; controls motor function, personality, and speech
2. **Parietal lobe:** Most superior portion of the cerebrum; receives and interprets nerve impulses from sensory receptors and interprets language
3. **Occipital lobe:** Most posterior portion of the cerebrum; controls vision
4. **Temporal lobe:** Left and right lateral portion of the cerebrum; controls hearing and smell

The diencephalon, located below the cerebrum, contains two of the most critical areas of the brain, the **thalamus** and the **hypothalamus**. The thalamus is composed of gray matter and acts as a center for relaying impulses from the eyes, ears, and skin to the cerebrum. Our pain perception is controlled by the thalamus. The hypothalamus, located just below the thalamus, controls body temperature, appetite, sleep, sexual desire, and emotions. The hypothalamus is actually responsible for controlling the autonomic nervous system, cardiovascular system, digestive system, and the release of hormones from the pituitary gland.

The cerebellum, the second largest portion of the brain, is located beneath the posterior part of the cerebrum. This part of the brain aids in coordinating voluntary body movements and maintaining balance and equilibrium. The cerebellum refines the muscular movement that is initiated in the cerebrum.

The final portion of the brain is the brain stem. This area has three components: **midbrain**, **pons**, and **medulla oblongata**. The midbrain acts as a pathway for impulses to be conducted between the brain and the spinal cord. The pons—a

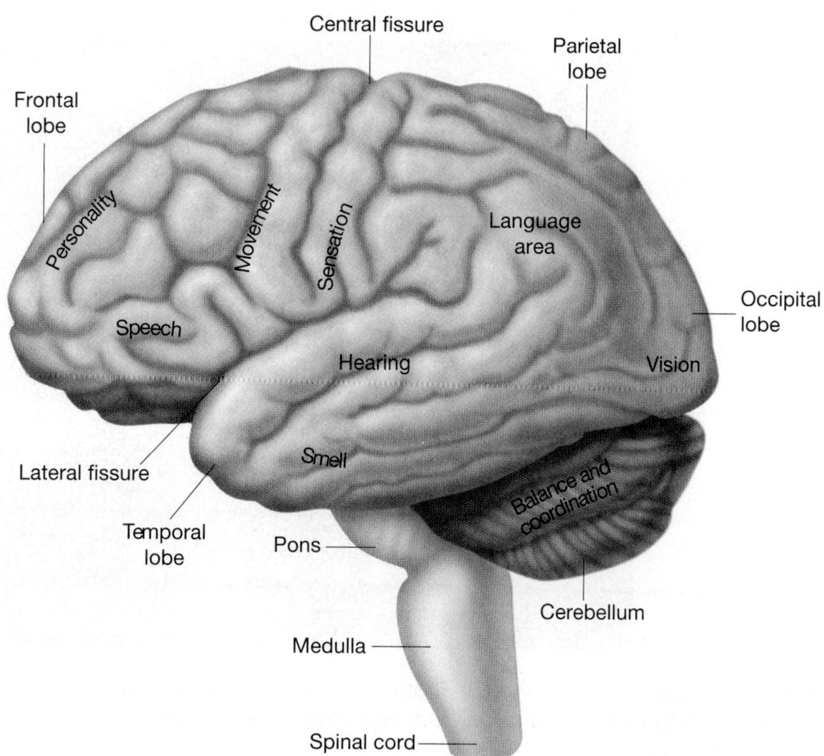

■ **Figure 12.4** The functional regions of the cerebrum.

term meaning "bridge"—connects the cerebellum to the rest of the brain. The medulla oblongata is the most inferior positioned portion of the brain; it connects the brain to the spinal cord. However, this vital area contains the centers that control respiration, heart rate, temperature, and blood pressure. Additionally, this is the site where nerve tracts cross from one side of the brain to control functions and movement on the other side of the body. In other words, with few exceptions, the left side of the brain controls the right side of the body and vice versa.

The brain has four interconnected cavities called **ventricles**: one in each cerebral hemisphere, one in the thalamus, and one in front of the cerebellum. These contain **cerebrospinal fluid** (CSF), which is the watery, clear fluid that provides protection from shock or sudden motion to the brain and spinal cord.

Spinal Cord

ascending tracts
central canal
descending tracts
spinal cavity
vertebral canal
vertebral column

The function of the spinal cord is to provide a pathway for impulses traveling to and from the brain. The spinal cord is actually a column of nervous tissue extending from the medulla oblongata of the brain down to the level of the second lumbar vertebra within the **vertebral column**. The 33 vertebrae of the backbone line up to form a continuous canal for the spinal cord called the **spinal cavity** or **vertebral canal** (see Figure 12.5■).

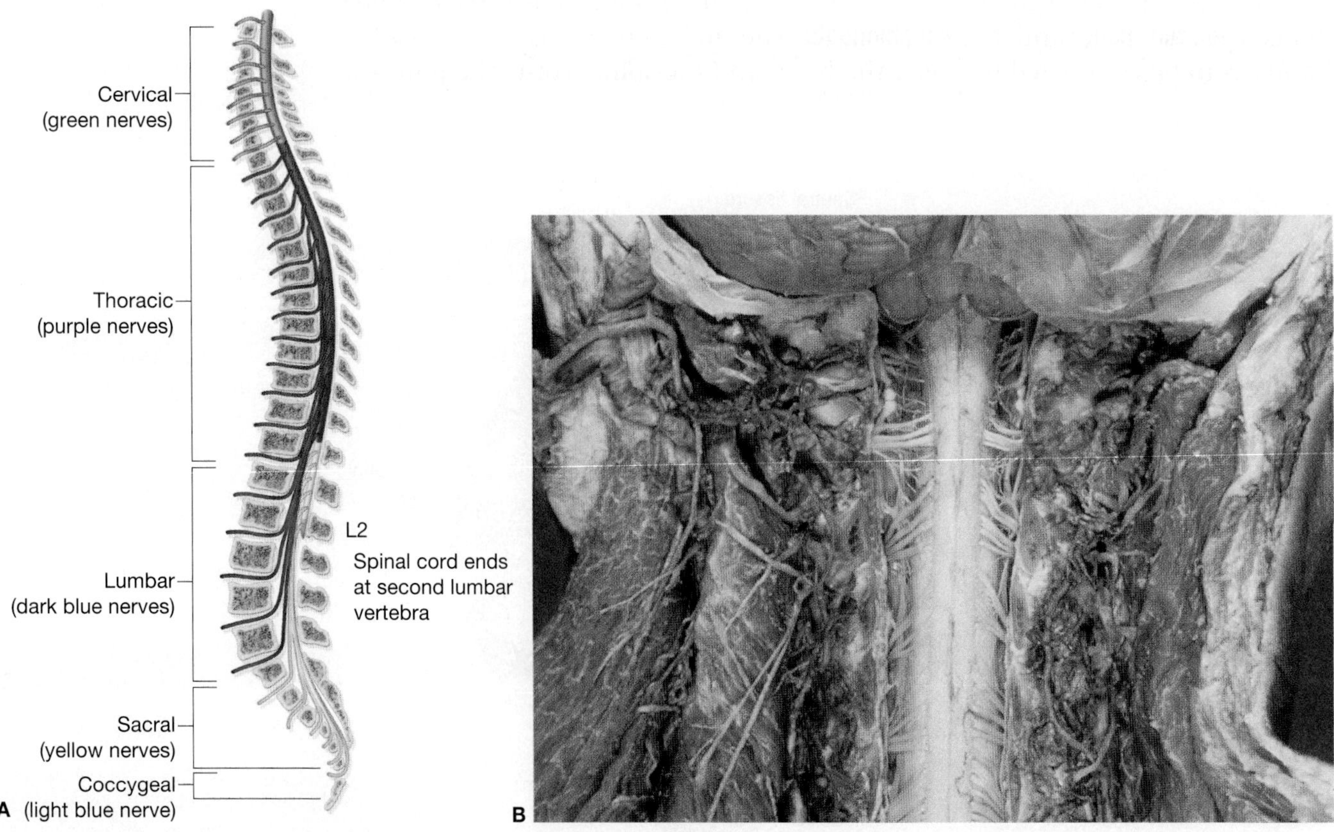

■ **Figure 12.5** A) The levels of the spinal cord and spinal nerves. B) Photograph of the spinal cord as it descends from the brain. The spinal nerve roots are clearly visible branching off from the spinal cord. *(VideoSurgery/Science Source)*

Similar to the brain, the spinal cord is also protected by cerebrospinal fluid. It flows down the center of the spinal cord within the **central canal**. The inner core of the spinal cord consists of cell bodies and dendrites of peripheral nerves and therefore is gray matter. The outer portion of the spinal cord is myelinated white matter. The white matter is either **ascending tracts** carrying sensory information up to the brain or **descending tracts** carrying motor commands down from the brain to a peripheral nerve.

Med Term Tip

Certain disease processes attack the gray matter and the white matter of the central nervous system. For instance, *poliomyelitis* is a viral infection of the gray matter of the spinal cord. The combining term *poli/o* means "gray matter." This disease has almost been eradicated, due to the polio vaccine.

Meninges

arachnoid layer (ah-RAK-noyd)
dura mater (DOO-rah / MATE-er)
pia mater (PEE-ah / MATE-er)
subarachnoid space (sub-ah-RAK-noyd)
subdural space (sub-DOO-ral)

What's In A Name?

Look for these word parts:
-oid = resembling
sub- = under

The meninges are three layers of connective tissue membranes surrounding the brain and spinal cord (see Figure 12.6■). Moving from external to internal, the meninges are:

1. **Dura mater:** Meaning "tough mother"; it forms a tough, fibrous sac around the central nervous system
2. **Subdural space:** Actual space between the dura mater and arachnoid layers
3. **Arachnoid layer:** Meaning "spiderlike"; it is a thin, delicate layer attached to the pia mater by weblike filaments
4. **Subarachnoid space:** Space between the arachnoid layer and the pia mater; it contains cerebrospinal fluid that cushions the brain from the outside
5. **Pia mater:** Meaning "soft mother"; it is the innermost membrane layer and is applied directly to the surface of the brain and spinal cord

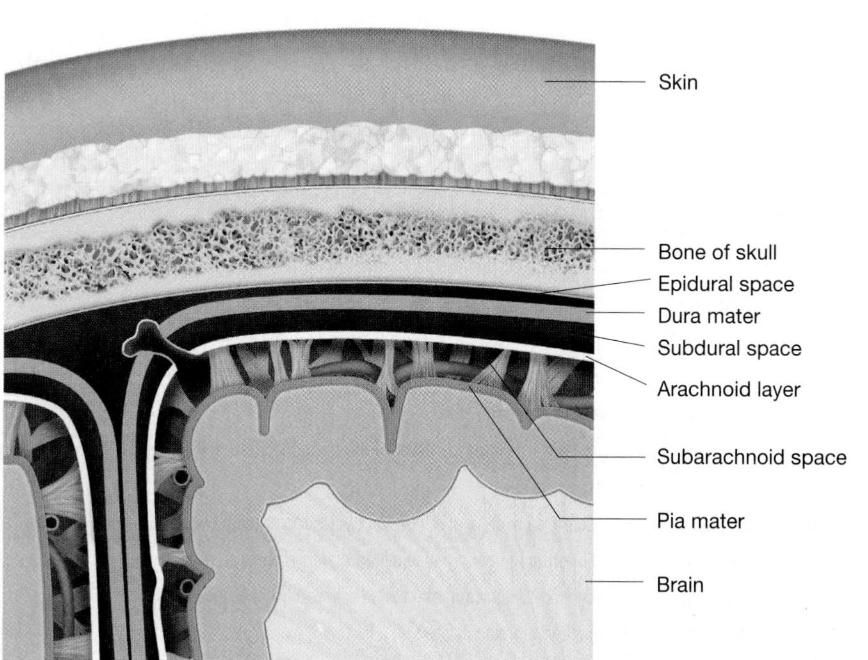

■ **Figure 12.6** The meninges. This figure illustrates the location and structure of each layer of the meninges and their relationship to the skull and brain.

What's In A Name?

Look for these word parts:
somat/o = body
-ic = pertaining to
auto- = self

Med Term Tip

Because nerve tracts cross from one side of the body to the other side of the brain, damage to one side of the brain results in symptoms appearing on the opposite side of the body. Since nerve cells that control the movement of the right side of the body are located in the left side of the medulla oblongata, a stroke that paralyzed the right side of the body would actually have occurred in the left side of the brain.

Peripheral Nervous System

afferent neurons (AFF-er-ent)
autonomic nervous system (aw-toh-NOM-ik)
efferent neurons (EFF-er-ent)
ganglion (GANG-lee-on)
motor neurons
nerve root
sensory neurons
somatic nerves

The peripheral nervous system (PNS) includes both the 12 pairs of cranial nerves and the 31 pairs of spinal nerves. A nerve is a group or bundle of axon fibers located outside the central nervous system that carries messages between the central nervous system and the various parts of the body. Whether a nerve is cranial or spinal is determined by where the nerve originates. Cranial nerves arise from the brain, mainly at the medulla oblongata. Spinal nerves split off from the spinal cord, and one pair (a left and a right) exits between each pair of vertebrae. The point where either type of nerve is attached to the central nervous system is called the **nerve root**. The names of most nerves reflect either the organ the nerve serves or the portion of the body the nerve is traveling through. The entire list of cranial nerves is found in Table 12.1 ■. Figure 12.7 ■ illustrates some of the major spinal nerves in the human body.

Although most nerves carry information to and from the central nervous system, individual neurons carry information in only one direction. **Afferent neurons**, also called **sensory neurons**, carry sensory information from a sensory receptor to the central nervous system. **Efferent neurons**, also called **motor neurons**, carry activity instructions from the central nervous system to muscles or glands out in the body (see Figure 12.8 ■). The nerve cell bodies of the neurons forming the nerve are grouped together in a knot-like mass, called a **ganglion**, located outside the central nervous system.

The nerves of the peripheral nervous system are subdivided into two divisions, the **autonomic nervous system** (ANS) and **somatic nerves**, each serving a different area of the body.

Med Term Tip

The term *autonomic* comes from the Latin word *autonomia*, meaning independent.

Autonomic Nervous System

parasympathetic branch (pair-ah-sim-pah-THET-ik)
sympathetic branch (sim-pah-THET-ik)

The autonomic nervous system is involved with the control of involuntary or unconscious bodily functions. It may increase or decrease the activity of the smooth muscle found in viscera and blood vessels, cardiac muscle, and glands.

Table 12.1 Cranial Nerves

Number	Name	Function
I	Olfactory	Transports impulses for sense of smell.
II	Optic	Carries impulses for sense of sight.
III	Oculomotor	Motor impulses for eye muscle movement and the pupil of the eye.
IV	Trochlear	Controls superior oblique muscle of eye on each side.
V	Trigeminal	Carries sensory facial impulses and controls muscles for chewing; branches into eyes, forehead, upper and lower jaw.
VI	Abducens	Controls an eyeball muscle to turn eye to side.
VII	Facial	Controls facial muscles for expression, salivation, and taste on two-thirds of tongue (anterior).
VIII	Vestibulocochlear	Responsible for impulses of equilibrium and hearing; also called *auditory nerve.*
IX	Glossopharyngeal	Carries sensory impulses from pharynx (swallowing) and taste on one-third of tongue.
X	Vagus	Supplies most organs in abdominal and thoracic cavities.
XI	Accessory	Controls the neck and shoulder muscles.
XII	Hypoglossal	Controls tongue muscles.

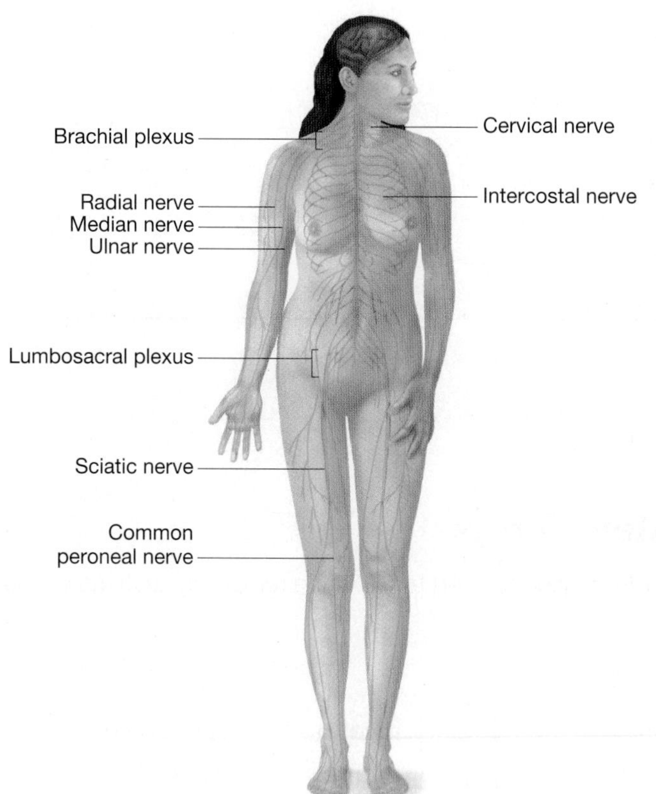

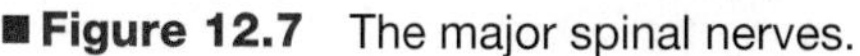
■ **Figure 12.7** The major spinal nerves.

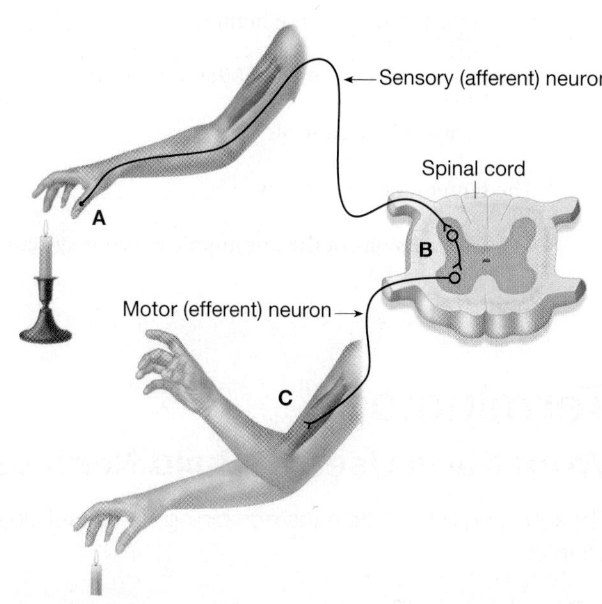

■ **Figure 12.8** The functional structure of the peripheral nervous system. A) Afferent or sensory neurons carry sensory information to the spinal cord. B) The spinal cord receives incoming sensory information and delivers motor messages. C) Efferent or motor neurons deliver motor commands to muscles and glands.

The autonomic nervous system is divided into two branches: **sympathetic branch** and **parasympathetic branch**. The sympathetic nerves control the "fight-or-flight" reaction during times of stress and crisis. These nerves increase heart rate, dilate airways, increase blood pressure, inhibit digestion, and stimulate the production of adrenaline during a crisis. The parasympathetic nerves serve as a counterbalance for the sympathetic nerves, the "rest-and-digest" reaction. Therefore, they cause heart rate to slow down, lower blood pressure, and stimulate digestion.

What's In A Name?

Look for these word parts:
-ic = pertaining to
para- = beside

Somatic Nerves

Somatic nerves serve the skin and skeletal muscles and are mainly involved with the conscious and voluntary activities of the body. The large variety of sensory receptors found in the dermis layer of the skin use somatic nerves to send their information, such as touch, temperature, pressure, and pain, to the brain. These are also the nerves that carry motor commands to skeletal muscles.

Practice As You Go

A. Complete the Statement

1. The organs of the nervous system are the ____________, ____________, and ____________.
2. The two divisions of the nervous system are the ____________ and ____________.
3. The neurons that carry impulses away from the brain and spinal cord are called ____________ neurons and the neurons that carry impulses to the brain and spinal cord are called ____________ neurons.

4. The largest portion of the brain is the ___________________.

5. The second largest portion of the brain is the ___________________.

6. The occipital lobe controls ___________________.

7. The temporal lobe controls ___________________ and ___________________.

8. The two divisions of the autonomic nervous system are the ___________________ and ___________________.

Terminology

Word Parts Used to Build Nervous System Terms

The following lists contain the combining forms, suffixes, and prefixes used to build terms in the remaining sections of this chapter.

Combining Forms

alges/o	sense of pain
angi/o	vessel
arteri/o	artery
astr/o	star
cephal/o	head
cerebell/o	cerebellum
cerebr/o	cerebrum
clon/o	rapid contracting and relaxing
concuss/o	to shake violently
crani/o	skull
cyt/o	cell
dur/o	dura mater
electr/o	electricity

encephal/o	brain
esthesi/o	sensation, feeling
gli/o	glue
hemat/o	blood
hem/o	blood
hydr/o	water
isch/o	to hold back
later/o	side
lumb/o	low back
medull/o	medulla oblongata
mening/o	meninges
meningi/o	meninges
ment/o	mind
my/o	muscle

myel/o	spinal cord
neur/o	nerve
poli/o	gray matter
pont/o	pons
radicul/o	nerve root
scler/o	hard
spin/o	spine
thalam/o	thalamus
thec/o	sheath
tom/o	to cut
ton/o	tone
vascul/o	blood vessel
ventricul/o	ventricle
vertebr/o	vertebra

Suffixes

-al	pertaining to
-algia	pain
-ar	pertaining to
-ary	pertaining to
-asthenia	weakness
-cele	protrusion
-eal	pertaining to
-ectomy	surgical removal
-gram	record
-graphy	process of recording

-ia	condition, state
-ic	pertaining to
-ine	pertaining to
-ion	action
-itis	inflammation
-logy	study of
-nic	pertaining to
-oma	tumor, mass
-osis	abnormal condition
-otomy	cutting into

-paresis	weakness
-pathy	disease
-phasia	speech
-plasty	surgical repair
-plegia	paralysis
-rrhaphy	suture
-taxia	muscle coordination
-tic	pertaining to
-trophic	pertaining to development

Prefixes

a-	without
an-	without
anti-	against
bi-	two
de-	without
dys-	abnormal, difficult
endo-	within

epi-	above
hemi-	half
hyper-	excessive
intra-	within
mono-	one
para-	abnormal, two like parts of a pair

poly-	many
quadri-	four
semi-	partial
sub-	under
un-	not

Adjective Forms of Anatomical Terms

Term	Word Parts	Definition
cerebellar (ser-eh-BELL-ar)	cerebell/o = cerebellum -ar = pertaining to	Pertaining to the cerebellum.
cerebral (seh-REE-bral)	cerebr/o = cerebrum -al = pertaining to	Pertaining to the cerebrum.
cerebrospinal (ser-eh-broh-SPY-nal)	cerebr/o = cerebrum spin/o = spine -al = pertaining to	Pertaining to the cerebrum and spine.
cranial (KRAY-nee-al)	crani/o = skull -al = pertaining to	Pertaining to the skull.
encephalic (EN-seh-FAL-ik)	encephal/o = brain -ic = pertaining to	Pertaining to the brain.
intracranial (in-tra-KRAY-nee-al)	intra- = within crani/o = skull -al = pertaining to	Pertaining to within the skull.
intrathecal (in-tra-THEE-kal)	intra- = within thec/o = sheath -al = pertaining to	Pertaining to within the meninges, specifically the subdural or subarachnoid space.
medullary (MED-yoo-lair-ee)	medull/o = medulla oblongata -ary = pertaining to	Pertaining to the medulla oblongata.
meningeal (meh-NIN-jee-all)	mening/o = meninges -eal = pertaining to	Pertaining to the meninges.
myelonic (MY-eh-LON-ik)	myel/o = spinal cord -nic = pertaining to	Pertaining to the spinal cord.
neural (NOO-rall)	neur/o = nerve -al = pertaining to	Pertaining to nerves.
neuroglial (noo-ROG-lee-al)	neur/o = nerve gli/o = glue -al = pertaining to	Pertaining to the support cells, glial cells, of nerves.
pontine (pon-TEEN)	pont/o = pons -ine = pertaining to	Pertaining to the pons.
spinal (SPY-nal)	spin/o = spine -al = pertaining to	Pertaining to the spine.
subdural (sub-DOO-ral)	sub- = under dur/o = dura mater -al = pertaining to	Pertaining to under the dura mater.

Adjective Forms of Anatomical Terms (continued)

Term	Word Parts	Definition
thalamic (tha-LAM-ik)	thalam/o = thalamus -ic = pertaining to	Pertaining to the thalamus.
ventricular (ven-TRIK-yoo-lar)	ventricul/o = ventricle -ar = pertaining to	Pertaining to the ventricles.
vertebral (VER-teh-bral)	vertebr/o = vertebra -al = pertaining to	Pertaining to the vertebrae.

Practice As You Go

B. Give the adjective form for each anatomical structure

1. The cerebrum and spinal cord ______________________________
2. The meninges ______________________________
3. Under the dura mater ______________________________
4. The brain ______________________________
5. A nerve ______________________________
6. Within the skull ______________________________

Pathology

Term	Word Parts	Definition
Medical Specialties		
anesthesiology (AN-es-thee-zee-OL-oh-jee)	an- = without esthesi/o = sensation, feeling -logy = study of	Branch of medicine specializing in all aspects of anesthesia, including for surgical procedures, resuscitation measures, and the management of acute and chronic pain. Physician is an *anesthesiologist.*
neurology (noo-ROL-oh-jee)	neur/o = nerve -logy = study of	Branch of medicine concerned with diagnosis and treatment of diseases and conditions of the nervous system. Physician is a *neurologist.*
neurosurgery (noo-roh-SIR-jury)	neur/o = nerve	Branch of medicine concerned with treating conditions and diseases of the nervous system by surgical means. Physician is a *neurosurgeon.*
Signs and Symptoms		
absence seizure		Type of epileptic seizure that lasts only a few seconds to half a minute, characterized by a loss of awareness and an absence of activity. It is also known as a *petit mal seizure.*
analgesia (an-al-JEE-zee-ah)	an- = without alges/o = sense of pain -ia = state	Absence of pain.

Pathology (continued)

Term	Word Parts	Definition
anesthesia (an-ess-THEE-zee-ah)	an- = without esthesi/o = feeling, sensation -ia = condition	Lack of feeling or sensation.
aphasia (ah-FAY-zee-ah)	a- = without -phasia = speech	Inability to communicate verbally or in writing due to damage of the speech or language centers in the brain.
ataxia (ah-TAK-see-ah)	a- = without -taxia = muscle coordination	Lack of muscle coordination.
aura (AW-ruh)		Sensations, such as seeing colors or smelling an unusual odor, that occur just prior to an epileptic seizure or migraine headache.
cephalalgia (seff-al-AL-jee-ah)	cephal/o = head -algia = pain	Headache (HA).
coma (COH-mah)		Profound unconsciousness resulting from an illness or injury.
conscious (KON-shus)		Condition of being awake and aware of surroundings.
convulsion (kon-VULL-shun)		Severe involuntary muscle contractions and relaxations. These have a variety of causes, such as epilepsy, fever, and toxic conditions.
delirium (dee-LEER-ee-um)	de- = without	Abnormal mental state characterized by confusion, disorientation, and agitation.
dementia (dee-MEN-she-ah)	de- = without ment/o = mind -ia = condition	Progressive impairment of intellectual function that interferes with performing activities of daily living. Patients have little awareness of their condition. Found in disorders such as Alzheimer's.
dysphasia (dis-FAY-zee-ah)	dys- = abnormal, difficult -phasia = speech	Difficulty communicating verbally or in writing due to damage of the speech or language centers in the brain.
focal seizure (FOE-kal)	-al = pertaining to	Localized seizure often affecting one limb.
hemiparesis (hem-ee-par-EE-sis)	hemi- = half -paresis = weakness	Weakness or loss of motion on one side of the body.
hemiplegia (hem-ee-PLEE-jee-ah)	hemi- = half -plegia = paralysis	Paralysis on only one side of the body.
hyperesthesia (high-per-ess-THEE-zee-ah)	hyper- = excessive esthesi/o = feeling, sensations -ia = condition	Abnormally heightened sense of feeling, sense of pain, or sensitivity to touch.
monoparesis (mon-oh-pah-REE-sis)	mono- = one -paresis = weakness	Muscle weakness in one limb.
monoplegia (mon-oh-PLEE-jee-ah)	mono- = one -plegia = paralysis	Paralysis of one limb.
neuralgia (noo-RAL-jee-ah)	neur/o = nerve -algia = pain	Nerve pain.
palsy (PAWL-zee)		Temporary or permanent loss of the ability to control movement.

Pathology (continued)

Term	Word Parts	Definition
paralysis (pah-RAL-ih-sis)		Temporary or permanent loss of function or voluntary movement.
paraplegia (pair-ah-PLEE-jee-ah)	para- = two like parts of a pair -plegia = paralysis	Paralysis of the lower portion of the body and both legs.
paresthesia (par-es-THEE-zee-ah)	para- = abnormal esthesi/o = sensation, feeling -ia = condition	Abnormal sensation such as burning or tingling.
quadriplegia (kwod-rih-PLEE-jee-ah)	quadri- = four -plegia = paralysis	Paralysis of all four limbs.
seizure (SEE-zyoor)		Sudden, uncontrollable onset of symptoms, such as in an epileptic seizure.
semiconscious (sem-ee-KON-shus)	semi- = partial	State of being aware of surroundings and responding to stimuli only part of the time.
syncope (SIN-koh-pee)		Fainting.
tonic-clonic seizure	ton/o = tone clon/o = rapid contracting and relaxing -ic = pertaining to	Type of severe epileptic seizure characterized by a loss of consciousness and convulsions. The seizure alternates between strong continuous muscle spasms (tonic) and rhythmic muscle contraction and relaxation (clonic). It is also known as a *grand mal seizure.*
tremor (TREM-or)		Involuntary, repetitive, alternating movement of a part of the body.
unconscious (un-KON-shus)	un- = not	State of being unaware of surroundings, with the inability to respond to stimuli.
Brain		
Alzheimer's disease (ALTS-high-merz)		Chronic, organic mental disorder consisting of dementia, which is more prevalent in adults after 65 years of age. Involves progressive disorientation, apathy, speech and gait disturbances, and loss of memory. Named for German neurologist Alois Alzheimer.
astrocytoma (ass-troh-sigh-TOH-mah)	astr/o = star cyt/o = cell -oma = tumor	Tumor of the brain or spinal cord composed of astrocytes, one type of neuroglial cells.
brain tumor ■ **Figure 12.9** Color-enhanced CT scan showing two malignant tumors in the brain. *(Scott Camazine/ Science Source)*	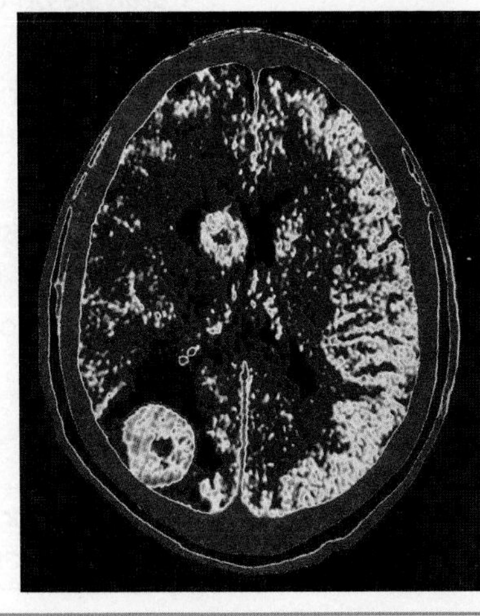	Intracranial mass, either benign or malignant. A benign tumor of the brain can still be fatal since it will grow and cause pressure on normal brain tissue.

Pathology (continued)

Term	Word Parts	Definition
cerebellitis (ser-eh-bell-EYE-tis)	cerebell/o = cerebellum -itis = inflammation	Inflammation of the cerebellum.
cerebral aneurysm (AN-yoo-rizm)	cerebr/o = cerebrum -al = pertaining to	Localized abnormal dilation of a blood vessel, usually an artery; the result of a congenital defect or weakness in the wall of the vessel. A ruptured aneurysm is a common cause of a hemorrhagic cerebrovascular accident.
cerebral contusion (kon-TOO-shun)	cerebr/o = cerebrum -al = pertaining to	Bruising of the brain from a blow or impact.
cerebral palsy (CP) (ser-REE-bral / PAWL-zee)	cerebr/o = cerebrum -al = pertaining to	Brain damage resulting from a defect, trauma, infection, or lack of oxygen before, during, or shortly after birth.
cerebrovascular accident (CVA) (ser-eh-broh-VASS-kyoo-lar)	cerebr/o = cerebrum vascul/o = blood vessel -ar = pertaining to	Development of an infarct due to loss in the blood supply to an area of the brain. Blood flow can be interrupted by a ruptured blood vessel (hemorrhage), a floating clot (embolus), a stationary clot (thrombosis), or compression. The extent of damage depends on the size and location of the infarct and often includes dysphasia and hemiplegia. Commonly called a *stroke.*

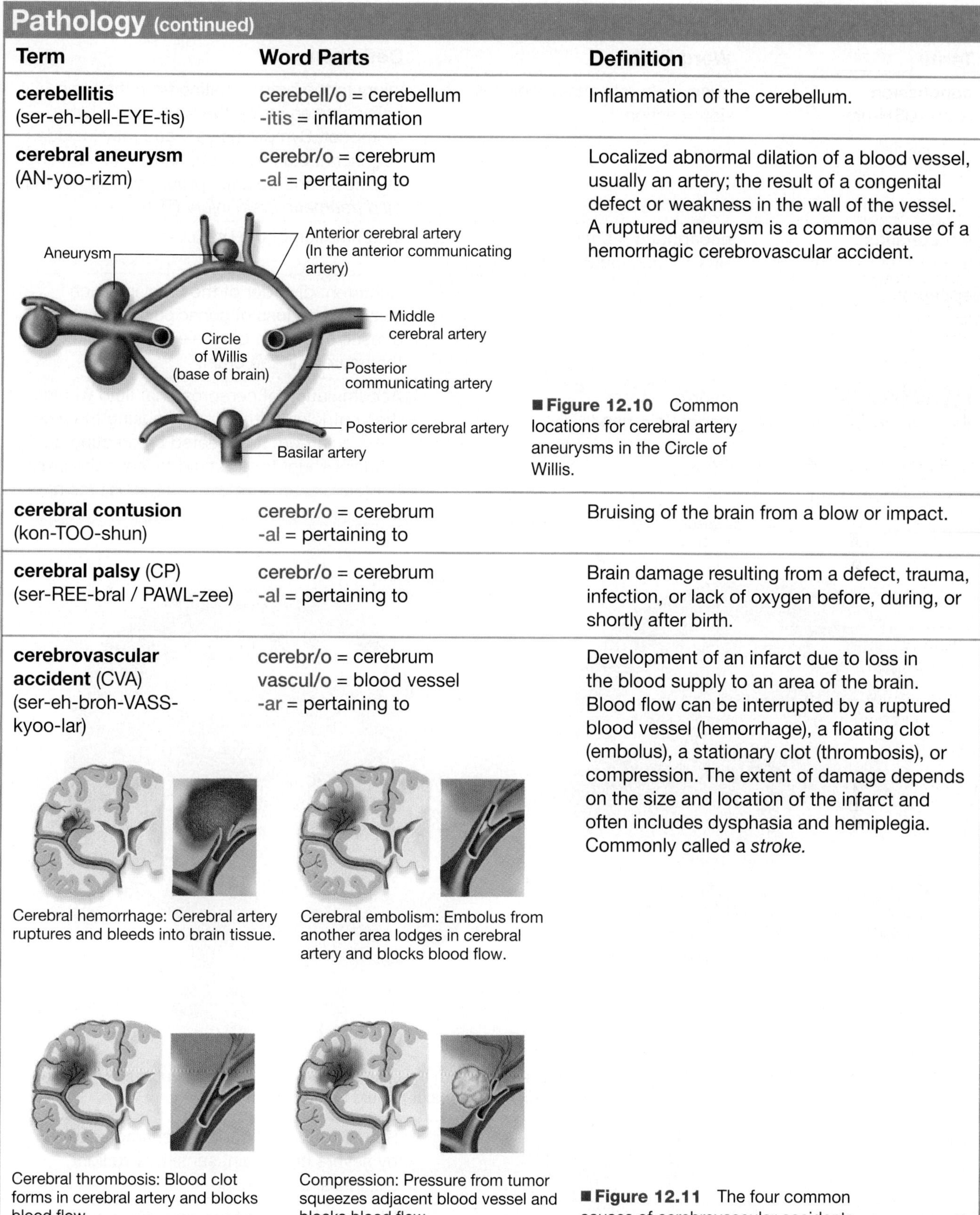

■ **Figure 12.10** Common locations for cerebral artery aneurysms in the Circle of Willis.

Cerebral hemorrhage: Cerebral artery ruptures and bleeds into brain tissue.

Cerebral embolism: Embolus from another area lodges in cerebral artery and blocks blood flow.

Cerebral thrombosis: Blood clot forms in cerebral artery and blocks blood flow.

Compression: Pressure from tumor squeezes adjacent blood vessel and blocks blood flow.

■ **Figure 12.11** The four common causes of cerebrovascular accidents.

Pathology (continued)

Term	Word Parts	Definition
concussion (kon-KUSH-un)	concuss/o = to shake violently -ion = action	Injury to the brain resulting from the brain being shaken inside the skull from a blow or impact. Symptoms vary and may include headache, blurred vision, nausea or vomiting, dizziness, and balance problems. Also called *mild traumatic brain injury* (TBI).
encephalitis (en-seff-ah-LYE-tis)	encephal/o = brain -itis = inflammation	Inflammation of the brain.
epilepsy (EP-ih-lep-see)		Recurrent disorder of the brain in which seizures and loss of consciousness occur as a result of uncontrolled electrical activity of the neurons in the brain.
hydrocephalus (high-droh-SEFF-ah-lus)	hydr/o = water cephal/o = head	Accumulation of cerebrospinal fluid within the ventricles of the brain, causing the head to be enlarged. It is treated by creating an artificial shunt for the fluid to leave the brain. If left untreated, it may lead to seizures and mental retardation.

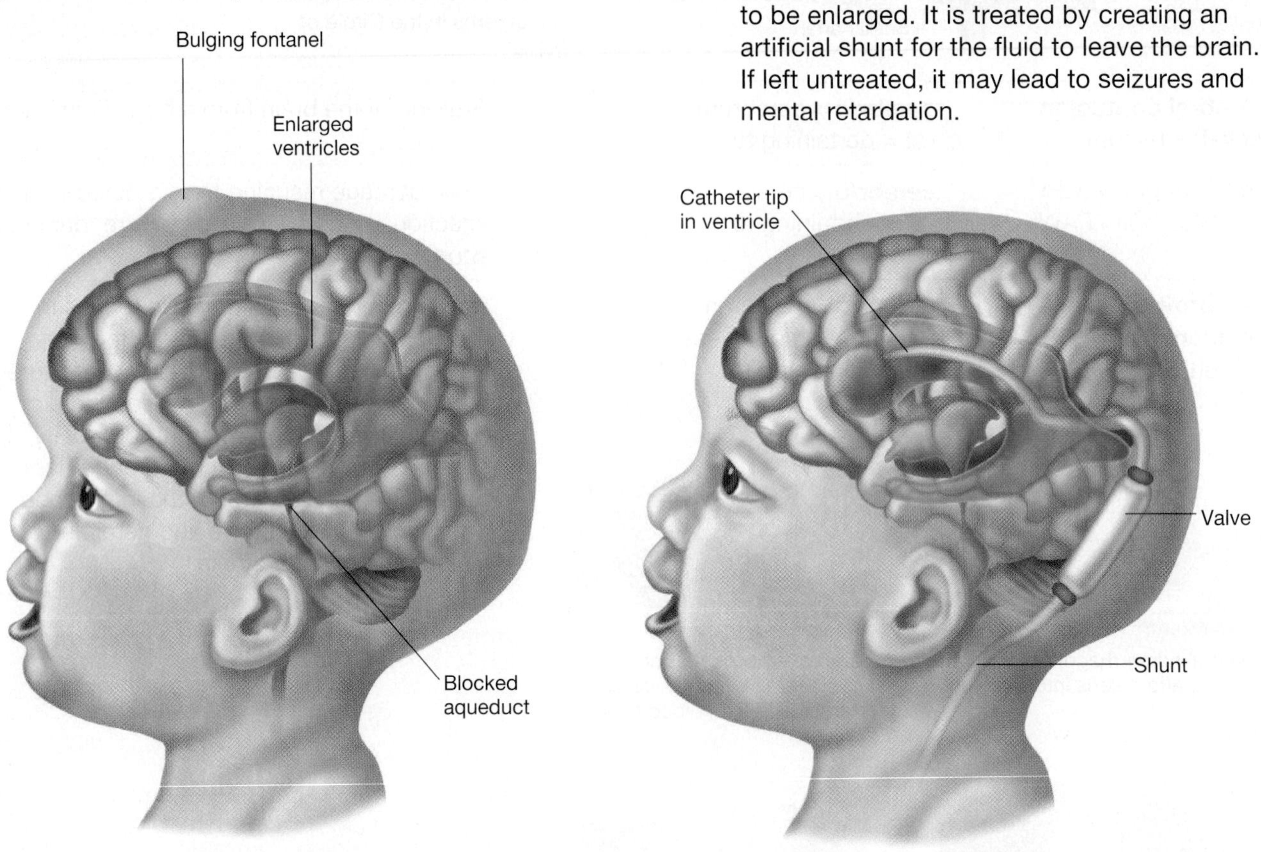

■ Figure 12.12 Hydrocephalus. The figure on the left is a child with the enlarged ventricles of hydrocephalus. The figure on the right is the same child with a shunt to send the excess cerebrospinal fluid to the abdominal cavity.

Term	Word Parts	Definition
migraine (MY-grain)		Specific type of headache characterized by severe head pain, sensitivity to light, dizziness, and nausea.
Parkinson's disease (PARK-in-sons)		Chronic disorder of the nervous system with fine tremors, muscular weakness, rigidity, and a shuffling gait. Named for British physician James Parkinson.

Pathology (continued)

Term	Word Parts	Definition
Reye's syndrome (RISE / SIN-drohm)		Combination of symptoms first recognized by Australian pathologist R. D. K. Reye that includes acute encephalopathy and damage to various organs, especially the liver. This occurs in children under age 15 who have had a viral infection. It is also associated with taking aspirin. For this reason, it's not recommended for children to use aspirin.
transient ischemic attack (TIA) (TRAN-shent / iss-KEM-ik)	isch/o = to hold back hem/o = blood -ic = pertaining to	Temporary interference with blood supply to the brain, causing neurological symptoms such as dizziness, numbness, and hemiparesis. May eventually lead to a full-blown stroke (cerebrovascular accident).
traumatic brain injury (TBI)	-tic = pertaining to	Damage to the brain resulting from impact (such as a car accident), blast waves (such as from an explosion), or a penetrating projectile (such as caused by a bullet). Symptoms may be mild, moderate, or severe and may include loss of consciousness, headache, vomiting, loss of motor coordination, and dizziness.
Spinal Cord		
amyotrophic lateral sclerosis (ALS) (ah-my-oh-TROFF-ik / LAT-er-al / skleh-ROH-sis)	a- = without my/o = muscle -trophic = pertaining to development later/o = side -al = pertaining to scler/o = hard -osis = abnormal condition	Disease with muscular weakness and atrophy due to degeneration of motor neurons of the spinal cord. Also called *Lou Gehrig's disease*, after the New York Yankees baseball player who died from the disease.
meningocele (men-IN-goh-seel)	mening/o = meninges -cele = protrusion	Congenital condition in which the meninges protrude through an opening in the vertebral column (see Figure 12.13A ■). See *spina bifida.*
myelitis (my-eh-LYE-tis)	myel/o = spinal cord -itis = inflammation	Inflammation of the spinal cord.
myelomeningocele (my-eh-loh-meh-NIN-goh-seel)	myel/o = spinal cord mening/o = meninges -cele = protrusion	Congenital condition in which the meninges and spinal cord protrude through an opening in the vertebral column (see Figure 12.13B ■). See *spina bifida.*
poliomyelitis (poh-lee-oh-my-eh-LYE-tis)	poli/o = gray matter myel/o = spinal cord -itis = inflammation	Viral inflammation of the gray matter of the spinal cord. Results in varying degrees of paralysis; may be mild and reversible or may be severe and permanent. This disease has been almost eliminated due to the discovery of a vaccine in the 1950s.

Pathology (continued)

Term	Word Parts	Definition
spina bifida (SPY-nah / BIFF-ih-dah)	spin/o = spine bi- = two	Congenital defect in the walls of the spinal canal in which the laminae of the vertebra do not meet or close (see Figure 12.13C ■). May result in a meningocele or a myelomeningocele—meninges or the spinal cord being pushed through the opening.

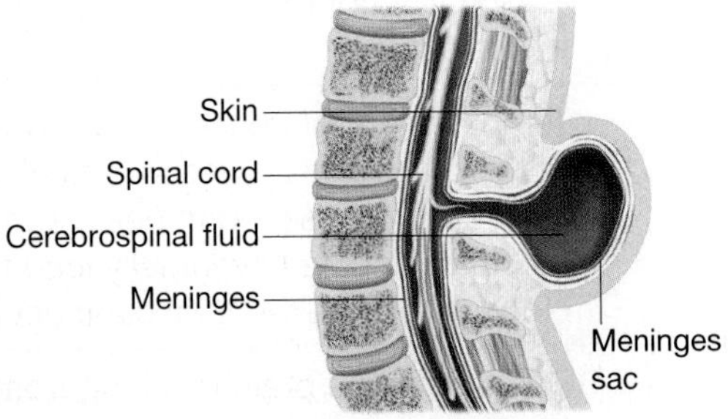

A. Meningocele

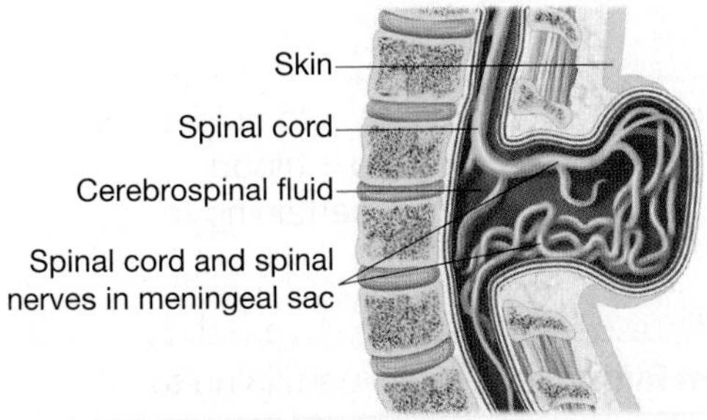

B. Myelomeningocele

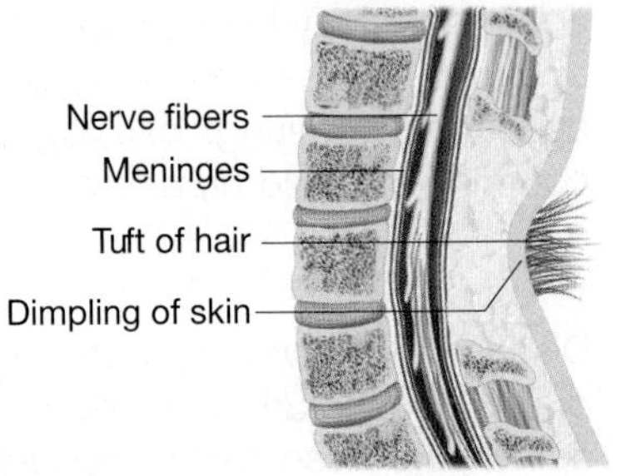

C. Spina bifida

■ **Figure 12.13** A) Meningocele, the meninges sac protrudes through the opening in the vertebra. B) Myelomeningocele, the meninges sac and spinal cord protrude through the opening in the vertebra. C) Spina bifida occulta, the vertebra is not complete, but there is not protrusion of nervous system structures.

Term	Word Parts	Definition
spinal cord injury (SCI)	spin/o = spine -al = pertaining to	Damage to the spinal cord as a result of trauma. Spinal cord may be bruised or completely severed.
Nerves		
Bell's palsy (BELLZ / PAWL-zee)		One-sided facial paralysis due to inflammation of the facial nerve, probably viral in nature. The patient cannot control salivation, tearing of the eyes, or expression, but most will eventually recover.
Guillain-Barré syndrome (GHEE-yan / bah-RAY)		Disease of the nervous system in which nerves lose their myelin covering. May be caused by an autoimmune reaction. Characterized by loss of sensation and/or muscle control starting in the legs. Symptoms then move toward the trunk and may even result in paralysis of the diaphragm.
multiple sclerosis (MS) (MULL-tih-pl / skleh-ROH-sis)	scler/o = hard -osis = abnormal condition	Inflammatory disease of the central nervous system in which there is extreme weakness and numbness due to loss of myelin insulation around nerves.

Pathology (continued)

Term	Word Parts	Definition
myasthenia gravis (my-ass-THEE-nee-ah / GRAV-iss)	my/o = muscle -asthenia = weakness	Disease with severe muscular weakness and fatigue due to insufficient neurotransmitter at a synapse.
neuroma (noo-ROH-mah)	neur/o = nerve -oma = tumor	Nerve tumor or tumor of the connective tissue sheath around a nerve.
neuropathy (noo-ROP-ah-thee)	neur/o = nerve -pathy = disease	General term for disease or damage to a nerve.
polyneuritis (pol-ee-noo-RYE-tis)	poly- = many neur/o = nerve -itis = inflammation	Inflammation of two or more nerves.
radiculitis (rah-dick-yoo-LYE-tis)	radicul/o = nerve root -itis = inflammation	Inflammation of a nerve root; may be caused by a herniated nucleus pulposus.
radiculopathy (rah-dick-yoo-LOP-ah-thee)	radicul/o = nerve root -pathy = disease	Refers to the condition that occurs when a herniated nucleus pulposus puts pressure on a nerve root. Symptoms include pain and numbness along the path of the affected nerve.
shingles (SHING-lz)		Eruption of painful blisters on the body along a nerve path. Thought to be caused by a *Herpes zoster* virus infection of the nerve root.
Meninges		
epidural hematoma (ep-ih-DOO-ral / hee-mah-TOH-mah)	epi- = above dur/o = dura mater -al = pertaining to hemat/o = blood -oma = mass	Mass of blood in the space outside the dura mater of the brain and spinal cord.
meningioma (meh-nin-jee-OH-mah)	meningi/o = meninges -oma = tumor	A tumor in the meninges.
meningitis (men-in-JYE-tis)	mening/o = meninges -itis = inflammation	Inflammation of the meninges around the brain or spinal cord caused by bacterial or viral infection. Symptoms include fever, headache, neck stiffness, lethargy, vomiting, irritability, and photophobia.

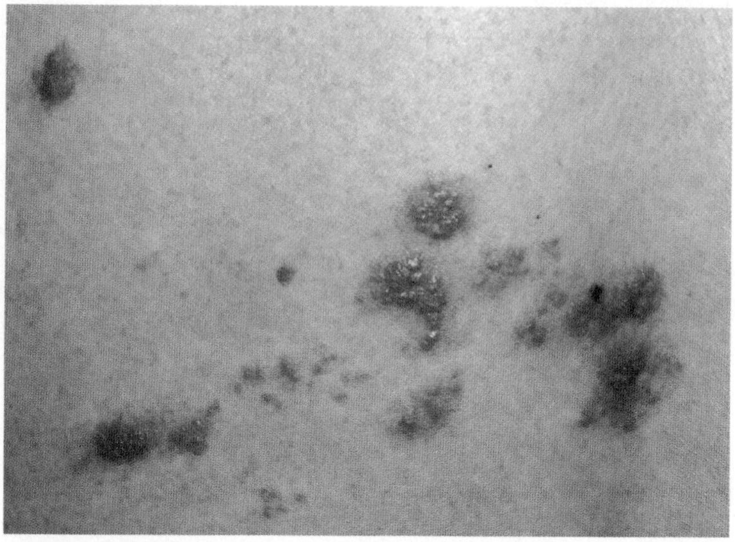

■ **Figure 12.14** Photograph of the skin eruptions associated with shingles. *(Stephen VanHorn/Shutterstock)*

Pathology (continued)

Term	Word Parts	Definition
subdural hematoma (sub-DOO-ral / hee-mah-TOH-mah)	sub- = under dur/o = dura mater -al = pertaining to hemat/o = blood -oma = mass	Mass of blood forming beneath the dura mater if the meninges are torn by trauma. May exert fatal pressure on the brain if the hematoma is not drained by surgery.

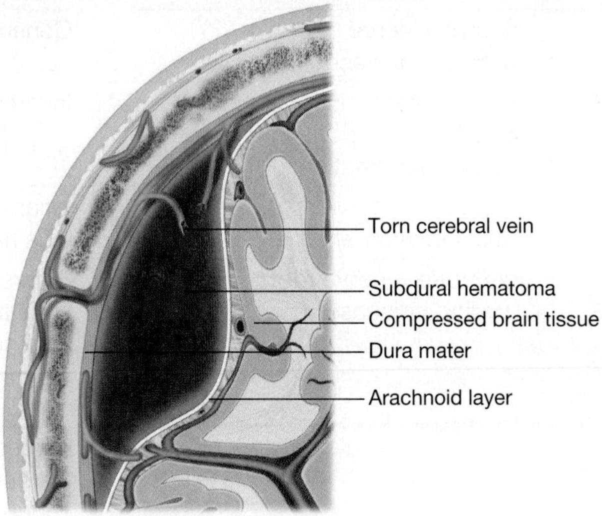

■ Figure 12.15 A subdural hematoma. A meningeal vein is ruptured and blood has accumulated in the subdural space, producing pressure on the brain.

Practice As You Go

C. Terminology Matching

Match each pathology to its definition.

1. ________ aura
2. ________ meningitis
3. ________ coma
4. ________ shingles
5. ________ syncope
6. ________ palsy
7. ________ absence seizure
8. ________ tonic-clonic seizure
9. ________ meningocele
10. ________ concussion

a. mild traumatic brain injury
b. sensations before a seizure
c. seizure with convulsions
d. congenital hernia of meninges
e. seizure without convulsion
f. inflammation of meninges
g. profound unconsciousness
h. *Herpes zoster* infection
i. fainting
j. loss of ability to control movement

Diagnostic Procedures

Term	Word Parts	Definition
Clinical Laboratory Tests		
cerebrospinal fluid analysis (ser-eh-broh-SPY-nal / an-NAL-ih-sis)	cerebr/o = cerebrum spin/o = spine -al = pertaining to	Laboratory examination of the clear, watery, colorless fluid from within the brain and spinal cord. Infections and the abnormal presence of blood can be detected in this test.
Diagnostic Imaging		
brain scan		Image of the brain taken after injection of radioactive isotopes into the circulation.
cerebral angiography (seh-REE-bral / an-jee-OG-rah-fee)	cerebr/o = cerebrum -al = pertaining to angi/o = vessel -graphy = process of recording	X-ray of the blood vessels of the brain after the injection of radiopaque dye.
echoencephalography (ek-oh-en-SEFF-ah-log-rah-fee)	encephal/o = brain -graphy = process of recording	Recording of the ultrasonic echoes of the brain. Useful in determining abnormal patterns of shifting in the brain.
myelogram (MY-eh-loh-gram)	myel/o = spinal cord -gram = record	X-ray record of the spinal cord.
myelography (my-eh-LOG-rah-fee)	myel/o = spinal cord -graphy = process of recording	Injection of radiopaque dye into the spinal canal. An X-ray is then taken to examine the normal and abnormal outlines made by the dye.
positron emission tomography (PET) (PAHZ-ih-tron / ee-MISH-un / toh-MOG-rah-fee)	tom/o = to cut -graphy = process of recording	Image of the brain produced by measuring gamma rays emitted from the brain after injecting glucose tagged with positively charged isotopes. Measurement of glucose uptake by the brain tissue indicates how metabolically active the tissue is.
Additional Diagnostic Tests		
Babinski's reflex (bah-BIN-skeez)		Reflex test developed by French neurologist Joseph Babinski to determine lesions and abnormalities in the nervous system. The Babinski reflex is present if the great toe extends instead of flexes when the lateral sole of the foot is stroked. The normal response to this stimulation is flexion of the toe.
electroencephalogram (EEG) (ee-lek-troh-en-SEFF-ah-loh-gram)	electr/o = electricity encephal/o = brain -gram = record	Record of the brain's electrical patterns.
electroencephalography (EEG) (ee-lek-troh-en-SEFF-ah-LOG-rah-fee)	electr/o = electricity encephal/o = brain -graphy = process of recording	Recording the electrical activity of the brain by placing electrodes at various positions on the scalp. Also used in sleep studies to determine if there is a normal pattern of activity during sleep.

Diagnostic Procedures (continued)

Term	Word Parts	Definition
lumbar puncture (LP) (LUM-bar / PUNK-chur)	lumb/o = low back -ar = pertaining to	Puncture with a needle into the lumbar area (usually the fourth intervertebral space) to withdraw fluid for examination and for the injection of anesthesia. Also called *spinal puncture* or *spinal tap.*
nerve conduction velocity		Test that measures how fast an impulse travels along a nerve. Can pinpoint an area of nerve damage.

■ **Figure 12.16** A lumbar puncture. The needle is inserted between the lumbar vertebrae and into the spinal canal.

Therapeutic Procedures

Term	Word Parts	Definition
Medical Procedures		
nerve block		Injection of regional anesthetic to stop the passage of sensory or pain impulses along a nerve path.
Surgical Procedures		
carotid endarterectomy (kah-ROT-id / end-ar-ter-EK-toh-mee)	endo- = within arteri/o = artery -ectomy = surgical removal	Surgical procedure for removing an obstruction within the carotid artery, a major artery in the neck that carries oxygenated blood to the brain. Developed to prevent strokes, but is found to be useful only in severe stenosis with transient ischemic attack.
cerebrospinal fluid shunts (ser-eh-bro-SPY-nal)	cerebr/o = cerebrum spin/o = spine -al = pertaining to	Surgical procedure in which a bypass is created to drain cerebrospinal fluid. It is used to treat hydrocephalus by draining the excess cerebrospinal fluid from the brain and diverting it to the abdominal cavity.
laminectomy (lam-ih-NEK-toh-mee)	-ectomy = surgical removal	Removal of a portion of a vertebra, called the *lamina*, in order to relieve pressure on a spinal nerve.
neurectomy (noo-REK-toh-mee)	neur/o = nerve -ectomy = surgical removal	Surgical removal of a nerve.
neuroplasty (NOOR-oh-plas-tee)	neur/o = nerve -plasty = surgical repair	Surgical repair of a nerve.

Therapeutic Procedures (continued)

Term	Word Parts	Definition
neurorrhaphy (noo-ROR-ah-fee)	neur/o = nerve -rrhaphy = suture	To suture a nerve back together. Actually refers to suturing the connective tissue sheath around the nerve.
tractotomy (track-TOT-oh-mee)	-otomy = cutting into	Surgical interruption of a nerve tract in the spinal cord. Used to treat intractable pain or muscle spasms.

Practice As You Go

D. Match each procedure term with its definition

1. ________ brain scan
2. ________ lumbar puncture
3. ________ cerebral angiography
4. ________ EEG
5. ________ PET scan
6. ________ nerve block
7. ________ neurorrhaphy
8. ________ myelogram

a. image made by measuring gamma rays
b. record of brain's electrical activity
c. obtains CSF from around spinal cord
d. regional injection of anesthetic
e. diagnostic image made with radioactive isotopes
f. X-ray of spinal cord
g. X-ray of brain's blood vessels
h. suture together sheath around a nerve

Pharmacology

Classification	Word Parts	Action	Examples
analgesic (an-al-JEE-zik)	an- = without alges/o = sense of pain -ic = pertaining to	Treats minor to moderate pain without loss of consciousness.	aspirin, Bayer, Ecotrin; acetaminophen, Tylenol; ibuprofen, Motrin
anesthetic (an-ess-THET-ik)	an- = without esthesi/o = feeling, sensation -tic = pertaining to	Produces a loss of sensation or a loss of consciousness.	lidocaine, Xylocaine; pentobarbital, Nembutal; propofol, Diprivan; procaine, Novocain
anticonvulsant (an-tye-kon-VULL-sant)	anti- = against	Reduces the excitability of neurons and therefore prevents the uncontrolled neuron activity associated with seizures.	carbamazepine, Tegretol; phenobarbital, Nembutal
dopaminergic drugs (dope-ah-men-ER-gik)	-ic = pertaining to	Treat Parkinson's disease by either replacing the dopamine that is lacking or increasing the strength of the dopamine that is present.	levodopa; L-dopa, Larodopa; levodopa/carbidopa, Sinemet

Pharmacology (continued)

Classification	Word Parts	Action	Examples
hypnotic (hip-NOT-tik)	-ic = pertaining to	Promotes sleep.	secobarbital, Seconal; temazepam, Restoril
narcotic analgesic (nar-KOT-tik)	-ic = pertaining to an- = without alges/o = sense of pain -ic = pertaining to	Treats severe pain; has the potential to be habit forming if taken for a prolonged time. Also called *opiate*.	morphine, MS Contin; oxycodone, OxyContin; meperidine, Demerol
sedative (SED-ah-tiv)		Has a relaxing or calming effect.	amobarbital, Amytal; butabarbital, Butisol

Abbreviations

ALS	amyotrophic lateral sclerosis	**ICP**	intracranial pressure
ANS	autonomic nervous system	**LP**	lumbar puncture
CNS	central nervous system	**MS**	multiple sclerosis
CP	cerebral palsy	**PET**	positron emission tomography
CSF	cerebrospinal fluid	**PNS**	peripheral nervous system
CVA	cerebrovascular accident	**SCI**	spinal cord injury
CVD	cerebrovascular disease	**TBI**	traumatic brain injury
EEG	electroencephalogram, electroencephalography	**TIA**	transient ischemic attack
HA	headache		

Practice As You Go

E. What's the Abbreviation?

1. cerebrospinal fluid ______
2. cerebrovascular disease ______
3. electroencephalogram ______
4. intracranial pressure ______
5. positron emission tomography ______
6. cerebrovascular accident ______
7. autonomic nervous system ______

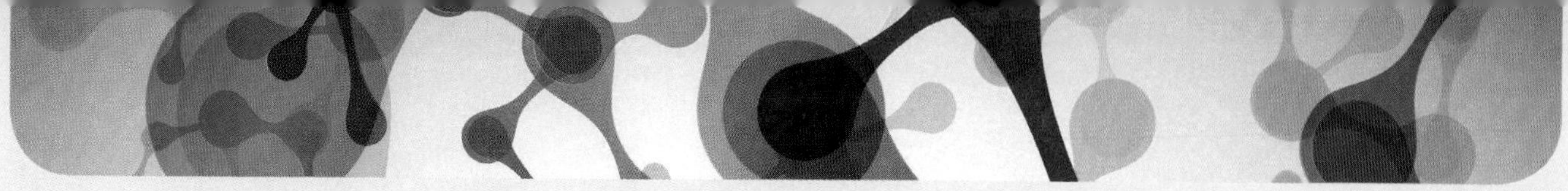

Chapter Review

Real-World Applications

Medical Record Analysis

This Discharge Summary contains 12 medical terms. Underline each term and write it in the list below the report. Then define each term.

Discharge Summary	
Admitting Diagnosis:	Paraplegia following motorcycle accident.
Final Diagnosis:	Comminuted L2 fracture with epidural hematoma and spinal cord injury resulting in complete paraplegia at the L2 level.
History of Present Illness:	Patient is a 23-year-old male who was involved in a motorcycle accident. He was unconscious for 35 minutes but was fully aware of his surroundings upon regaining consciousness. He was immediately aware of total anesthesia and paralysis below the waist.
Summary of Hospital Course:	CT scan revealed extensive bone destruction at the fracture site and that the spinal cord was severed. Patient was unable to voluntarily contract any lower extremity muscles and was not able to feel touch or pinpricks. Lumbar laminectomy with spinal fusion was performed to stabilize the fracture and remove the epidural hematoma. The immediate postoperative recovery period proceeded normally. Patient began physical therapy and occupational therapy. After two months, X-rays indicated full healing of the spinal fusion and patient was transferred to a rehabilitation institute.
Discharge Plans:	Patient was transferred to a rehabilitation institute to continue intensive PT and OT.

	Term	Definition
1.	______________	______________________________
2.	______________	______________________________
3.	______________	______________________________
4.	______________	______________________________
5.	______________	______________________________
6.	______________	______________________________
7.	______________	______________________________
8.	______________	______________________________
9.	______________	______________________________
10.	______________	______________________________
11.	______________	______________________________
12.	______________	______________________________

Chart Note Transcription

The chart note below contains 11 phrases that can be reworded with a medical term that you learned in this, or an earlier, chapter. Each phrase is identified with an underline. Determine the medical term and write your answers in the space provided.

Pearson General Hospital Consultation Report

Task Edit View Time Scale Options Help Download Archive Date: 17 May 2015

Current Complaint: Patient is a 38-year-old female referred to the specialist in the treatment of diseases of the nervous system **1** by her family physician with complaints of difficulty with speech, **2** loss of motion on one side of the body, **3** and severe involuntary muscle contractions. **4**

Past History: Patient is married and nulliparous. Has been well prior to current symptoms.

Signs and Symptoms: Her husband reports he first noted loss of motion on one side of the body when she began to drag her left foot. It has progressed to involve both left upper and lower extremities, with approximately a 50% loss in control of left lower extremity and a 25% loss of control in left upper extremity. Difficulty with speech is mild and mainly with recalling the names of common objects. Severe involuntary muscle contractions appear to be triggered by stress and last approximately two minutes. Results of a recording of the electrical activity of the brain **5** and a puncture with a needle into the low back to withdraw fluid for examination **6** were normal. However, an injection with radioactive isotopes **7** revealed the presence of a mass in the right outer layer of the largest section of the brain. **8**

Diagnosis: Astrocyte tumor **9** in the right outer layer of the largest section of the brain. **8**

Treatment: A right skull incision **10** was performed to permit the surgical use of extreme cold **11** to destroy the tumor. Patient experienced moderate improvement in loss of motion on one side of the body **3** and severe involuntary muscle contractions, **4** but difficulty with speech **2** was unchanged.

1. ______________________
2. ______________________
3. ______________________
4. ______________________
5. ______________________
6. ______________________
7. ______________________
8. ______________________
9. ______________________
10. ______________________
11. ______________________

Case Study

Below is a case study presentation of a patient with a condition covered in this chapter. Read the case study and answer the questions below. Some questions will ask for information not included within this chapter. Use your text, a medical dictionary, or any other reference material you choose to answer these questions.

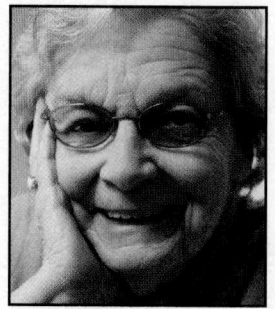

(iofoto/Shutterstock)

Anna Moore, an 83-year-old female, is admitted to the ER with aphasia, hemiparesis on her left side, syncope, and delirium. Her daughter called the ambulance after discovering her mother in this condition at home. Mrs. Moore has a history of hypertension, atherosclerosis, and diabetes mellitus. She was admitted to the hospital after a brain scan revealed an infarct in the right cerebral hemisphere leading to a diagnosis of CVA of the middle cerebral artery.

Questions

1. What pathological condition does Ms. Moore have? Look this condition up in a reference source and include a short description of it.

____

____

2. List and define each of the patient's presenting symptoms in the ER.

____

____

3. The patient has a history of three significant conditions. Describe each in your own words.

____

____

4. What diagnostic test did the physician perform? Describe this test and the results in your own words.

____

____

5. What is an infarct and what causes it?

____

____

6. List and describe the four common causes of a CVA.

____

____

Practice Exercises

A. Terminology Matching

Match each cranial nerve to its function.

1.	_______ olfactory	a. carries facial sensory impulses
2.	_______ optic	b. turns eye to side
3.	_______ oculomotor	c. controls tongue muscles
4.	_______ trochlear	d. controls eye muscles and pupils
5.	_______ trigeminal	e. swallowing
6.	_______ abducens	f. controls facial muscles
7.	_______ facial	g. controls oblique eye muscles
8.	_______ vestibulocochlear	h. smell
9.	_______ glossopharyngeal	i. controls neck and shoulder muscles
10.	_______ vagus	j. hearing and equilibrium
11.	_______ accessory	k. vision
12.	_______ hypoglossal	l. organs in lower body cavities

B. Word Building Practice

The combining form **neur/o** refers to the nerve. Use it to write a term that means:

1. inflammation of the nerve _______________
2. specialist in nerves _______________
3. pain in the nerve _______________
4. inflammation of many nerves _______________
5. removal of a nerve _______________
6. surgical repair of a nerve _______________
7. nerve tumor _______________
8. suture of a nerve _______________

The combining form **mening/o** refers to the meninges or membranes. Use it to write a term that means:

9. inflammation of the meninges _______________
10. protrusion of the meninges _______________
11. protrusion of the spinal cord and the meninges _______________

The combining form **encephal/o** refers to the brain. Use it to write a term that means:

12. X-ray record of the brain ______________________________

13. disease of the brain ______________________________

14. inflammation of the brain ______________________________

15. protrusion of the brain ______________________________

The combining form **cerebr/o** refers to the cerebrum. Use it to write a term that means:

16. pertaining to the cerebrum and spinal cord ______________________________

17. pertaining to the cerebrum ______________________________

C. What Does it Stand For?

1. TIA ______________________________
2. MS ______________________________
3. SCI ______________________________
4. CNS ______________________________
5. PNS ______________________________
6. HA ______________________________
7. CP ______________________________
8. LP ______________________________
9. ALS ______________________________

D. Define the Procedures and Tests

1. myelography ______________________________
2. cerebral angiography ______________________________
3. Babinski's reflex ______________________________
4. nerve conduction velocity ______________________________
5. cerebrospinal fluid analysis ______________________________
6. PET scan ______________________________
7. echoencephalography ______________________________
8. lumbar puncture ______________________________

E. Define the Suffix

	Definition	Example from Chapter
1. **-plegia**	____________	____________
2. **-taxia**	____________	____________
3. **-trophic**	____________	____________
4. **-paresis**	____________	____________
5. **-phasia**	____________	____________

F. Define the Combining Form

	Definition	Example from Chapter
1. **mening/o**	____________	____________
2. **encephal/o**	____________	____________
3. **cerebell/o**	____________	____________
4. **myel/o**	____________	____________
5. **cephal/o**	____________	____________
6. **thalam/o**	____________	____________
7. **neur/o**	____________	____________
8. **radicul/o**	____________	____________
9. **cerebr/o**	____________	____________
10. **pont/o**	____________	____________

G. Define the Term

1. astrocytoma ____________
2. epilepsy ____________
3. anesthesia ____________
4. hemiparesis ____________
5. neurosurgeon ____________
6. analgesia ____________
7. focal seizure ____________
8. quadriplegia ____________
9. subdural hematoma ____________
10. intrathecal ____________

H. Terminology Matching

Match each term to its definition.

1.	________ neurologist	a.	sudden attack
2.	________ cerebrovascular accident	b.	a type of severe headache
3.	________ concussion	c.	loss of intellectual ability
4.	________ aphasia	d.	physician who treats nerve problems
5.	________ migraine	e.	stroke
6.	________ seizure	f.	mild traumatic brain injury
7.	________ dementia	g.	loss of ability to speak
8.	________ ataxia	h.	congenital anomaly
9.	________ spina bifida	i.	state of being unaware
10.	________ unconscious	j.	lack of muscle coordination

I. Fill in the Blank

Parkinson's disease	**transient ischemic attack**	**cerebral palsy**	**cerebrospinal fluid shunt**
Bell's palsy	**subdural hematoma**	**amyotrophic lateral sclerosis**	**nerve conduction velocity**
delirium	**cerebral aneurysm**		

1. Dr. Martin noted that a 96-year-old patient suffered from ________________________ when she determined that he was confused, disoriented, and agitated.
2. Lucinda's ____________ resulted in increasing muscle weakness as the motor neurons in her spinal cord degenerated.
3. The diagnosis of ______________________ was correct because the weakness affected only one side of Charles's face.
4. A cerebral angiogram was ordered because Dr. Larson suspected Mrs. Constantine had a(n) ____________________.
5. Roberta's symptoms included fine tremors, muscular weakness, rigidity, and a shuffling gait, leading to a diagnosis of ________________________________.
6. Matthew's hydrocephalus required the placement of a(n) ____.
7. Because Mae's hemiparesis was temporary, the final diagnosis was ____.
8. Following a car accident, a CT scan showed a(n) _______________________ was putting pressure on the brain, necessitating immediate neurosurgery.
9. Birth trauma resulted in the newborn developing ____.
10. A(n) _________________________ test was performed in order to pinpoint the exact position of the nerve damage.

J. Pharmacology Challenge

Fill in the classification for each drug description, then match the brand name.

Drug Description	Classification	Brand Name
1. ________ produces loss of sensation	____________________	a. L-Dopa
2. ________ treats Parkinson's disease	____________________	b. Amytal
3. ________ promotes sleep	____________________	c. OxyContin
4. ________ medication for mild pain	____________________	d. Seconal
5. ________ produces a calming effect	____________________	e. Xylocaine
6. ________ treats severe pain	____________________	f. Tegretol
7. ________ treats seizures	____________________	g. Motrin

Labeling Exercise

Image A

Write the labels for this figure on the numbered lines provided.

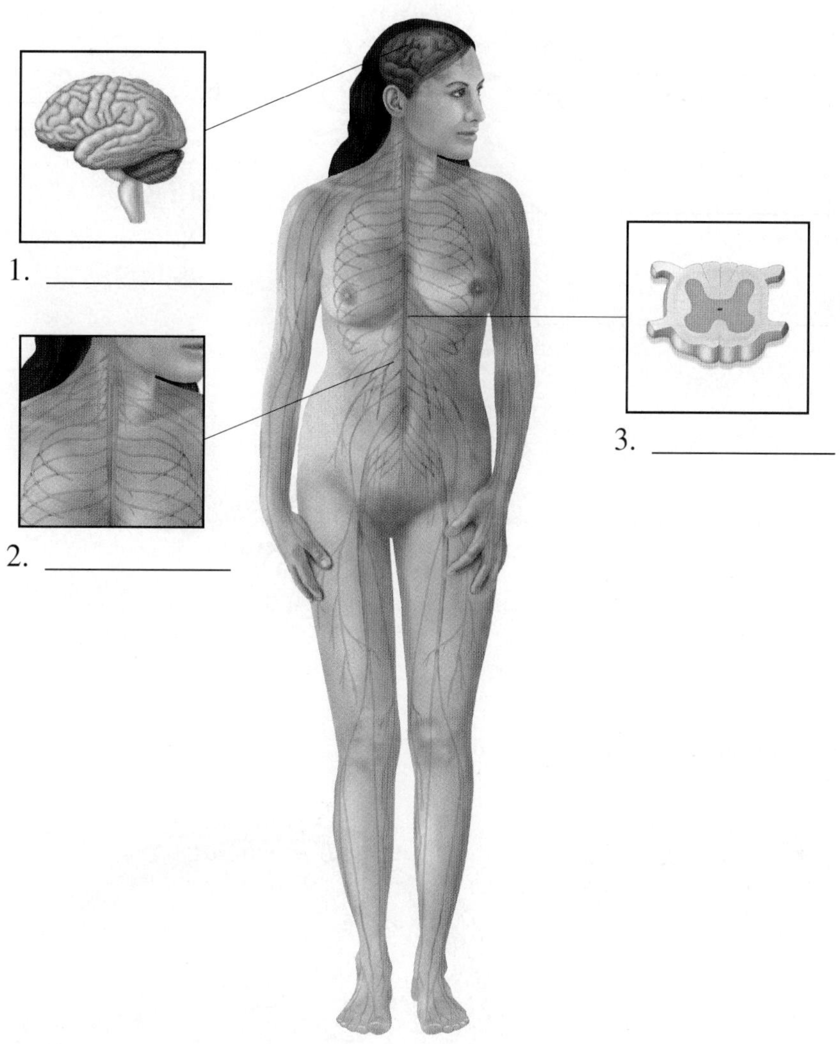

Image B

Write the labels for this figure on the numbered lines provided.

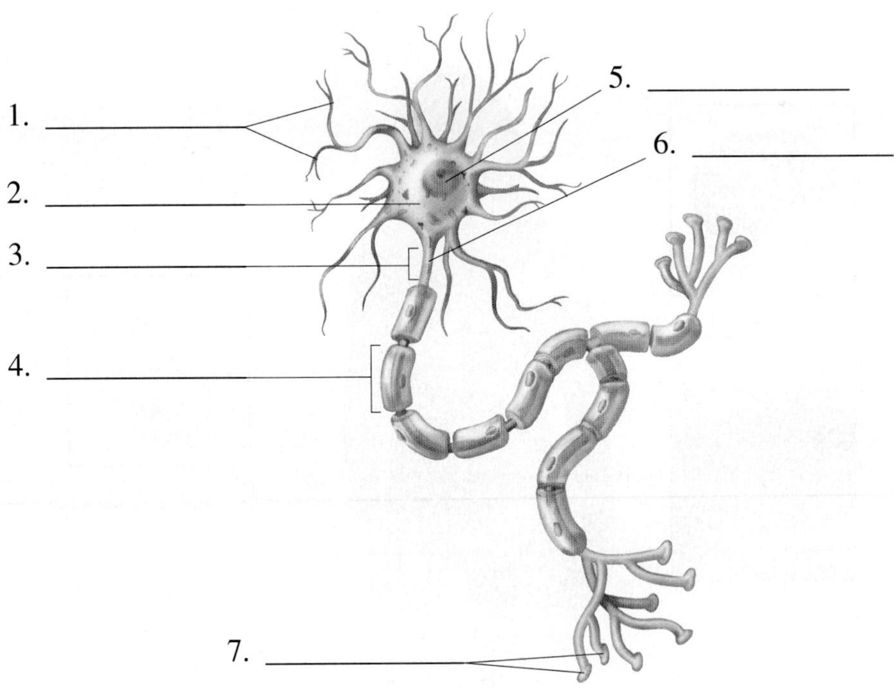

Image C

Write the labels for this figure on the numbered lines provided.

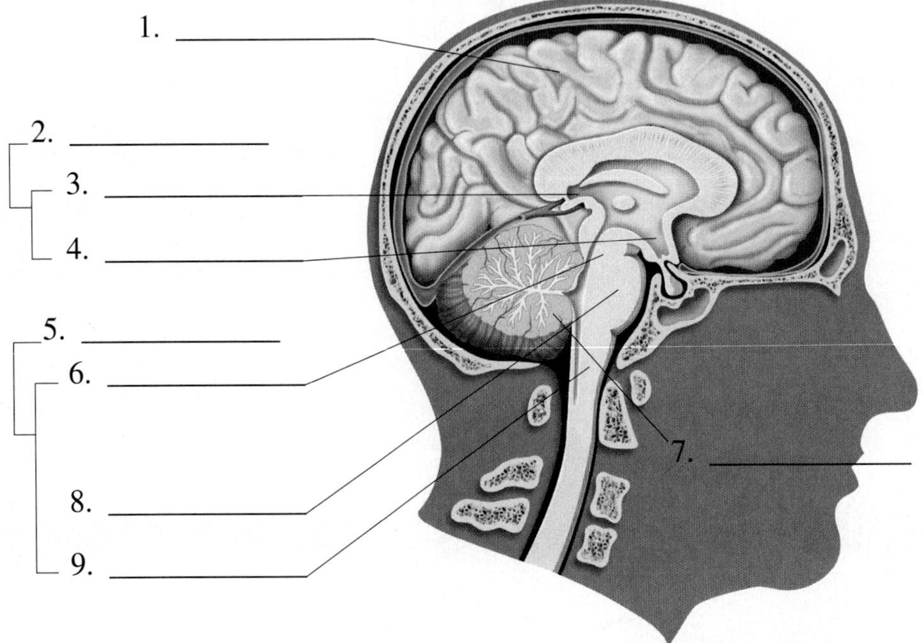

13

Special Senses: The Eye and Ear

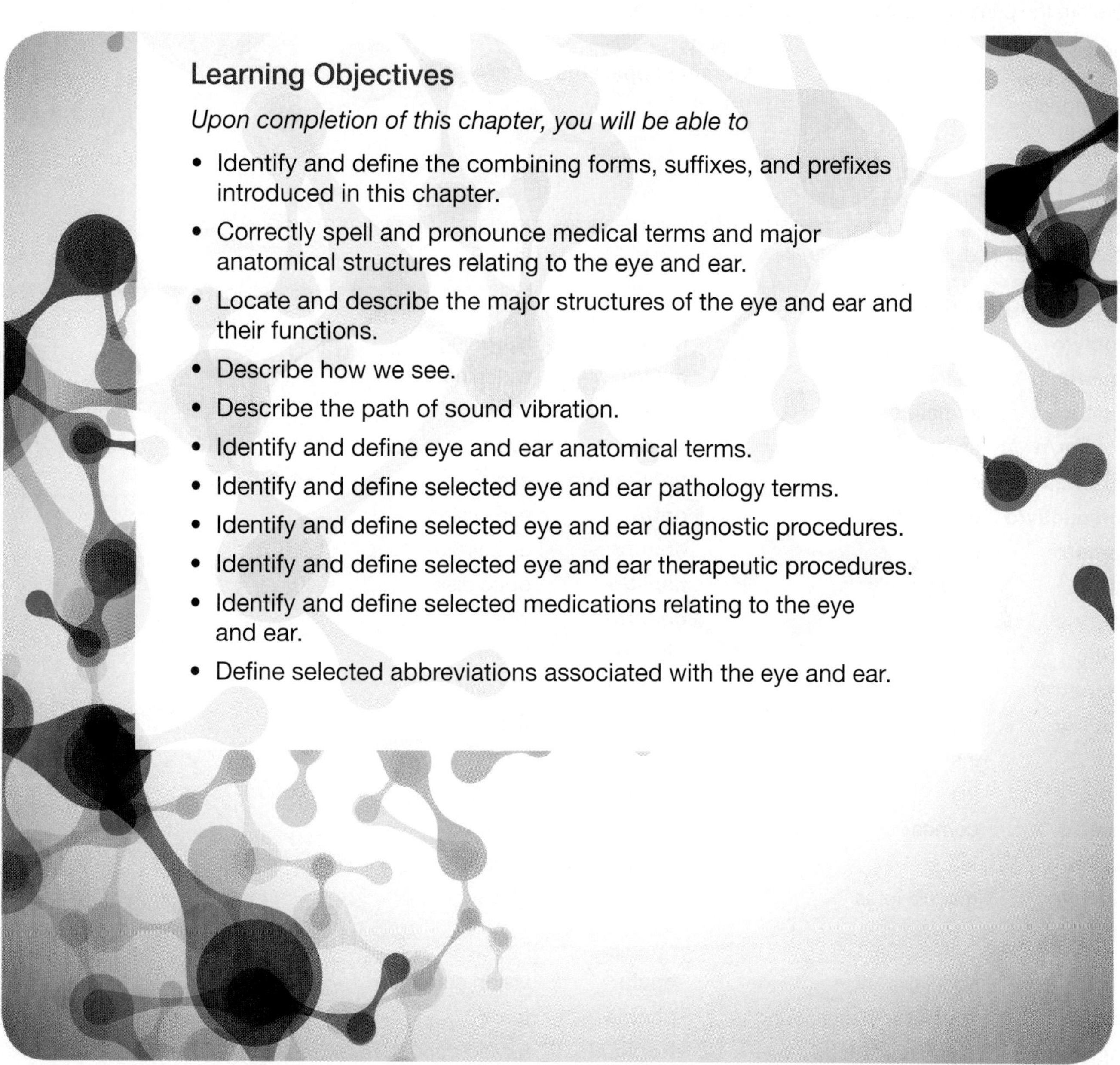

Learning Objectives

Upon completion of this chapter, you will be able to

- Identify and define the combining forms, suffixes, and prefixes introduced in this chapter.
- Correctly spell and pronounce medical terms and major anatomical structures relating to the eye and ear.
- Locate and describe the major structures of the eye and ear and their functions.
- Describe how we see.
- Describe the path of sound vibration.
- Identify and define eye and ear anatomical terms.
- Identify and define selected eye and ear pathology terms.
- Identify and define selected eye and ear diagnostic procedures.
- Identify and define selected eye and ear therapeutic procedures.
- Identify and define selected medications relating to the eye and ear.
- Define selected abbreviations associated with the eye and ear.

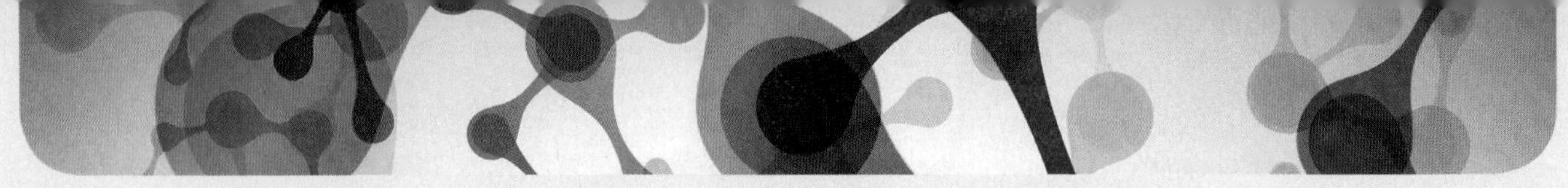

Section I: The Eye at a Glance

Function

The eye contains the sensory receptor cells for vision.

Structures

Here are the primary structures that comprise the eye:

choroid
conjunctiva
eye muscles
eyeball
eyelids
lacrimal apparatus
retina
sclera

Word Parts

Here are the most common word parts (with their meanings) used to build eye terms. For a more comprehensive list, refer to the Terminology section of this chapter.

Combining Forms

ambly/o	dull, dim
aque/o	water
blast/o	immature
blephar/o	eyelid
chromat/o	color
conjunctiv/o	conjunctiva
corne/o	cornea
cycl/o	ciliary body
dacry/o	tears
dipl/o	double
emmetr/o	correct, proper
glauc/o	gray
ir/o	iris
irid/o	iris
kerat/o	cornea
lacrim/o	tears
macul/o	macula lutea
mi/o	lessening
mydr/i	widening
nyctal/o	night
ocul/o	eye
ophthalm/o	eye
opt/o	eye, vision
optic/o	eye, vision
papill/o	optic disk
phac/o	lens
phot/o	light
presby/o	old age
pupill/o	pupil
retin/o	retina
scler/o	sclera
stigmat/o	point
uve/o	choroid
vitre/o	glassy

Suffixes

-ician	specialist
-metrist	specialist in measuring
-opia	vision condition
-opsia	vision condition
-phobia	fear
-tropia	turned condition

Prefixes

eso-	inward
exo-	outward
myo-	to shut

The Eye Illustrated

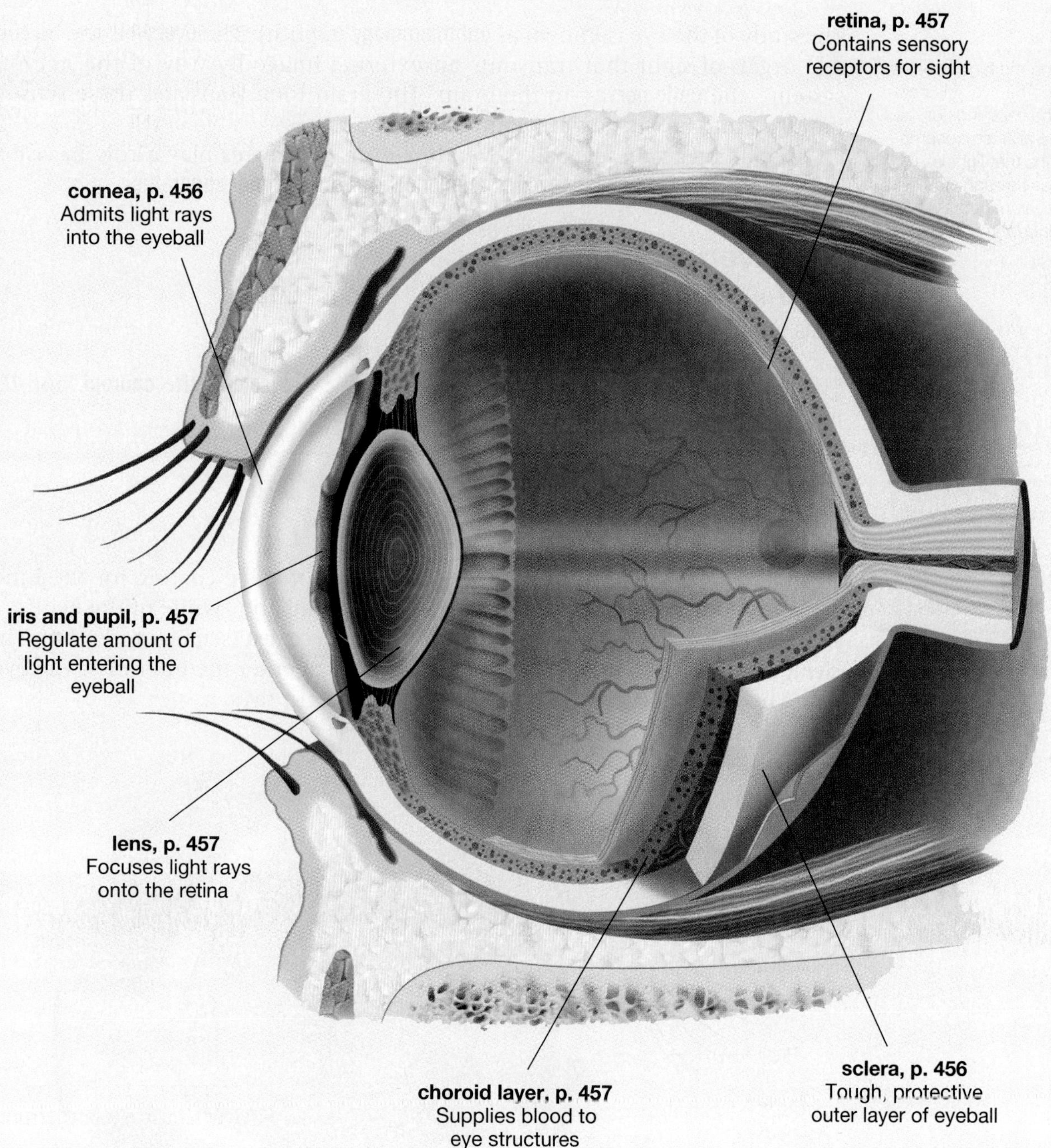

retina, p. 457
Contains sensory receptors for sight
cornea, p. 456
Admits light rays into the eyeball
iris and pupil, p. 457
Regulate amount of light entering the eyeball
lens, p. 457
Focuses light rays onto the retina
choroid layer, p. 457
Supplies blood to eye structures
sclera, p. 456
Tough, protective outer layer of eyeball

Anatomy and Physiology of the Eye

conjunctiva (kon-JUNK-tih-vah)
eye muscles
eyeball
eyelids
lacrimal apparatus (LAK-rim-al)
ophthalmology (off-thal-MALL-oh-gee)
optic nerve (OP-tik)

Med Term Tip

When studying the functions and terminology of the eye, it is helpful to know the meanings of the terms *opaque* and *transparent.* Opaque means that light is unable to pass through. Transparent, however, means that light is permitted through.

The study of the eye is known as **ophthalmology** (Ophth). The **eyeball** is the incredible organ of sight that transmits an external image by way of the nervous system—the **optic nerve**—to the brain. The brain then translates these sensory impulses into an image with computer-like accuracy.

In addition to the eyeball, several external structures play a role in vision. These are the **eye muscles**, **eyelids**, **conjunctiva**, and **lacrimal apparatus**.

The Eyeball

choroid (KOR-oyd)
retina (RET-in-ah)
sclera (SKLAIR-ah)

The actual eyeball is composed of three layers: the **sclera**, the **choroid**, and the **retina**.

Med Term Tip

The color of the sclera may indicate the presence of disease. For instance, a yellowish cast to the sclera can be present in liver disease and certain anemias.

Sclera

cornea (COR-nee-ah)
refracts

The outer layer, the sclera, provides a tough protective coating for the inner structures of the eye. Another term for the sclera is the "white of the eye."

The anterior portion of the sclera is called the **cornea** (see Figure 13.1 ■). This clear, transparent area of the sclera allows light to enter the interior of the eyeball. The cornea actually bends, or **refracts**, the light rays.

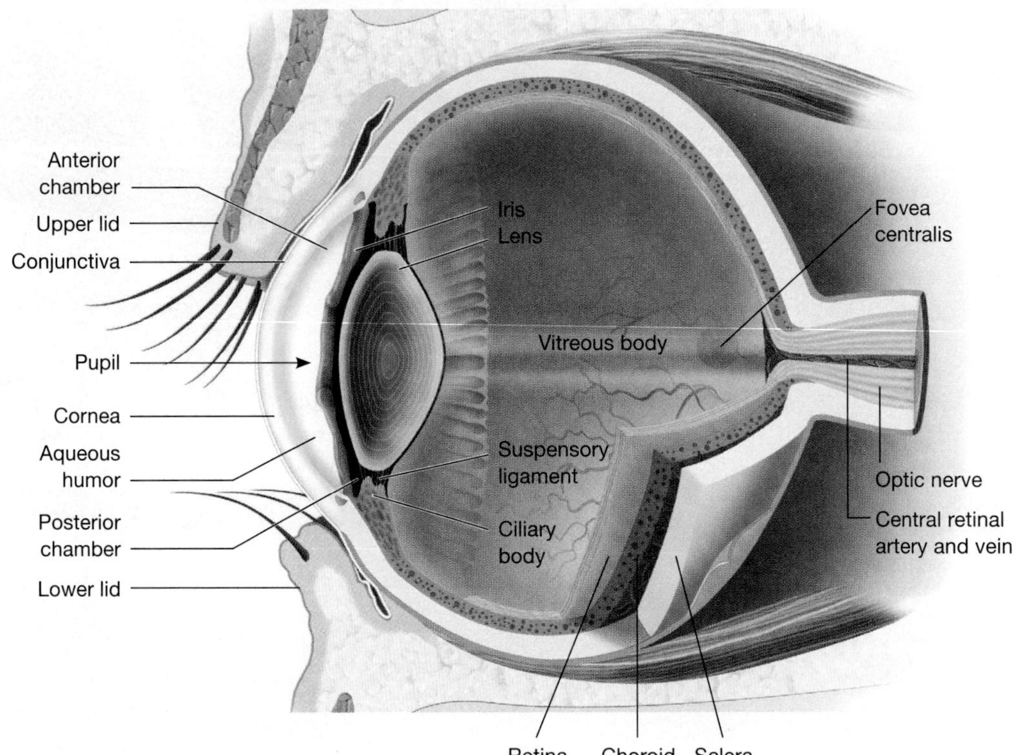

■ **Figure 13.1** The internal structures of the eye.

Choroid

ciliary body (SIL-ee-air-ee)
iris
lens
pupil

The second or middle layer of the eyeball is called the choroid. This opaque layer provides the blood supply for the eye.

The anterior portion of the choroid layer consists of the **iris**, **pupil**, and **ciliary body** (see again Figure 13.1). The iris is the colored portion of the eye and contains smooth muscle. The pupil is the opening in the center of the iris that allows light rays to enter the eyeball. The iris muscles contract or relax to change the size of the pupil, thereby controlling how much light enters the interior of the eyeball. Immediately posterior to the iris is the ciliary body. This is a ring of smooth muscle. Sitting in the center of the ring is the **lens**. The lens is not actually part of the choroid layer, but it is attached to the ciliary body by many thin ligaments called *suspensory ligaments*. The muscular ciliary body contracts or relaxes to pull on the edge of the lens, changing the shape of the lens so it can focus incoming light onto the retina.

Med Term Tip

The function of the choroid, to provide the rest of the eyeball with blood, is responsible for an alternate name for this layer—*uvea*. The combining form *uve/o* means "vascular."

Med Term Tip

The term *ciliary* comes from the Latin word *cilium*, which is taken to refer to the eyelashes (or hair-like structures). In this case, the ciliary body received its name because of the many, very fine ligaments extending from it and attaching to the edge of the lens.

Retina

aqueous humor (AY-kwee-us)
cones
fovea centralis (FOH-vee-ah / sen-TRAH-lis)
macula lutea (MAK-yoo-lah / loo-TEE-ah)
optic disk
retinal blood vessels (RET-in-al)
rods
vitreous humor (VIT-ree-us)

What's In A Name?

aque/o = water
centr/o = center
vitre/o = glassy
-ous = pertaining to

The third and innermost layer of the eyeball is the retina. It contains the sensory receptor cells (**rods** and **cones**) that respond to light rays. Rods are active in dim light and help us to see in gray tones. Cones are active only in bright light and are responsible for color vision. When someone looks directly at an object, the image falls on an area called the **macula lutea**, or "yellow spot" (see again Figure 13.1). In the center of the macula lutea is a depression called the **fovea centralis**, meaning "central pit." This pit contains a high concentration of sensory receptor cells and, therefore, is the point of clearest vision. Also visible on the retina is the **optic disk**. This is the point where the **retinal blood vessels** enter and exit the eyeball and where the optic nerve leaves the eyeball (see Figure 13.2 ■). There are no sensory receptor cells in the optic disk and therefore it causes a blind spot in each eye's field of vision. The interior spaces of the eyeball are not empty. The spaces between the cornea and lens are filled with **aqueous humor**, a watery fluid, and the large open area between the lens and retina contains **vitreous humor**, a semisolid gel.

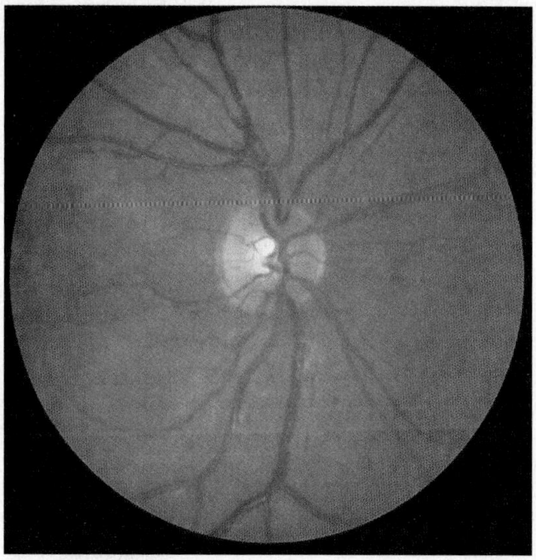

■ **Figure 13.2** Photograph of the retina of the eye. The optic disk appears yellow and the retinal arteries radiate out from it. *(Science Source)*

Muscles of the Eye

oblique muscles (oh-BLEEK) **rectus muscles** (REK-tus)

Med Term Tip

Like many other muscles, the names *rectus* and *oblique* provide clues regarding the direction of their fibers, or their *line of pull.* Rectus means straight and oblique means slanted. Rectus muscles have a straight line of pull. Since the fibers of an oblique muscle are slanted on an angle, they produce rotation.

Six muscles connect the actual eyeball to the skull (see Figure 13.3 ■). These muscles allow for change in the direction of each eye's sightline. In addition, they provide support for the eyeball in the eye socket. Children may be born with a weakness in some of these muscles and may require treatments such as eye exercises or even surgery to correct this problem, commonly referred to as crossed eyes or *strabismus* (see Figure 13.4 ■). The muscles involved are the four **rectus** and two **oblique muscles.** Rectus (meaning "straight") muscles pull the eye up, down, left, or right in a straight line. Oblique muscles are on an angle and produce diagonal eye movement.

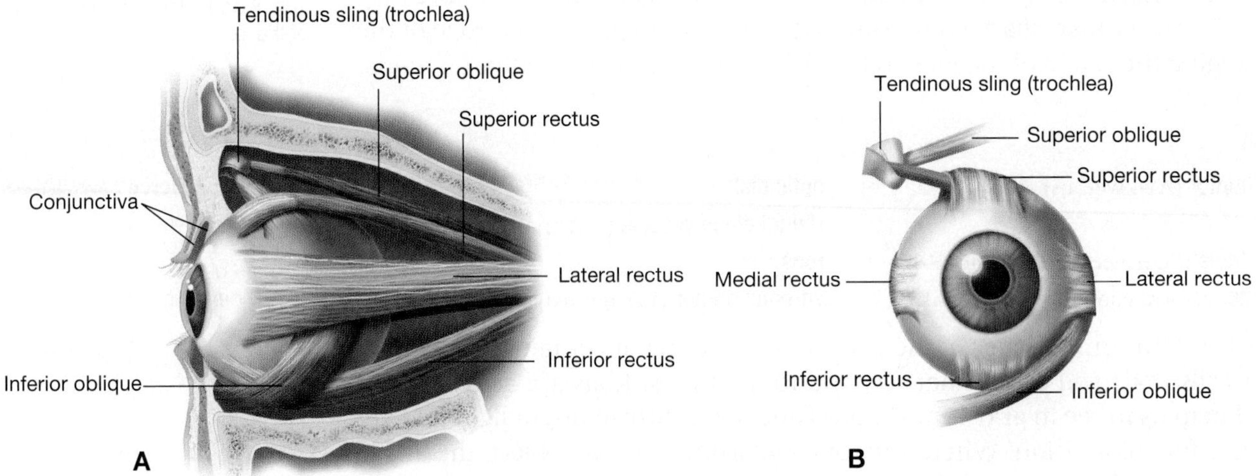

■ **Figure 13.3** The arrangement of the external eye muscles, A) lateral and B) anterior views.

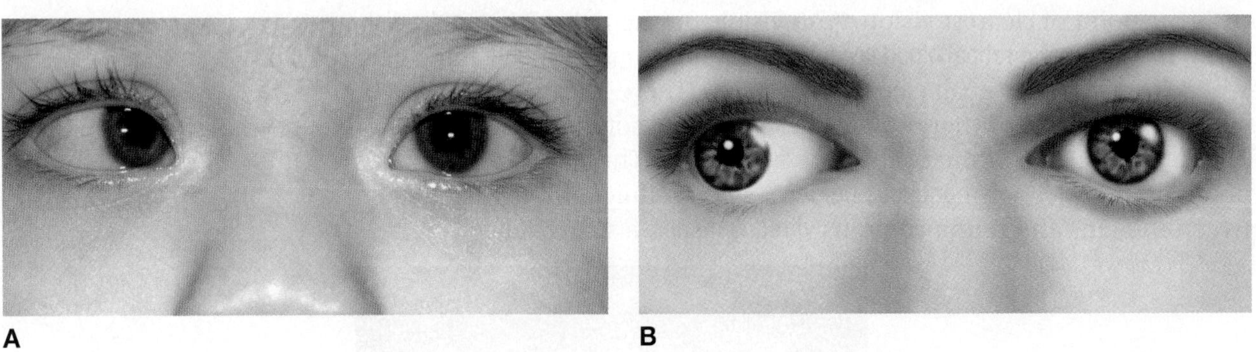

■ **Figure 13.4** Examples of common forms of strabismus. A) Esotropia with the right eye turning inward. *(Biophoto Associates/Science Source)* B) Exotropia with the right eye turning outward. *(Gwen Shockey/Science Source)*

The Eyelids

cilia (SIL-ee-ah) **sebaceous glands** (see-BAY-shus)
eyelashes

What's In A Name?

seb/o = oil
-ous = pertaining to

A pair of eyelids over each eyeball provides protection from foreign particles, injury from the sun and intense light, and trauma (see again Figure 13.1). Both the upper and lower edges of the eyelids have **eyelashes**, or **cilia**, that protect the eye from foreign particles. In addition, **sebaceous glands** located in the eyelids secrete lubricating oil onto the eyeball.

Conjunctiva

mucous membrane

The conjunctiva of the eye is a **mucous membrane** lining. It forms a continuous covering on the underside of each eyelid and across the anterior surface of each eyeball (see again Figure 13.1). This serves as protection for the eye by sealing off the eyeball in the socket.

What's In A Name?
muc/o = mucus
-ous = pertaining to

Lacrimal Apparatus

lacrimal ducts
lacrimal gland
nasal cavity
nasolacrimal duct (naz-oh-LAK-rim-al)
tears

The **lacrimal gland** is located under the outer upper corner of each eyelid. These glands produce **tears**. Tears serve the important function of washing and lubricating the anterior surface of the eyeball. **Lacrimal ducts**, located in the inner corner of the eye socket, then collect the tears and drain them into the **nasolacrimal duct**. This duct ultimately drains the tears into the **nasal cavity** (see Figure 13.5 ■).

What's In A Name?
lacrim/o = tears
nas/o = nose
-al = pertaining to

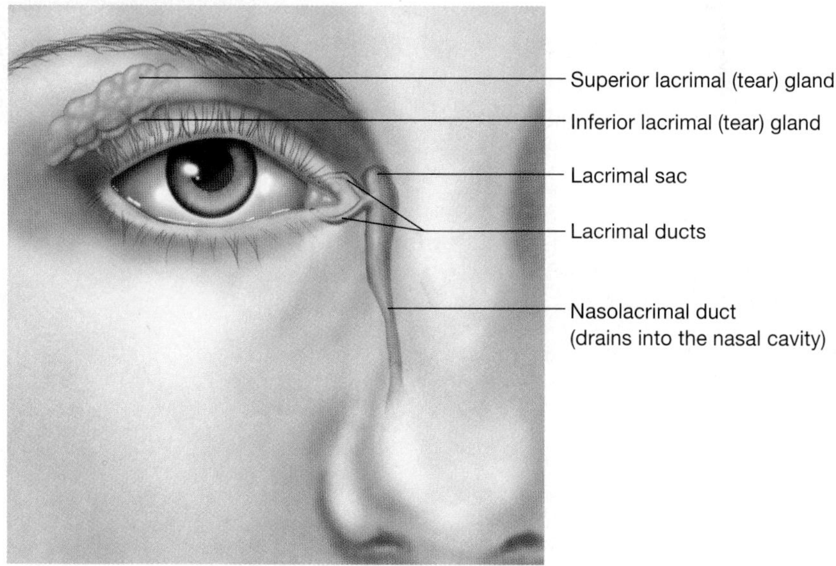

■ **Figure 13.5** The structure of the lacrimal apparatus.

How We See

When light rays strike the eye, they first pass through the cornea, pupil, aqueous humor, lens, and vitreous humor (see Figure 13.6 ■). They then strike the retina and stimulate the rods and cones. When the light rays hit the retina, an upside-down image is sent along nerve impulses to the optic nerve (see Figure 13.7 ■). The optic nerve transmits these impulses to the brain, where the upside-down image is translated into the right-side-up image we are looking at.

Vision requires proper functioning of four mechanisms:

1. Coordination of the external eye muscles so that both eyes move together.
2. The correct amount of light admitted by the pupil.
3. The correct focus of light on the retina by the lens.
4. The optic nerve transmitting sensory images to the brain.

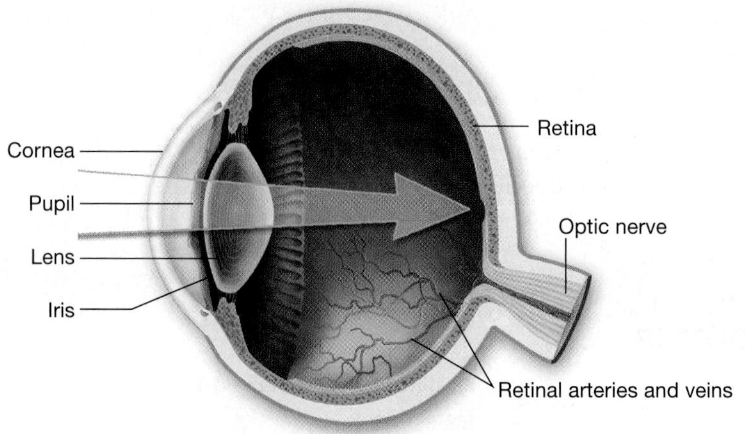

■ **Figure 13.6** The path of light through the cornea, iris, lens, and striking the retina.

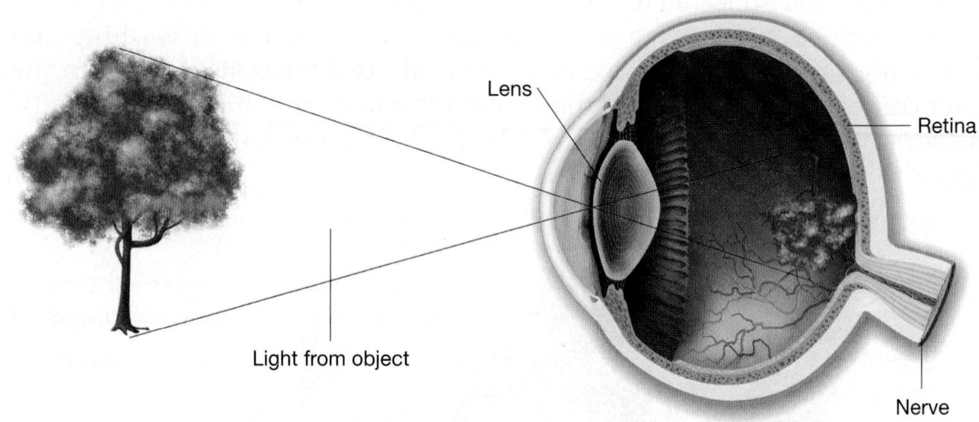

■ **Figure 13.7** The image formed on the retina is inverted. The brain rights the image as part of the interpretation process.

Practice As You Go

A. Complete the Statement

1. The study of the eye is ____________________.
2. Another term for eyelashes is ____________________.
3. The glands responsible for tears are called ____________________ glands.
4. The clear, transparent portion of the sclera is called the ____________________.
5. The innermost layer of the eye, which is composed of sensory receptors, is the ____________________.
6. The pupil of the eye is actually a hole in the ____________________.

Terminology

Word Parts Used to Build Eye Terms

The following lists contain the combining forms, suffixes, and prefixes used to build terms in the remaining sections of this chapter.

Combining Forms

aden/o	gland
ambly/o	dull, dim
angi/o	vessel
bi/o	life
blast/o	immature
blephar/o	eyelid
chromat/o	color
conjunctiv/o	conjunctiva
corne/o	cornea
cry/o	cold
cycl/o	ciliary body
cyst/o	sac
dacry/o	tears
dipl/o	double

emmetr/o	correct, proper
esthesi/o	sensation, feeling
glauc/o	gray
ir/o	iris
irid/o	iris
kerat/o	cornea
lacrim/o	tears
macul/o	macula lutea
mi/o	lessening
myc/o	fungus
mydr/i	widening
nyctal/o	night
ocul/o	eye
ophthalm/o	eye

opt/o	eye, vision
optic/o	eye, vision
papill/o	optic disk
phac/o	lens
phot/o	light
presby/o	old age
pupill/o	pupil
retin/o	retina
scler/o	sclera
stigmat/o	point
ton/o	tone
uve/o	choroid
xer/o	dry

Suffixes

-al	pertaining to
-algia	pain
-ar	pertaining to
-ary	pertaining to
-atic	pertaining to
-ectomy	surgical removal
-edema	swelling
-graphy	process of recording
-ia	condition
-ic	pertaining to
-ician	specialist
-ism	state of
-itis	inflammation
-logist	one who studies

-logy	study of
-malacia	abnormal softening
-meter	instrument to measure
-metrist	specialist in measuring
-metry	process of measuring
-oma	tumor; mass
-opia	vision condition
-opsia	vision condition
-osis	abnormal condition
-otomy	cutting into
-pathy	disease

-pexy	surgical fixation
-phobia	fear
-plasty	surgical repair
-plegia	paralysis
-ptosis	drooping
-rrhagia	abnormal flow condition
-scope	instrument for viewing
-scopy	process of visually examining
-tic	pertaining to
-tropia	turned condition

Prefixes

a-	without
an-	without
anti-	against
de-	without
eso-	inward

exo-	outward
extra-	outside of
hemi-	half
hyper-	excessive
intra-	within

micro-	small
mono-	one
myo-	to shut

Adjective Forms of Anatomical Terms

Term	Word Parts	Definition
conjunctival (kon-JUNK-tih-vall)	conjunctiv/o = conjunctiva -al = pertaining to	Pertaining to the conjunctiva.
corneal (KOR-nee-all)	corne/o = cornea -al = pertaining to **Word Watch** Be careful using the combining forms *core/o* meaning "pupil" and *corne/o* meaning "cornea."	Pertaining to the cornea.
extraocular (EKS-truh-OCK-yoo-lar)	extra- = outside of ocul/o = eye -ar = pertaining to	Pertaining to being outside the eyeball; for example, the extraocular eye muscles.
intraocular (in-trah-OCK-yoo-lar)	intra- = within ocul/o = eye -ar = pertaining to	Pertaining to within the eye.
iridal (ir-id-al)	irid/o = iris -al = pertaining to	Pertaining to the iris.
lacrimal (LAK-rim-al)	lacrim/o = tears -al = pertaining to	Pertaining to tears.
macular (MACK-yoo-lar)	macul/o = macula lutea -ar = pertaining to	Pertaining to the macula lutea.
ocular (OCK-yoo-lar)	ocul/o = eye -ar = pertaining to	Pertaining to the eye.
ophthalmic (off-THAL-mik)	ophthalm/o = eye -ic = pertaining to	Pertaining to the eye.
optic (OP-tik)	opt/o = eye, vision -ic = pertaining to	Pertaining to the eye or vision.
optical (OP-tih-kal)	optic/o = eye, vision -al = pertaining to	Pertaining to the eye or vision.
pupillary (PYOO-pih-lair-ee)	pupill/o = pupil -ary = pertaining to	Pertaining to the pupil.
retinal (RET-in-al)	retin/o = retina -al = pertaining to	Pertaining to the retina.
scleral (SKLAIR-all)	scler/o = sclera -al = pertaining to	Pertaining to the sclera.
uveal (YOO-vee-al)	uve/o = choroid -al = pertaining to	Pertaining to the choroid layer of the eye.

Practice As You Go

B. Give the adjective form for each anatomical structure

1. The pupil ______________________
2. The eye or vision ______________________ or ______________________
3. The retina ______________________
4. Tears ______________________
5. Within the eye ______________________
6. Outside of the eye ______________________

Pathology

Term	Word Parts	Definition
Medical Specialties		
ophthalmologist (opf-thal-MOLL-oh-jist)	ophthalm/o = eye -logist = one who studies	Medical doctor who has specialized in the diagnosis and treatment of eye conditions and diseases.
ophthalmology (Ophth.) (opf-thal-MOLL-oh-jee)	ophthalm/o = eye -logy = study of	Branch of medicine involving the diagnosis and treatment of conditions and diseases of the eye and surrounding structures.
optician (op-TISH-an)	opt/o = vision -ician = specialist	Person trained in grinding and fitting corrective lenses.
optometrist (op-TOM-eh-trist)	opt/o = vision -metrist = specialist in measuring	Doctor of optometry.
optometry (op-TOM-eh-tree)	opt/o = vision -metry = process of measuring	Medical profession specializing in examining the eyes, testing visual acuity, and prescribing corrective lenses.
Signs and Symptoms		
blepharoptosis (blef-ah-rop-TOH-sis)	blephar/o = eyelid -ptosis = drooping	Drooping eyelid.
cycloplegia (sigh-kloh-PLEE-jee-ah)	cycl/o = ciliary body -plegia = paralysis	Paralysis of the ciliary body. This affects changing the shape of the lens to bring images into focus.
diplopia (dip-LOH-pee-ah)	dipl/o = double -opia = vision condition	Condition of seeing double.
emmetropia (EM) (em-eh-TROH-pee-ah)	emmetr/o = correct, proper -opia = vision condition	State of normal vision.
iridoplegia (ir-id-oh-PLEE-jee-ah)	irid/o = iris -plegia = paralysis	Paralysis of the iris. This affects changing the size of the pupil to regulate the amount of light entering the eye.

Pathology (continued)

Term	Word Parts	Definition
nyctalopia (nik-tah-LOH-pee-ah)	nyctal/o = night -opia = vision condition	Difficulty seeing in dim light; also called *night blindness.* Usually due to damaged rods.
	Med Term Tip The simple translation of *nyctalopia* is "night vision." However, it is used to mean "night blindness."	
ophthalmalgia (off-thal-MAL-jee-ah)	ophthalm/o = eye -algia = pain	Eye pain.
ophthalmoplegia (off-thal-moh-PLEE-jee-ah)	ophthalm/o = eye -plegia = paralysis	Paralysis of one or more of the extraocular eye muscles.
ophthalmorrhagia (off-thal-moh-RAH-jee-ah)	ophthalm/o = eye -rrhagia = abnormal flow condition	Bleeding from the eye.
papilledema (pah-pill-eh-DEEM-ah)	papill/o = optic disk -edema = swelling	Swelling of the optic disk. Often as a result of increased intraocular pressure. Also called *choked disk.*
photophobia (foh-toh-FOH-bee-ah)	phot/o = light -phobia = fear	Although the term translates into *fear of light*, it actually means a strong sensitivity to bright light.
presbyopia (prez-bee-OH-pee-ah)	presby/o = old age -opia = vision condition	Visual loss due to old age, resulting in difficulty in focusing for near vision (such as reading).
scleromalacia (sklair-oh-mah-LAY-she-ah)	scler/o = sclera -malacia = abnormal softening	Softening of the sclera.
xerophthalmia (zeer-of-THAL-mee-ah)	xer/o = dry ophthalm/o = eye -ia = condition	Dry eyes.
Eyeball		
achromatopsia (ah-kroh-mah-TOP-see-ah)	a- = without chromat/o = color -opsia = vision condition	Severe, congenital deficiency in color vision; complete color blidness; more common in males.
amblyopia (am-blee-OH-pee-ah)	ambly/o = dull, dim -opia = vision condition	Loss of vision not as a result of eye pathology. Usually occurs in patients who see two images. In order to see only one image, the brain will no longer recognize the image being sent to it by one of the eyes. May occur if strabismus is not corrected. This condition is not treatable with a prescription lens. Commonly referred to as *lazy eye.*
astigmatism (Astigm) (ah-STIG-mah-tizm)	a- = without stigmat/o = point -ism = state of	Condition in which light rays are focused unevenly on the retina, causing a distorted image, due to an abnormal curvature of the cornea.

Pathology (continued)

Term	Word Parts	Definition
cataract (KAT-ah-rakt) ■ **Figure 13.8** Photograph of a person with a cataract in the right eye. *(ARZTSAMUI/Shutterstock)*	Med Term Tip The term *cataract* comes from the Latin word meaning "waterfall." This refers to how a person with a cataract sees the world—as if looking through a waterfall. 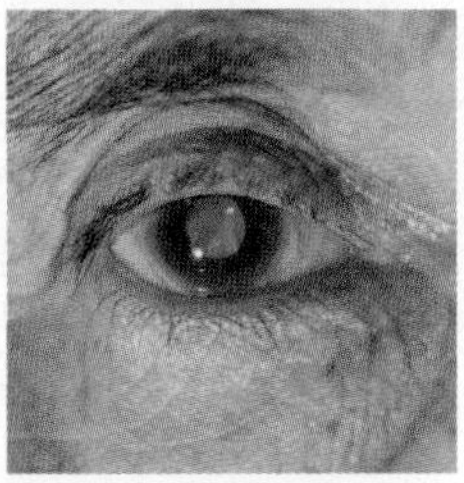	Damage to the lens causing it to become opaque or cloudy, resulting in diminished vision. Treatment is usually surgical removal of the cataract or replacement of the lens.
corneal abrasion	corne/o = cornea -al = pertaining to	Scraping injury to the cornea. If it does not heal, it may develop into an ulcer.
glaucoma (glau-KOH-mah)	glauc/o = gray -oma = mass	Increase in intraocular pressure, which, if untreated, may result in atrophy (wasting away) of the optic nerve and blindness. Glaucoma is treated with medication and surgery. There is an increased risk of developing glaucoma in persons over age 60, those of African ancestry, people who have sustained a serious eye injury, or anyone with a family history of diabetes or glaucoma.
hyperopia (high-per-OH-pee-ah) ■ **Figure 13.9** Hyperopia (farsightedness). In the uncorrected top figure, the image would come into focus behind the retina, making the image on the retina blurry. The bottom image shows how a biconvex lens corrects this condition.	hyper- = excessive -opia = vision condition 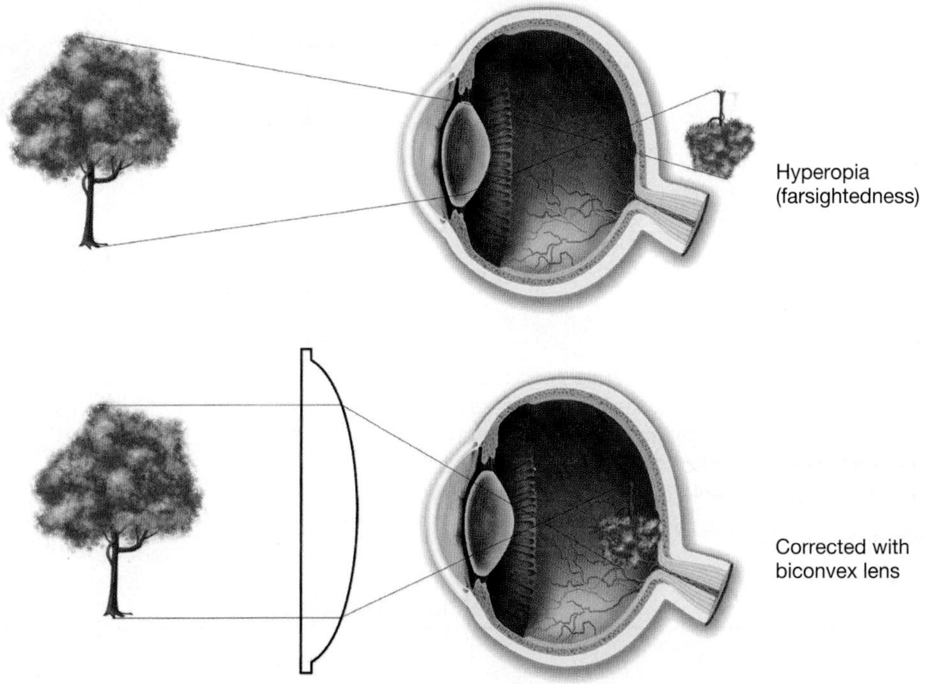 Hyperopia (farsightedness) Corrected with biconvex lens	With this condition a person can see things in the distance but has trouble reading material at close range. Also known as *farsightedness.* This condition is corrected with converging or biconvex lenses.

Pathology (continued)

Term	Word Parts	Definition
iritis (eye-RYE-tis)	ir/o = iris -itis = inflammation	Inflammation of the iris.
keratitis (kair-ah-TYE-tis)	kerat/o = cornea -itis = inflammation Word Watch Be careful using the combining form *kerat/o*, which means both "cornea" and the "hard protein keratin."	Inflammation of the cornea.
legally blind		Describes a person who has severely impaired vision. Usually defined as having visual acuity of 20/200 that cannot be improved with corrective lenses or having a visual field of less than 20 degrees.
macular degeneration (MAK-yoo-lar)	macul/o = macula lutea -ar = pertaining to	Deterioration of the macular area of the retina of the eye. May be treated with laser surgery to destroy the blood vessels beneath the macula.
monochromatism (mon-oh-KROH-mah-tizm)	mono- = one chromat/o = color -ism = state of	Unable to perceive one color.
myopia (MY) (my-OH-pee-ah) Med Term Tip The term *myopia* appears to use the combining form my/o, which means "muscle." This combining form comes from the Greek word *mys*. But in this case the term uses the prefix myo-, which comes from the Greek word *myo* or *myein*, meaning "to shut."	myo- = to shut -opia = vision condition	With this condition a person can see things close up but distance vision is blurred. Also known as *nearsightedness*. This condition is corrected with diverging or biconcave lenses. Named because persons with myopia often partially shut their eyes, squint, in order to see better.

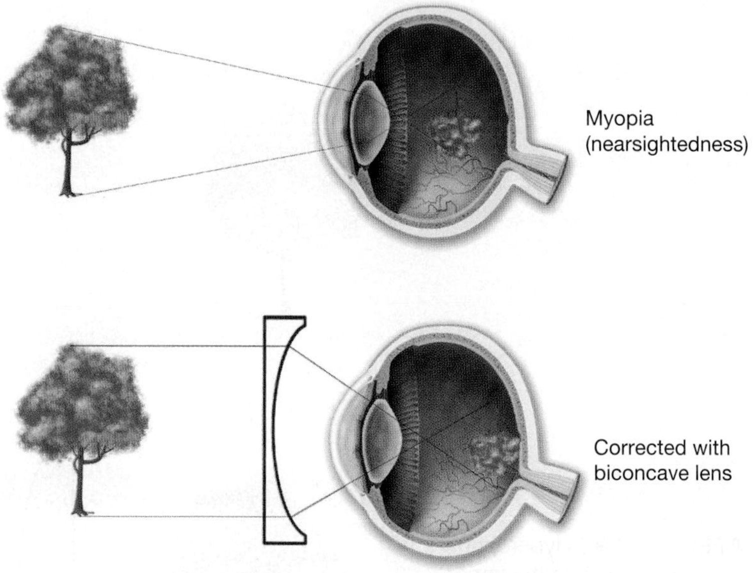

■ **Figure 13.10** Myopia (nearsightedness). In the uncorrected top figure, the image comes into focus in front of the lens, making the image on the retina blurry. The bottom image shows how a biconcave lens corrects this condition.

Term	Word Parts	Definition
oculomycosis (ock-yoo-loh-my-KOH-sis)	ocul/o = eye myc/o = fungus -osis = abnormal condition	Fungus infection of the eye.

Pathology (continued)

Term	Word Parts	Definition
retinal detachment (RET-in-al)	retin/o = retina -al = pertaining to	Occurs when the retina becomes separated from the choroid layer. This separation seriously damages blood vessels and nerves, resulting in blindness. May be treated with surgical or medical procedures to stabilize the retina and prevent separation.
retinitis pigmentosa (ret-in-EYE-tis / pig-men-TOH-sah)	retin/o = retina -itis = inflammation	Progressive disease of the eye resulting in the retina becoming hard (sclerosed), pigmented (colored), and atrophied (wasting away). There is no known cure for this condition.
retinoblastoma (RET-in-noh-blast-OH-mah)	retin/o = retina blast/o = immature -oma = tumor	Malignant eye tumor occurring in children, usually under the age of 3. Requires enucleation.
retinopathy (ret-in-OP-ah-thee)	retin/o = retina -pathy = disease	General term for disease affecting the retina.
scleritis (skler-EYE-tis)	scler/o = sclera -itis = inflammation	Inflammation of the sclera.
uveitis (yoo-vee-EYE-tis)	uve/o = choroid -itis = inflammation	Inflammation of the choroid layer.
Conjunctiva		
conjunctivitis (kon-junk-tih-VYE-tis)	conjunctiv/o = conjunctiva -itis = inflammation	Inflammation of the conjunctiva usually as the result of a bacterial infection. Commonly called *pinkeye*.
pterygium (teh-RIJ-ee-um)		Hypertrophied conjunctival tissue in the inner corner of the eye.
Eyelids		
blepharitis (blef-ah-RYE-tis)	blephar/o = eyelid -itis = inflammation	Inflammation of the eyelid.
hordeolum (hor-DEE-oh-lum)		Refers to a *stye* (or *sty*), a small purulent inflammatory infection of a sebaceous gland of the eyelid; treated with hot compresses and/or surgical incision.
Lacrimal Apparatus		
dacryoadenitis (dak-ree-oh-ad-eh-NYE-tis)	dacry/o = tears aden/o = gland -itis = inflammation	Inflammation of the lacrimal gland.
dacryocystitis (dak-ree-oh-sis-TYE-tis)	dacry/o = tears cyst/o = sac -itis = inflammation	Inflammation of the lacrimal sac.
Eye Muscles		
esotropia (ST) (ess-oh-TROH-pee-ah)	eso- = inward -tropia = turned condition	Inward turning of the eye; also called *cross-eyed.* An example of a form of strabismus (muscle weakness of the eye).
exotropia (XT) (eks-oh-TROH-pee-ah)	exo- = outward -tropia = turned condition	Outward turning of the eye; also called *wall-eyed.* Also an example of strabismus (muscle weakness of the eye).

Pathology (continued)

Term	Word Parts	Definition
strabismus (strah-BIZ-mus)		Eye muscle weakness commonly seen in children resulting in the eyes looking in different directions at the same time. May be corrected with glasses, eye exercises, and/or surgery.
Brain-Related Vision Pathologies		
hemianopia (hem-ee-ah-NOP-ee-ah)	hemi- = half an- = without -opia = vision condition	Loss of vision in half of the visual field. A stroke patient may suffer from this disorder.
nystagmus (niss-TAG-mus)		Jerky-appearing involuntary eye movements, usually left and right. Often an indication of brain injury.

Practice As You Go

C. Terminology Matching

Match each term to its definition.

1. ________ emmetropia — a. opacity of the lens
2. ________ hyperopia — b. a form of strabismus
3. ________ cataract — c. nearsightedness
4. ________ astigmatism — d. due to abnormal curvature of cornea
5. ________ esotropia — e. lazy eye
6. ________ xerophthalmia — f. involuntary movements of the eye
7. ________ myopia — g. farsightedness
8. ________ nystagmus — h. normal vision
9. ________ amblyopia — i. dry eyes
10. ________ presbyopia — j. old-age vision loss

Diagnostic Procedures

Term	Word Parts	Definition
Eye Examination Tests		
color vision tests ■ **Figure 13.11** An example of color blindness test. A person with red-green color blindness would not be able to distinguish the green 27 from the surrounding red circles.		Use of polychromic (multicolored) charts to determine the ability of the patient to recognize color.
fluorescein angiography (floo-oh-RESS-ee-in / an-jee-OG-rah-fee)	angi/o = vessel -graphy = process of recording	Process of injecting a dye (fluorescein) to observe the movement of blood and detect lesions in the macular area of the retina. Used to determine if there is a detachment of the retina.
fluorescein staining (floo-oh-RESS-ee-in)		Application of dye eyedrops of a bright green fluorescent color used to look for corneal abrasions or ulcers.
keratometer kair-ah-TOM-eh-ter	kerat/o = cornea -meter = instrument to measure	An instrument used to measure the curvature of the cornea.
keratometry (kair-ah-TOM-eh-tree)	kerat/o = cornea -metry = process of measuring	Measurement of the curvature of the cornea using an instrument called a *keratometer.*
ophthalmoscope (off-THAL-moh-scope)	ophthalm/o = eye -scope = instrument for viewing	Instrument used to examine the inside of the eye through the pupil.
ophthalmoscopy (off-thal-MOSS-koh-pee)	ophthalm/o = eye -scopy = process of visually examining	Examination of the interior of the eyes using an instrument called an *ophthalmoscope* (see Figure 13.12 ■). The physician dilates the pupil in order to see the cornea, lens, and retina. Used to identify abnormalities in the blood vessels of the eye and some systemic diseases.

Diagnostic Procedures (continued)

Term	Word Parts	Definition
■ **Figure 13.12** Examination of the interior of the eye using an ophthalmoscope. *(Monkey Business Images/Shutterstock)*	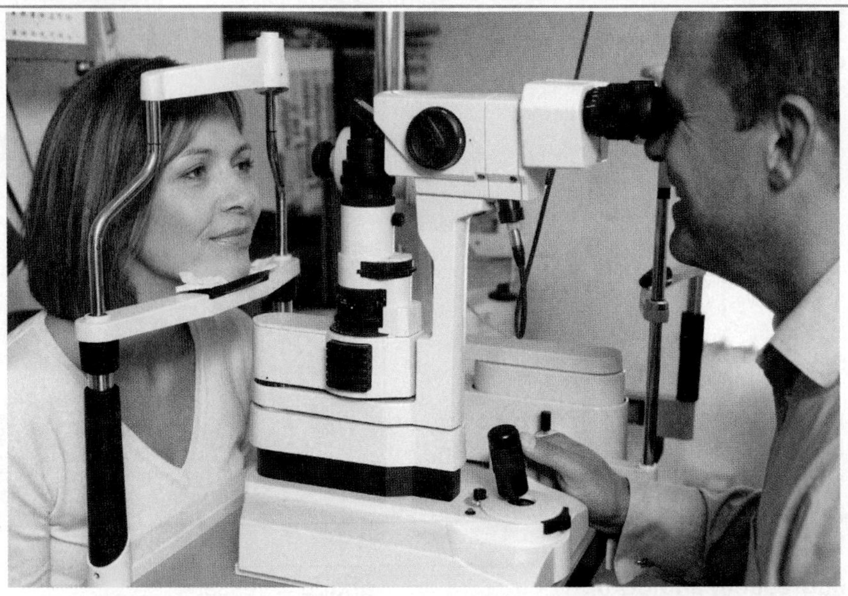	
optometer (op-TOM-eh-ter)	opt/o = vision -meter = instrument to measure	Instrument used to measure how well the eye is able to focus images clearly on the retina.
refractive error test (ree-FRAK-tiv)		Vision test for a defect in the ability of the eye to accurately focus the image that is hitting it. Refractive errors result in myopia and hyperopia.
slit lamp microscopy	micro- = small -scopy = process of visually examining	Examining the conjunctiva, cornea, iris, and lens of the eye.
Snellen chart (SNEL-en)		Chart used for testing distance vision named for Dutch ophthalmologist Herman Snellen. It contains letters of varying sizes and is administered from a distance of 20 feet. A person who can read at 20 feet what the average person can read at this distance is said to have 20/20 vision.
tonometry (tohn-OM-eh-tree)	ton/o = tone -metry = process of measuring	Measurement of the intraocular pressure of the eye using a *tonometer* to check for the condition of glaucoma. Generally part of a normal eye exam for adults.
visual acuity (VA) **test** (VIZH-oo-al / ah-KYOO-ih-tee)	-al = pertaining to	Measurement of the sharpness of a patient's vision. Usually, a Snellen chart is used for this test in which the patient identifies letters from a distance of 20 feet.

Therapeutic Procedures

Terms	Word Parts	Definition
Surgical Procedures		
blepharectomy (blef-ah-REK-toh-mee)	blephar/o = eyelid -ectomy = surgical removal	Surgical removal of all or part of the eyelid.
blepharoplasty (BLEF-ah-roh-plass-tee)	blephar/o = eyelid -plasty = surgical repair	Surgical repair of the eyelid. A common plastic surgery to correct blepharoptosis.
conjunctivoplasty (kon-junk-tih-VOH-plas-tee)	conjunctiv/o = conjunctiva -plasty = surgical repair	Surgical repair of the conjunctiva.
cryoextraction (cry-oh-eks-TRAK-shun)	cry/o = cold	Procedure in which cataract is lifted from the lens with an extremely cold probe.
cryoretinopexy (cry-oh-RET-ih-noh-pek-see)	cry/o = cold retin/o = retina -pexy = surgical fixation	Surgical fixation of the retina by using extreme cold.
enucleation (ee-new-klee-AY-shun)		Surgical removal of an eyeball.
iridectomy (ir-id-EK-toh-mee)	irid/o = iris -ectomy = surgical removal	Surgical removal of a small portion of the iris.
iridosclerotomy (ir-ih-doh-skleh-ROT-oh-mee)	irid/o = iris scler/o = sclera -otomy = cutting into	To cut into the iris and sclera.
keratoplasty (KAIR-ah-toh-plass-tee)	kerat/o = cornea -plasty = surgical repair	Surgical repair of the cornea is the simple translation of this term that is utilized to mean corneal transplant.
laser-assisted in situ keratomileusis (LASIK) (in-SIH-tyoo / kair-ah-toh-mih-LOO-sis) ■ **Figure 13.13** LASIK surgery uses a laser to reshape the cornea. *(mehmetcan/Shutterstock)*	kerat/o = cornea	Correction of myopia using laser surgery to remove corneal tissue.
laser photocoagulation (LAY-zer / foh-toh-koh-ag-yoo-LAY-shun)	phot/o = light	Use of a laser beam to destroy very small precise areas of the retina. May be used to treat retinal detachment or macular degeneration.

Therapeutic Procedures (continued)

Terms	Word Parts	Definition
phacoemulsification (fak-oh-ee-mull-sih-fih-KAY-shun)	phac/o = lens	Use of high-frequency sound waves to emulsify (liquefy) a lens with a cataract, which is then aspirated (removed by suction) with a needle.
photorefractive keratectomy (PRK) (foh-toh-ree-FRAK-tiv / kair-ah-TEK-toh-mee)	phot/o = light kerat/o = cornea -ectomy = surgical removal	Use of a laser to reshape the cornea and correct errors of refraction.
prosthetic lens implant (pros-THET-ik)		Use of an artificial lens to replace the lens removed during cataract surgery.
radial keratotomy (RK) (RAY-dee-all / kair-ah-TOT-oh-mee)	-al = pertaining to kerat/o = cornea -otomy = cutting into	Spokelike incisions around the cornea that result in it becoming flatter. A surgical treatment for myopia.
retinopexy (ret-ih-noh-PEX-ee)	retin/o = retina -pexy = surgical fixation	Surgical fixation of the retina. One treatment for a detaching retina.
scleral buckling (SKLAIR-al)	scler/o = sclera -al = pertaining to	Placing a band of silicone around the outside of the sclera that stabilizes a detaching retina.
sclerotomy (skleh-ROT-oh-mee)	scler/o = sclera -otomy = cutting into	To cut into the sclera.
strabotomy (strah-BOT-oh-mee)	-otomy = cutting into	Incision into the eye muscles in order to correct strabismus.

Practice As You Go

D. Terminology Matching

Match each term to its definition.

1. ________ fluorescein staining
2. ________ ophthalmoscopy
3. ________ tonometry
4. ________ enucleation
5. ________ keratoplasty
6. ________ phacoemulsification

a. examining the interior of the eyeball
b. used to mean corneal transplant
c. liquefies a cataract
d. looks for corneal abrasions or ulcers
e. surgical removal of the eyeball
f. measures intraocular pressure

Pharmacology

Classification	Word Parts	Action	Examples
anesthetic ophthalmic solution (off-THAL-mik)	an- = without esthesi/o = sensation, feeling -tic = pertaining to ophthalm/o = eye -ic = pertaining to	Eyedrops for pain relief associated with eye infections, corneal abrasions, or surgery.	proparacain, Ak-Taine, Ocu-Caine; tetracaine, Opticaine, Pontocaine
antibiotic ophthalmic solution (off-THAL-mik)	anti- = against bi/o = life -tic = pertaining to ophthalm/o = eye -ic = pertaining to	Eyedrops for the treatment of bacterial eye infections.	erythromycin, Del-Mycin, Ilotycin Ophthalmic
antiglaucoma medications (an-tye-glau-KOH-mah)	anti- = against glauc/o = gray -oma = mass	Reduce intraocular pressure by lowering the amount of aqueous humor in the eyeball. May achieve this by either reducing the production of aqueous humor or increasing its outflow.	timolol, Betimol, Timoptic; acetazolamide, Ak-Zol, Dazamide; prostaglandin analogs, Lumigan, Xalatan
artificial tears		Medications, many of them over-the-counter, to treat dry eyes.	buffered isotonic solutions, Akwa Tears, Refresh Plus, Moisture Eyes
miotic drops (my-OT-ik)	mi/o = lessening -tic = pertaining to	Any substance that causes the pupil to constrict. These medications may also be used to treat glaucoma.	physostigmine, Eserine Sulfate, Isopto Eserine; carbachol, Carbastat, Miostat
mydriatic drops (mid-ree-AT-ik)	mydr/i = widening -atic = pertaining to	Any substance that causes the pupil to dilate by paralyzing the iris and/or ciliary body muscles. Particularly useful during eye examinations and eye surgery.	atropine sulfate, Atropine-Care Ophthalmic, Atropisol Ophthalmic
ophthalmic decongestants	ophthalm/o = eye -ic = pertaining to de- = without	Over-the-counter medications that constrict the arterioles of the eye and reduce redness and itching of the conjunctiva.	tetrahydrozoline, Visine, Murine

Abbreviations

ARMD	age-related macular degeneration	**EM**	emmetropia
Astigm	astigmatism	**EOM**	extraocular movement
c.gl.	correction with glasses	**ICCE**	intracapsular cataract extraction
D	diopter (lens strength)	**IOP**	intraocular pressure
DVA	distance visual acuity	**LASIK**	laser-assisted in situ keratomileusis
ECCE	extracapsular cataract extraction	**OD**	right eye
EENT	eye, ear, nose, and throat	**Ophth.**	ophthalmology

Abbreviations (continued)

OS	left eye	**s.gl.**	without correction or glasses
OU	each eye/both eyes	**SMD**	senile macular degeneration
PERRLA	pupils equal, round, react to light and accommodation	**ST**	esotropia
PRK	photorefractive keratectomy	**VA**	visual acuity
REM	rapid eye movement	**VF**	visual field
RK	radial keratotomy	**XT**	exotropia

Med Term Tip

The abbreviations for right eye (OD) and left eye (OS) are easy to remember when we know their origins. OD stands for *oculus* (eye) *dexter* (right). OS has its origin in *oculus* (eye) *sinister* (left). At one time in history it was considered to be sinister if a person looked at another from only the left side. Hence the term *oculus sinister* means "left eye."

Practice As You Go

E. What's the Abbreviation?

1. pressure equalizing tube ______
2. emmetropia ______
3. exotropia ______
4. left eye ______
5. extraocular movement ______
6. visual acuity ______

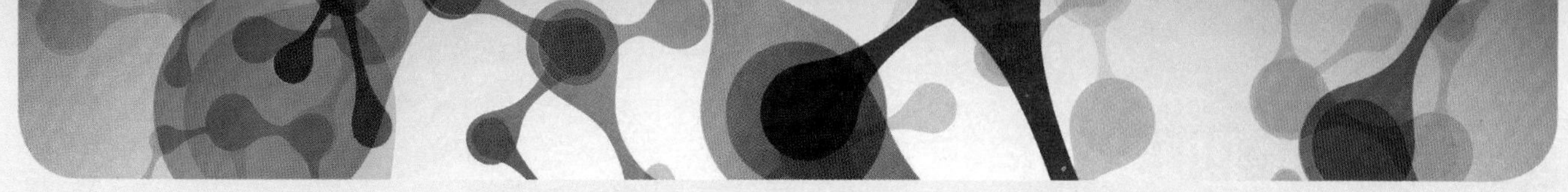

Section II: The Ear at a Glance

Function

The ear contains the sensory receptors for hearing and equilibrium (balance).

Structures

Here are the primary structures that comprise the ear:

auricle	**inner ear**
external ear	**middle ear**

Word Parts

Here are the most common word parts (with their meanings) used to build ear terms. For a more comprehensive list, refer to the Terminology section of this chapter.

Combining Forms

acous/o	hearing	**labyrinth/o**	labyrinth (inner ear)
audi/o	hearing	**myring/o**	tympanic membrane
audit/o	hearing	**ot/o**	ear
aur/o	ear	**salping/o**	auditory tube (eustachian tube)
auricul/o	ear	**staped/o**	stapes
cerumin/o	cerumen	**tympan/o**	tympanic membrane
cochle/o	cochlea	**vestibul/o**	vestibule

Suffixes

-cusis	hearing
-otia	ear condition

The Ear Illustrated

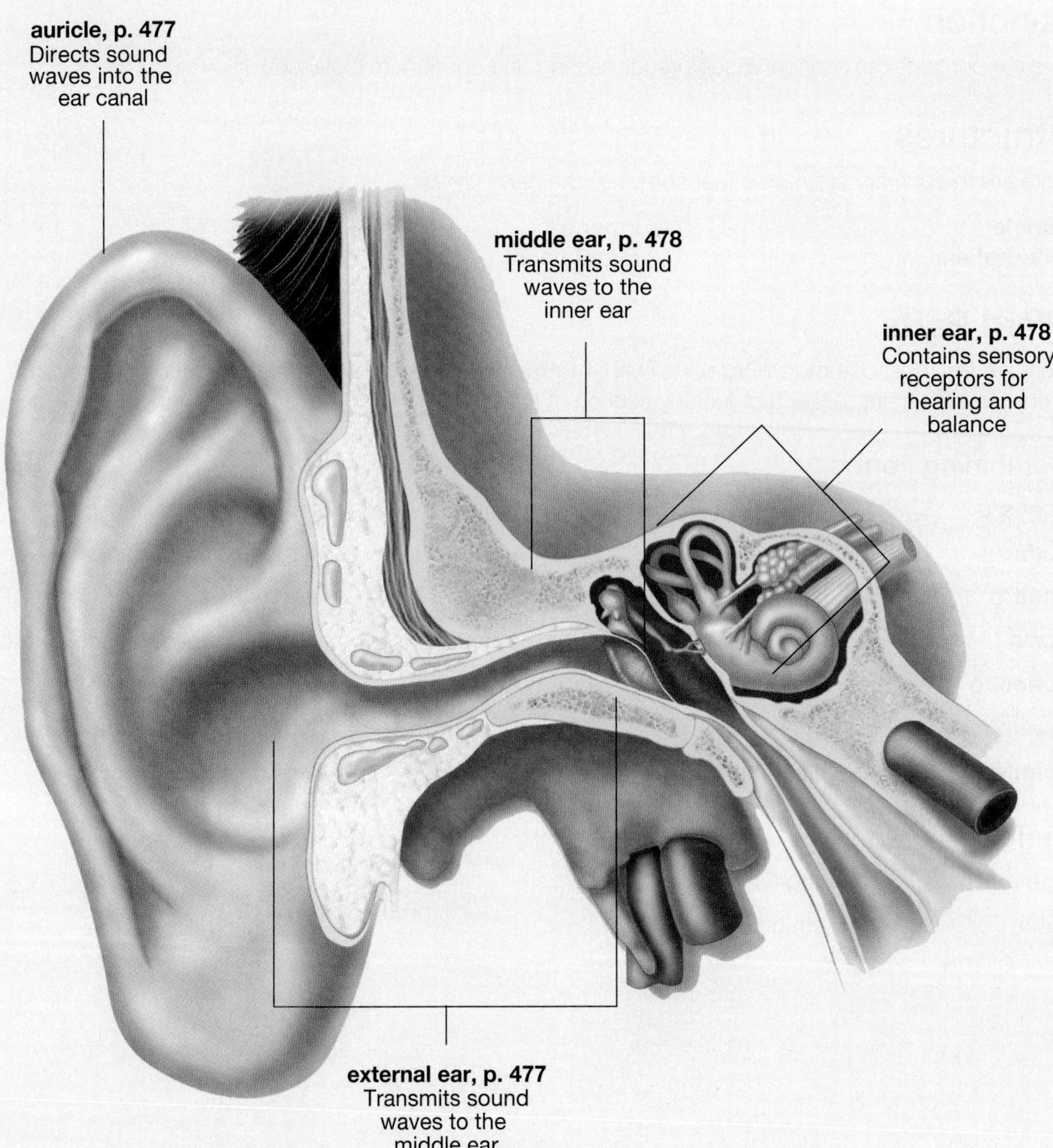

auricle, p. 477
Directs sound waves into the ear canal
middle ear, p. 478
Transmits sound waves to the inner ear
inner ear, p. 478
Contains sensory receptors for hearing and balance
external ear, p. 477
Transmits sound waves to the middle ear

Anatomy and Physiology of the Ear

audiology (aw-dee-OL-oh-jee)
cochlear nerve (KOK-lee-ar)
equilibrium (ee-kwih-LIB-ree-um)
external ear
hearing
inner ear
middle ear
otology (oh-TOL-oh-jee)
vestibular nerve (ves-TIB-yoo-lar)
vestibulocochlear nerve (ves-tib-yoo-loh-KOK-lee-ar)

The study of the ear is referred to as **otology** (Oto), and the study of hearing disorders is called **audiology.** While there is a large amount of overlap between these two areas, there are also examples of ear problems that do not affect hearing. The ear is responsible for two senses: **hearing** and **equilibrium**, or our sense of balance. Hearing and equilibrium sensory information is carried to the brain by cranial nerve VIII, the **vestibulocochlear nerve.** This nerve is divided into two major branches. The **cochlear nerve** carries hearing information, and the **vestibular nerve** carries equilibrium information.

What's In A Name?
cochle/o = cochlea
vestibul/o = vestibule
-al = pertaining to
-ar = pertaining to
ex- = outward

The ear is subdivided into three areas: **external ear**, **middle ear**, and **inner ear.**

External Ear

auditory canal (AW-dih-tor-ee)
auricle (AW-rih-kl)
cerumen (seh-ROO-men)
external auditory meatus (AW-dih-tor-ee / me-A-tus)
pinna (PIN-ah)
tympanic membrane (tim-PAN-ik)

The external ear consists of three parts: the **auricle**, the **auditory canal**, and the **tympanic membrane** (see Figure 13.14■). The auricle or **pinna** is what is commonly referred to as the *ear* because this is the only visible portion. The auricle with its earlobe has a unique shape in each person and functions like a funnel to capture sound waves as they go past the outer ear and channel them through the **external auditory meatus.** The sound then moves along the auditory canal and causes the

What's In A Name?
-al = pertaining to
ex- = outward

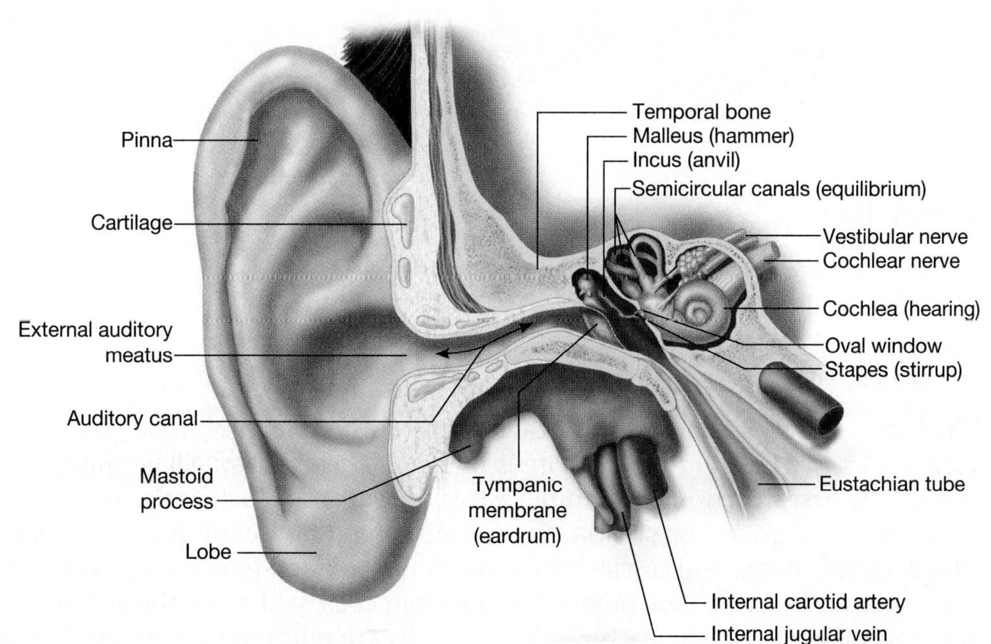

■ **Figure 13.14** The internal structures of the outer, middle, and inner ear.

Med Term Tip

The term *tympanic membrane* comes from the Greek word for "drumhead." The tympanic membrane or eardrum vibrates to sound waves like a drum head.

tympanic membrane (eardrum) to vibrate. The tympanic membrane actually separates the external ear from the middle ear. Earwax or **cerumen** is produced in oil glands in the auditory canal. This wax helps to protect and lubricate the ear. It is also just barely liquid at body temperature. This causes cerumen to slowly flow out of the auditory canal, carrying dirt and dust with it. Therefore, the auditory canal is self-cleaning.

Middle Ear

auditory tube (AW-dih-tor-ee)
eustachian tube (yoo-STAY-she-en)
incus (ING-kus)
malleus (MAL-ee-us)
ossicles (OSS-ih-kls)
oval window
stapes (STAY-peez)

Med Term Tip

The three bones in the middle ear are referred to by terms that are similar to their shape. Thus, the malleus is called the hammer, the incus is the anvil, and the stapes is the stirrup (see again Figure 13.15).

The middle ear is located in a small cavity in the temporal bone of the skull. This air-filled cavity contains three tiny bones called **ossicles** (see Figure 13.15 ■). These three bones—the **malleus**, **incus**, and **stapes**—are vital to the hearing process. They amplify the vibrations in the middle ear and transmit them to the inner ear from the malleus to the incus and finally to the stapes. The stapes, the last of the three ossicles, is attached to a very thin membrane that covers the opening to the inner ear called the **oval window.**

The **eustachian tube** or **auditory tube** connects the nasopharynx with the middle ear (see again Figure 13.14). Each time you swallow the eustachian tube opens. This connection allows pressure to equalize between the middle ear cavity and the atmospheric pressure.

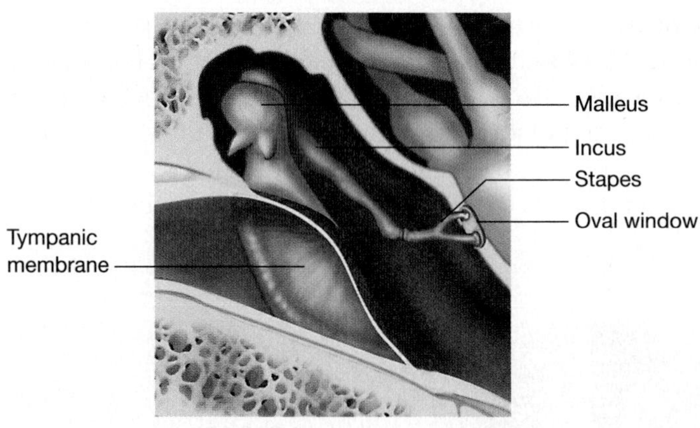

■ **Figure 13.15**
Close-up view of the ossicles within the middle ear. These three bones extend from the tympanic membrane to the oval window.

What's In A Name?
-ar = pertaining to
-ule = small
semi- = partial

Inner Ear

cochlea (KOK-lee-ah)
labyrinth (LAB-ih-rinth)
organs of Corti (KOR-tee)
saccule (SAK-yool)
semicircular canals
utricle (YOO-trih-kl)
vestibule (VES-tih-byul)

Med Term Tip

The term *vestibule* comes from the Latin word *vestibulum*, meaning "entrance." It received this name because it is the entryway into the inner ear.

The inner ear is also located in a cavity within the temporal bone (see again Figure 13.14). This fluid-filled cavity is referred to as the **labyrinth** because of its shape. The first structure of the inner ear is the **vestibule.** Each of the remaining inner ear structures—the **cochlea** (the sensory organ for hearing) and the **semicircular canals, utricle,** and **saccule** (the sensory organs for equilibrium)—open off the vestibule. Each of these organs contains hair cells, which are the actual sensory receptor cells. In the cochlea, the hair cells are referred to as **organs of Corti.**

How We Hear

conductive hearing loss (kon-DUK-tiv)
sensorineural hearing loss (sen-soh-ree-NOO-ral)

Figure 13.16 ■ outlines the path of sound through the outer ear and middle ear and into the cochlea of the inner ear. Sound waves traveling down the external auditory canal strike the eardrum, causing it to vibrate. The ossicles conduct these vibrations across the middle ear from the eardrum to the oval window. Oval window movements initiate vibrations in the fluid that fills the cochlea. As the fluid vibrations strike a hair cell, they bend the small hairs and stimulate the nerve ending. The nerve ending then sends an electrical impulse to the brain on the cochlear portion of the vestibulocochlear nerve.

Hearing loss can be divided into two main categories: **conductive hearing loss** and **sensorineural hearing loss**. Conductive refers to disease or malformation of the outer or middle ear. All sound is weaker and muffled in conductive hearing loss since it is not conducted correctly to the inner ear. Sensorineural hearing loss is the result of damage or malformation of the inner ear (cochlea) or the cochlear nerve. In this hearing loss, some sounds are distorted and heard incorrectly. There can also be a combination of both conductive and sensorineural hearing loss.

What's In A Name?
neur/o = nerve
-al = pertaining to

Med Term Tip
Hearing impairment is becoming a greater problem for the general population for several reasons. First, people are living longer. Hearing loss can accompany old age, and there are a greater number of people over age 50 requiring hearing assistance. In addition, sound technology has produced music quality that was never available before. However, listening to loud music either naturally or through earphones can cause gradual damage to the hearing mechanism.

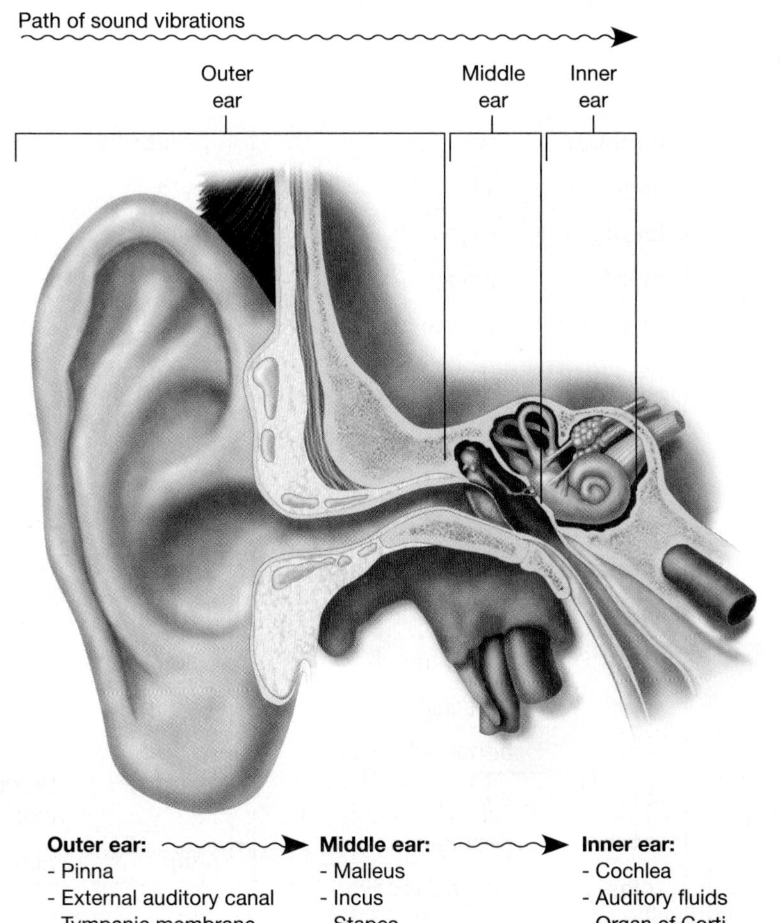

■ **Figure 13.16** The path of sound waves through the outer, middle, and inner ear.

Practice As You Go

F. Complete the Statement

1. The three bones in the middle ear are the ____________, ____________, and ____________.
2. The study of the ear is called ____________.
3. Another term for the eardrum is ____________.
4. ____________ is produced in the oil glands in the auditory canal.
5. The ____________ tube connects the nasopharynx with the middle ear.
6. The ____________ is responsible for conducting impulses from the ear to the brain.

Terminology

Word Parts Used to Build Ear Terms

The following lists contain the combining forms, suffixes, and prefixes used to build terms in the remaining sections of this chapter.

Combining Forms

acous/o	hearing
audi/o	hearing
audit/o	hearing
aur/o	ear
auricul/o	ear
bi/o	life
cerumin/o	cerumen

cochle/o	cochlea
labyrinth/o	labyrinth
laryng/o	larynx
myc/o	fungus
myring/o	tympanic membrane
neur/o	nerve
ot/o	ear

presby/o	old age
py/o	pus
rhin/o	nose
salping/o	auditory tube
staped/o	stapes
tympan/o	tympanic membrane
vestibul/o	vestibule

Suffixes

-al	pertaining to
-algia	pain
-ar	pertaining to
-cusis	hearing
-ectomy	surgical removal
-emetic	pertaining to vomiting
-gram	record
-ic	pertaining to
-itis	inflammation

-logy	study of
-meter	instrument to measure
-metry	process of measuring
-oma	mass; tumor
-ory	pertaining to
-osis	abnormal condition
-otia	ear condition
-otomy	cutting into
-plasty	surgical repair

-rrhagia	abnormal flow
-rrhea	discharge
-rrhexis	rupture
-sclerosis	hardening
-scope	instrument to visually examine
-scopy	process of visually examining
-tic	pertaining to

Prefixes

an-	without
anti-	against
bi-	two
macro-	large
micro-	small
mono-	one

Adjective Forms of Anatomical Terms

Term	Word Parts	Definition
acoustic (ah-KOOS-tik)	acous/o = hearing -tic = pertaining to	Pertaining to hearing.
auditory (AW-dih-tor-ee)	audit/o = hearing -ory = pertaining to	Pertaining to hearing.
aural (AW-ral)	aur/o = ear -al = pertaining to **Word Watch** Be careful when using two terms that sound the same—*aural* meaning "pertaining to the ear" and *oral* meaning "pertaining to the mouth."	Pertaining to the ear.
auricular (aw-RIK-cu-lar)	auricul/o = ear -ar = pertaining to	Pertaining to the ear.
binaural (bin-AW-rall)	bi- = two aur/o = ear -al = pertaining to	Pertaining to both ears.
cochlear (KOK-lee-ar)	cochle/o = cochlea -ar = pertaining to	Pertaining to the cochlea.
monaural (mon-AW-rall)	mono- = one aur/o = ear -al = pertaining to	Pertaining to one ear.
otic (OH-tik)	ot/o = ear -ic = pertaining to	Pertaining to the ear.
tympanic (tim-PAN-ik)	tympan/o = tympanic membrane -ic = pertaining to	Pertaining to the tympanic membrane.
vestibular (ves-TIB-you-lar)	vestibul/o = vestibule -ar = pertaining to	Pertaining to the vestibule.

Practice As You Go

G. Give the adjective form for each anatomical structure

1. The cochlea ____________________
2. The ear ____________________, ____________________, or ____________________
3. The vestibule ____________________
4. Hearing ____________________ or ____________________
5. One ear ____________________

Pathology

Term	Word Parts	Definition
Medical Specialties		
audiology (aw-dee-OL-oh-jee)	audi/o = hearing -logy = study of	Medical specialty involved with measuring hearing function and identifying hearing loss. Specialist is an *audiologist.*
otorhinolaryngology (ENT) (oh-toh-rye-noh-lair-in-GOL-oh-jee)	ot/o = ear rhin/o = nose laryng/o = larynx -logy = study of	Branch of medicine involving the diagnosis and treatment of conditions and diseases of the ear, nose, and throat. Also referred to as *ENT.* Physician is an *otorhinolaryngologist.*
Signs and Symptoms		
macrotia (mah-KROH-she-ah)	macro- = large -otia = ear condition	Condition of having abnormally large ears.
microtia (my-KROH-she-ah)	micro- = small -otia = ear condition	Condition of having abnormally small ears.
otalgia (oh-TAL-jee-ah)	ot/o = ear -algia = pain	Ear pain.
otopyorrhea (oh-toh-pye-oh-REE-ah)	ot/o = ear py/o = pus -rrhea = discharge	Discharge of pus from the ear.
otorrhagia (oh-toh-RAH-jee-ah)	ot/o = ear -rrhagia = abnormal flow	Bleeding from the ear.
presbycusis (pres-bih-KOO-sis)	presby/o = old age -cusis = hearing condition	Normal loss of hearing that can accompany the aging process.
residual hearing (rih-ZID-joo-al)	-al = pertaining to	Amount of hearing that is still present after damage has occurred to the auditory mechanism.
tinnitus (tin-EYE-tus)		Ringing in the ears.
tympanorrhexis (tim-pan-oh-REK-sis)	tympan/o = tympanic membrane -rrhexis = rupture	Rupture of the tympanic membrane.
vertigo (VER-tih-goh)		Dizziness caused by the sensation that the room is spinning.
Hearing Loss		
anacusis (an-ah-KOO-sis)	an- = without -cusis = hearing	Total absence of hearing; inability to perceive sound. Also called *deafness.*
deafness		Inability to hear or having some degree of hearing impairment.
External Ear		
ceruminoma (seh-roo-men-OH-ma)	cerumin/o = cerumen -oma = mass	Excessive accumulation of earwax resulting in a hard wax plug. Sound becomes muffled.

Pathology (continued)

Term	Word Parts	Definition
otitis externa (OE) (oh-TYE-tis / ex-TERN-ah)	ot/o = ear -itis = inflammation	External ear infection. May be caused by bacteria or fungus. Also called *otomycosis* and commonly referred to as *swimmer's ear.*
otomycosis (oh-toh-my-KOH-sis)	ot/o = ear myc/o = fungus -osis = abnormal condition	Fungal infection of the ear. One type of otitis externa.
Middle Ear		
myringitis (mir-ing-JYE-tis)	myring/o = tympanic membrane -itis = inflammation	Inflammation of the tympanic membrane.
otitis media (OM) (oh-TYE-tis / MEE-dee-ah)	ot/o = ear -itis = inflammation	Seen frequently in children; commonly referred to as a *middle ear infection.* Often preceded by an upper respiratory infection during which pathogens move from the pharynx to the middle ear via the eustachian tube. Fluid accumulates in the middle ear cavity. The fluid may be watery, *serous otitis media*, or full of pus, *purulent otitis media.*
otosclerosis (oh-toh-sklair-OH-sis)	ot/o = ear -sclerosis = hardening	Loss of mobility of the stapes bone, leading to progressive hearing loss.
salpingitis (sal-pin-JIGH-tis)	salping/o = auditory tube -itis = inflammation **Word Watch** Be careful using the combining form *salping/o*, which can mean either "eustachian tube" or "fallopian tube."	Inflammation of the auditory tube.
tympanitis (tim-pan-EYE-tis)	tympan/o = tympanic membrane -itis = inflammation	Inflammation of the tympanic membrane.
Inner Ear		
acoustic neuroma (ah-KOOS-tik / noor-OH-mah)	acous/o = hearing -tic = pertaining to neur/o = nerve -oma = tumor	Benign tumor of the eighth cranial nerve sheath. The pressure causes symptoms such as tinnitus, headache, dizziness, and progressive hearing loss.
labyrinthitis (lab-ih-rin-THIGH-tis)	labyrinth/o = labyrinth -itis = inflammation	May affect both the hearing and equilibrium portions of the inner ear. Also referred to as an *inner ear infection.*
Ménière's disease (may-nee-AIRZ)		Abnormal condition within the labyrinth of the inner ear that can lead to a progressive loss of hearing. The symptoms are vertigo, hearing loss, and tinnitus (ringing in the ears). Named for French physician Prosper Ménière.

Practice As You Go

H. Terminology Matching

Match each term to its definition.

1. ________ anacusis	a. small ears
2. ________ otitis externa	b. dizziness
3. ________ microtia	c. ringing in the ears
4. ________ otopyorrhea	d. a fungal infection
5. ________ labyrinthitis	e. absence of hearing
6. ________ tinnitus	f. ruptured eardrum
7. ________ otosclerosis	g. pus discharge from the ear
8. ________ vertigo	h. swimmer's ear
9. ________ otomycosis	i. loss of mobility of stapes
10. ________ tympanorrhexis	j. inner ear infection

Diagnostic Procedures

Term	Word Parts	Definition
Audiology Tests		
audiogram (AW-dee-oh-gram)	audi/o = hearing -gram = record	Graphic record that illustrates the results of audiometry.
audiometer (aw-dee-OM-eh-ter)	audi/o = hearing -meter = instrument to measure	Instrument to measure hearing.
audiometry (aw-dee-OM-eh-tree)	audi/o = hearing -metry = process of measuring	Test of hearing ability by determining the lowest and highest intensity (decibels) and frequencies (hertz) that a person can distinguish. The patient may sit in a soundproof booth and receive sounds through earphones as the technician decreases the sound or lowers the tones.

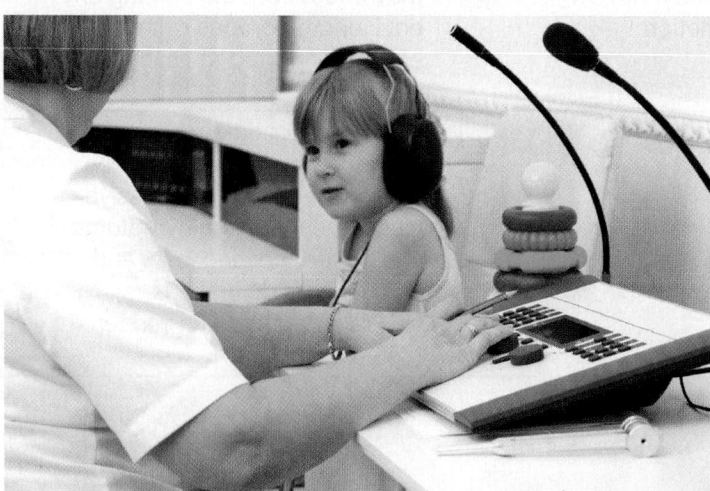

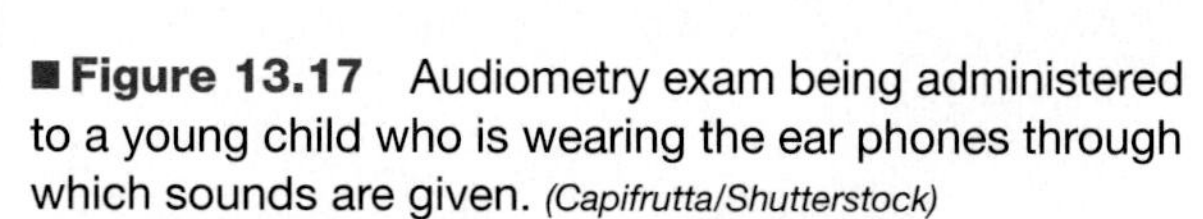

■ **Figure 13.17** Audiometry exam being administered to a young child who is wearing the ear phones through which sounds are given. *(Capifrutta/Shutterstock)*

Diagnostic Procedures (continued)

Term	Word Parts	Definition
decibel (dB) (DES-ih-bel)		Measures the intensity or loudness of a sound. Zero decibels is the quietest sound measured and 120 dB is the loudest sound commonly measured.
hertz (Hz)		Measurement of the frequency or pitch of sound. The lowest pitch on an audiogram is 250 Hz. The measurement can go as high as 8000 Hz, which is the highest pitch measured.
Rinne and Weber tuning-fork tests (RIN-eh)		Tests that assess both nerve and bone conduction of sound. The physician holds a tuning fork, an instrument that produces a constant pitch when it is struck, against or near the bones on the side of the head.
Otology Tests		
otoscope (OH-toh-scope)	ot/o = ear -scope = instrument to visually examine	Instrument to view inside the ear canal.
otoscopy (oh-TOSS-koh-pee)	ot/o = ear -scopy = process of visually examining	Examination of the ear canal, eardrum, and outer ear using an *otoscope.* **Med Term Tip** Small children are prone to placing objects in their ears. In some cases, as with peas and beans, these become moist in the ear canal and swell, which makes removal difficult. *Otoscopy*, or the examination of the ear using an *otoscope*, can aid in identifying and removing the cause of hearing loss if it is due to foreign bodies.
■ **Figure 13.18** An otoscope, used to visually examine the external auditory ear canal and tympanic membrane. *(Patrick Watson, Pearson Education)*		
tympanogram (TIM-pah-no-gram)	tympan/o = tympanic membrane -gram = record	Graphic record that illustrates the results of tympanometry.
tympanometer (tim-pah-NOM-eh-ter)	tympan/o = tympanic membrane -meter = instrument to measure	Instrument used to measure the movement of the tympanic membrane.
tympanometry (tim-pah-NOM-eh-tree)	tympan/o = tympanic membrane -metry = process of measuring	Measurement of the movement of the tympanic membrane. Can indicate the presence of pressure in the middle ear.

Diagnostic Procedures (continued)

Term	Word Parts	Definition
Balance Tests		
falling test		Test used to observe balance and equilibrium. The patient is observed balancing on one foot, then with one foot in front of the other, and then walking forward with eyes open. The same test is conducted with the patient's eyes closed. Swaying and falling with the eyes closed can indicate an ear and equilibrium malfunction.

Therapeutic Procedures

Term	Word Parts	Definition
Audiology Procedures		
American Sign Language (ASL)		Nonverbal method of communicating in which the hands and fingers are used to indicate words and concepts. Used by both persons who are deaf and persons with speech impairments.

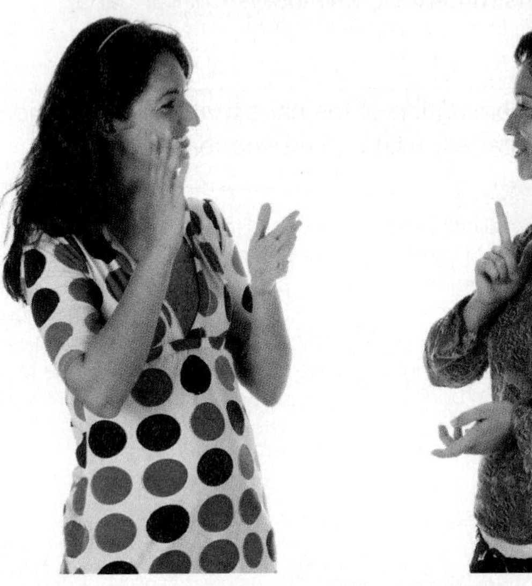

■ **Figure 13.19** Two women having a conversation using American Sign Language. *(Vladimir Mucibabic/ Shutterstock)*

Term	Word Parts	Definition
hearing aid		Apparatus or mechanical device used by persons with impaired hearing to amplify sound. Also called an *amplification device.*
Surgical Procedures		
cochlear implant (KOK-lee-ar)	cochle/o = cochlea -ar = pertaining to	Mechanical device surgically placed under the skin behind the outer ear (pinna) that converts sound signals into magnetic impulses to stimulate the auditory nerve. Can be beneficial for those with profound sensorineural hearing loss.

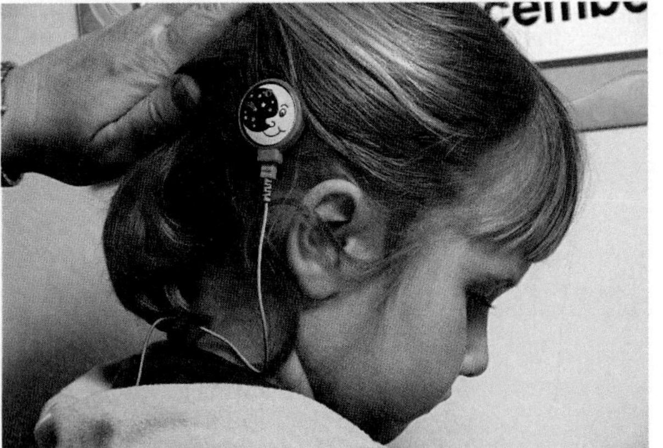

■ **Figure 13.20** Photograph of a child with a cochlear implant. This device sends electrical impulses directly to the brain. *(George Dodson, Pearson Education)*

Therapeutic Procedures (continued)

Term	Word Parts	Definition
labyrinthectomy (lab-ih-rin-THEK-toh-mee)	labyrinth/o = labyrinth -ectomy = surgical removal	Surgical removal of the labyrinth.
labyrinthotomy (lab-ih-rinth-OT-oh-mee)	labyrinth/o = labyrinth -otomy = cutting into	To cut into the labyrinth.
myringectomy (mir-in-GEK-toh-mee)	myring/o = tympanic membrane -ectomy = surgical removal	Surgical removal of the tympanic membrane.
myringoplasty (mir-IN-goh-plass-tee)	myring/o = tympanic membrane -plasty = surgical repair	Surgical repair of the tympanic membrane.
myringotomy (mir-in-GOT-oh-mee)	myring/o = tympanic membrane -otomy = cutting into	Surgical puncture of the eardrum with removal of fluid and pus from the middle ear to eliminate a persistent ear infection and excessive pressure on the tympanic membrane. A pressure equalizing tube is placed in the tympanic membrane to allow for drainage of the middle ear cavity; this tube typically falls out on its own.
otoplasty (OH-toh-plas-tee)	ot/o = ear -plasty = surgical repair	Surgical repair of the external ear.
pressure equalizing tube (PE tube)		Small tube surgically placed in a child's eardrum to assist in drainage of trapped fluid and to equalize pressure between the middle ear cavity and the atmosphere.
salpingotomy (sal-pin-GOT-oh-mee)	salping/o = auditory tube -otomy = cutting into	To cut into the auditory tube.
stapedectomy (stay-pee-DEK-toh-mee)	staped/o = stapes -ectomy = pertaining to	Removal of the stapes bone to treat otosclerosis (hardening of the bone). A prosthesis or artificial stapes may be implanted.
tympanectomy (tim-pan-EK-toh-mee)	tympan/o = tympanic membrane -ectomy = surgical removal	Surgical removal of the tympanic membrane.
tympanoplasty (tim-pan-oh-PLASS-tee)	tympan/o = tympanic membrane -plasty = surgical repair	Surgical repair of the tympanic membrane.
tympanotomy (tim-pan-OT-oh-mee)	tympan/o = tympanic membrane -otomy = cutting into	To cut into the tympanic membrane.

Practice As You Go

I. Terminology Matching

Match each term to its definition.

1. ________ myringotomy
2. ________ tympanoplasty
3. ________ otoplasty
4. ________ stapedectomy
5. ________ Rinne & Weber
6. ________ falling test
7. ________ PE tube
8. ________ cochlear implant

a. removal of stapes bone
b. reconstruction of eardrum
c. surgical puncture of eardrum
d. repairs external ear
e. drains off fluid
f. treats sensorineural hearing loss
g. tuning-fork tests
h. balance test

Pharmacology

Classification	Word Parts	Action	Examples
antibiotic otic solution (OH-tik)	anti- = against bi/o = life -tic = pertaining to ot/o = ear -ic = pertaining to	Eardrops to treat otitis externa.	Neomycin, polymyxin B and hydrocortisone solution, Otocort, Cortisporin, Otic Care
antiemetic (an-tyeee-MIT-tik)	anti- = against -emetic = pertaining to vomiting	Effective in treating the nausea associated with vertigo.	meclizine, Antivert, Meni-D; prochlorperazine, Compazine
anti-inflammatory otic solution (OH-tik)	anti- = against -ory = pertaining to ot/o = ear -ic = pertaining to	Reduces inflammation, itching, and edema associated with otitis externa.	antipyrine and benzoaine, A/B Otic
wax emulsifiers		Substances used to soften earwax to prevent buildup within the external ear canal.	carbamide peroxide, Debrox Drops, Murine Ear Wax Removal Drops

Abbreviations

AD	right ear	**Hz**	hertz
AS	left ear	**OE**	otitis externa
ASL	American Sign Language	**OM**	otitis media
AU	both ears	**Oto**	otology
BC	bone conduction	**PE tube**	pressure equalizing tube
Db	decibel	**PORP**	partial ossicular replacement prosthesis
EENT	eye, ear, nose, throat	**SOM**	serous otitis media
ENT	ear, nose, and throat	**TORP**	total ossicular replacement prosthesis
HEENT	head, ear, eye, nose, throat		

Practice As You Go

J. What's the Abbreviation?

1. otitis externa ______
2. eye, ear, nose, and throat ______
3. bone conduction ______
4. both ears ______
5. otitis media ______

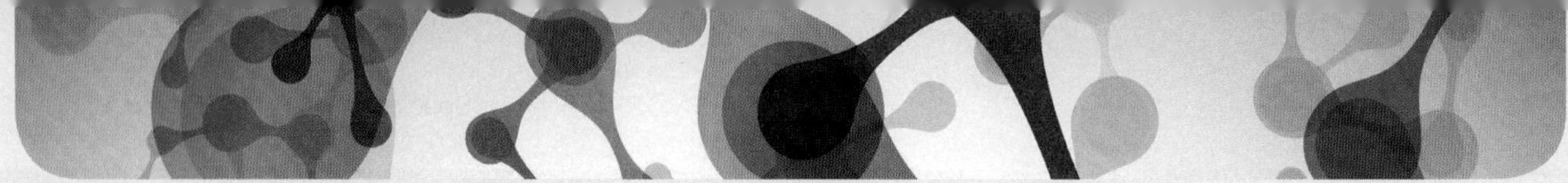

Chapter Review

Real-World Applications

Medical Record Analysis

This Ophthalmology Consultation Report contains 11 medical terms. Underline each term and write it in the list below the report. Then define each term.

Ophthalmology Consultation Report

Reason for Consultation:	Evaluation of progressive loss of vision in right eye.
History of Present Illness:	Patient is a 79-year-old female who has noted gradual deterioration of vision and increasing photophobia during the past year, particularly in the right eye. She states that it feels like there is a film over her right eye. She denies any change in vision in her left eye. Patient has used corrective lenses her entire adult life for hyperopia.
Results of Physical Examination:	Visual acuity test showed no change in this patient's long-standing hyperopia. The pupils react properly to light. Intraocular pressure is normal. Ophthalmoscopy after application of mydriatic drops revealed presence of large opaque cataract in lens of right eye. There is a very small cataract forming in the left eye. There is no evidence of retinopathy, macular degeneration, or keratitis.
Assessment:	Diminished vision in right eye secondary to cataract.
Recommendations:	Phacoemulsification of cataract followed by prosthetic lens implant.

	Term	Definition
1.	____________	____________
2.	____________	____________
3.	____________	____________
4.	____________	____________
5.	____________	____________
6.	____________	____________
7.	____________	____________
8.	____________	____________
9.	____________	____________
10.	____________	____________
11.	____________	____________

Chart Note Transcription

The chart note below contains 10 phrases that can be reworded with a medical term that you learned in this chapter. Each phrase is identified with an underline. Determine the medical term and write your answers in the space provided.

Pearson General Hospital Consultation Report

Task Edit View Time Scale Options Help Download Archive Date: 17 May 2015

Current Complaint:	An eight-year-old female was referred to the specialist in the treatment of diseases of the ear, nose, and throat **1** by her pediatrician for evaluation of chronic left middle ear infection. **2**
Past History:	Patient's mother reports that her daughter began to experience recurrent ear infections at approximately six months of age. Frequency of the infections has increased during the past two years, and she is missing school. Mother also reports the child's teacher feels she is having difficulty hearing in the classroom.
Signs and Symptoms:	Both ears **3** visual examination of the external ear canal and eardrum **4** revealed that the membrane between the external ear canal and middle ear **5** is normal on the right and bulging on the left. An excessive amount of earwax **6** was noted in both ears. **3** Measurement of the movement of the eardrum **7** indicates that there is a buildup of fluid in the left middle ear. Tests of hearing ability **8** report normal hearing on the right and loss of hearing as a result of the blocking of sound transmission in the middle ear **9** on the left. Patient also noted to have acute pharyngitis with purulent drainage at time of evaluation.
Diagnosis:	Hearing loss secondary to chronic left middle ear infection.
Treatment:	Left eardrum incision **10** with placement of pressure equalizing tube for drainage.

1. ____________________

2. ____________________

3. ____________________

4. ____________________

5. ____________________

6. ____________________

7. ____________________

8. ____________________

9. ____________________

10. ____________________

Case Study

Below is a case study presentation of a patient with a condition covered in this chapter. Read the case study and answer the questions below. Some questions will ask for information not included within this chapter. Use your text, a medical dictionary, or any other reference material you choose to answer these questions.

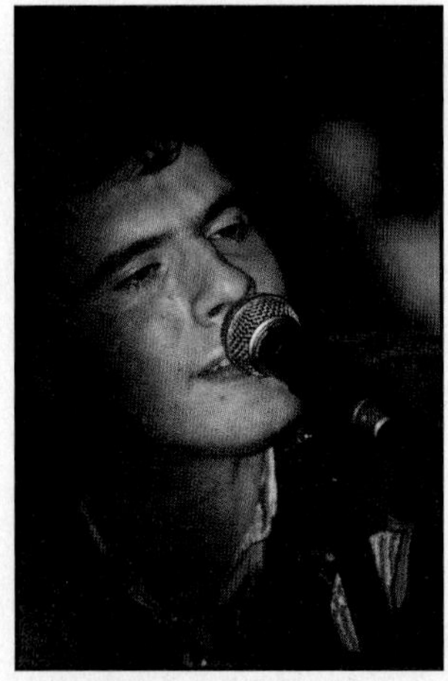
(© MY-Music/Alamy)

This 35-year-old male musician was seen in the EENT clinic complaining of a progressive hearing loss over the past 15 years. He is now unable to hear what is being said if there is any environmental noise present. He states that he has played with a group of musicians using amplified instruments and no earplugs for the past 20 years. External ear structures appear normal bilaterally with otoscopy. Tympanometry is normal bilaterally. Audiometry reveals diminished hearing bilaterally. Rinne and Weber tuning-fork tests indicate that the patient has a moderate amount of conductive hearing loss but rule out sensorineural hearing loss. Diagnosis is moderate bilateral conductive hearing loss as a result of prolonged exposure to loud noise. Patient is referred for evaluation for a hearing aid.

Questions

1. Which type of hearing loss does this patient appear to have? Look this condition up in a reference source and include a short description of it.

____

____

2. Explain how the other type of hearing loss (the type ruled out by the Rinne and Weber tuning-fork tests) is different from what this patient has.

____

____

3. What diagnostic tests did the physician perform? Describe them in your own words.

____

____

4. Explain the difference between a hearing aid and a cochlear implant.

____

____

5. How do you think this patient could have avoided this hearing loss?

____

____

Practice Exercises

A. Pharmacology Challenge

Fill in the classification for each drug description, then match the brand name.

	Drug Description	Classification	Brand Name
1.	________ treats dry eyes	________________	a. Atropine-Care
2.	________ reduces intraocular pressure	________________	b. A/B Otic
3.	________ eardrops for ear infection	________________	c. Timoptic
4.	________ dilates pupil	________________	d. Opticaine
5.	________ treats nausea from vertigo	________________	e. Debrox Drops
6.	________ eyedrops for bacterial infection	________________	f. Eserine Sulfate
7.	________ treats ear itching	________________	g. Antivert
8.	________ constricts pupil	________________	h. Refresh Plus
9.	________ softens cerumen	________________	i. Otocort
10.	________ eyedrops for pain	________________	j. Del-Mycin

B. Word Building Practice

The combining form **blephar/o** refers to the eyelid. Use it to write a term that means:

1. inflammation of the eyelid ________________
2. surgical repair of the eyelid ________________
3. drooping of the upper eyelid ________________

The combining form **retin/o** refers to the retina. Use it to write a term that means:

4. a disease of the retina ________________
5. surgical fixation of the retina ________________

The combining form **ophthalm/o** refers to the eye. Use it to write a term that means:

6. the study of the eye ________________
7. pertaining to the eye ________________
8. an eye examination using a scope ________________

The combining form **irid/o** refers to the iris. Use it to write a term that means:

9. iris paralysis ________________
10. removal of the iris ________________

The combining form **ot/o** refers to the ear. Write a word that means:

11. ear surgical repair ____________________
12. pus flow from the ear ____________________
13. pain in the ear ____________________
14. inflammation of the ear ____________________

The combining form **tympan/o** refers to the eardrum. Write a word that means:

15. eardrum rupture ____________________
16. eardrum incision ____________________
17. eardrum inflammation ____________________

The combining form **audi/o** refers to hearing. Write a word that means:

18. record of hearing ____________________
19. instrument to measure hearing ____________________
20. study of hearing ____________________

C. Name That Suffix

	Suffix	Example from Chapter
1. to turn	____________________	____________________
2. vision	____________________	____________________
3. inflammation of	____________________	____________________
4. the study of	____________________	____________________
5. cutting into	____________________	____________________
6. surgical repair	____________________	____________________
7. surgical fixation	____________________	____________________
8. pain	____________________	____________________
9. ear condition	____________________	____________________
10. hearing	____________________	____________________

D. Define the Combining Form

	Definition	Example from Chapter
1. **dacry/o**	____________________	____________________
2. **uve/o**	____________________	____________________

	Definition	Example from Chapter
3. **aque/o**	___	___
4. **phot/o**	___	___
5. **kerat/o**	___	___
6. **vitre/o**	___	___
7. **dipl/o**	___	___
8. **glauc/o**	___	___
9. **presby/o**	___	___
10. **ambly/o**	___	___
11. **aur/o**	___	___
12. **staped/o**	___	___
13. **acous/o**	___	___
14. **salping/o**	___	___
15. **myring/o**	___	___

E. Answer the Question

1. Describe the difference between conductive hearing loss and sensorineural hearing loss. ___

   ___
2. List in order the eyeball structures light rays pass through. ___,

   ___, ___, ___
3. Describe the role of the conjunctiva. ___
4. List the ossicles and what they do. ___

F. What Does it Stand For?

1. Oto ___
2. OU ___
3. REM ___
4. Hz ___
5. SMD ___
6. PERRLA ___
7. IOP ___

8. dB ____________________

9. OD ____________________

10. VF ____________________

G. Fill in the Blank

emmetropia	tonometry	Ménière's disease
hyperopia	cataract	hordeolum
acoustic neuroma	strabismus	myopia
otorhinolaryngologist	presbycusis	
conjunctivitis	inner ear	

1. Cheri is having a regular eye checkup. The pressure reading test that the physician will do to detect glaucoma is ____________________.

2. Carlos's ophthalmologist tells him that he has normal vision. This is called ____________________.

3. Ana has been given an antibiotic eye ointment for pinkeye. The medical term for this condition is ____________________.

4. Adrian is nearsighted and cannot read signs in the distance. This is called ____________________.

5. Ivan is scheduled to have surgery to have the opaque lens of his right eye removed. This condition is a(n) ____________________.

6. Roberto has developed a stye on the corner of his left eye. He has been told to treat it with hot compresses. This condition is called a(n) ____________________.

7. Judith has twin boys with crossed eyes that will require surgical correction. The medical term for this condition is ____________________.

8. Beth is farsighted and has difficulty reading textbooks. Her eyeglass correction will be for ____________________.

9. Grace was told by her physician that her hearing loss was a part of the aging process. The term for this is ____________________.

10. Stacey is having frequent middle ear infections and wishes to be treated by a specialist. She would go to a(n) ____________________.

11. Warren was told that his dizziness may be caused by a problem in the ____________________ area.

12. Shantel is suffering from an abnormal condition of the inner ear, vertigo, and tinnitus. She may have ____________________.

13. Keisha was told that her tumor of the eighth cranial nerve was benign, but she still experienced a hearing loss as a result of the tumor. This tumor is called a(n) ____________________.

H. Define the Term

1. amblyopia ____________________
2. diplopia ____________________
3. mydriatic ____________________
4. miotic ____________________
5. presbyopia ____________________
6. tinnitus ____________________
7. stapes ____________________
8. tympanometry ____________________
9. eustachian tube ____________________
10. labyrinth ____________________
11. audiogram ____________________
12. otitis media ____________________

Labeling Exercise

Image A

Write the labels for this figure on the numbered lines provided.

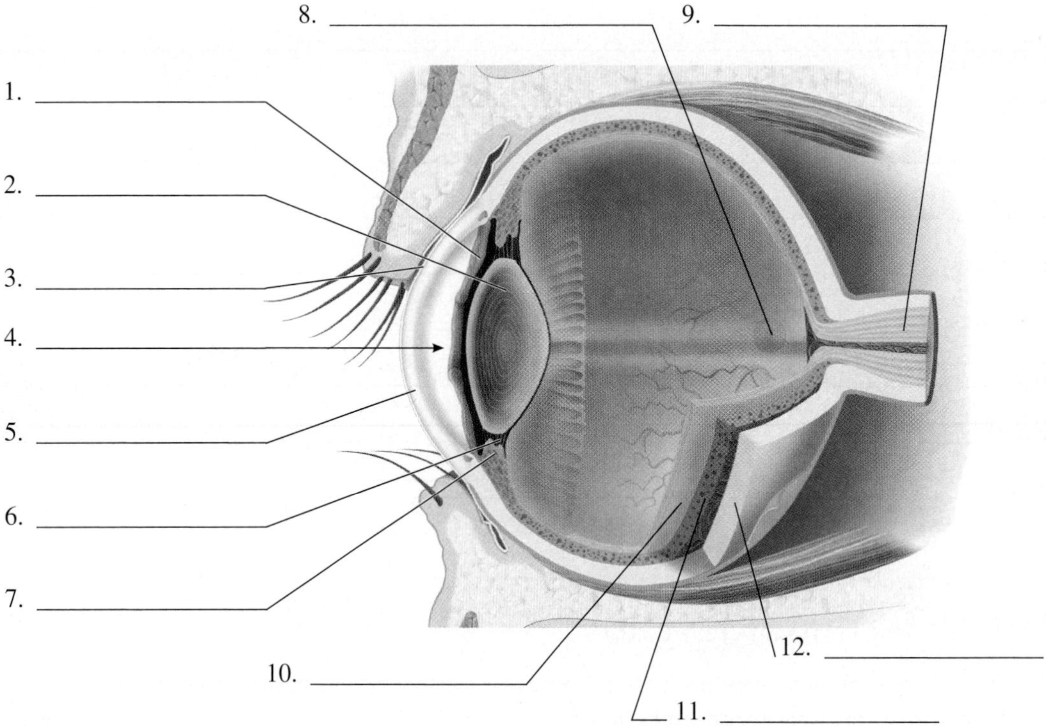

Image B

Write the labels for this figure on the numbered lines provided.

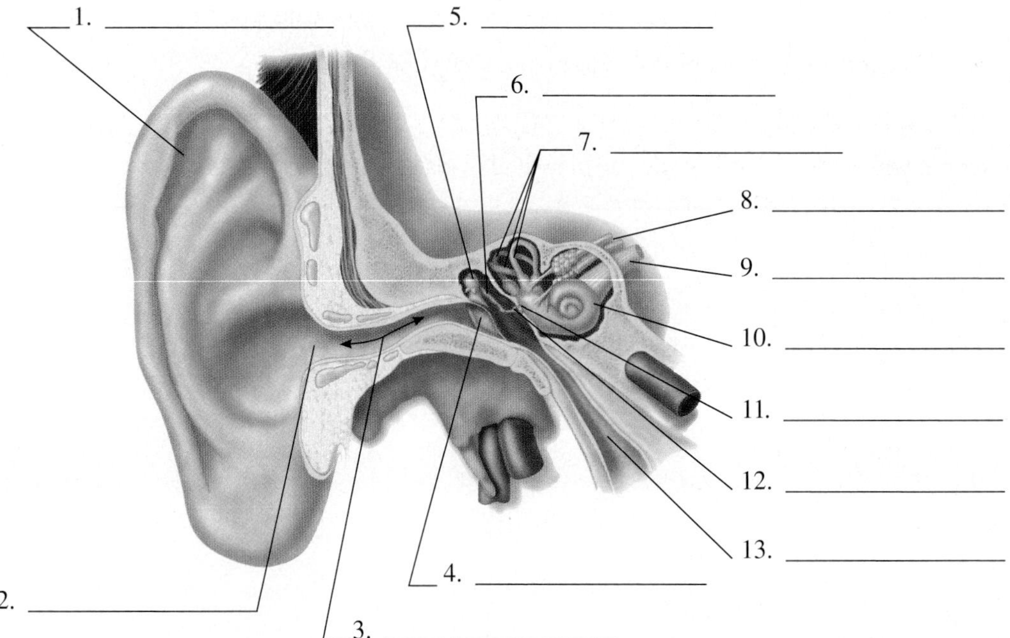

14

Special Topics

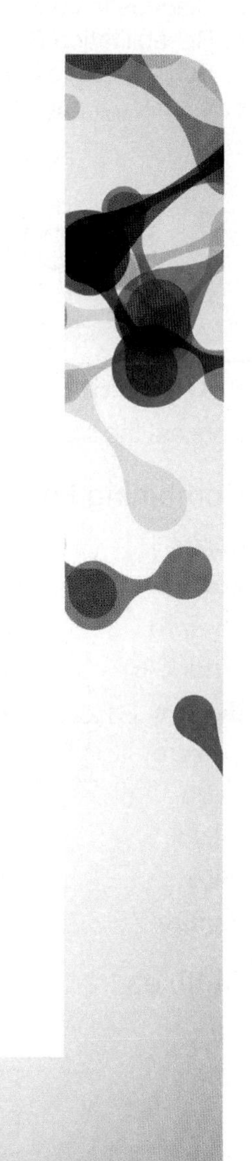

Learning Objectives

Upon completion of this chapter, you will be able to

- Identify and define the combining forms, suffixes, and prefixes introduced in this chapter.
- Correctly spell and pronounce medical terms relating to the medical fields introduced in this chapter.
- Describe pertinent information relating to pharmacology.
- Describe pertinent information relating to mental health.
- Describe pertinent information relating to diagnostic imaging.
- Describe pertinent information relating to rehabilitation services.
- Describe pertinent information relating to surgery.
- Describe pertinent information relating to oncology.
- Identify and define vocabulary terms relating to the topics.
- Identify and define selected pathology terms relating to the topics.
- Identify and define selected diagnostic procedures relating to the topics.
- Identify and define selected therapeutic procedures relating to the topics.
- Define selected abbreviations associated with the topics.

Introduction

There are many specialized areas within medicine, and each has medical terms relating to that field. This chapter presents medical terminology from six of these fields:

Section I: Pharmacology at a Glance

Word Parts

Here are the most common word parts (with their meanings) used to build pharmacology terms.

Combining Forms

aer/o air
bucc/o cheek
chem/o drug
cutane/o skin
derm/o skin
enter/o intestine
hal/o to breathe
iatr/o physician, medicine, treatment
idi/o distinctive
lingu/o tongue
muscul/o muscle
or/o mouth
pharmac/o drug
rect/o rectum
thec/o sheath (meninges)
topic/o a specific area
toxic/o poison
vagin/o vagina
ven/o vein

Suffixes

-al pertaining to
-ar pertaining to
-ary pertaining to
-genic produced by
-ical pertaining to
-ist specialist
-logy study of
-ous pertaining to
-phylaxis protection

Prefixes

anti- against
contra- against
in- inward
intra- within
non- not
para- beside
pro- before
sub- under
trans- across

Pharmacology

pharmacology (far-ma-KALL-oh-jee)

Pharmacology is the study of the origin, characteristics, and effects of drugs. Drugs are obtained from many different sources. Some drugs, such as vitamins, are found naturally in the foods we eat. Others, such as hormones, are obtained from animals. Penicillin and some of the other antibiotics are developed from mold, which is a fungus. Plants have been the source of many of today's drugs. Many drugs, such as those used in chemotherapy, are synthetic, meaning they are developed by artificial means in a laboratory.

Drug Names

brand name
chemical name
generic name
nonproprietary name (non-prah-PRYE-ah-tair-ee)
pharmaceutical (far-mih-SOO-tih-kal)
pharmacist (FAR-mah-sist)
proprietary name (proh-PRYE-ah-tair-ee)
trademark

Med Term Tip

The terms *drug* and *medication* have the same meaning. However, the general public often uses the term *drug* to refer to a narcotic type of medication. The term can also mean illegal chemical substances. For purposes of medical terminology, use of the word *drug* means medication.

All drugs are chemicals. The **chemical name** describes the chemical formula or molecular structure of a particular drug. For example, the chemical name for ibuprofen, an over-the-counter pain medication, is 2-*p*-isobutylphenyl propionic acid. Just as in this case, chemical names are usually very long, so a shorter name is given to the drug. This name is the **generic** or **nonproprietary name**, and it is recognized and accepted as the official name for a drug.

Each drug has only one generic name, such as ibuprofen, and this name is not subject to copyright protection, so any **pharmaceutical** manufacturer may use it. However, the pharmaceutical company that originally developed the drug has exclusive rights to produce it for 17 years. After that time, any manufacturer may produce and sell the drug. When a company manufactures a drug for sale, it must choose a **brand name**, or **proprietary name**, for its product. This is the company's **trademark** for the drug. For example, ibuprofen is known by several brand names, including Motrin™, Advil™, and Nuprin™. All three contain the same ibuprofen; they are just marketed by different pharmaceutical companies. (See Table 14.1 ■ for examples of different drug names.)

Generic drugs are usually priced lower than brand name drugs. A physician can indicate on the prescription if the **pharmacist** may substitute a generic drug for a brand name. The physician may prefer that a particular brand name drug be used if he or she believes it to be more effective than the generic drug.

What's In A Name?

Look for these word parts:
chem/o = drug
pharmac/o = drug
-ary = pertaining to
-ical = pertaining to
-ist = specialist
-logy = study of
non- = not

Table 14.1 Examples of Different Drug Names

Chemical Name	Generic Name	Brand Names
2-*p*-isobutylphenyl propionic acid	Ibuprofen	Motrin™
		Advil™
		Nuprin™
Acetylsalicylic acid	Aspirin	Anacin™
		Bufferin™
		Excedrin™
S-2-[1-(methylamino) ethyl] benzenemethanol hydrochloride	Pseudoephedrine hydrochloride	Sudafed™
		Actifed™
		Nucofed™

Legal Classification of Drugs

controlled substances
Drug Enforcement Agency
over-the-counter drug
prescription (prih-SKRIP-shun)
prescription drug (prih-SKRIP-shun)

A **prescription drug** can only be ordered by licensed healthcare practitioners such as physicians, dentists, or physician assistants. These drugs must include the words "Caution: Federal law prohibits dispensing without prescription" on their labels. Antibiotics, such as penicillin, and heart medications, such as digoxin, are available only by prescription. A **prescription** is the written explanation to the pharmacist regarding the name of the medication, the dosage, and the times of administration. A licensed practitioner can also give a prescription order orally to a pharmacist.

Med Term Tip

It is critical that patients receive the correct drug, but it is not possible to list or remember all the drug names. You must acquire the habit of looking up any drug name you do not recognize in the *Physician's Desk Reference (PDR)*. Every medical office or medical facility should have a copy of this book.

A drug that does not require a prescription is referred to as an **over-the-counter** (OTC) **drug**. Many medications or drugs can be purchased without a prescription, for example, aspirin, antacids, and antidiarrheal medications. However, taking aspirin along with an anticoagulant, such as coumadin, can cause internal bleeding in some people, and OTC antacids interfere with the absorption of the prescription drug tetracycline into the body. It is better for the physician or pharmacist to advise the patient on the proper OTC drugs to use with prescription drugs.

Certain drugs are **controlled substances** if they have a potential for being addictive (habit forming) or can be abused. The **Drug Enforcement Agency** (DEA) enforces the control of these drugs. Some of the more commonly prescribed controlled substances are:

- butabarbital
- chloral hydrate
- codeine
- diazepam
- oxycontin
- morphine
- phenobarbital
- secobarbital

Controlled drugs are classified as Schedule I through Schedule V, indicating their potential for abuse. The differences between each schedule are listed in Table 14.2■.

Table 14.2 Schedule for Controlled Substances

Classification	Meaning
Schedule I	Drugs with the highest potential for addiction and abuse. They are not accepted for medical use. Examples are heroin and LSD.
Schedule II	Drugs with a high potential for addiction and abuse accepted for medical use in the United States. Examples are codeine, cocaine, morphine, opium, and secobarbital.
Schedule III	Drugs with a moderate to low potential for addiction and abuse. Examples are butabarbital, anabolic steroids, and acetaminophen with codeine.
Schedule IV	Drugs with a lower potential for addiction and abuse than Schedule III drugs. Examples are chloral hydrate, phenobarbital, and diazepam.
Schedule V	Drugs with a low potential for addiction and abuse. An example is low-strength codeine combined with other drugs to suppress coughing.

How to Read a Prescription

A prescription is not difficult to read once you understand the symbols that are used. Symbols and abbreviations based on Latin and Greek words are used to save time for the physician. For example, the abbreviation po, meaning to be taken by mouth, comes from the Latin term *per os*, which means "by mouth."

See Figure 14.1 ■ for an example of a prescription. In this example, the prescribed medication (Rx) is Tagamet (a medication to reduce stomach acid) in the 800 milligram (mg) size. The instructions on the label are to say (Sig) to take 1 (ṫ)by mouth (po) every (q) bedtime (hs). The pharmacist is to dispense (disp) 30 tablets (#30). The prescription concludes by informing the pharmacist to refill the prescription two times, and he or she may substitute with another

Med Term Tip

Many abbreviations have multiple meanings, such as od, which can mean overdose (od) or right eye (OD), depending on whether the letters are lowercase or uppercase. Care must be taken when reading abbreviations since some may be written too quickly, making them difficult to decipher. Never create your own abbreviations.

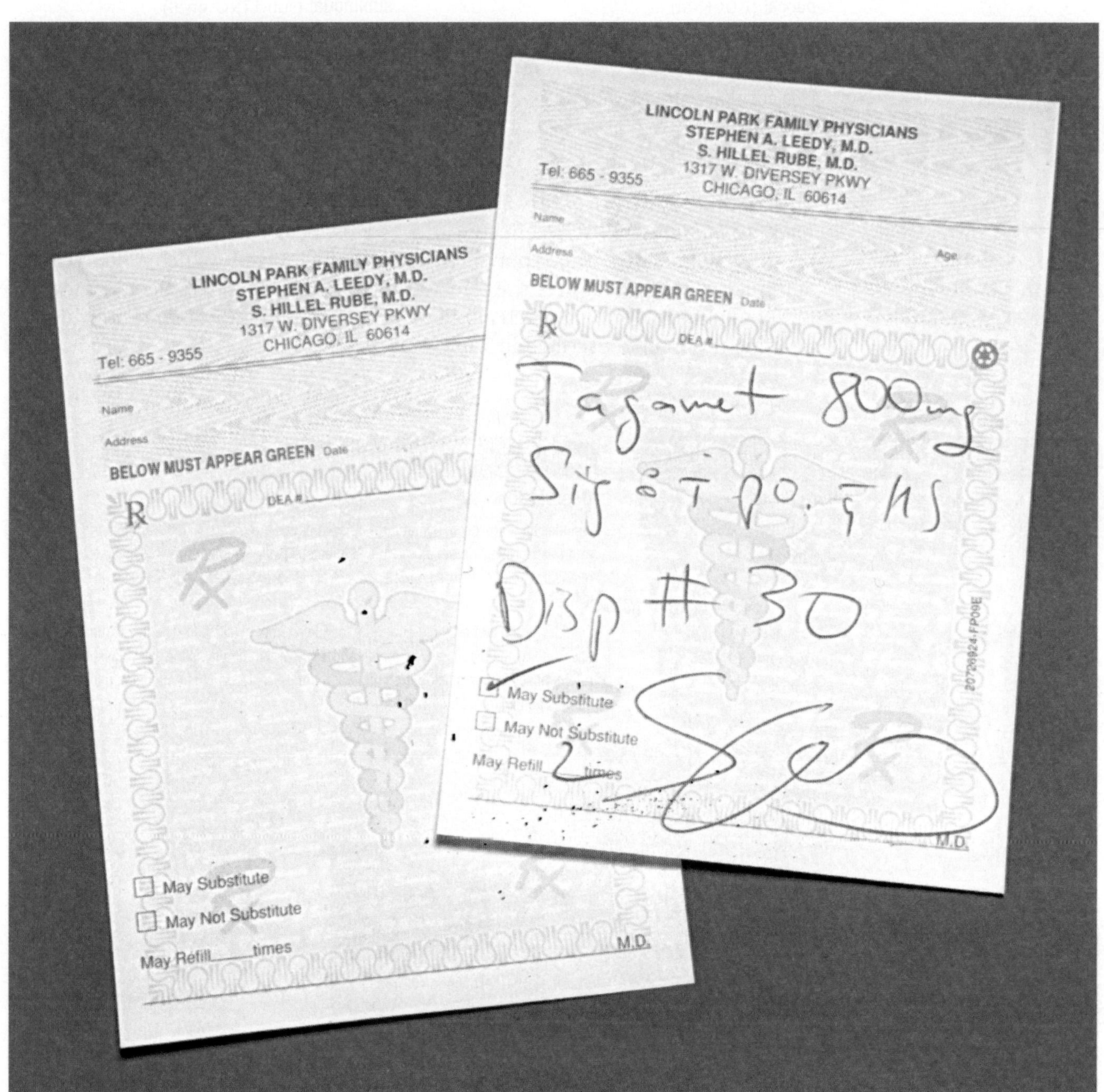

■ **Figure 14.1** A sample prescription written by a physician. *(Michal Heron, Pearson Education)*

medication. Each prescription must contain the date, physician's name, address, and Drug Enforcement Agency number as well as the patient's name and date of birth. The physician must also sign his or her name at the bottom of the prescription. A blank prescription cannot be handed to a patient.

The physician's instruction to the patient will be placed on the label. The pharmacist will also include instructions about the medication and alert the patient to side effects that may need to be reported to the physician. Additionally, any special instructions regarding the medication (i.e., take with meals, do not take along with dairy products, etc.) are supplied by the pharmacist.

Routes and Methods of Drug Administration

aerosol (AIR-oh-sol)
buccal (BUCK-al)
eardrops
eyedrops
inhalation (in-hah-LAY-shun)
oral (OR-al)
parenteral (par-EN-ter-al)
rectal (REK-tal)
sublingual (sub-LING-gwal)
suppositories (suh-POZ-ih-tor-ees)
topical (TOP-ih-kal)
transdermal (tranz-DER-mal)
vaginal (VAJ-in-al)

The method by which a drug is introduced into the body is referred to as the *route of administration*. To be effective, drugs must be administered by a particular route. In some cases, there may be a variety of routes by which a drug can be administered. For instance, the female hormone estrogen can be administered orally in pill form or by a patch applied to the skin. The most common routes of administration are described in Table 14.3 ■.

Table 14.3 Common Routes of Drug Administration

Method	Word Parts	Description
oral	or/o = mouth -al = pertaining to	Includes all drugs given by mouth. The advantages are ease of administration and a slow rate of absorption via the stomach and intestinal wall. The disadvantages include slowness of absorption and destruction of some chemical compounds by gastric juices. In addition, some medications, such as aspirin, can have a corrosive action on the stomach lining.
sublingual	sub- = under lingu/o = tongue -al = pertaining to	Includes drugs that are held under the tongue and not swallowed. The medication is absorbed by the blood vessels on the underside of the tongue as the saliva dissolves it. The rate of absorption is quicker than the oral route. Nitroglycerin to treat angina pectoris (chest pain) is administered by this route.

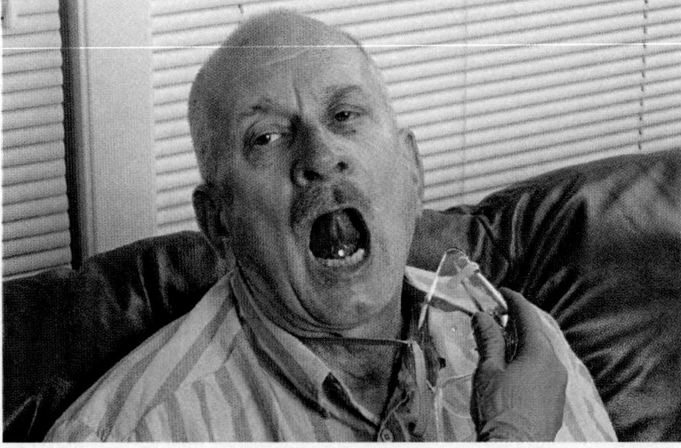

■ **Figure 14.2** Sublingual medication administration. Photograph of a male patient placing a nitroglycerin tablet under his tongue. *(Michal Heron, Pearson Education)*

Table 14.3 Common Routes of Drug Administration (continued)

Method	Word Parts	Description
inhalation	in- = inward hal/o = to breathe	Includes drugs inhaled directly into the nose and mouth. **Aerosol** (aer/o = air) sprays are administered by this route.

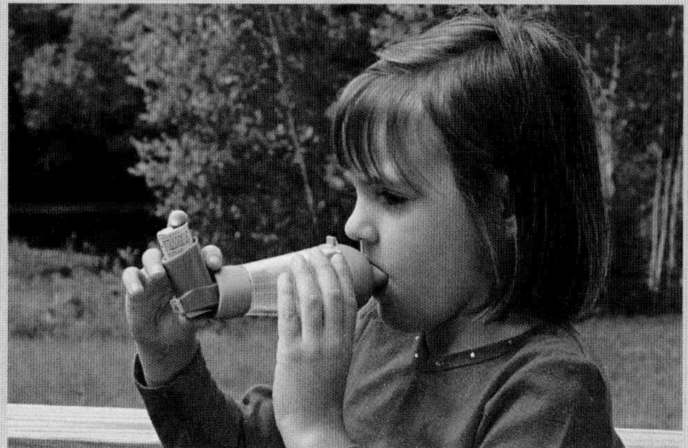

■ **Figure 14.3** Inhalation medication administration. Photograph of a young girl using a metered dose inhaler. *(Michal Heron, Pearson Education)*

Method	Word Parts	Description
parenteral	para- = beside enter/o = intestine -al = pertaining to	An invasive method of administering drugs as it requires the skin to be punctured by a needle. The needle with syringe attached is introduced either under the skin or into a muscle, vein, or body cavity.
intracavitary (in-trah-KAV-ih-tair-ee)	intra- = within -ary = pertaining to	Injection into a body cavity such as the peritoneal cavity or the chest cavity. One type of parenteral route of administration.
intradermal (ID) (in-trah-DER-mal)	intra- = within derm/o = skin -al = pertaining to	Very shallow injection just under the top layer of the skin. Commonly used in skin testing for allergies and tuberculosis testing. One type of parenteral route of administration.

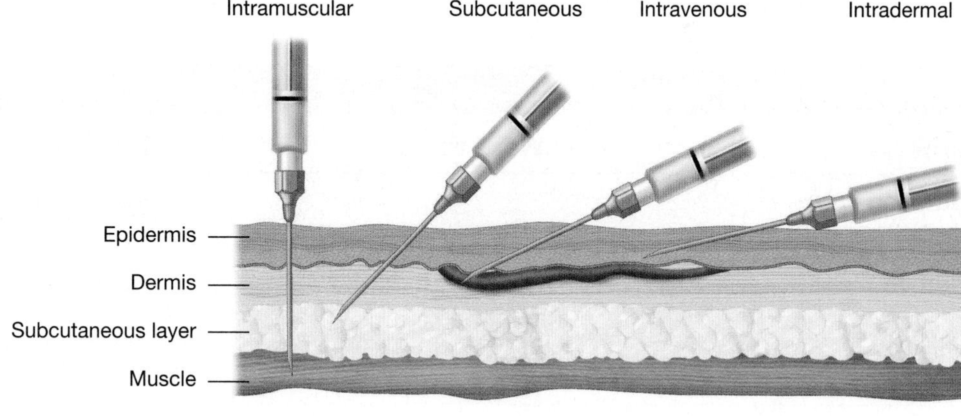

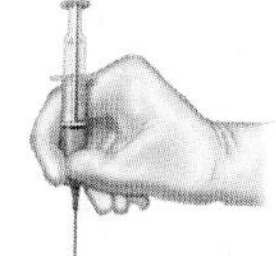

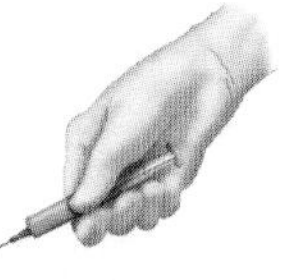

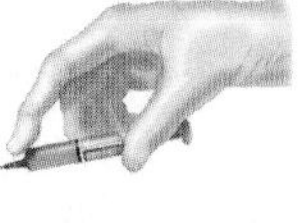

■ **Figure 14.4** Parenteral medication administration. The angle of needle insertion for four different types of parenteral injections.

Method	Word Parts	Description
intramuscular (IM) (in-trah-MUSS-kyoo-lar)	intra- = within muscul/o = muscle -ar = pertaining to	Injection directly into the muscle of the buttocks, thigh, or upper arm. Used when there is a large amount of medication or it is irritating (see again Figure 14.4). One type of parenteral route of administration.
intrathecal (in-trah-THEE-kal)	intra- = within thec/o = sheath (meninges) -al = pertaining to	Injection into the meningeal space surrounding the brain and spinal cord. One type of parenteral route of administration.

Table 14.3 Common Routes of Drug Administration (continued)

Method	Word Parts	Description
intravenous (IV) (in-trah-VEE-nus)	intra- = within ven/o = vein -ous = pertaining to	Injection into the veins. This route may be set up to deliver medication very quickly or to deliver a continuous drip of medication (see again Figure 14.4). One type of parenteral route of administration.
subcutaneous (Subc, Subq) (sub-kyoo-TAY-nee-us)	sub- = under cutane/o = skin -ous = pertaining to	Injection into the subcutaneous layer of the skin, usually the upper, outer arm or abdomen (see again Figure 14.4); for example, insulin injection. One type of parenteral route of administration.
transdermal	trans- = across derm/o = skin -al = pertaining to	Includes medications that coat the underside of a patch, which is applied to the skin where it is then absorbed. Examples include birth control patches, nicotine patches, and sea sickness patches.
rectal	rect/o = rectum -al = pertaining to	Includes medications introduced directly into the rectal cavity in the form of **suppositories** or solution. Drugs may have to be administered by this route if the patient is unable to take them by mouth due to nausea, vomiting, or surgery.
topical	topic/o = a specific area -al = pertaining to	Includes medications applied directly to the skin or mucous membranes. They are distributed in ointment, cream, or lotion form, and are used to treat skin infections and eruptions.
vaginal	vagin/o = vagina -al = pertaining to	Includes tablets and suppositories that may be inserted vaginally to treat vaginal yeast infections and other irritations.
eyedrops		Includes drops used during eye examinations to dilate the pupil of the eye for better examination of the interior of the eye. They are also placed into the eye to control eye pressure in glaucoma and treat infections.
eardrops		Includes drops placed directly into the ear canal for the purpose of relieving pain or treating infection.
buccal	bucc/o = cheek -al = pertaining to	Includes drugs that are placed under the lip or between the cheek and gum.

Pharmacology Terms

Term	Word Parts	Definition
addiction (ah-DICK-shun)		Acquired dependence on a drug.
additive		Sum of the action of two (or more) drugs given. In this case, the total strength of the medications is equal to the sum of the strength of each individual drug.
antidote (AN-tih-doht)	anti- = against	Substance that will neutralize poisons or their side effects.
broad spectrum		Ability of a drug to be effective against a wide range of microorganisms.
contraindication (kon-trah-in-dih-KAY-shun)	contra- = against	Condition in which a particular drug should not be used.
cumulative action		Action that occurs in the body when a drug is allowed to accumulate or stay in the body.

Pharmacology Terms (continued)

Term	Word Parts	Definition
drug interaction		Occurs when the effect of one drug is altered because it was taken at the same time as another drug.
drug tolerance		Decrease in susceptibility to a drug after continued use of the drug.
habituation (hah-bich-yoo-AY-shun)		Development of an emotional dependence on a drug due to repeated use.
iatrogenic (eye-ah-troh-JEN-ik)	iatr/o = medicine -genic = produced by	Usually an unfavorable response resulting from taking a medication.
idiosyncrasy (id-ee-oh-SIN-krah-see)	idi/o = distinctive	Unusual or abnormal response to a drug or food.
placebo (plah-SEE-boh)		Inactive, harmless substance used to satisfy a patient's desire for medication. This is also used in research when given to a control group of patients in a study in which another group receives a drug. The effect of the placebo versus the drug is then observed.
potentiation (poe-ten-chee-AY-shun)		Giving a patient a second drug to boost (potentiate) the effect of another drug. The total strength of the drugs is greater than the sum of the strength of the individual drugs.
prophylaxis (proh-fih-LAK-sis)	pro- = before -phylaxis = protection	Prevention of disease. For example, an antibiotic can be used to prevent the occurrence of a disease.
side effect		Response to a drug other than the effect desired. Also called an *adverse reaction.*
tolerance (TAHL-er-ans)		Development of a capacity for withstanding a large amount of a substance, such as foods, drugs, or poison, without any adverse effect. A decreased sensitivity to further doses will develop.
toxicity (tok-SISS-ih-tee)	toxic/o = poison	Extent or degree to which a substance is poisonous.
unit dose		Drug dosage system that provides prepackaged, prelabeled, individual medications that are ready for immediate use by the patient.

Abbreviations			
@	at	**non rep**	do not repeat
ā	before	**NPO, npo**	nothing by mouth
ac	before meals	**NS**	normal saline
ad lib	as desired	**od**	overdose
ante	before	**oint**	ointment
APAP	acetaminophen (Tylenol™)	**OTC**	over-the-counter
aq	aqueous (water)	**oz**	ounce
ASA	aspirin	**p̄**	after
bid	twice a day	**pc**	after meals
c̄	with	**PCA**	patient-controlled administration
cap(s)	capsule(s)	**PDR**	*Physician's Desk Reference*
d	day	**per**	with
d/c, DISC	discontinue	**po**	by mouth
DC, disc	discontinue	**prn**	as needed
DEA	Drug Enforcement Agency	**pt**	patient
dil	dilute	**q**	every
disp	dispense	**qam**	every morning
dtd	give of such a dose	**qh**	every hour
Dx	diagnosis	**qhs**	at bedtime
et	and	**qid**	four times a day
FDA	Federal Drug Administration	**qs**	quantity sufficient
gm	gram	**Rx**	take
gr	grain	**s̄**	without
gt	drop	**Sig**	label as follows/directions
gtt	drops	**sl**	under the tongue
hs	at bedtime	**sol**	solution
i̇̄	one	**s̄s̄**	one-half
ID	intradermal	**stat**	at once/immediately
i̇̄i̇̄	two	**Subc, Subq**	subcutaneous
i̇̄i̇̄i̇̄	three	**suppos, supp**	suppository
IM	intramuscular	**susp**	suspension
inj	injection	**syr**	syrup
IV	intravenous	**T, tbsp**	tablespoon
kg	kilogram	**t, tsp**	teaspoon
L	liter	**tab**	tablet
mcg	microgram	**tid**	three times a day
mEq	milliequivalent	**TO**	telephone order
mg	milligram	**top**	apply topically
mL	milliliter	**VO**	verbal order
no sub	no substitute	**wt**	weight
noc	night	**x**	times

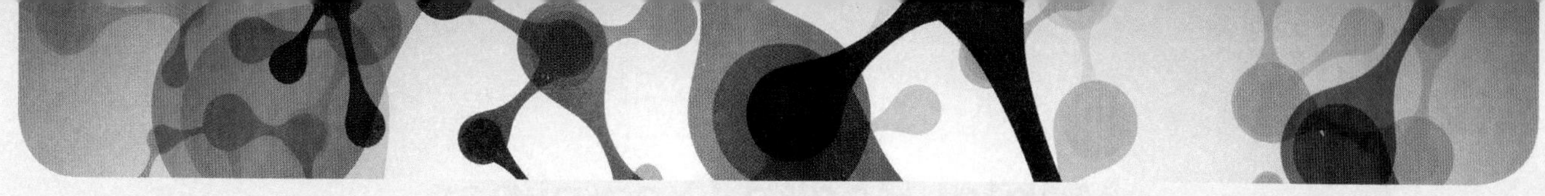

Section II: Mental Health at a Glance

Word Parts

Here are the most common word parts (with their meanings) used to build mental health terms.

Combining Forms

amnes/o	forgetfulness
anxi/o	fear, worry
compuls/o	drive, compel
delus/o	false belief
depress/o	to press down
electr/o	electricity
hallucin/o	imagined perception
klept/o	to steal
ment/o	mind
narc/o	stupor, sleep
neur/o	nerve
obsess/o	besieged by thoughts
ped/o	child
pharmac/o	drug
phob/o	irrational fear
phren/o	mind
psych/o	mind
pyr/o	fire
schiz/o	split
soci/o	society
somat/o	body
somn/o	sleep
vers/o	to turn

Suffixes

-al	pertaining to
-ar	pertaining to
-ia	state, condition
-iatric	pertaining to medical treatment
-iatrist	physician
-iatry	medical treatment
-ic	pertaining to
-ile	pertaining to
-ism	state of
-lepsy	seizure
-logist	one who studies
-logy	study of
-mania	frenzy
-orexia	appetite
-philic	pertaining to being attracted to
-phoria	condition to bear
-therapy	treatment
-tic	pertaining to

Prefixes

an-	without
anti-	against
auto-	self
bi-	two
de-	without
dis-	apart
dys-	difficult
ex-	outward
hyper-	excessive
in-	not
para-	abnormal
post-	after
pre-	before

Mental Health Disciplines

Psychology

abnormal psychology
clinical psychologist (sigh-KALL-oh-jist)
normal psychology
psychology (sigh-KALL-oh-jee)

Med Term Tip

All social interactions pose some problems for some people. These problems are not necessarily abnormal. One means of judging if behavior is abnormal is to compare one person's behavior with others in the community. Also, if a person's behavior interferes with the activities of daily living, it is often considered abnormal.

Psychology is the study of human behavior and thought processes. This behavioral science is primarily concerned with understanding how human beings interact with their physical environment and with each other. Behavior can be divided into two categories: normal and abnormal. The study of **normal psychology** includes how the personality develops, how people handle stress, and the stages of mental development. In contrast, **abnormal psychology** studies and treats behaviors that are outside of normal and that are detrimental to the person or society. These maladaptive behaviors range from occasional difficulty coping with stress, to bizarre actions and beliefs, to total withdrawal. A **clinical psychologist**, though not a physician, is a specialist in evaluating and treating persons with mental and emotional disorders.

Psychiatry

psychiatric nurse (sigh-kee-AT-rik)
psychiatric social worker
psychiatrist (sigh-KIGH-ah-trist)
psychiatry (sigh-KIGH-ah-tree)

What's In A Name?

Look for these word parts:
psych/o = mind
-iatric = pertaining to medical treatment
-iatrist = physician
-iatry = medical treatment
-logist = one who studies
-logy = study of

Psychiatry is the branch of medicine that deals with the diagnosis, treatment, and prevention of mental disorders. A **psychiatrist** is a medical physician specializing in the care of patients with mental, emotional, and behavioral disorders. Other health professions also have specialty areas in caring for clients with mental illness. Good examples are **psychiatric nurses** and **psychiatric social workers**.

Pathology

The legal definition of mental disorder is "impaired judgment and lack of self-control." The guide for terminology and classifications relating to psychiatric disorders is the *Diagnostic and Statistical Manual of Mental Disorders, Fifth Edition* (DSM-5), which is published by the American Psychiatric Association (2013). The DSM organizes mental disorders into 19 major diagnostic categories of disorders. These categories and examples of conditions included in each are described below.

Med Term Tip

Mental disorders are sometimes more simply characterized by whether they are a *neurosis* or a *psychosis.* Neuroses are inappropriate coping mechanisms to handle stress, such as phobias and panic attacks. Psychoses involve extreme distortions of reality and disorganization of a person's thinking, including bizarre behaviors, hallucinations, and delusions. Schizophrenia is an example of a psychosis.

Term	Word Parts	Definition
Anxiety Disorders	anxi/o = fear, worry dis- = apart	Characterized by persistent worry and apprehension.
panic disorder	-ic = pertaining to dis- = apart	Feeling of intense apprehension, terror, or sense of impending danger.
general anxiety disorder (ang-ZY-eh-tee)	anxi/o = fear, worry dis- = apart	Feeling of dread in the absence of a clearly identifiable stress trigger.
phobias (FOH-bee-ahs)	phob/o = irrational fear -ia = state, condition	Irrational fear, such as *arachnophobia*, or fear of spiders.
Obsessive–Compulsive and Related Disorders	dis- = apart	Characterized by obsessive preoccupations and repetitive behaviors.
obsessive–compulsive disorder (OCD) (ob-SESS-iv / kom-PUHL-siv)	obsess/o = besieged by thoughts compuls/o = drive, compel dis- = apart	Performing repetitive rituals to reduce anxiety.

Pathology (continued)

Term	Word Parts	Definition
Neurocognitive Disorders	neur/o = nerve dis- = apart	Deterioration of mental functions due to temporary or permanent brain dysfunction.
dementia (dee-MEN-she-ah)	de- = without ment/o = mind -ia = state, condition	Progressive confusion and disorientation.
Alzheimer's disease (AD) (ALTS-high-merz)	dis- = apart	Degenerative brain disorder with gradual loss of cognitive abilities.
Neurodevelopmental Disorders	neur/o = nerve -al = pertaining to dis- = apart	Impairment in the growth or development of the central nervous system.
intellectual development disorder	-al = pertaining to dis- = apart	Below average intellectual functioning.
attention-deficit/hyperactivity disorder (ADHD)	hyper- = excessive dis- = apart	Inattention and impulsive behavior.
autism spectrum disorder (AW-tizm)	auto- = self -ism = state of dis- = apart	Range of conditions involving deficits in social interaction, communication skills, and restricted patterns of behavior.
Dissociative Disorders	dis- = apart soci/o = society	Disorders in which severe emotional conflict is so repressed that a split in the personality may occur or the person may lose memory.
dissociative amnesia (am-NEE-zee-ah)	dis- = apart soci/o = society amnes/o = forgetfulness -ia = state, condition	Loss of memory.
dissociative identity disorder	dis- = apart soci/o = society	Having two or more distinct personalities.
Feeding and Eating Disorders		Abnormal behaviors related to eating.
anorexia nervosa (an-oh-REK-see-ah / ner-VOH-sah)	an- = without -orexia = appetite	Disorder characterized by distorted body image, a pathological fear of becoming fat, and severe weight loss due to excessive dieting.

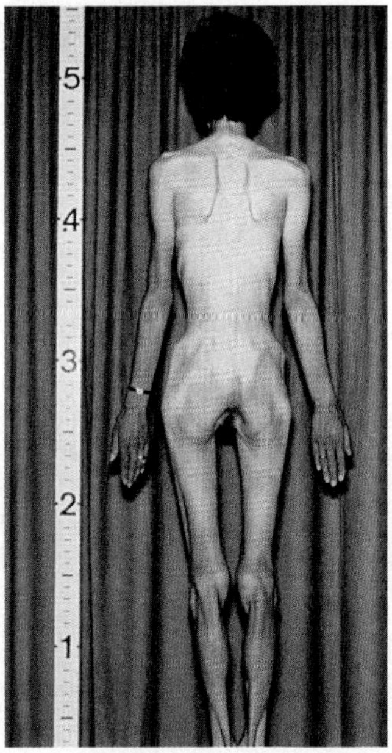

■ **Figure 14.5** Photograph of a young woman suffering from anorexia nervosa, posterior view. *(© Wellcome Image Library/Custom Medical Stock Photo, Inc.)*

Pathology (continued)

Term	Word Parts	Definition
bulimia (boo-LIM-ee-ah)	-ia = state, condition	Binge eating and intentional vomiting.
Disruptive, Impulse Control, and Conduct Disorders	dis- = apart	Inability to resist an impulse to perform some act that is harmful to the individual or others.
kleptomania (klep-toh-MAY-nee-ah)	klept/o = to steal -mania = frenzy	Stealing.
pyromania (pie-roh-MAY-nee-ah)	pyr/o = fire -mania = frenzy	Setting fires.
explosive disorder	ex- = outward dis- = apart	Violent rages.
Depressive Disorders	depress/o = to press down dis- = apart	Characterized by instability in mood.
major depressive disorder	depress/o = to press down dis- = apart	Feelings of hopelessness, helplessness, worthlessness; lack of pleasure in any activity; potential for suicide.
mania (MAY-nee-ah)	-mania = frenzy	Extreme elation.
Bipolar and Related Disorders	bi- = two -ar = pertaining to dis- = apart	
bipolar disorder (BPD)	bi- = two -ar = pertaining to **Med Term Tip** The healthcare professional must take all threats of suicide from patients seriously. Psychologists tell us that there is no clear suicide type, which means that we cannot predict who will actually take his or her own life. Always tell the physician about any discussion a patient has concerning suicide. If you believe a patient is in danger of suicide, do not be afraid to ask, "Are you thinking about suicide?"	Alternation between periods of deep depression and mania.
Personality Disorders	dis- = apart	Inflexible or maladaptive behavior patterns that affect a person's ability to function in society.
paranoid personality disorder	dis- = apart	Exaggerated feelings of persecution.
narcissistic personality disorder (nar-sis-SIST-ik)	dis- = apart	Abnormal sense of self-importance.
antisocial personality disorder	anti- = against soci/o = society -al = pertaining to dis- = apart	Behaviors that are against legal or social norms.
Schizophrenia Spectrum and Other Psychotic Disorders	schiz/o = split phren/o = mind -ia = state, condition	Mental disorders characterized by distortions of reality.
delusional disorder (dee-LOO-zhun-al)	delus/o = false belief -al = pertaining to dis- = apart	A false belief held even in the face of contrary evidence.
hallucination (hah-loo-sih-NAY-shun)	hallucin/o = imagined perception	Perceiving something that is not there.

Pathology (continued)

Term	Word Parts	Definition
Paraphilic Disorders	para- = abnormal -philic = pertaining to being attracted to dis- = apart	Disorders include aberrant sexual activity and sexual dysfunction.
pedophilic disorder (pee-doh-FILL-ik)	ped/o = child -philic = pertaining to being attracted to dis- = apart	Sexual interest in children.
sexual masochism disorder (MAS-oh-kizm)	-al = pertaining to -ism = state of dis- = apart	Gratification derived from being hurt or abused.
voyeuristic disorder (VOY-er-iss-tick)	-tic = pertaining to	Gratification derived from observing others engaged in sexual acts.
Sleep–Wake Disorders	dis- = apart	Disorders relating to either sleeping or wakefulness.
insomnia disorder (in-SOM-nee-ah)	in- = not somn/o = sleep -ia = state, condition	Inability to sleep.
narcolepsy (NAR-koh-lep-see)	narc/o = stupor, sleep -lepsy = seizure	Recurring episodes of sleeping during the daytime and often difficulty sleeping at night.
Somatic Symptom and Related Disorders	somat/o = body -ic = pertaining to dis- = apart	Patient has physical symptoms for which no physical disease can be determined.
somatic symptom disorder (SSD)	somat/o = body -ic = pertaining to dis- = apart	Having physical symptoms that cause distress and disrupt daily life. Includes a preoccupation with the symptoms and behaviors based on the symptoms.
conversion disorder	vers/o = to turn dis- = apart	Anxiety is transformed into physical symptoms such as heart palpitations, paralysis, or blindness.
Substance Use and Addictive Disorders	dis- = apart	
substance use disorders	dis- = apart	Overindulgence or dependence on chemical substances including alcohol, illegal drugs, and prescription drugs.
gambling disorder	dis- = apart	Inability to stop gambling.
Gender Dysphoria	dys- = abnormal -phoria = condition to bear	
gender dysphoria (dis-FOR-ee-ah)	dys- = abnormal -phoria = condition to bear	Occurs when birth gender is contrary to the gender a person identifies as. Includes both male to female (MTF) and female to male (FTM).
Trauma- and Stressor-Related Disorders	dis- = apart	
posttraumatic stress disorder (PTSD)	post- = after -ic = pertaining to dis- = apart	Results from exposure to actual or implied death, serious injury, or sexual violence. Condition impairs person's social interactions and capacity to work.

Pathology (continued)

Term	Word Parts	Definition
Elimination Disorders	dis- = apart	
enuresis		Act of voiding urine in inappropriate places after toilet training.
encopresis		Act of voiding feces in inappropriate places after toilet training.
Sexual Dysfunctions	-al = pertaining to dys- = abnormal, difficult	Having difficulty during any stage of normal sexual activity that negatively impacts quality of life.
erectile dysfunction	-ile = pertaining to dys- = difficult	The inability to achieve or maintain an erection.
premature ejaculation	pre- = before	Ejaculation of semen before or shortly after penetration.

Therapeutic Procedures

Term	Word Parts	Definition
electroconvulsive therapy (ECT) (ee-lek-troh-kon-VULL-siv)	electr/o = electricity	Procedure occasionally used for cases of prolonged major depression. This controversial treatment involves placement of an electrode on one or both sides of the patient's head and a current is turned on, briefly causing a convulsive seizure. A low level of voltage is used in modern electroconvulsive therapy, and the patient is administered a muscle relaxant and anesthesia. Advocates of this treatment state that it is a more effective way to treat severe depression than using drugs. It is not effective with disorders other than depression, such as schizophrenia and alcoholism.
Psychopharmacology (sigh-koh-far-mah-KALL-oh-jee)	psych/o = mind pharmac/o = drug -logy = study of	Study of the effects of drugs on the mind and particularly the use of drugs in treating mental disorders. The main classes of drugs for the treatment of mental disorders are:
antipsychotic drugs	anti- = against psych/o = mind -tic = pertaining to	These major tranquilizers include chlorpromazine (Thorazine™), haloperidol (Haldol™), clozapine (Clozaril™), and risperidone. These drugs have transformed the treatment of patients with psychoses and schizophrenia by reducing patient agitation and panic and shortening schizophrenic episodes. One of the side effects of these drugs is involuntary muscle movements, which approximately one-fourth of all adults who take the drugs develop.
antidepressant drugs	anti- = against depress/o = to press down	Classified as stimulants; alter the patient's mood by affecting levels of neurotransmitters in the brain. Antidepressants, such as serotonin norepinephrine reuptake inhibitors, are nonaddictive but they can produce unpleasant side effects such as dry mouth, weight gain, blurred vision, and nausea.
minor tranquilizers		Include Valium™ and Xanax™. These are also classified as central nervous system depressants and are prescribed for anxiety.
lithium		Special category of drug used successfully to calm patients who suffer from bipolar disorder (depression alternating with manic excitement).

Therapeutic Procedures (continued)

Term	Word Parts	Definition
Psychotherapy (sigh-koh-THAIR-ah-pee)	psych/o = mind -therapy = treatment	A method of treating mental disorders by mental rather than chemical or physical means. It includes:
psychoanalysis	psych/o = mind	Method of obtaining a detailed account of the past and present emotional and mental experiences from the patient to determine the source of the problem and eliminate the effects. It is a system developed by Sigmund Freud that encourages the patient to discuss repressed, painful, or hidden experiences with the hope of eliminating or minimizing the problem.
humanistic psychotherapy	-tic = pertaining to psych/o = mind -therapy = treatment	Therapist does not delve into the patients' past when using these methods. Instead, it is believed that patients can learn how to use their own internal resources to deal with their problems. The therapist creates a therapeutic atmosphere, which builds patient self-esteem and encourages discussion of problems, thereby gaining insight in how to handle them. Also called *client-centered* or *nondirective psychotherapy.*
family and group psychotherapy	psych/o = mind -therapy = treatment	Often described as solution focused, the therapist places minimal emphasis on patient past history and strong emphasis on having patient state and discuss goals and then find a way to achieve them.

Abbreviations

AD	Alzheimer's disease	**MA**	mental age
ADD	attention-deficit disorder	**MMPI**	Minnesota Multiphasic Personality Inventory
ADHD	attention-deficit/hyperactivity disorder	**MTF**	male to female
BPD	bipolar disorder	**OCD**	obsessive–compulsive disorder
CA	chronological age	**PTSD**	posttraumatic stress disorder
DSM	*Diagnostic and Statistical Manual of Mental Disorders*	**SAD**	seasonal affective disorder
ECT	electroconvulsive therapy	**SSD**	somatic symptom disorder
FTM	female to male		

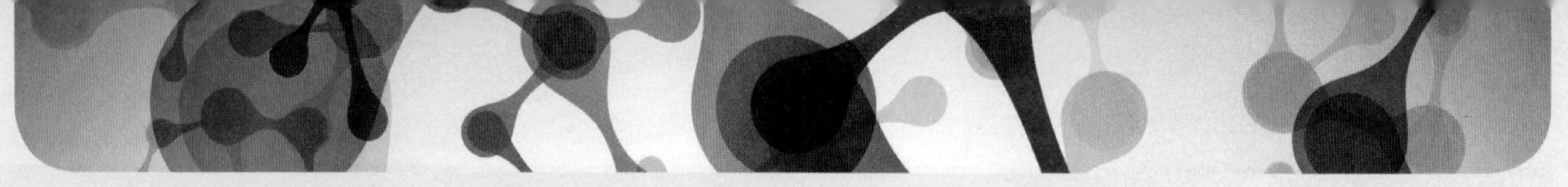

Section III: Diagnostic Imaging at a Glance

Word Parts

Here are the most common word parts (with their meanings) used to build diagnostic imaging terms.

Combining Forms

anter/o	front
fluor/o	fluorescence, luminous
later/o	side
nucle/o	nucleus
poster/o	back
radi/o	ray (X-ray)
roentgen/o	X-ray
son/o	sound
tom/o	to cut

Suffixes

-al	pertaining to
-ar	pertaining to
-graphy	process of recording
-ic	pertaining to
-ior	pertaining to
-logist	one who studies
-logy	study of
-lucent	to shine through
-opaque	nontransparent
-scopy	process of visually examining

Prefix

ultra-	beyond

Diagnostic Imaging

roentgenology (rent-gen-ALL-oh-jee) **X-rays**

Diagnostic imaging is the medical specialty that uses a variety of methods to produce images of the internal structures of the body. These images are then used to diagnose disease. This area of medicine began as **roentgenology** (**roentgen/o** = X-ray; **-logy** = study of), named after German physicist Wilhelm Roentgen who discovered roentgen rays in 1895. This discovery, now commonly known as **X-rays**, revolutionized the diagnosis of disease.

What's In A Name?
Look for these word parts:
roentgen/o = X-ray
-logy = study of

Diagnostic Imaging Terms

Term	Word Parts	Definition
anteroposterior view (AP view)	**anter/o** = front **poster/o** = back **-ior** = pertaining to	Positioning the patient so that the X-rays pass through the body from the anterior side to the posterior side.
barium (Ba) (BAH-ree-um)		Soft metallic element from the earth used as a radiopaque X-ray dye.
film		Thin sheet of cellulose material coated with a light-sensitive substance that is used in taking photographs. There is a special photographic film that is sensitive to X-rays.
film badge		Badge containing film that is sensitive to X-rays. This is worn by all personnel in radiology to measure the amount of X-rays to which they are exposed.
lateral view	**later/o** = side **-al** = pertaining to	Positioning of the patient so that the side of the body faces the X-ray machine.
oblique view (oh-BLEEK)		Positioning of the patient so that the X-rays pass through the body on an angle.
posteroanterior view (PA view)	**poster/o** = back **anter/o** = front **-ior** = pertaining to	Positioning of the patient so that the X-rays pass through the body from the posterior side to the anterior side.
radiography (ray-dee-OG-rah-fee)	**radi/o** = X-ray **-graphy** = process of recording	Making of X-ray pictures.
radioisotope (ray-dee-oh-EYE-soh-tohp)	**radi/o** = X-ray	Radioactive form of an element.
radiologist (ray-dee-ALL-oh-jist)	**radi/o** = X-ray **-logist** = one who studies	Physician who uses images to diagnose abnormalities and radiant energy to treat various conditions such as cancer.
radiolucent (ray-dee-oh-LOO-cent)	**radi/o** = X-ray **-lucent** = to shine through	Structures that allow X-rays to pass through, expose the photographic plate, and appear as black areas on the X-ray.
radiopaque (ray-dee-oh-PAYK)	**radi/o** = X-ray **-opaque** = nontransparent	Structures that are impenetrable to X-rays, appearing as a light area on the radiograph (X-ray).

Diagnostic Imaging Terms (continued)

Term	Word Parts	Definition
roentgen (RENT-gen)	roentgen/o = X-ray	Unit for describing an exposure dose of radiation.
scan		Recording on a photographic plate the emission of radioactive waves after a substance has been injected into the body.
■ **Figure 14.6** Nuclear medicine. Bone scan produced after injection of radioactive substance into the body. *(Photodisc/Getty Images)*		
shield		Device used to protect against radiation.
tagging		Attaching a radioactive material to a chemical, and tracing it as it moves through the body.
uptake		Absorption of radioactive material and medicines into an organ or tissue.
X-ray		High-energy wave that can penetrate most solid matter and present the image on photographic film.

Diagnostic Imaging Procedures

Term	Word Parts	Definition
computed tomography scan (CT scan) (toh-MOG-rah-fee)	tom/o = to cut -graphy = process of recording	Imaging technique that is able to produce a cross-sectional view of the body. X-ray pictures are taken at multiple angles through the body. A computer then uses all these images to construct a composite cross-section. Refer back to Figure 12.9 in Chapter 12 for an example of a computed tomography scan showing a brain tumor.

Diagnostic Imaging Procedures (continued)

Term	Word Parts	Definition
contrast studies ■ **Figure 14.7** Contrast study. X-ray of cerebral blood vessels taken after injection of radiopaque substance into the bloodstream. *(Neil Goldstein, Pearson Education)*	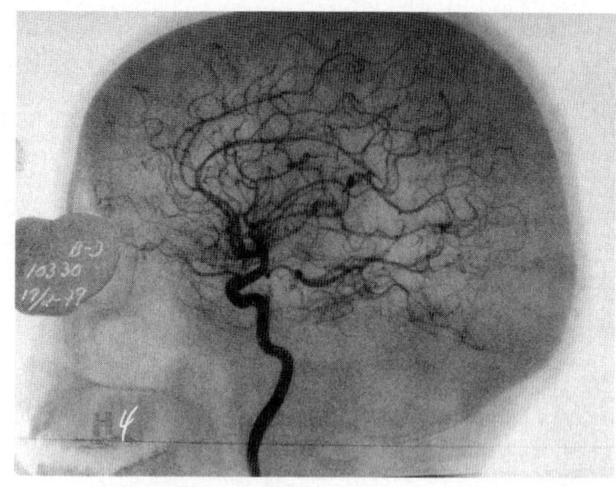	Radiopaque substance is injected or swallowed. X-rays are then taken that will outline the body structure containing the radiopaque substance. For example, angiograms and myelograms.
Doppler ultrasonography	ultra- = beyond son/o = sound -graphy = process of recording	Use of ultrasound to record the velocity of blood flowing through blood vessels. Used to detect blood clots and blood vessel obstructions.
fluoroscopy (floo-or-OS-koh-pee)	fluor/o = luminous -scopy = process of visually examining	X-rays strike a fluorescing screen rather than a photographic plate, causing it to glow. The glowing screen changes from minute to minute; therefore movement, such as the heart beating or the digestive tract moving, can be seen.
magnetic resonance imaging (MRI) (REZ-oh-nence) 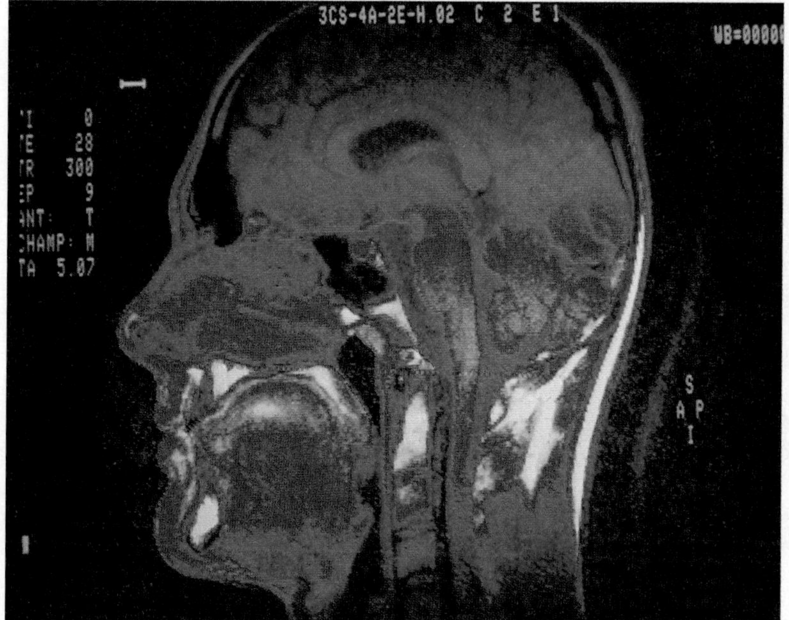	-ic = pertaining to	Use of electromagnetic energy to produce an image of soft tissues in any plane of the body. Atoms behave differently when placed in a strong magnetic field. When the body is exposed to this magnetic field the nuclei of the body's atoms emit radio-frequency signals that can be used to create an image. ■ **Figure 14.8** Color-enhanced magnetic resonance image (MRI), showing a sagittal view of the head. *(Science Source)*

Diagnostic Imaging Procedures (continued)

Term	Word Parts	Definition
nuclear medicine scan	nucle/o = nucleus -ar = pertaining to	Use of radioactive substances to diagnose diseases. A radioactive substance known to accumulate in certain body tissues is injected or inhaled. After waiting for the substance to travel to the body area of interest, the radioactivity level is recorded. Commonly referred to as a *scan* (see again Figure 14.6). See Table 14.4 ■ for examples of the radioactive substances used in nuclear medicine.

Table 14.4 Substances Used to Visualize Various Body Organs in Nuclear Medicine

Organ	Substance
bone	technetium (^{99m}Tc)–labeled phosphate
tumors	gallium (^{67}Ga)
lungs	xenon (^{133}Xe)
liver	technetium (^{99m}Tc)–labeled sulfur
heart	thallium (^{201}Tl)
thyroid	iodine (^{131}I)

Term	Word Parts	Definition
positron emission tomography (PET) (POS-ih-tron / eh-MIS-shun / toh-MOG-rah-fee)	tom/o = to cut -graphy = process of recording	Image is produced following the injection of radioactive glucose. The glucose will accumulate in areas of high metabolic activity. Therefore, this process will highlight areas that are consuming a large quantity of glucose. This may show an active area of the brain or a tumor.

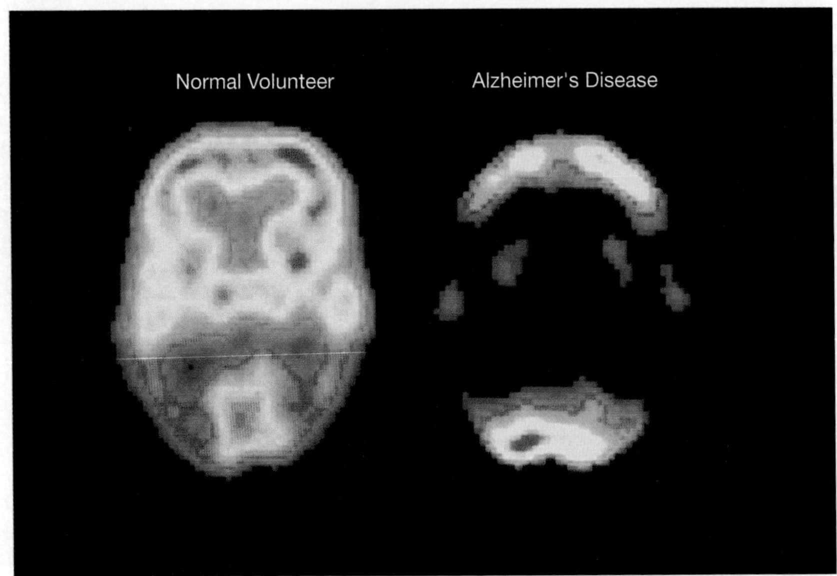

■ **Figure 14.9** Positron emission tomography (PET) image, showing the difference in the metabolic activity of the brain of a person with Alzheimer's disease and that of a healthy person. *(Science Source)*

Term	Word Parts	Definition
radiology (ray-dee-ALL-oh-jee)	radi/o = X-ray -logy = study of	Use of high-energy radiation, X-rays, to expose a photographic plate. The image is a black-and-white picture with radiopaque structures such as bone appearing white and radiolucent tissue such as muscles appearing dark.

Diagnostic Imaging Procedures (continued)

Term	Word Parts	Definition
ultrasound (US) (ULL-trah-sound)	ultra- = beyond	Use of high-frequency sound waves to produce an image. Sound waves directed into the body from a transducer will bounce off internal structures and echo back to the transducer. The speed of the echo is dependent on the density of the tissue. A computer is able to correlate speed of echo with density and produce an image. Used to visualize internal organs, heart valves, and fetuses.

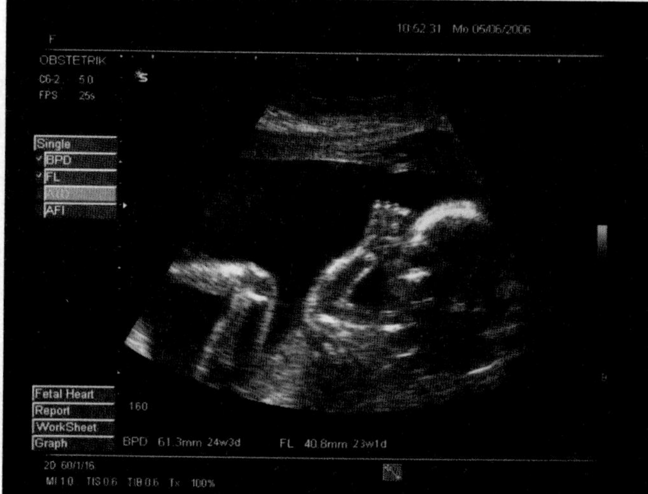

■ **Figure 14.10** Ultrasound showing the outline of a fetus. *(Mikael Damkier/Shutterstock)*

Abbreviations

^{67}Ga	radioactive gallium	**IVP**	intravenous pyelogram
^{99m}Tc	radioactive technetium	**KUB**	kidneys, ureters, bladder
^{131}I	radioactive iodine	**LAT**	lateral
^{201}Tl	radioactive thallium	**LGI**	lower gastrointestinal series
^{133}Xe	radioactive xenon	**LL**	left lateral
Angio	angiography	**mA**	milliampere
AP	anteroposterior	**mCi**	millicurie
Ba	barium	**MRA**	magnetic resonance angiography
BaE	barium enema	**MRI**	magnetic resonance imaging
CAT	computerized axial tomography	**NMR**	nuclear magnetic resonance
Ci	curie	**PA**	posteroanterior
CT	computerized tomography	**PET**	positron emission tomography
CXR	chest X-ray	**PTC**	percutaneous transhepatic cholangiography
decub	lying down	**R**	roentgen
DI	diagnostic imaging	**Ra**	radium
DSA	digital subtraction angiography	**rad**	radiation-absorbed dose
ERCP	endoscopic retrograde cholangiopancreatography	**RL**	right lateral
Fx, FX	fracture	**RRT**	registered radiologic technologist
GB	gallbladder X-ray	**UGI**	upper gastrointestinal series
IVC	intravenous cholangiogram	**US**	ultrasound

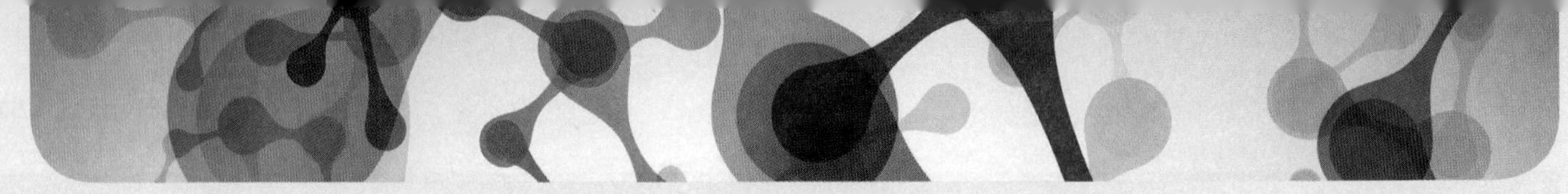

Section IV: Rehabilitation Services at a Glance

Word Parts

Here are the most common word parts (with their meanings) used to build rehabilitation services terms.

Combining Forms

cry/o	cold
cutane/o	skin
electr/o	electricity
erg/o	work
habilitat/o	ability
hydr/o	water
my/o	muscle
orth/o	straight, correct
phon/o	sound
physic/o	body
prosthet/o	addition
therm/o	heat

Suffixes

-al	pertaining to
-graphy	process of recording
-ic	pertaining to
-nomics	pertaining to laws
-ous	pertaining to
-phoresis	carrying
-therapy	treatment
-tic	pertaining to

Prefixes

re-	again
trans-	across
ultra-	beyond

Rehabilitation Services

occupational therapy **physical therapy**

The goal of rehabilitation is to prevent disability and restore as much function as possible following disease, illness, or injury. Rehabilitation services include the healthcare specialties of **physical therapy** (PT) and **occupational therapy** (OT).

What's In A Name?
Look for these word parts:
physic/o = body
-al = pertaining to

Physical Therapy

Physical therapy (PT) involves treating disorders using physical means and methods. Physical therapy personnel assess joint motion, muscle strength and endurance, function of heart and lungs, performance of activities required in daily living, and the ability to carry out other responsibilities. Physical therapy treatment includes gait training, therapeutic exercise, massage, joint and soft tissue mobilization, thermotherapy, cryotherapy, electrical stimulation, ultrasound, and hydrotherapy. These methods strengthen muscles, improve motion and circulation, reduce pain, and increase function.

Occupational Therapy

Occupational therapy (OT) assists patients to regain, develop, and improve skills that are important for independent functioning (activities of daily living). Occupational therapy personnel work with people who, because of illness, injury, or developmental or psychological impairments, require specialized training in skills that will enable them to lead independent, productive, and satisfying lives in regard to personal care, work, and leisure. Occupational therapists instruct patients in the use of adaptive equipment and techniques, body mechanics, and energy conservation. They also employ modalities such as heat, cold, and therapeutic exercise.

Rehabilitation Services Terms

Term	Word Parts	Definition
activities of daily living (ADLs)		Activities usually performed in the course of a normal day, such as eating, dressing, and washing.

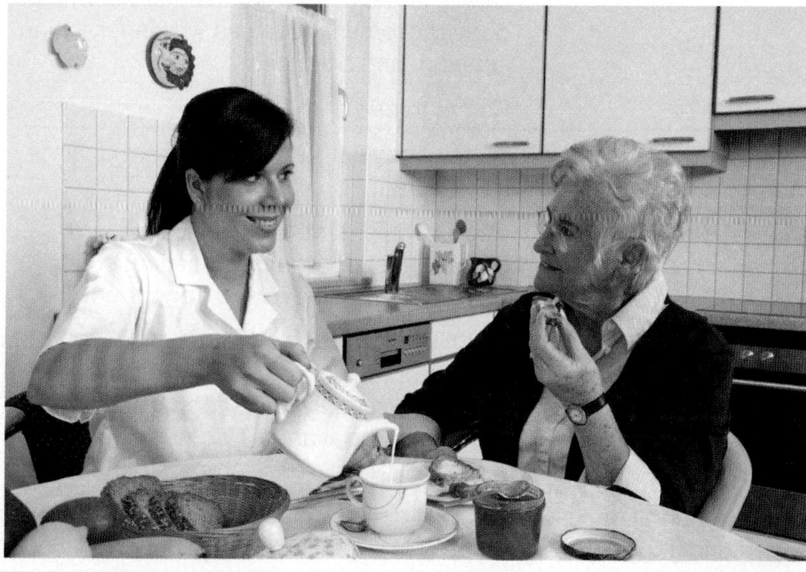

■ **Figure 14.11** Photograph of an occupational therapist assisting a patient with learning independence in activities of daily living (ADLs). *(Gina Sanders/ Shutterstock)*

Rehabilitation Services Terms (continued)

Term	Word Parts	Definition
adaptive equipment	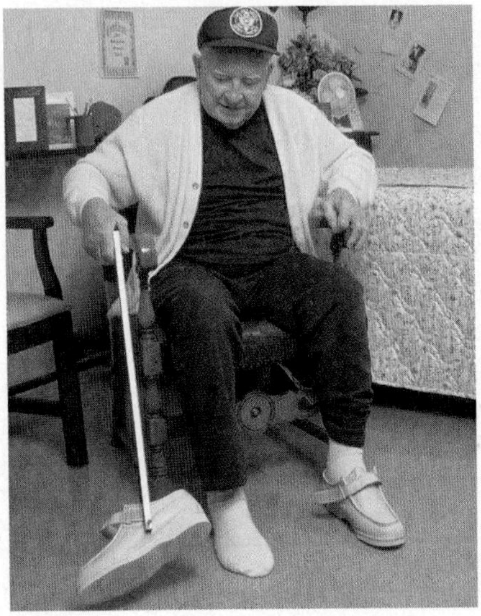	Modification of equipment or devices to improve the function and independence of a person with a disability. 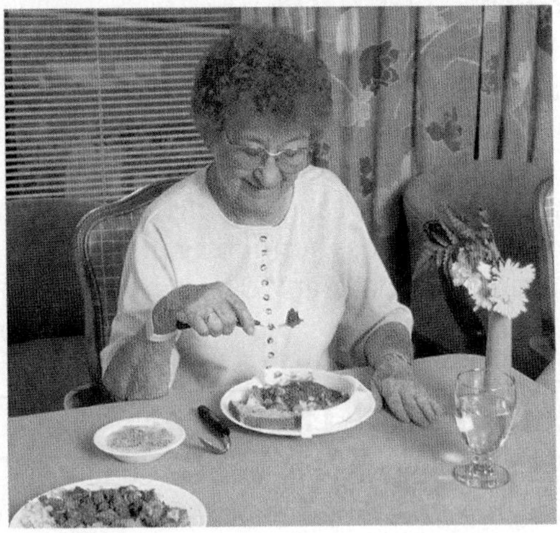
body mechanics	-ic = pertaining to	Use of good posture and position while performing activities of daily living to prevent injury and stress on body parts.
ergonomics (er-goh-NOM-iks)	erg/o = work -nomics = pertaining to laws	Study of human work including how the requirements for performing work and the work environment affect the musculoskeletal and nervous systems.
fine motor skills		Use of precise and coordinated movements in such activities as writing, buttoning, and cutting.
gait (GAYT)		Manner of walking.
gross motor skills		Use of large muscle groups that coordinate body movements such as walking, running, jumping, and balance.
lower extremity (LE)		Refers to one of the legs.
mobility		State of having normal movement of all body parts.
orthotics (or-THOT-iks)	orth/o = straight -tic = pertaining to	Use of equipment, such as splints and braces, to support a paralyzed muscle, promote a specific motion, or correct musculoskeletal deformities.
physical medicine	physic/o = body -al = pertaining to	Branch of medicine focused on restoring function. Primarily cares for patients with musculoskeletal and nervous system disorders. Physician is a *physiatrist.*
prosthetics (pros-THET-iks)	prosthet/o = addition -ic = pertaining to	Artificial devices, such as limbs and joints, that replace a missing body part.

■ **Figure 14.12** Using adaptive equipment. A) Male putting on shoe. B) Female eating one handed. *(Michal Heron, Pearson Education)*

A

B

Rehabilitation Services Terms (continued)

Term	Word Parts	Definition
range of motion (ROM)		Range of movement of a joint, from maximum flexion through maximum extension. It is measured as degrees of a circle.
rehabilitation	re- = again habilitat/o = ability	Process of treatment and exercise that can help a person with a disability attain maximum function and well-being.
upper extremity (UE)		Refers to one of the arms.

Therapeutic Procedures

Term	Word Parts	Definition
active exercises		Exercises that a patient performs without assistance.
active range of motion (AROM)		Range of motion for joints that a patient is able to perform without assistance from someone else.
active-resistive exercises		Exercises in which the patient works against resistance applied to a muscle, such as a weight. Used to increase strength.
cryotherapy (cry-oh-THAIR-ah-pee)	cry/o = cold -therapy = treatment	Using cold for therapeutic purposes.
debridement (day-breed-MON)		Removal of dead or damaged tissue from a wound. Commonly performed for burn therapy.
electromyography (EMG) (ee-LEK-troh-my-OG-rah-fee)	electr/o = electricity my/o = muscle -graphy = process of recording	The recording of a muscle's response to electrical stimulation. The graphic record produced is an *electromyogram.*
gait training		Assisting a patient to learn to walk again or how to use an assistive device to walk.

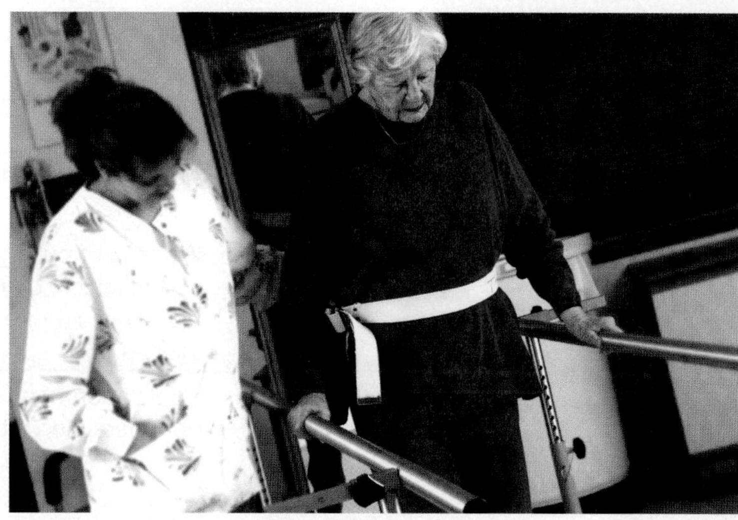

■ Figure 14.13 Physical therapist assisting a patient to walk in the parallel bars. *(auremat/Shutterstock)*

Therapeutic Procedures (continued)

Term	Word Parts	Definition
hydrotherapy (high-droh-THAIR-ah-pee)	hydr/o = water -therapy = treatment	Application of warm water as a therapeutic treatment. Can be done in baths, swimming pools, and whirlpools.
massage		Kneading or applying pressure by hands to a part of the patient's body to promote muscle relaxation and reduce tension.
mobilization		Treatments such as exercise and massage to restore movement to joints and soft tissue.
moist hot packs		Applying moist warmth to a body part to produce a slight dilation of blood vessels in the skin. Causes muscle relaxation in the deeper regions of the body and increases circulation, which aids healing.
nerve conduction velocity		Test to determine if nerves have been damaged by recording the rate at which an electrical impulse travels along a nerve. If the nerve is damaged, the velocity will be decreased.
pain control		Managing pain through a variety of means, including medications, biofeedback, and mechanical devices.
passive range of motion (PROM)		Therapist putting a patient's joints through available range of motion without assistance from the patient.
phonophoresis (foh-noh-foh-REE-sis)	phon/o = sound -phoresis = carrying	Use of ultrasound waves to introduce medication across the skin and into the subcutaneous tissues.
postural drainage with clapping	-al = pertaining to	Draining secretions from the bronchi or a lung cavity by having the patient lie so that gravity allows drainage to occur. Clapping is using the hand in a cupped position to perform percussion on the chest. Assists in loosening secretions and mucus.
therapeutic exercise (thair-ah-PEW-tik)	-ic = pertaining to	Exercise planned and carried out to achieve a specific physical benefit, such as improved range of motion, muscle strength, or cardiovascular function.
thermotherapy (ther-moh-THAIR-ah-pee)	therm/o = heat -therapy = treatment	Applying heat to the body for therapeutic purposes.
traction		Process of pulling or drawing, usually with a mechanical device. Used in treating orthopedic (bone and joint) problems and injuries.
transcutaneous electrical nerve stimulation (TENS) (tranz-kyoo-TAY-nee-us)	trans- = across cutane/o = skin -ous = pertaining to electr/o = electricity -al = pertaining to	Application of an electric current to a peripheral nerve to relieve pain.

Therapeutic Procedures (continued)

Term	Word Parts	Definition
ultrasound (US)	ultra- = beyond	Use of high-frequency sound waves to create heat in soft tissues under the skin. It is particularly useful for treating injuries to muscles, tendons, and ligaments, as well as muscle spasms.
whirlpool		Bath in which there are continuous jets of hot water reaching the body surfaces.

■ **Figure 14.14** Patient receiving ultrasound treatment to the left elbow. *(GWImages/Shutterstock)*

Abbreviations

AAROM	active assistive range of motion	**PROM**	passive range of motion
ADLs	activities of daily living	**PT**	physical therapy
AROM	active range of motion	**ROM**	range of motion
EMG	electromyogram	**TENS**	transcutaneous electrical nerve stimulation
e-stim	electrical stimulation	**UE**	upper extremity
LE	lower extremity	**US**	ultrasound
OT	occupational therapy		

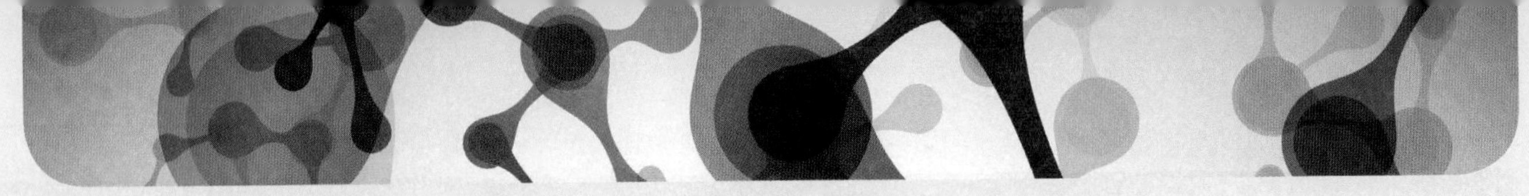

Section V: Surgery at a Glance

Word Parts

Here are the most common word parts (with their meanings) used to build surgical terms.

Combining Forms

alges/o	pain
aspir/o	to breathe in
cis/o	to cut
cry/o	cold
cutane/o	skin
dilat/o	to widen
electr/o	electricity
esthesi/o	sensation, feeling
hal/o	to breathe
hem/o	blood
later/o	side
lith/o	stone
recumb/o	to lie back
sect/o	to cut
specul/o	to look at
tenacul/o	to hold
topic/o	a specific area
ven/o	vein

Suffixes

-al	pertaining to
-ia	state, condition
-ic	pertaining to
-ion	action
-ist	specialist
-logist	one who studies
-otomy	to cut into
-ous	pertaining to
-scopic	pertaining to visually examining
-stasis	standing still
-stat	to keep from moving

Prefixes

an-	without
dis-	apart
endo-	within
ex-	outward
in-	inward
intra-	within
peri-	around
post-	after
pre-	before
re-	again
sub-	under

Surgery

operative report
surgeon
surgery

Surgery is the branch of medicine dealing with operative procedures to correct deformities and defects, repair injuries, and diagnose and cure diseases. A **surgeon** is a physician who has completed additional training of five years or more in a surgical specialty area. These specialty areas include orthopedics; neurosurgery; gynecology; ophthalmology; urology; and thoracic, vascular, cardiac, plastic, and general surgery. The surgeon must complete an **operative report** for every procedure that he or she performs. This is a detailed description that includes:

- Preoperative diagnosis
- Indication for the procedure
- Name of the procedure
- Surgical techniques employed
- Findings during surgery
- Postoperative diagnosis
- Name of the surgeon

This report also includes information pertaining to the patient such as name, address, age, patient number, and date of the procedure.

Surgical terminology includes terms related to anesthesiology, surgical instruments, surgical procedures, incisions, and suture materials. Specific surgical procedures are frequently named by using the combining form for the body part being operated on and adding a suffix that describes the procedure. For example, an incision into the chest is a *thoracotomy*, removal of the stomach is *gastrectomy*, and surgical repair of the skin is *dermatoplasty*. A list of the most frequently used surgical suffixes is found in Chapter 1 and common surgical procedures are defined in each system chapter.

Anesthesia

anesthesia (an-ess-THEE-zee-ah)
anesthesiologist (an-es-thee-zee-OL-oh-jist)
general anesthesia
inhalation (in-hah-LAY-shun)
intravenous (in-trah-VEE-nus)
local anesthesia
nurse anesthetist (ah-NES-the-tist)
regional anesthesia
subcutaneous (sub-kyoo-TAY-nee-us)
topical anesthesia

An **anesthesiologist** is a physician who specializes in the practice of administering anesthetics. A **nurse anesthetist** is a registered nurse who has received additional training and education in the administration of anesthetic medications. **Anesthesia** results in the loss of feeling or sensation. The most common types of anesthesia are general, regional, local, and topical anesthesia (see Table 14.5 ■).

What's In A Name?
Look for these word parts:
an- = without
esthesi/o = sensation, feeling
-ist = specialist
-logist = one who studies

Surgical Instruments

Physicians have developed surgical instruments since the time of the early Egyptians. Instruments include surgical knives, saws, clamps, drills, and needles. Some of the more commonly used surgical instruments are listed in Table 14.6 ■ and are shown in Figure 14.15 ■.

Table 14.5 Types of Anesthesia

Type	Word Parts	Description
general anesthesia (GA)	an- = without esthesi/o = sensation, feeling -ia = state, condition	Produces a loss of consciousness including an absence of pain sensation. The patient's vital signs (VS)—heart rate, breathing rate, pulse, and blood pressure—are carefully monitored when using a general anesthetic.
intravenous (IV)	intra- = within ven/o = vein -ous = pertaining to	Route for administering general anesthesia via injection into a vein.
inhalation	in- = inward hal/o = to breathe	Route for administering general anesthesia by breathing it in.
regional anesthesia	-al = pertaining to an- = without esthesi/o = sensation, feeling -ia = state, condition	Also referred to as a *nerve block*. This anesthetic interrupts a patient's pain sensation in a particular region of the body, such as the arm. The anesthetic is injected near the nerve that will be blocked from sensation. The patient usually remains conscious.
local anesthesia	-al = pertaining to an- = without esthesi/o = sensation, feeling -ia = state, condition	Produces a loss of sensation in one localized part of the body. The patient remains conscious.
subcutaneous	sub- = under cutane/o = skin -ous = pertaining to	Method of applying local anesthesia involving injecting the anesthetic under the skin. This type of anesthetic is used to deaden the skin prior to suturing a laceration.
topical	topic/o = a specific area -al = pertaining to	Method of applying local anesthesia involving placing a liquid or gel directly onto a specific area of skin. This type of anesthetic is used on the skin, the cornea, and the mucous membranes in dental work.

Table 14.6 Common Surgical Instruments

Instrument	Word Parts	Use
aspirator (AS-pih-ray-tor)	aspir/o = to breathe in	Suctions fluid
clamp		Grasps tissue; controls bleeding
curette (kyoo-RET)		Scrapes and removes tissue
dilator (dye-LAY-tor)	dilat/o = to widen	Enlarges an opening by stretching
forceps (FOR-seps)		Grasps tissue
hemostat (HEE-moh-stat)	hem/o = blood -stat = to keep from moving	Forceps to grasp blood vessel to control bleeding
probe		Explores tissue
scalpel		Cuts and separates tissue
speculum (SPEK-yoo-lum)	specul/o = to look at	Spreads apart walls of a cavity
tenaculum (teh-NAK-yoo-lum)	tenacul/o = to hold	Long-handled clamp
trephine (treh-FINE)		Saw that removes disk-shaped piece of tissue or bone

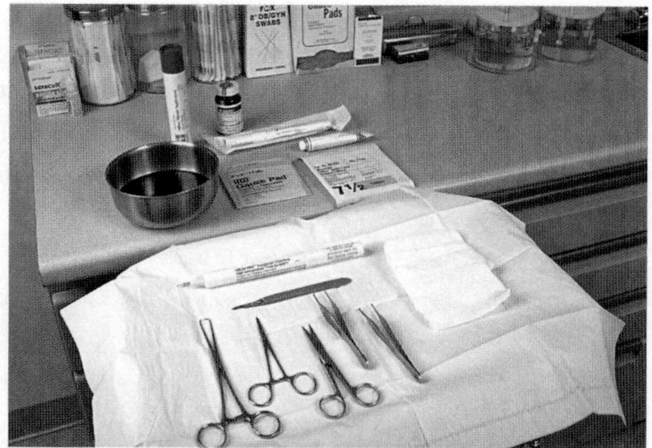

■ **Figure 14.15** Surgical instruments prepared for a procedure. *(Brian Warling, Pearson Education)*

Surgical Positions

Patients are placed in specific positions so the surgeon is able to reach the area that is to be operated on. Table 14.7 ■ describes and Figure 14.16 ■ illustrates some common surgical positions.

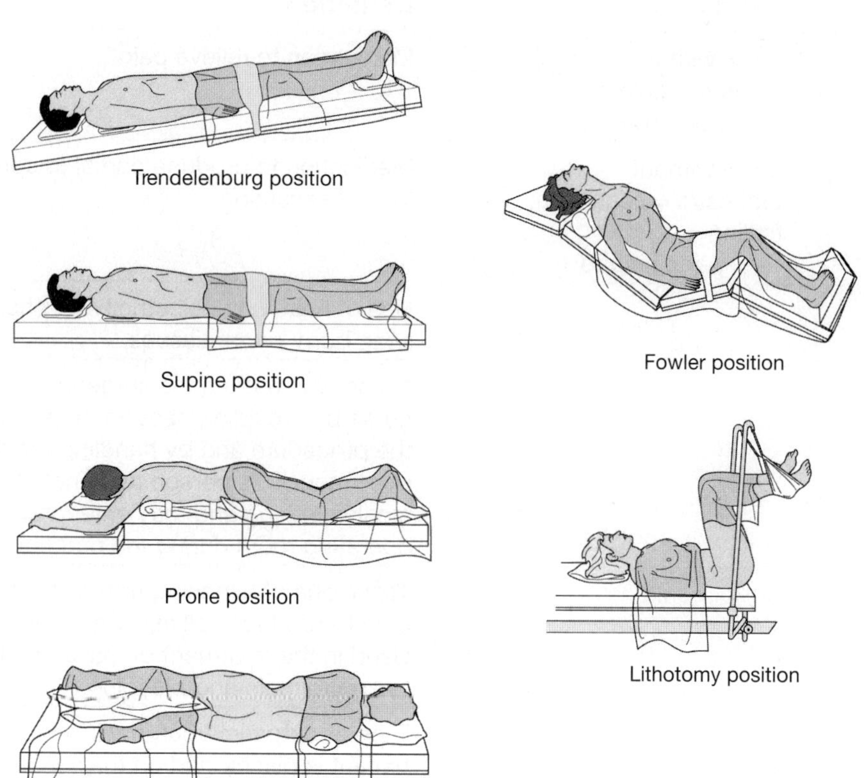

■ **Figure 14.16** Examples of common surgical positions.

Table 14.7 Common Surgical Positions

Position	Word Parts	Description
Fowler		Sitting with back positioned at a 45° angle
lateral recumbent (ree-KUM-bent)	later/o = side -al = pertaining to recumb/o = to lie back	Lying on either the left or right side
lithotomy (lith-OT-oh-mee)	lith/o = stone -otomy = to cut into	Lying face up with hips and knees bent at 90° angles
prone (PROHN)		Lying horizontal and face down
supine (soo-PINE)		Lying horizontal and face up; also called *dorsal recumbent*
Trendelenburg (TREN-deh-len-berg)		Lying face up and on an incline with head lower than legs

Surgery Terms

Term	Word Parts	Definition
analgesic (an-al-JEE-zik)	an- = without alges/o = pain -ic = pertaining to	Medication to relieve pain.
anesthetic (an-ess-THET-ik)	an- = without esthesi/o = sensation, feeling -ic = pertaining to	Medication to produce partial to complete loss of sensation.
cauterization (kaw-ter-ih-ZAY-shun)		Use of heat, cold, electricity, or chemicals to scar, burn, or cut tissues.
circulating nurse		Nurse who assists the surgeon and scrub nurse by providing needed materials during the procedure and by handling the surgical specimen. This person does not wear sterile clothing and may enter and leave the operating room during the procedure.
cryosurgery (cry-oh-SER-jer-ee)	cry/o = cold	Technique of exposing tissues to extreme cold to produce cell injury and destruction. Used in the treatment of malignant tumors or to control pain and bleeding.
day surgery		Type of outpatient surgery in which the patient is discharged on the same day he or she is admitted; also called *ambulatory surgery.*
dissection (dih-SEK-shun)	dis- = apart sect/o = to cut	Surgical cutting of parts for separation and study.
draping		Process of covering the patient with sterile cloths that allow only the operative site to be exposed to the surgeon.

Surgery Terms (continued)

Term	Word Parts	Definition
electrocautery (ee-lek-troh-KAW-ter-ee)	electr/o = electricity	Use of an electric current to stop bleeding by coagulating blood vessels.
endoscopic surgery (en-doh-SKOP-ik)	endo- = within -scopic = pertaining to visually examining	Use of a lighted instrument to examine the interior of a cavity.
excision (ek-SIZH-un)	ex- = outward cis/o = to cut -ion = action	To cut out. The surgical removal of part or all of an organ or structure.
hemostasis (hee-moh-STAY-sis)	hem/o = blood -stasis = standing still	Stopping the flow of blood using instruments, pressure, and/or medication.
incision (in-SIZH-un)	in- = inward cis/o = to cut -ion = action	To cut into or to cut open an organ or structure.
intraoperative (in-trah-OP-er-ah-tiv)	intra- = within	Period of time during surgery.
laser surgery		Use of a controlled beam of light for cutting, hemostasis, or tissue destruction.
perioperative (per-ee-OP-er-ah-tiv)	peri- = around	Period of time that includes before, during, and after a surgical procedure.
postoperative (post-op) (post-OP-er-ah-tiv)	post- = after	Period of time immediately following surgery.
preoperative (preop) (pree-OP-er-ah-tiv)	pre- = before	Period of time preceding surgery.
resection (ree-SEK-shun)	re- = again sect/o = to cut	To surgically cut out or remove; excision.
scrub nurse		Surgical assistant who hands instruments to the surgeon. This person wears sterile clothing and maintains the sterile operative field.
suture material (SOO-cher)		Used to close a wound or incision. Examples are cotton, catgut, silk thread, or staples. They may or may not be removed when the wound heals, depending on the type of material that is used.

Abbreviations

D & C	dilation and curettage	**PARR**	postanesthetic recovery room
Endo	endoscopy	**post-op**	postoperative
EUA	exam under anesthesia	**preop, pre-op**	preoperative
GA	general anesthesia	**prep**	preparation, prepared
I & D	incision and drainage	**T & A**	tonsillectomy and adenoidectomy
MUA	manipulation under anesthesia	**TAH**	total abdominal hysterectomy
OR	operating room	**TURP**	transurethral resection of prostate

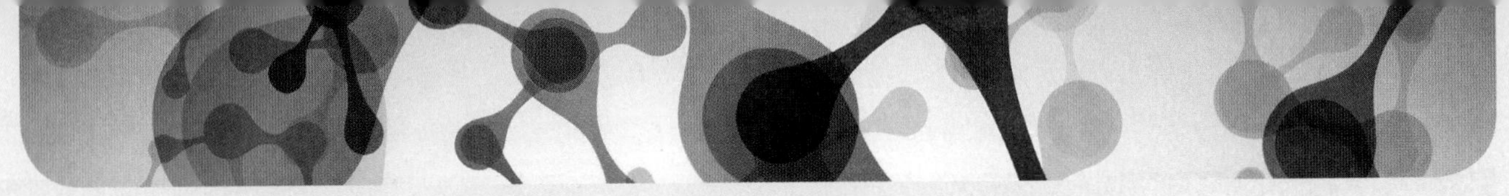

Section VI: Oncology at a Glance

Word Parts

Here are the most common word parts (with their meanings) used to build oncology terms.

Combining Forms

bi/o	life	**morbid/o**	ill
capsul/o	to box	**mort/o**	death
carcin/o	cancerous	**mutat/o**	to change
chem/o	drug	**onc/o**	tumor
cyt/o	cell	**path/o**	disease
immun/o	protection	**radic/o**	root
lapar/o	abdomen	**radi/o**	radiation
laps/o	to slide back	**tox/o**	poison
miss/o	to send back		

Suffixes

-al	pertaining to	**-opsy**	view of
-gen	that which produces	**-otomy**	to cut into
-genic	producing	**-plasia**	formation of cells
-logic	pertaining to studying	**-plasm**	formation
-logist	one who studies	**-stasis**	standing still
-logy	study of	**-therapy**	treatment
-oma	tumor		

Prefixes

en-	inward	**meta-**	beyond
hyper-	excessive	**neo-**	new
in-	inward	**re-**	again

Oncology

benign (bee-NINE)
carcinoma (kar-sin-NOH-mah)
malignant (mah-LIG-nant)
oncology (ong-KALL-oh-jee)
protocol (PROH-toh-kall)
tumors

Oncology is the branch of medicine dealing with **tumors**. A tumor can be classified as **benign** or **malignant**. A benign tumor is one that is generally not progressive or recurring. Often, a benign tumor will have the suffix *-oma* at the end of the term. However, a malignant tumor indicates that there is a cancerous growth present (see Figure 14.17■). These terms will usually have the word *carcinoma* added. The medical specialty of oncology primarily treats patients who have cancer.

The treatment for cancer can consist of a variety or a combination of treatments. The **protocol** (prot) for a particular patient will consist of the actual plan of care, including the medications, surgeries, and treatments such as chemotherapy and radiation therapy. Often, the entire healthcare team, including the physician, oncologist, radiologist, nurse, patient, and family, will assist in designing the treatment plan.

What's In A Name?

Look for these word parts:
carcin/o = cancer
onc/o = tumor
-logy = study of
-oma = tumor

Med Term Tip

Carcinoma or cancer (Ca) can affect almost every organ in the body. The medical term reflects the area of the body affected as well as the type of tumor cell. For example, there can be an esophageal carcinoma, gastric adenocarcinoma, or adenocarcinoma of the uterus.

Staging Tumors

grade
metastases (meh-TASS-tah-seez)
pathologist (path-ALL-oh-jist)
staging

The process of classifying tumors based on their degree of tissue invasion and the potential response to therapy is referred to as **staging**. The TNM staging system is frequently used, with the *T* referring to the tumor's size and invasion, the *N* referring to lymph node involvement, and the *M* referring to the presence of **metastases** (mets) of the tumor cells (see Figure 14.18■).

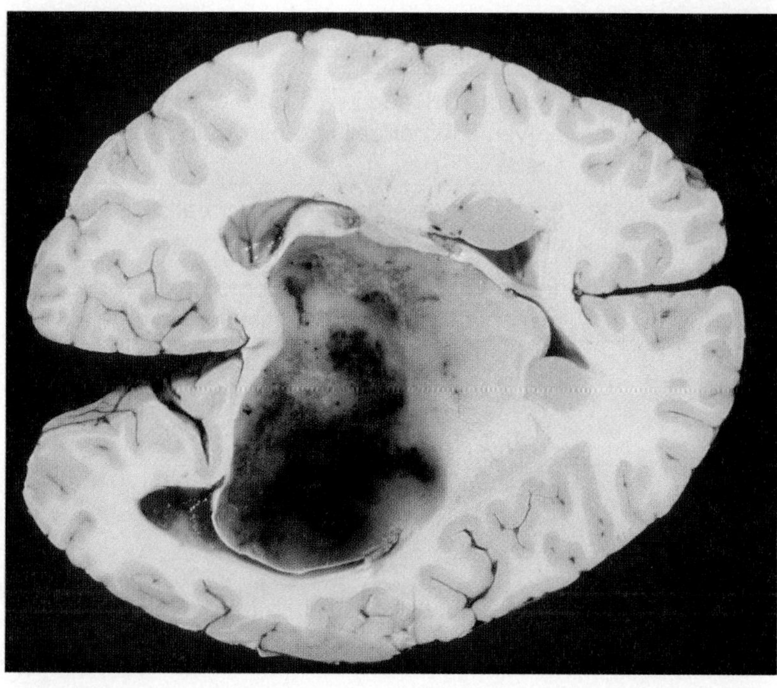

■ **Figure 14.17** Photograph of a brain specimen with a large malignant tumor. *(Biophoto Associates/Photo Researchers, Inc.)*

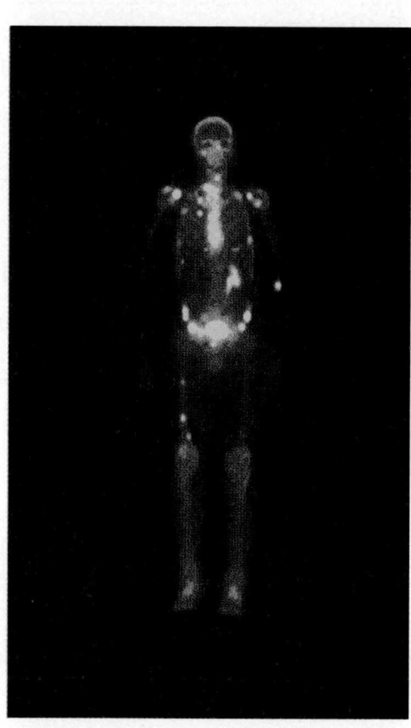

■ **Figure 14.18** Nuclear medicine bone scan showing metastatic tumors in the skeleton. *(Medical Body Scans/Science Source)*

What's In A Name?

Look for these word parts:
path/o = disease
-logist = one who studies
meta- = beyond

In addition, a tumor can be graded from grade I through grade IV. The **grade** is based on the microscopic appearance of the tumor cells. The **pathologist** rates or grades the cells based on whether the tumor resembles the normal tissue. The classification system is illustrated in Table 14.8 ■. The cells in a grade I tumor are well differentiated, which makes it easier to treat than the more advanced grades.

Table 14.8 Tumor Grade Classification

Grade	Meaning
GX	Grade cannot be determined
GI	Cells are well differentiated
GII	Cells are moderately differentiated
GIII	Cells are poorly differentiated
GIV	Cells are undifferentiated

Oncology Terms

Term	Word Parts	Definition
carcinogen (kar-SIN-oh-jen)	carcin/o = cancer -gen = that which produces	Substance or chemical agent that produces or increases the risk of developing cancer. For example, cigarette smoke and insecticides are considered to be carcinogens.
	Med Term Tip The term *benign* comes from the Latin term *bene*, which means "kind or good." On the other hand, the term *malignant* comes from the Latin term *mal*, meaning "bad or malicious."	
carcinoma in situ (CIS) (kar-sin-NOH-mah)	carcin/o = cancer -oma = tumor	Malignant tumor whose cells have not spread beyond the original site.
encapsulated (en-CAP-soo-lay-ted)	en- = inward capsul/o = to box	Growth enclosed in a sheath of tissue that prevents tumor cells from invading surrounding tissue.
hyperplasia (high-per-PLAY-zee-ah)	hyper- = excessive -plasia = formation of cells	Excessive development of normal cells within an organ.
invasive disease (in-VAY-siv)	in- = inward	Tendency of a malignant tumor to spread to immediately surrounding tissue and organs.

Oncology Terms (continued)

Term	Word Parts	Definition
metastasis (mets) (meh-TASS-tah-sis)	meta- = beyond -stasis = standing still	Movement and spread of cancer cells from one part of the body to another. Metastases is the plural.

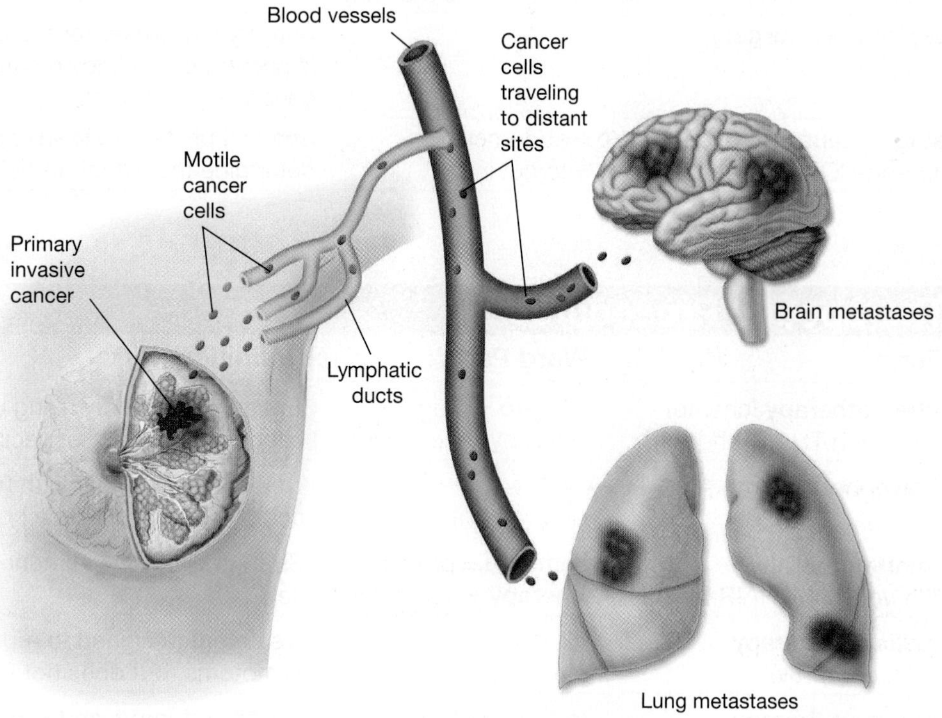

■ **Figure 14.19** Illustration showing how the primary breast tumor metastasized through the lymphatic and blood vessels to secondary sites in the brain and lungs.

Term	Word Parts	Definition
morbidity (mor-BID-ih-tee)	morbid/o = ill	Number representing the sick persons in a particular population.
mortality (mor-TAL-ih-tee)	mort/o = death	Number representing the deaths in a particular population.
mutation (mew-TAY-shun)	mutat/o = to change	Change or transformation from the original.
neoplasm (NEE-oh-plazm)	neo- = new -plasm = formation	New and abnormal growth or tumor. These can be benign or malignant.
oncogenic (ong-koh-JEN-ik)	onc/o = tumor -genic = producing	Cancer causing.
primary site		Term used to designate where a malignant tumor first appeared.
relapse (REE-laps)	re- = again laps/o = to slide back	Return of disease symptoms after a period of improvement.
remission (rih-MISH-un)	re- = again miss/o = to send back	Period during which the symptoms of a disease or disorder leave. Can be temporary.

Diagnostic Procedures

Term	Word Parts	Definition
biopsy (BX, bx) (BYE-op-see)	bi/o = life -opsy = view of	Excision of a small piece of tissue for microscopic examination to assist in determining a diagnosis.
cytologic testing (sigh-toh-LAH-jik)	cyt/o = cell -logic = pertaining to studying	Examination of cells to determine their structure and origin. Pap smears are considered a form of cytologic testing.
exploratory surgery		Surgery performed for the purpose of determining if cancer is present or if a known cancer has spread. Biopsies are generally performed.
staging laparotomy (lap-ah-ROT-oh-mee)	lapar/o = abdomen -otomy = to cut into	Surgical procedure in which the abdomen is entered to determine the extent and staging of a tumor.

Therapeutic Procedures

Term	Word Parts	Definition
chemotherapy (chemo) (kee-moh-THAIR-ah-pee)	chem/o = drug -therapy = treatment	Treating disease by using chemicals that have a toxic effect on the body, especially cancerous tissue.
hormone therapy		Treatment of cancer with natural hormones or with chemicals that produce hormone-like effects.
immunotherapy (im-yoo-noh-THAIR-ah-pee)	immun/o = protection -therapy = treatment	Strengthening the immune system to attack cancerous cells.
palliative therapy (PAL-ee-ah-tiv)		Treatment designed to reduce the intensity of painful symptoms, but does not produce a cure.
radiation therapy	radi/o = radiation	Exposing tumors and surrounding tissues to X-rays, gamma rays, neutrons, protons, and other sources to kill cancer cells and shrink tumors.
radical surgery	radic/o = root -al = pertaining to	Extensive surgery to remove as much tissue associated with a tumor as possible.
radioactive implant (ray-dee-oh-AK-tiv)	radi/o = radiation	Embedding a radioactive source directly into tissue to provide a highly localized radiation dosage to damage nearby cancerous cells. Also called *brachytherapy.*

Abbreviations

BX, bx	biopsy	**mets**	metastases
Ca	cancer	**MTX**	methotrexate
chemo	chemotherapy	**prot**	protocol
CIS	carcinoma in situ	**st**	stage
5-FU	5-fluorouracil	**TNM**	tumor, nodes, metastases
GA	gallium		

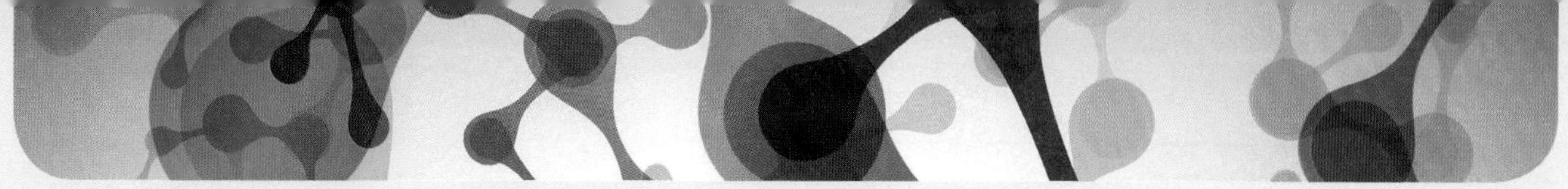

Chapter Review

Real-World Applications

Chart Note Transcription

The chart note below contains 11 phrases that can be reworded with a medical term that you learned in this chapter. Each phrase is identified with an underline. Determine the medical term and write your answers in the space provided.

Current Complaint:	A 56-year-old male was referred to a specialist in the treatment of cancer **1** for treatment of a suspicious right kidney mass discovered by his internist on a CT scan.
Past History:	Patient had been aware of right side pain, difficulty urinating, and weight loss during the past six months.
Signs and Symptoms:	Surgery to determine if cancer is present **2** was performed and small samples of tissue removed for examination under a microscope **3** were taken from the suspicious right kidney mass. After it was determined to be cancerous with a tendency to grow worse, **4** a right nephrectomy was performed. Reports indicate that the new and abnormal growth **5** was graded to be moderately differentiated **6** and well enclosed in a sheath of tissue **7** with no signs of spreading to another part of the body. **8**
Diagnosis:	Cancerous tumor of the right kidney. **9**
Treatment:	Post surgery the patient began a plan of treatment **10** of the use of chemical agents with a specific toxic effect. **11**

1. ______
2. ______
3. ______
4. ______
5. ______
6. ______
7. ______
8. ______
9. ______
10. ______
11. ______

Case Study

Below is a case study presentation of a patient with a condition covered by this chapter. Read the case study and answer the questions below. Some questions will ask for information not included within this chapter. Use your text, a medical dictionary, or any other reference material you choose to answer these questions.

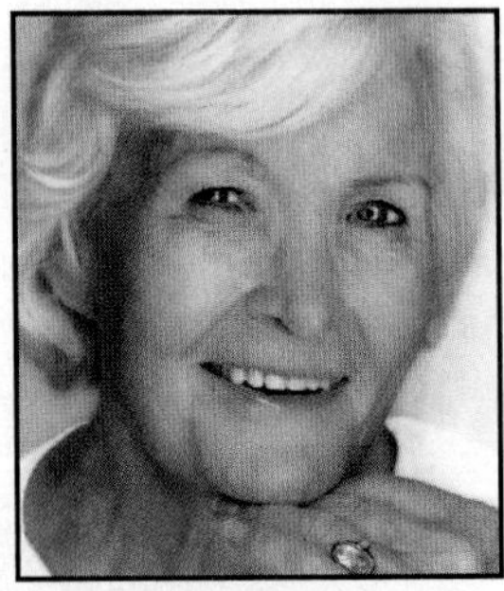

(Martina Ebel/Shutterstock)

Patient is a 72-year-old female complaining of increasing dyspnea with activity during the past six months. She now has a frequent harsh cough producing thick sputum and occasional hemoptysis. Patient is thin and short of stature. She is not SOB sitting in examination room. CT scan of the bronchial tree confirmed the presence of a mass in the right lung. Sputum was collected for sputum culture and sensitivity and sputum cytology. Sputum specimen was negative for the presence of bacteria. Sputum cytology revealed bronchogenic carcinoma. Patient will be referred to thoracic surgeon for consultation regarding lobectomy. Following recovery from this surgery she is to return to oncology clinic for chemotherapy and to determine if the tumor has metastasized.

Questions

1. What is this patient's diagnosis? Look it up and write a short description.

____

____

2. The patient had three complaints. List the three complaints and describe each in your own words.

____

____

3. Describe in your own words the diagnostic imaging procedure used on this patient and the results.

____

____

4. List and describe in your own words the clinical laboratory diagnostic tests run on this patient and the results of each test.

____

____

5. What surgical procedure will this patient undergo? Describe it in your own words.

____

____

6. What does the term *metastasized* mean?

____

____

Practice Exercises

A. Complete the Statement

1. The reference book containing important information regarding medications is the ______________________.
2. A person specializing in the dispensing of medications is a ______________________.
3. The accepted official name for a drug is the ______________________ name.
4. The trade name for a drug is the ______________________ name.
5. What does the chemical name represent? ______________________
6. What federal agency enforces controls over the use of drugs causing dependency? ______________________

B. Drug Administration Practice

Name the route of drug administration for the following descriptions.

1. under the tongue ______________________
2. into the anus or rectum ______________________
3. applied to the skin ______________________
4. injected under the first layer of skin ______________________
5. injected into a muscle ______________________
6. injected into a vein ______________________
7. by mouth ______________________

C. Define the Term

1. idiosyncrasy ______________________
2. parenteral ______________________
3. placebo ______________________
4. toxicity ______________________
5. side effect ______________________
6. unit dose ______________________
7. habituation ______________________
8. antidote ______________________
9. contraindication ______________________
10. prophylaxis ______________________

D. What Does it Stand For?

1. gr
2. bid
3. tid
4. ad lib
5. prn
6. ante
7. OTC
8. gt
9. Sig
10. stat
11. mg
12. aq
13. noc
14. NPO
15. hs
16. IV
17. TO
18. gtt
19. pc
20. d/c

E. Prescription Practice

Write out the following prescription instructions in the space provided.

1. Pravachol, 20 mg, Sig. ī – daily hs, 30, refill 3x, no sub.
2. Lanoxin, 0.125 mg, Sig. i̅i̅i̅ — stat, then i̅i̅ q AM, 100, refills prn.
3. Synthroid, 0.075 mg, Sig. ī – daily, 100, refill x4.
4. Norvasc, 5 mg, ī – q am, 60, refillable.

F. Terminology Matching

Match each term to its definition.

1.	________ neurocognitive disorder	a.	conversion disorder
2.	________ elimination disorder	b.	kleptomania
3.	________ dissociative disorder	c.	pedophilic disorder
4.	________ eating disorder	d.	narcissistic personality
5.	________ sleep–wake disorder	e.	insomnia
6.	________ depressive disorder	f.	mania
7.	________ impulse control disorder	g.	panic attacks
8.	________ somatic symptom disorder	h.	amnesia
9.	________ personality disorder	i.	dementia
10.	________ paraphilic disorder	j.	anorexia nervosa
11.	________ anxiety disorder	k.	enuresis

G. Name the Treatment

Identify each mental health treatment from its description.

1. depressant drugs prescribed for anxiety ________________________________
2. client-centered psychotherapy ________________________________
3. drug used to calm patients with bipolar disorder ________________________________
4. reduces patient agitation and panic and shortens schizophrenic episodes ________________________________
5. obtains a detailed account of the past and present emotional and mental experiences ________________________________
6. stimulants that alter the patient's mood by affecting neurotransmitter levels ________________________________

H. Name the Anesthesia

Identify the type of anesthesia for each description.

1. produces loss of consciousness and absence of pain ________________________________
2. produces loss of sensation in one localized part of the body ________________________________
3. anesthetic applied directly onto a specific skin area ________________________________
4. also referred to as a nerve block ________________________________

I. Terminology Matching

Match the term to its definition.

1. _______ ultrasound
2. _______ MRI
3. _______ Doppler US
4. _______ nuclear medicine scan
5. _______ CT scan
6. _______ contrast study
7. _______ fluoroscopy
8. _______ radiography
9. _______ PET scan

a. radiopaque substances used to outline hollow structures
b. records velocity of blood flowing through vessels
c. image created by electromagnetic energy
d. glowing screen shows movement
e. making an X-ray
f. multiple-angle X-rays compiled into a cross-section
g. uses radioactive substances
h. image of internal organs using sound waves
i. indicates metabolic activity

J. What Does it Stand For?

1. ROM _______________
2. OT _______________
3. ADLs _______________
4. LE _______________
5. EMG _______________
6. TENS _______________
7. PT _______________
8. PROM _______________
9. e-stim _______________
10. US _______________

K. Name the Procedure Described

Identify the rehabilitation procedure described by each phrase.

1. kneading or applying pressure by hands _______________
2. removal of dead and damaged tissue from a wound _______________
3. using water for treatment purposes _______________
4. drainage of secretions from the bronchi _______________
5. exercises performed by a patient without resistance _______________
6. medication introduced by ultrasound waves _______________
7. use of cold for therapeutic purposes _______________
8. pulling with a mechanical device _______________

L. Terminology Matching

Match each term to its definition.

1. ________ forceps	a.	scrapes and removes tissue
2. ________ tenaculum	b.	cuts and separates tissue
3. ________ Trendelenburg	c.	lying horizontal and face up
4. ________ lithotomy	d.	lying on either the left or right side
5. ________ curette	e.	long-handled clamp
6. ________ aspirator	f.	explores tissue
7. ________ supine	g.	lying face up with hips and knees bent at 90° angles
8. ________ probe	h.	grasps tissue
9. ________ scalpel	i.	suctions fluid
10. ________ lateral recumbent	j.	lying face up on an incline, head lower than legs

M. What Does it Stand For?

1. MRI ________________________________
2. Ba ________________________________
3. AP ________________________________
4. CT ________________________________
5. RL ________________________________
6. PA ________________________________
7. LL ________________________________
8. PET ________________________________
9. UGI ________________________________
10. KUB ________________________________

N. Terminology Matching

Match each term to its definition.

1. ________ oncogenic
2. ________ benign
3. ________ encapsulated
4. ________ relapse
5. ________ primary site
6. ________ protocol
7. ________ staging laparotomy
8. ________ cytologic testing
9. ________ radioactive implant
10. ________ bx

a. examine cells to determine their structure and origin
b. the plan for care for any individual patient
c. biopsy
d. growth that is not recurrent or progressive
e. placing a radioactive substance directly into the tissue
f. where the malignant tumor first appeared
g. growth is enclosed in a tissue sheath
h. cancer causing
i. abdominal surgery to determine extent of tumor
j. return of disease symptoms

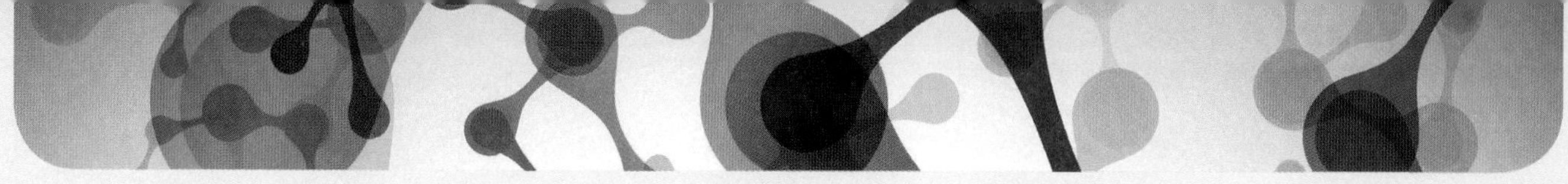

Appendices

Appendix I

Word Parts Arranged Alphabetically and Defined

The word parts that have been presented in this textbook are summarized here with their definitions for quick reference. Prefixes are listed first, followed by combining forms and suffixes.

Prefix	Definition
a-	without
ab-	away from
ad-	toward
allo-	other, different from usual
an-	without
ante-	before, in front of
anti-	against
auto-	self
bi-	two
brady-	slow
circum-	around
contra-	against
de-	without
di-	two
dis-	apart
dys-	painful; difficult; abnormal
e-	outward
en-	inward
endo-	within; inner
epi-	above
eso-	inward
eu-	normal
ex-	outward
exo-	outward
extra-	outside of
hemi-	half
hetero-	different
homo-	same
hyper-	excessive
hypo-	below; insufficient
in-	not; inward
inter-	between
intra-	within
macro-	large
meta-	beyond
micro-	small
mono-	one
multi-	many
myo-	to shut
neo-	new
non-	not
nulli-	none
pan-	all
para-	beside; abnormal; two like parts of a pair
per-	through
peri-	around
poly-	many
post-	after
pre-	before
primi-	first
pro-	before
pseudo-	false
quadri-	four
re-	again
retro-	backward; behind
semi-	partial
sub-	under
tachy-	fast
tetra-	four
trans-	across
tri-	three
ultra-	beyond
un-	not
xeno-	foreign

Combining Form	Definition
abdomin/o	abdomen
acous/o	hearing
acr/o	extremities
aden/o	gland
adenoid/o	adenoids
adip/o	fat
adren/o	adrenal glands
adrenal/o	adrenal glands
aer/o	air
agglutin/o	clumping

Combining Form	Definition
albin/o	white
alges/o	pain, sense of pain
alveol/o	alveolus
ambly/o	dull, dim
amnes/o	forgetfulness
amni/o	amnion
an/o	anus
andr/o	male
angi/o	vessel
ankyl/o	stiff joint
anter/o	front
anthrac/o	coal
anxi/o	fear, worry
aort/o	aorta
append/o	appendix
appendic/o	appendix
aque/o	water
arteri/o	artery
arthr/o	joint
articul/o	joint
aspir/o	to breathe in
astr/o	star
atel/o	incomplete
ather/o	fatty substance
atri/o	atrium
audi/o	hearing
audit/o	hearing
aur/o	ear
auricul/o	ear
axill/o	axilla, underarm
azot/o	nitrogenous waste
bacteri/o	bacteria
balan/o	glans penis
bar/o	weight
bas/o	base
bi/o	life
blast/o	immature
blephar/o	eyelid
brachi/o	arm
bronch/o	bronchus
bronchi/o	bronchus
bronchiol/o	bronchiole
bucc/o	cheek
burs/o	sac, bursa
calc/o	calcium
capsul/o	to box
carcin/o	cancer
cardi/o	heart
carp/o	carpus
caud/o	tail
cauter/o	to burn
cec/o	cecum
centr/o	center
cephal/o	head
cerebell/o	cerebellum
cerebr/o	cerebrum
cerumin/o	cerumen
cervic/o	neck, cervix
chem/o	chemical, drug
chol/e	bile, gall
cholangi/o	bile duct
cholecyst/o	gallbladder
choledoch/o	common bile duct
chondr/o	cartilage
chori/o	chorion
chrom/o	color
chromat/o	color
cirrh/o	yellow
cis/o	to cut
clavicul/o	clavicle
cleid/o	clavicle
clon/o	rapid contracting and relaxing
coagul/o	clotting
coccyg/o	coccyx
cochle/o	cochlea
col/o	colon
colon/o	colon
colp/o	vagina
compuls/o	drive, compel
concuss/o	to shake violently
coni/o	dust
conjunctiv/o	conjunctiva
core/o	pupil
corne/o	cornea
coron/o	heart
corpor/o	body
cortic/o	outer layer
cost/o	rib
crani/o	skull
crin/o	to secrete
crur/o	leg
cry/o	cold
crypt/o	hidden
culd/o	cul-de-sac
cutane/o	skin
cyan/o	blue
cycl/o	ciliary body
cyst/o	sac, urinary bladder, pouch
cyt/o	cell
dacry/o	tears
delus/o	false belief
dent/o	tooth
depress/o	to press down
derm/o	skin
dermat/o	skin
diaphor/o	profuse sweating
diaphragmat/o	diaphragm
dilat/o	to widen

Combining Form	Definition
dipl/o	double
dist/o	away from
diverticul/o	pouch
dors/o	back
duct/o	to bring
duoden/o	duodenum
dur/o	dura mater
electr/o	electricity
embol/o	plug
embry/o	embryo
emmetr/o	correct, proper
encephal/o	brain
enter/o	small intestine
eosin/o	rosy red
epididym/o	epididymis
epiglott/o	epiglottis
episi/o	vulva
epitheli/o	epithelium
erg/o	work
erythr/o	red
esophag/o	esophagus
esthesi/o	sensation, feeling
estr/o	female
extens/o	to stretch out
fasci/o	fibrous band
femor/o	femur
fet/o	fetus
fibr/o	fibers
fibrin/o	fibers
fibul/o	fibula
flex/o	to bend
fluor/o	fluorescence, luminous
fus/o	pouring
gastr/o	stomach
genit/o	genital
gingiv/o	gums
glauc/o	gray
gli/o	glue
glomerul/o	glomerulus
gloss/o	tongue
gluc/o	glucose
glute/o	buttock
glyc/o	sugar
glycos/o	sugar, glucose
gonad/o	sex glands
granul/o	granules
gynec/o	woman, female
habilitat/o	ability
hal/o	to breathe
hallucin/o	imagined perception
hem/o	blood
hemat/o	blood
hepat/o	liver
hidr/o	sweat
hist/o	tissue
home/o	sameness
humer/o	humerus
hydr/o	water
hymen/o	hymen
hyster/o	uterus
iatr/o	physician, medicine, treatment
ichthy/o	scaly, dry
idi/o	distinctive
ile/o	ileum
ili/o	ilium
immun/o	immunity, protection
infer/o	below
inguin/o	groin region
iod/o	iodine
ir/o	iris
irid/o	iris
isch/o	to hold back
ischi/o	ischium
jejun/o	jejunum
kal/i	potassium
kerat/o	hard, horny, cornea
ket/o	ketones
keton/o	ketones
kinesi/o	movement
klept/o	to steal
kyph/o	hump
labi/o	lip
labyrinth/o	labyrinth (inner ear)
lacrim/o	tears
lact/o	milk
lamin/o	lamina (part of vertebra)
lapar/o	abdomen
laps/o	to slide back
laryng/o	larynx
later/o	side
leuk/o	white
lingu/o	tongue
lip/o	fat
lith/o	stone
lob/o	lobe
lord/o	bent backward
lumb/o	loin (low back between ribs and pelvis)
lymph/o	lymph
lymphaden/o	lymph node
lymphangi/o	lymph vessel
macul/o	macula lutea
mamm/o	breast
mandibul/o	mandible
mast/o	breast
maxill/o	maxilla
meat/o	meatus
medi/o	middle

Combining Form	Definition
medull/o	inner region, medulla oblongata
melan/o	black
men/o	menses, menstruation
mening/o	meninges
meningi/o	meninges
ment/o	mind
metacarp/o	metacarpus
metatars/o	metatarsus
metr/o	uterus
mi/o	lessening
mineral/o	minerals, electrolytes
miss/o	to send back
morbid/o	ill
morph/o	shape
mort/o	death
muc/o	mucus
muscul/o	muscle
mutat/o	to change
my/o	muscle
myc/o	fungus
mydr/i	widening
myel/o	bone marrow, spinal cord
myocardi/o	heart muscle
myos/o	muscle
myring/o	tympanic membrane
narc/o	stupor, sleep
nas/o	nose
nat/o	birth
natr/o	sodium
necr/o	death
nephr/o	kidney
neur/o	nerve
neutr/o	neutral
noct/i	night
nucle/o	nucleus
nyctal/o	night
o/o	egg
obsess/o	besieged by thoughts
ocul/o	eye
odont/o	tooth
olig/o	scanty
onc/o	tumor
onych/o	nail
oophor/o	ovary
ophthalm/o	eye
opt/o	eye, vision
optic/o	eye, vision
or/o	mouth
orch/o	testes
orchi/o	testes
orchid/o	testes
orth/o	straight, upright, correct
oste/o	bone

Combining Form	Definition
ot/o	ear
ov/o, ov/i	ovum
ovari/o	ovary
ox/o, ox/i	oxygen
palat/o	palate
pancreat/o	pancreas
papill/o	optic disk
parathyroid/o	parathyroid gland
pariet/o	cavity wall
patell/o	patella
path/o	disease
pector/o	chest
ped/o	child; foot
pedicul/o	lice
pelv/o	pelvis
pen/o	penis
perine/o	perineum
peripher/o	away from center
peritone/o	peritoneum
phac/o	lens
phag/o	eat, swallow
phalang/o	phalanges
pharmac/o	drug
pharyng/o	pharynx
phleb/o	vein
phob/o	irrational fear
phon/o	sound
phot/o	light
phren/o	mind
physic/o	body
pineal/o	pineal gland
pituitar/o	pituitary gland
plant/o	sole of foot
pleur/o	pleura
pneum/o	lung, air
pneumon/o	lung, air
pod/o	foot
poli/o	gray matter
polyp/o	polyp
pont/o	pons
poster/o	back
presby/o	old age
proct/o	rectum and anus
prostat/o	prostate gland
prosthet/o	addition
protein/o	protein
proxim/o	near to
psych/o	mind
pub/o	genital region, pubis
pulmon/o	lung
pupill/o	pupil
py/o	pus
pyel/o	renal pelvis
pylor/o	pylorus

Combining Form	Definition
pyr/o	fire
radi/o	radius; ray (X-ray), radiation
radic/o	root
radicul/o	nerve root
rect/o	rectum
recumb/o	to lie back
ren/o	kidney
retin/o	retina
rhin/o	nose
rhytid/o	wrinkle
roentgen/o	X-ray
rotat/o	to revolve
sacr/o	sacrum
salping/o	uterine (fallopian) tubes, auditory tube (eustachian tube)
sanguin/o	blood
sarc/o	flesh
scapul/o	scapula
schiz/o	split
scler/o	hard, sclera
scoli/o	crooked
seb/o	oil
sect/o	to cut
sept/o	wall
septic/o	infection
sialaden/o	salivary gland
sigmoid/o	sigmoid colon
sinus/o	sinus
soci/o	society
somat/o	body
somn/o	sleep
son/o	sound
specul/o	to look at
spermat/o	sperm
sphygm/o	pulse
spin/o	spine
spir/o	breathing
splen/o	spleen
spondyl/o	vertebrae
staped/o	stapes
stern/o	sternum
steth/o	chest
stigmat/o	point
super/o	above
synov/o, synovi/o	synovial membrane
system/o	system
tars/o	tarsus
ten/o	tendon

Combining Form	Definition
tenacul/o	to hold
tend/o, tendin/o	tendon
testicul/o	testicle
thalam/o	thalamus
thec/o	sheath (meninges)
theli/o	nipple
therm/o	heat
thorac/o	chest
thromb/o	clot
thym/o	thymus gland
thyr/o	thyroid gland
thyroid/o	thyroid gland
tibi/o	tibia
tom/o	to cut
ton/o	tone
tonsill/o	tonsils
topic/o	a specific area
tox/o, toxic/o	poison
trache/o	trachea
trich/o	hair
tuss/o	cough
tympan/o	tympanic membrane
uln/o	ulna
ungu/o	nail
ur/o	urine
ureter/o	ureter
urethr/o	urethra
urin/o	urine
uter/o	uterus
uve/o	choroid
vagin/o	vagina
valv/o	valve
valvul/o	valve
varic/o	dilated vein
vas/o	vessel, vas deferens
vascul/o	blood vessel
ven/o	vein
ventr/o	belly
ventricul/o	ventricle
vers/o	to turn
vertebr/o	vertebra
vesic/o	sac, bladder
vesicul/o	seminal vesicle
vestibul/o	vestibule
viscer/o	internal organ
vitre/o	glassy
vulv/o	vulva
xer/o	dry

Suffix	Definition
-ac	pertaining to
-al	pertaining to
-algia	pain
-an	pertaining to

Suffix	Definition
-apheresis	removal, carry away
-ar	pertaining to
-arche	beginning
-ary	pertaining to

Suffix	Definition
-asthenia	weakness
-atic	pertaining to
-blast	immature
-capnia	carbon dioxide
-cardia	heart condition
-cele	protrusion
-centesis	puncture to withdraw fluid
-cide	to kill
-clasia	to surgically break
-crit	separation of
-cusis	hearing
-cyesis	state of pregnancy
-cyte	cell
-cytic	pertaining to cells
-cytosis	more than the normal number of cells
-derma	skin condition
-desis	to fuse
-dipsia	thirst
-dynia	pain
-eal	pertaining to
-ectasis	dilation
-ectomy	surgical removal
-edema	swelling
-emesis	vomit
-emetic	pertaining to vomiting
-emia	blood condition
-emic	pertaining to a blood condition
-gen	that which produces
-genesis	produces
-genic	producing
-globin	protein
-globulin	protein
-gram	record or picture
-graphy	process of recording
-gravida	pregnancy
-ia	state, condition
-iac	pertaining to
-iasis	abnormal condition
-iatric	pertaining to medical treatment
-iatrist	physician
-iatry	medical treatment
-ic	pertaining to
-ical	pertaining to
-ician	specialist
-ile	pertaining to
-ine	pertaining to
-ion	action
-ior	pertaining to
-ism	state of
-ist	specialist
-istry	specialty of
-itis	inflammation
-kinesia	movement

Suffix	Definition
-lepsy	seizure
-listhesis	slipping
-lith	stone
-lithiasis	condition of stones
-logic	pertaining to study of
-logist	one who studies
-logy	study of
-lucent	to shine through
-lysis	to destroy (to break down)
-lytic	destruction
-malacia	abnormal softening
-mania	frenzy
-manometer	instrument to measure pressure
-megaly	enlarged
-meter	instrument for measuring
-metrist	specialist in measuring
-metry	process of measuring
-nic	pertaining to
-nomics	pertaining to laws
-oid	resembling
-ole	small
-oma	tumor, mass
-opaque	nontransparent
-opia	vision condition
-opsia	vision condition
-opsy	view of
-orexia	appetite
-ory	pertaining to
-ose	pertaining to
-osis	abnormal condition
-osmia	smell
-ostomy	surgically create an opening
-otia	ear condition
-otomy	cutting into
-ous	pertaining to
-para	to bear (offspring)
-paresis	weakness
-partum	childbirth
-pathy	disease
-penia	abnormal decrease, too few
-pepsia	digestion
-pexy	surgical fixation
-phage	to eat
-phagia	eat, swallow
-phasia	speech
-phil	attracted to
-philia	condition of being attracted to
-philic	pertaining to being attracted to
-phobia	fear
-phonia	voice
-phoresis	carrying
-phoria	condition to bear
-phylaxis	protection

Suffix	Definition
-plasia	formation of cells
-plasm	formation
-plastic	pertaining to formation
-plastin	formation
-plasty	surgical repair
-plegia	paralysis
-pnea	breathing
-poiesis	formation
-porosis	porous
-prandial	pertaining to a meal
-pressin	to press down
-ptosis	drooping
-ptysis	spitting
-rrhage	excessive, abnormal flow
-rrhagia	abnormal flow condition
-rrhagic	pertaining to abnormal flow
-rrhaphy	to suture
-rrhea	discharge
-rrhexis	rupture
-salpinx	uterine tube
-sclerosis	hardening
-scope	instrument for viewing
-scopic	pertaining to visually examining
-scopy	process of visually examining
-spasm	involuntary muscle contraction
-spermia	condition of sperm
-stasis	standing still
-stat	to keep from moving
-stenosis	narrowing
-taxia	muscle coordination
-tension	pressure
-therapy	treatment
-thorax	chest
-tic	pertaining to
-tocia	labor, childbirth
-tome	instrument to cut
-tonia	tone
-tonic	pertaining to tone
-toxic	pertaining to poison
-tripsy	surgical crushing
-trophic	pertaining to development
-trophy	development
-tropia	turned condition
-tropic	pertaining to stimulating
-tropin	to stimulate
-ule	small
-uria	condition of the urine

Appendix II

Word Parts Arranged Alphabetically by Definition

The definitions of the word parts that have been presented in this textbook are presented here and are arranged alphabetically. Prefixes are listed first, followed by combining forms and suffixes.

Definition	Prefix
abnormal	**dys-, para-**
above	**epi-**
across	**trans-**
after	**post-**
again	**re-**
against	**anti-, contra-**
all	**pan-**
apart	**dis-**
around	**circum-, peri-**
away from	**ab-**
backward; behind	**retro-**
before	**pre-, pro-**
before, in front of	**ante-**
below; insufficient	**hypo-**
beside; abnormal; two like parts of a pair	**para-**
between	**inter-**
beyond	**meta-, ultra-**
different	**hetero-**
excessive	**hyper-**
false	**pseudo-**
fast	**tachy-**
first	**primi-**
foreign	**xeno-**
four	**quadri-, tetra-**
half	**hemi-**
inward	**en-**
inward	**eso-**
large	**macro-**
many	**multi-, poly-**
new	**neo-**
none	**nulli-**
normal	**eu-**
not	**non-, un-**
not; inward	**in-**
one	**mono-**
other, different from usual	**allo-**
outside of	**extra-**
outward	**e-, ex-, exo-**
painful; difficult; abnormal	**dys-**
partial	**semi-**
same	**homo-**
self	**auto-**
to shut	**myo-**
slow	**brady-**
small	**micro-**
three	**tri-**
through	**per-**
toward	**ad-**
two	**bi-, di-**
under	**sub-**
within	**intra-**
within; inner	**endo-**
without	**a-, an-, de-**

Definition	Combining Form
ability	**habilitat/o**
above	**super/o**
addition	**prosthet/o**
adenoids	**adenoid/o**
adrenal glands	**adren/o, adrenal/o**
air	**aer/o**
alveolus	**alveol/o**
amnion	**amni/o**
anus	**an/o**
aorta	**aort/o**
appendix	**append/o, appendic/o**
arm	**brachi/o**
artery	**arteri/o**
atrium	**atri/o**
auditory tube (eustachian tube)	**salping/o**
away from	**dist/o**
away from center	**peripher/o**
axilla, underarm	**axill/o**
back	**dors/o, poster/o**
bacteria	**bacteri/o**
base	**bas/o**
belly	**ventr/o**
below	**infer/o**
to bend	**flex/o**
bent backward	**lord/o**
besieged by thoughts	**obsess/o**
bile duct	**cholangi/o**
bile, gall	**chol/e**
birth	**nat/o**
black	**melan/o**
blood	**hem/o, hemat/o, sanguin/o**
blood vessel	**vascul/o**

Definition	Combining Form
blue	**cyan/o**
body	**corpor/o, physic/o, somat/o**
bone	**oste/o**
bone marrow, spinal cord	**myel/o**
to box	**capsul/o**
brain	**encephal/o**
breast	**mamm/o, mast/o**
to breathe	**hal/o**
to breathe in	**aspir/o**
breathing	**spir/o**
to bring	**duct/o**
bronchiole	**bronchiol/o**
bronchus	**bronch/o, bronchi/o**
to burn	**cauter/o**
buttock	**glute/o**
calcium	**calc/o**
cancer	**carcin/o**
carpus	**carp/o**
cartilage	**chondr/o**
cavity wall	**pariet/o**
cecum	**cec/o**
cell	**cyt/o**
center	**centr/o**
cerebellum	**cerebell/o**
cerebrum	**cerebr/o**
cerumen	**cerumin/o**
to change	**mutat/o**
cheek	**bucc/o**
chemical, drug	**chem/o**
chest	**pector/o, steth/o, thorac/o**
child; foot	**ped/o**
chorion	**chori/o**
choroid	**uve/o**
ciliary body	**cycl/o**
clavicle	**clavicul/o, cleid/o**
clot	**thromb/o**
clotting	**coagul/o**
clumping	**agglutin/o**
coal	**anthrac/o**
coccyx	**coccyg/o**
cochlea	**cochle/o**
cold	**cry/o**
colon	**col/o, colon/o**
color	**chrom/o, chromat/o**
common bile duct	**choledoch/o**
conjunctiva	**conjunctiv/o**
cornea	**corne/o**
correct, proper	**emmetr/o**
cough	**tuss/o**
crooked	**scoli/o**
cul-de-sac	**culd/o**
to cut	**cis/o, sect/o, tom/o**

Definition	Combining Form
death	**mort/o, necr/o**
diaphragm	**diaphragmat/o**
dilated vein	**varic/o**
disease	**path/o**
distinctive	**idi/o**
double	**dipl/o**
drive, compel	**compuls/o**
drug	**pharmac/o**
dry	**xer/o**
dull, dim	**ambly/o**
duodenum	**duoden/o**
dura mater	**dur/o**
dust	**coni/o**
ear	**aur/o, auricul/o, ot/o**
eat, swallow	**phag/o**
egg	**o/o**
electricity	**electr/o**
embryo	**embry/o**
epididymis	**epididym/o**
epiglottis	**epiglott/o**
epithelium	**epitheli/o**
esophagus	**esophag/o**
extremities	**acr/o**
eye	**ocul/o, ophthalm/o**
eye, vision	**opt/o, optic/o**
eyelid	**blephar/o**
false belief	**delus/o**
fat	**adip/o, lip/o**
fatty substance	**ather/o**
fear, worry	**anxi/o**
female	**estr/o, gynec/o**
femur	**femor/o**
fetus	**fet/o**
fibers	**fibr/o, fibrin/o**
fibrous band	**fasci/o**
fibula	**fibul/o**
fire	**pyr/o**
flesh	**sarc/o**
fluorescence, luminous	**fluor/o**
foot	**pod/o**
forgetfulness	**amnes/o**
front	**anter/o**
fungus	**myc/o**
gallbladder	**cholecyst/o**
genital	**genit/o**
genital region, pubis	**pub/o**
gland	**aden/o**
glans penis	**balan/o**
glassy	**vitre/o**
glomerulus	**glomerul/o**
glucose	**gluc/o**
glue	**gli/o**
granules	**granul/o**
gray	**glauc/o**

Definition	Combining Form
gray matter	**poli/o**
groin region	**inguin/o**
gums	**gingiv/o**
hair	**trich/o**
hard, horny, cornea	**kerat/o**
hard, sclera	**scler/o**
head	**cephal/o**
hearing	**acous/o, audi/o, audit/o**
heart	**cardi/o, coron/o**
heart muscle	**myocardi/o**
heat	**therm/o**
hidden	**crypt/o**
to hold	**tenacul/o**
to hold back	**isch/o**
humerus	**humer/o**
hump	**kyph/o**
hymen	**hymen/o**
ileum	**ile/o**
ilium	**ili/o**
ill	**morbid/o**
imagined perception	**hallucin/o**
immature	**blast/o**
immunity, protection	**immun/o**
incomplete	**atel/o**
infection	**septic/o**
inner region, medulla oblongata	**medull/o**
internal organ	**viscer/o**
iodine	**iod/o**
iris	**ir/o, irid/o**
irrational fear	**phob/o**
ischium	**ischi/o**
jejunum	**jejun/o**
joint	**arthr/o, articul/o**
ketones	**ket/o, keton/o**
kidney	**nephr/o, ren/o**
labyrinth (inner ear)	**labyrinth/o**
lamina (part of vertebra)	**lamin/o**
larynx	**laryng/o**
leg	**crur/o**
lens	**phac/o**
lessening	**mi/o**
lice	**pedicul/o**
to lie back	**recumb/o**
life	**bi/o**
light	**phot/o**
lip	**labi/o**
liver	**hepat/o**
lobe	**lob/o**
loin (low back between ribs and pelvis)	**lumb/o**
to look at	**specul/o**
lung	**pulmon/o**
lung, air	**pneum/o, pneumon/o**
lymph	**lymph/o**
lymph node	**lymphaden/o**
lymph vessel	**lymphangi/o**
macula lutea	**macul/o**
male	**andr/o**
mandible	**mandibul/o**
maxilla	**maxill/o**
meatus	**meat/o**
meninges	**mening/o, meningi/o**
menses, menstruation	**men/o**
metacarpus	**metacarp/o**
metatarsus	**metatars/o**
middle	**medi/o**
milk	**lact/o**
mind	**ment/o, phren/o, psych/o**
minerals, electrolytes	**mineral/o**
mouth	**or/o**
movement	**kinesi/o**
mucus	**muc/o**
muscle	**muscul/o, my/o, myos/o**
nail	**onych/o, ungu/o**
near to	**proxim/o**
neck, cervix	**cervic/o**
nerve	**neur/o**
nerve root	**radicul/o**
neutral	**neutr/o**
night	**noct/i, nyctal/o**
nipple	**theli/o**
nitrogenous waste	**azot/o**
nose	**nas/o, rhin/o**
nucleus	**nucle/o**
oil	**seb/o**
old age	**presby/o**
optic disk	**papill/o**
outer layer	**cortic/o**
ovary	**oophor/o, ovari/o**
ovum	**ov/o, ov/i**
oxygen	**ox/o, ox/i**
pain, sense of pain	**alges/o**
palate	**palat/o**
pancreas	**pancreat/o**
parathyroid gland	**parathyroid/o**
patella	**patell/o**
pelvis	**pelv/o**
penis	**pen/o**
perineum	**perine/o**
peritoneum	**peritone/o**
phalanges	**phalang/o**
pharynx	**pharyng/o**
physician, medicine, treatment	**iatr/o**
pineal gland	**pineal/o**
pituitary gland	**pituitar/o**

Definition	Combining Form
pleura	**pleur/o**
plug	**embol/o**
point	**stigmat/o**
poison	**tox/o, toxic/o**
polyp	**polyp/o**
pons	**pont/o**
potassium	**kal/i**
pouch	**diverticul/o**
pouring	**fus/o**
to press down	**depress/o**
profuse sweating	**diaphor/o**
prostate gland	**prostat/o**
protein	**protein/o**
pulse	**sphygm/o**
pupil	**core/o, pupill/o**
pus	**py/o**
pylorus	**pylor/o**
radius; ray (X-ray), radiation	**radi/o**
rapid contracting and relaxing	**clon/o**
rectum	**rect/o**
rectum and anus	**proct/o**
red	**erythr/o**
renal pelvis	**pyel/o**
retina	**retin/o**
to revolve	**rotat/o**
rib	**cost/o**
root	**radic/o**
rosy red	**eosin/o**
sac, bladder	**vesic/o**
sac, bursa	**burs/o**
sac, urinary bladder, pouch	**cyst/o**
sacrum	**sacr/o**
salivary gland	**sialaden/o**
sameness	**home/o**
scaly, dry	**ichthy/o**
scanty	**olig/o**
scapula	**scapul/o**
to secrete	**crin/o**
seminal vesicle	**vesicul/o**
to send back	**miss/o**
sensation, feeling	**esthesi/o**
sex glands	**gonad/o**
to shake violently	**concuss/o**
shape	**morph/o**
sheath (meninges)	**thec/o**
side	**later/o**
sigmoid colon	**sigmoid/o**
sinus	**sinus/o**
skin	**cutane/o, derm/o, dermat/o**
skull	**crani/o**
sleep	**somn/o**
to slide back	**laps/o**
small intestine	**enter/o**
society	**soci/o**
sodium	**natr/o**
sole of foot	**plant/o**
sound	**phon/o, son/o**
specific area	**topic/o**
sperm	**spermat/o**
spine	**spin/o**
spleen	**splen/o**
split	**schiz/o**
stapes	**staped/o**
star	**astr/o**
to steal	**klept/o**
sternum	**stern/o**
stiff joint	**ankyl/o**
stomach	**gastr/o**
stone	**lith/o**
straight, upright, correct	**orth/o**
to stretch out	**extens/o**
stupor, sleep	**narc/o**
sugar	**glyc/o**
sugar, glucose	**glycos/o**
sweat	**hidr/o**
synovial membrane	**synov/o, synovi/o**
system	**system/o**
tail	**caud/o**
tarsus	**tars/o**
tears	**dacry/o, lacrim/o**
tendon	**ten/o, tend/o, tendin/o**
testes	**orch/o, orchi/o, orchid/o**
testicle	**testicul/o**
thalamus	**thalam/o**
thymus gland	**thym/o**
thyroid gland	**thyr/o, thyroid/o**
tibia	**tibi/o**
tissue	**hist/o**
tone	**ton/o**
tongue	**gloss/o, lingu/o**
tonsils	**tonsill/o**
tooth	**dent/o, odont/o**
trachea	**trache/o**
tumor	**onc/o**
to turn	**vers/o**
tympanic membrane	**myring/o, tympan/o**
ulna	**uln/o**
ureter	**ureter/o**
urethra	**urethr/o**
urine	**ur/o, urin/o**
uterine (fallopian) tubes	**salping/o**
water	**hydr/o**
to widen	**dilat/o**
woman	**gynec/o**
yellow	**cirrh/o**

Definition	Suffix	Definition	Suffix
abnormal condition	**-iasis, -osis**	hardening	**-sclerosis**
abnormal decrease, too few	**-penia**	hearing	**-cusis**
abnormal flow (pertaining to)	**-rrhagic**	heart condition	**-cardia**
abnormal flow condition	**-rrhagia**	immature	**-blast**
abnormal softening	**-malacia**	inflammation	**-itis**
action	**-ion**	instrument for measuring	**-meter**
appetite	**-orexia**	instrument for viewing	**-scope**
attracted to	**-phil**	instrument to cut	**-tome**
to bear (offspring)	**-para**	instrument to measure pressure	**-manometer**
beginning	**-arche**		
being attracted to (condition of)	**-philia**	involuntary muscle contraction	**-spasm**
being attracted to (pertaining to)	**-philic**	to keep from moving	**-stat**
blood condition	**-emia**	to kill	**-cide**
blood condition (pertaining to a)	**-emic**	labor, childbirth	**-tocia**
breathing	**-pnea**	laws (pertaining to)	**-nomics**
carbon dioxide	**-capnia**	meal (pertaining to a)	**-prandial**
carrying	**-phoresis**	measure pressure (instrument to)	**-manometer**
cell	**-cyte**		
cells (pertaining to)	**-cytic**	measuring (instrument for)	**-meter**
chest	**-thorax**	measuring (process of)	**-metry**
childbirth	**-partum**	medical treatment	**-iatry**
condition (abnormal)	**-iasis, -osis**	medical treatment (pertaining to)	**-iatric**
condition of being attracted to	**-philia**	more than the normal number of cells	**-cytosis**
condition of sperm	**-spermia**		
condition of stones	**-lithiasis**	movement	**-kinesia**
condition of the urine	**-uria**	muscle coordination	**-taxia**
condition to bear	**-phoria**	narrowing	**-stenosis**
crushing (surgical)	**-tripsy**	nontransparent	**-opaque**
cut (instrument to)	**-tome**	one who studies	**-logist**
cutting into	**-otomy**	opening (surgically create an)	**-ostomy**
decrease, too few (abnormal)	**-penia**	pain	**-algia**
to destroy (to break down)	**-lysis**	pain	**-dynia**
destruction	**-lytic**	paralysis	**-plegia**
development	**-trophy**	pertaining to	**-ac, -al, -an, -ar, -ary, -atic, -eal, -ia, -iac, -ic, -ical, -ile, -ine, -ior, -nic, -ory, -ose, -ous, -tic**
development (pertaining to)	**-trophic**		
digestion	**-pepsia**		
dilation	**-ectasis**		
discharge	**-rrhea**		
disease	**-pathy**	pertaining to a blood condition	**-emic**
drooping	**-ptosis**	pertaining to a meal	**-prandial**
ear condition	**-otia**	pertaining to abnormal flow	**-rrhagic**
to eat	**-phage**	pertaining to being attracted to	**-philic**
eat, swallow	**-phagia**	pertaining to cells	**-cytic**
enlarged	**-megaly**	pertaining to development	**-trophic**
excessive, abnormal flow	**-rrhage**	pertaining to formation	**-plastic**
fear	**-phobia**	pertaining to laws	**-nomics**
fixation (surgical)	**-pexy**	pertaining to medical treatment	**-iatric**
flow condition (abnormal)	**-rrhagia**	pertaining to poison	**-toxic**
formation	**-plasm, -plastin, -poiesis**	pertaining to stimulating	**-tropic**
		pertaining to study of	**-logic**
formation (pertaining to)	**-plastic**	pertaining to tone	**-tonic**
formation of cells	**-plasia**	pertaining to visually examining	**-scopic**
frenzy	**-mania**	pertaining to vomiting	**-emetic**
to fuse	**-desis**	physician	**-iatrist**

Definition	Suffix
poison (pertaining to)	-toxic
porous	-porosis
pregnancy	-gravida
to press down	-pressin
pressure	-tension
process of measuring	-metry
process of recording	-graphy
process of visually examining	-scopy
produces	-genesis
producing	-genic
protection	-phylaxis
protein	-globin, -globulin
protrusion	-cele
puncture to withdraw fluid	-centesis
recording (process of)	-graphy
record or picture	-gram
removal, carry away	-apheresis
removal (surgical)	-ectomy
repair (surgical)	-plasty
resembling	-oid
rupture	-rrhexis
seizure	-lepsy
separation of	-crit
to shine through	-lucent
skin condition	-derma
slipping	-listhesis
small	-ole, -ule
smell	-osmia
softening (abnormal)	-malacia
specialist	-ician, -ist
specialist in measuring	-metrist
specialty of	-istry
speech	-phasia
sperm (condition of)	-spermia
spitting	-ptysis
standing still	-stasis
state of	-ism
state of pregnancy	-cyesis
state, condition	-ia
to stimulate	-tropin
stimulating (pertaining to)	-tropic

Definition	Suffix
stone	-lith
stones (condition of)	-lithiasis
study of	-logy
study of (pertaining to)	-logic
surgical crushing	-tripsy
surgical fixation	-pexy
to surgically break	-clasia
surgical removal	-ectomy
surgical repair	-plasty
surgically create an opening	-ostomy
to suture	-rrhaphy
swelling	-edema
that which produces	-gen
thirst	-dipsia
to bear (offspring)	-para
to destroy (to break down)	-lysis
to eat	-phage
to fuse	-desis
to kill	-cide
to press down	-pressin
to shine through	-lucent
to stimulate	-tropin
to surgically break	-clasia
to suture	-rrhaphy
tone	-tonia
tone (pertaining to)	-tonic
treatment	-therapy
tumor, mass	-oma
turned condition	-tropia
the urine (condition of)	-uria
uterine tube	-salpinx
view of	-opsy
viewing (instrument for)	-scope
vision condition	-opia, -opsia
visually examining (pertaining to)	-scopic
visually examining (process of)	-scopy
voice	-phonia
vomit	-emesis
vomiting (pertaining to)	-emetic
weakness	-asthenia, -paresis

Appendix III

Abbreviations

Abbreviation	Meaning
i̇	one
i̇i̇	two
i̇i̇i̇	three
@	at
5-FU	5-fluorouracil
^{67}Ga	radioactive gallium
^{99m}Tc	radioactive technetium
^{131}I	radioactive iodine
^{133}Xe	radioactive xenon
^{201}Tl	radioactive thallium
α	alpha
ā	before
AAROM	active assistive range of motion
AB	abortion
ABGs	arterial blood gases
ac	before meals
ACTH	adrenocorticotropic hormone
AD	Alzheimer's disease, right ear
ad lib	as desired
ADD	attention-deficit disorder
ADH	antidiuretic hormone
ADHD	attention-deficit/hyperactivity disorder
ADL	activities of daily living
AE	above elbow
AED	automated external defibrillator
AF	atrial fibrillation
AGN	acute glomerulonephritis
AI	artificial insemination
AIDS	acquired immunodeficiency syndrome
AK	above knee
ALL	acute lymphocytic leukemia
ALS	amyotrophic lateral sclerosis
ALT	alanine transaminase
AMI	acute myocardial infarction
AML	acute myelogenous leukemia
Angio	angiography
ANS	autonomic nervous system
ante	before
AP	anteroposterior
APAP	acetaminophen (Tylenol™)
aq	aqueous (water)
ARC	AIDS-related complex
ARDS	adult (or acute) respiratory distress syndrome
ARF	acute renal failure
ARMD	age-related macular degeneration
AROM	active range of motion
AS	arteriosclerosis, left ear

Abbreviation	Meaning
ASA	aspirin
ASD	atrial septal defect
ASHD	arteriosclerotic heart disease
ASL	American Sign Language
AST	aspartate transaminase
Astigm	astigmatism
ATN	acute tubular necrosis
AU	both ears
AV, A-V	atrioventricular
β	beta
Ba	barium
BaE	barium enema
basos	basophils
BBB	bundle branch block (L for left; R for right)
BC	bone conduction
BCC	basal cell carcinoma
BDT	bone density testing
BE	barium enema, below elbow
bid	twice a day
BK	below knee
BM	bowel movement
BMR	basal metabolic rate
BMT	bone marrow transplant
BNO	bladder neck obstruction
BP	blood pressure
BPD	bipolar disorder
BPH	benign prostatic hyperplasia
bpm	beats per minute
Bronch	bronchoscopy
BS	bowel sounds
BSE	breast self-examination
BUN	blood urea nitrogen
bx, BX	biopsy
c̄	with
C&S	culture and sensitivity
c.gl.	correction with glasses
C1, C2, etc.	first cervical vertebra, second cervical vertebra, etc.
Ca	calcium, cancer
CA	chronological age
CABG	coronary artery bypass graft
CAD	coronary artery disease
cap(s)	capsule(s)
CAPD	continuous ambulatory peritoneal dialysis
CAT	computerized axial tomography
cath	catheterization
CBC	complete blood count
CBD	common bile duct

Abbreviation	Meaning
CC	cardiac catheterization, chief complaint, clean catch urine specimen
CCU	coronary care unit
CF	cystic fibrosis
chemo	chemotherapy
CHF	congestive heart failure
Ci	curie
CIS	carcinoma in situ
Cl^-	chloride
CLL	chronic lymphocytic leukemia
CML	chronic myelogenous leukemia
CNS	central nervous system
CO_2	carbon dioxide
CoA	coarctation of the aorta
COPD	chronic obstructive pulmonary disease
CP	cerebral palsy, chest pain
CPK	creatine phosphokinase
CPR	cardiopulmonary resuscitation
CRF	chronic renal failure
CS, C-section	cesarean section
CSD	congenital septal defect
CSF	cerebrospinal fluid
CT	calcitonin, computerized tomography
CTA	clear to auscultation
CTS	carpal tunnel syndrome
CV	cardiovascular
CVA	cerebrovascular accident
CVD	cerebrovascular disease
CVS	chorionic villus sampling
Cx	cervix
CXR	chest X-ray
cysto	cystoscopy
D	diopter (lens strength)
d	day
D & C	dilation and curettage
Db	decibel
d/c, DISC	discontinue
DC, disc	discontinue
DEA	Drug Enforcement Agency
decub	decubitus ulcer, lying down
Derm, derm	dermatology
DI	diabetes insipidus, diagnostic imaging
diff	differential
dil	dilute
disp	dispense
DJD	degenerative joint disease
DM	diabetes mellitus
DOE	dyspnea on exertion
DPT	diphtheria, pertussis, tetanus injection
DRE	digital rectal exam
DSA	digital subtraction angiography
DSM	*Diagnostic and Statistical Manual of Mental Disorders*

Abbreviation	Meaning
dtd	give of such a dose
DTR	deep tendon reflex
DVA	distance visual acuity
DVT	deep vein thrombosis
Dx	diagnosis
DXA	dual-energy absorptiometry
ECC	extracorporeal circulation
ECCE	extracapsular cataract extraction
ECG, EKG	electrocardiogram
ECHO	echocardiogram
ECT	electroconvulsive therapy
ED	erectile dysfunction
EDC	estimated date of confinement
EEG	electroencephalogram, electroencephalography
EENT	eye, ear, nose, and throat
EGD	esophagogastroduodenoscopy
ELISA	enzyme-linked immunosorbent assay
EM	emmetropia
EMB	endometrial biopsy
EMG	electromyogram
Endo	endoscopy
ENT	ear, nose, and throat
EOM	extraocular movement
eosins, eos	eosinophils
ERCP	endoscopic retrograde cholangiopancreatography
ERT	estrogen replacement therapy
ERV	expiratory reserve volume
ESR, SR, sed rate	erythrocyte sedimentation rate
ESRD	end-stage renal disease
e-stim	electrical stimulation
ESWL	extracorporeal shockwave lithotripsy
et	and
EU	excretory urography
EUA	exam under anesthesia
FBS	fasting blood sugar
FDA	Federal Drug Administration
FEKG	fetal electrocardiogram
FHR	fetal heart rate
FHT	fetal heart tone
flu	influenza
FOBT	fecal occult blood test
FRC	functional residual capacity
FS	frozen section
FSH	follicle-stimulating hormone
FTM	female to male
FTND	full-term normal delivery
Fx, FX	fracture
GA	general anesthesia, gallium
GB	gallbladder X-ray
GC	gonorrhea
GERD	gastroesophageal reflux disease
GH	growth hormone

Abbreviation	Meaning
GI	gastrointestinal
GI, grav I	first pregnancy
gm	gram
GOT	glutamic oxaloacetic transaminase
gr	grain
gt	drop
GTT	glucose tolerance test
gtt	drops
GU	genitourinary
GVHD	graft versus host disease
GYN	gynecology
H_2O	water
HA	headache
HAV	hepatitis A virus
HBV	hepatitis B virus
HCG, hCG	human chorionic gonadotropin
HCl	hydrochloric acid
HCO_3^-	bicarbonate
HCT, Hct, crit	hematocrit
HCV	hepatitis C virus
HD	Hodgkin's disease, hemodialysis
HDN	hemolytic disease of the newborn
HDV	hepatitis D virus
HEENT	head, ear, eye, nose, throat
HEV	hepatitis E virus
Hgb, Hb, HGB	hemoglobin
HIV	human immunodeficiency virus
HMD	hyaline membrane disease
HNP	herniated nucleus pulposus
HPV	human papilloma virus
HRT	hormone replacement therapy
hs	at bedtime
HSG	hysterosalpingography
HSV-1	herpes simplex virus type 1
HTN	hypertension
Hz	hertz
I&D	incision and drainage
I&O	intake and output
IBD	inflammatory bowel disease
IBS	irritable bowel syndrome
IC	inspiratory capacity
ICCE	intracapsular cataract extraction
ICD	implantable cardioverter-defibrillator
ICP	intracranial pressure
ICU	intensive care unit
ID	intradermal
IDDM	insulin-dependent diabetes mellitus
Ig	immunoglobulins (IgA, IgD, IgE, IgG, IgM)
IM	intramuscular
inj	injection
IOP	intraocular pressure
IPD	intermittent peritoneal dialysis
IPPB	intermittent positive pressure breathing
IRDS	infant respiratory distress syndrome
IRV	inspiratory reserve volume
IUD	intrauterine device
IV	intravenous
IVC	intravenous cholangiography
IVF	*in vitro* fertilization
IVP	intravenous pyelogram
JRA	juvenile rheumatoid arthritis
K^+	potassium
kg	kilogram
KS	Kaposi's sarcoma
KUB	kidneys, ureters, bladder
L	liter
L1, L2, etc.	first lumbar vertebra, second lumbar vertebra, etc.
LASIK	laser-assisted in situ keratomileusis
lat	lateral
LBW	low birth weight
LE	lower extremity
LGI	lower gastrointestinal series
LH	luteinizing hormone
LL	left lateral
LLE	left lower extremity
LLL	left lower lobe
LLQ	left lower quadrant
LMP	last menstrual period
LP	lumbar puncture
LUE	left upper extremity
LUL	left upper lobe
LUQ	left upper quadrant
LVH	left ventricular hypertrophy
lymphs	lymphocytes
MA	mental age
mA	milliampere
mcg	microgram
mCi	millicurie
MD	muscular dystrophy
MDI	metered-dose inhaler
mEq	milliequivalent
mets	metastases
mg	milligram
MI	myocardial infarction, mitral insufficiency
mL	milliliter
MM	malignant melanoma
mm Hg	millimeters of mercury
MMPI	Minnesota Multiphasic Personality Inventory
mono	mononucleosis
monos	monocytes
MR	mitral regurgitation
MRA	magnetic resonance angiography
MRI	magnetic resonance imaging
MS	musculoskeletal, mitral stenosis, multiple sclerosis
MSH	melanocyte-stimulating hormone
MTF	male to female

Abbreviation	Meaning
MTX	methotrexate
MUA	manipulation under anesthesia
MVP	mitral valve prolapse
n&v	nausea and vomiting
Na^+	sodium
NB	newborn
NG	nasogastric (tube)
NHL	non-Hodgkin's lymphoma
NIDDM	non-insulin-dependent diabetes mellitus
NK	natural killer cells
NMR	nuclear magnetic resonance
no sub	no substitute
noc	night
non rep	do not repeat
NPH	neutral protamine Hagedorn (insulin)
NPO	nothing by mouth
NS	nephrotic syndrome, normal saline
NSAID	nonsteroidal anti-inflammatory drug
O&P	ova and parasites
O_2	oxygen
OA	osteoarthritis
OB	obstetrics
OCD	obsessive–compulsive disorder
OCPs	oral contraceptive pills
OD	right eye
od	overdose
OE	otitis externa
oint	ointment
OM	otitis media
Ophth.	ophthalmology
OR	operating room
ORIF	open reduction–internal fixation
Orth, ortho	orthopedics
OS	left eye
OT	occupational therapy
OTC	over the counter
Oto	otology
OU	each eye/both eyes
oz	ounce
$\bar{p}$	after
P	phosphorus, pulse
PA	posteroanterior, pernicious anemia
PAC	premature atrial contraction
Pap	Papanicolaou test
PARR	postanesthetic recovery room
PBI	protein-bound iodine
pc	after meals
PCA	patient-controlled administration
PCP	pneumocystis pneumonia
PCV	packed cell volume
PDA	patent ductus arteriosus
PDR	*Physician's Desk Reference*
PE tube	pressure equalizing tube

Abbreviation	Meaning
per	through
PERRLA	pupils equal, round, react to light and accommodation
PET	positron emission tomography
PFT	pulmonary function test
pH	acidity or alkalinity of urine
PI, para I	first delivery
PID	pelvic inflammatory disease
PIH	pregnancy-induced hypertension
PMN, polys	polymorphonuclear neutrophil
PMS	premenstrual syndrome
PNS	peripheral nervous system
PO	by mouth
PORP	partial ossicular replacement prosthesis
post-op	postoperative
pp	postprandial
PPD	purified protein derivative
preop, pre-op	preoperative
prep	preparation, prepare
PRK	photorefractive keratectomy
PRL	prolactin
prn	as needed
PROM	passive range of motion
prot	protocol
PSA	prostate-specific antigen
pt	patient
PT	physical therapy
PT, pro-time	prothrombin time
PTC	percutaneous transhepatic cholangiography
PTCA	percutaneous transluminal coronary angioplasty
PTH	parathyroid hormone
PTSD	posttraumatic stress disorder
PUD	peptic ulcer disease
PVC	premature ventricular contraction
q	every
qam	every morning
qh	every hour
qhs	at bedtime
qid	four times a day
qs	quantity sufficient
R	respiration, roentgen
RA	rheumatoid arthritis, room air
Ra	radium
rad	radiation-absorbed dose
RAI	radioactive iodine
RBC	red blood cell
RDS	respiratory distress syndrome
REM	rapid eye movement
Rh+	Rh-positive
Rh–	Rh-negative
RIA	radioimmunoassay
RK	radial keratotomy

Abbreviation	Meaning
RL	right lateral
RLE	right lower extremity
RLL	right lower lobe
RLQ	right lower quadrant
RML	right middle lobe
ROM	range of motion
RP	retrograde pyelogram
RPR	rapid plasma reagin (test for syphilis)
RRT	registered respiratory therapist, registered radiologic technologist
RUE	right upper extremity
RUL	right upper lobe
RUQ	right upper quadrant
RV	reserve volume
Rx	take
$\bar{s}$	without
$\overline{ss}$	one-half
s.gl.	without correction or glasses
S1	first heart sound
S2	second heart sound
SA, S-A	sinoatrial
SAD	seasonal affective disorder
SARS	severe acute respiratory syndrome
SCC	squamous cell carcinoma
SCI	spinal cord injury
SCIDS	severe combined immunodeficiency syndrome
segs	segmented neutrophils
SG	skin graft
SG, sp. gr.	specific gravity
SIDS	sudden infant death syndrome
Sig	label as follows/directions
SK	streptokinase
sl	under the tongue
SLE	systemic lupus erythematosus
SMAC	sequential multiple analyzer computer
SMD	senile macular degeneration
SOB	shortness of breath
sol	solution
SOM	serous otitis media
SPP	suprapubic prostatectomy
SSD	somatic symptom disorder
ST	esotropia
st	stage
stat	at once/immediately
STD	sexually transmitted disease
STI	sexually transmitted infection
STSG	split-thickness skin graft
Subc, Subq	subcutaneous
suppos, supp	suppository
susp	suspension
syr	syrup
T & A	tonsillectomy and adenoidectomy
T, tbsp	tablespoon
t, tsp	teaspoon
T1, T2, etc.	first thoracic vertebra, second thoracic vertebra, etc.
T_3	triiodothyronine
T_4	thyroxine
tab	tablet
TAH	total abdominal hysterectomy
TAH-BSO	total abdominal hysterectomy–bilateral salpingo-oophorectomy
TB	tuberculosis
TBI	traumatic brain injury
TENS	transcutaneous electrical nerve stimulation
TFT	thyroid function test
THA	total hip arthroplasty
THR	total hip replacement
TIA	transient ischemic attack
tid	three times a day
TKA	total knee arthroplasty
TKR	total knee replacement
TLC	total lung capacity
TNM	tumor, nodes, metastases
TO	telephone order
top	apply topically
TORP	total ossicular replacement prosthesis
tPA	tissue plasminogen activator
TPN	total parenteral nutrition
TPR	temperature, pulse, and respiration
TSH	thyroid-stimulating hormone
TSS	toxic shock syndrome
TUR	transurethral resection
TURP	transurethral resection of the prostate
TV	tidal volume
U/A, UA	urinalysis
UC	urine culture, uterine contractions
UE	upper extremity
UGI	upper gastrointestinal series
URI	upper respiratory infection
US	ultrasound
UTI	urinary tract infection
UV	ultraviolet
V fib	ventricular fibrillation
VA	visual acuity
VC	vital capacity
VCUG	voiding cystourethrography
VD	venereal disease
VF	visual field
VO	verbal order
VSD	ventricular septal defect
VT	ventricular tachycardia
WBC	white blood cell
wt	weight
x	times
XT	exotropia

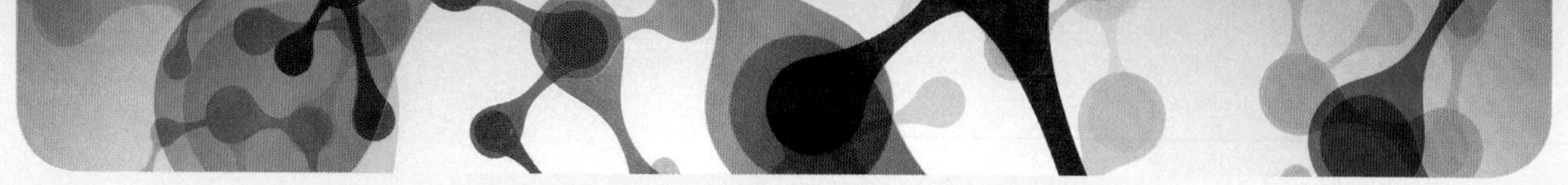

Answer Keys

Chapter 1 Answers

Practice As You Go

A. **1.** word root, combining vowel, prefix, suffix **2.** combining form **3.** o **4.** suffix **5.** prefix

B. **1.** cardiology **2.** gastrology **3.** dermatology **4.** ophthalmology **5.** immunology **6.** nephrology **7.** hematology **8.** gynecology **9.** neurology **10.** pathology

C. **1.** tachy-, fast **2.** pseudo-, false **3.** hypo-, insufficient **4.** inter-, between **5.** eu-, normal **6.** post-, after **7.** mono-, one **8.** sub-, under

D. **1.** pulmonology **2.** rhinorrhea **3.** nephromalacia **4.** cardiomegaly **5.** gastrotomy **6.** dermatitis **7.** laryngectomy **8.** arthroplasty

E. **1.** metastases **2.** ova **3.** diverticula **4.** atria **5.** diagnoses **6.** vertebrae

Practice Exercises

A. **1.** l **2.** e **3.** j **4.** f **5.** d **6.** k **7.** m **8.** o **9.** g **10.** n **11.** b **12.** h **13.** a **14.** c **15.** i

B. **1.** surgical repair **2.** narrowing **3.** inflammation **4.** pertaining to **5.** pain **6.** cutting into **7.** enlarged **8.** surgical removal **9.** excessive, abnormal flow **10.** puncture to remove fluid **11.** record or picture **12.** pertaining to **13.** abnormal softening **14.** state of **15.** to suture **16.** surgically create an opening **17.** surgical fixation **18.** discharge **19.** process of visually examining **20.** tumor, mass

C. **1.** endo- **2.** macro- **3.** pre- **4.** peri- **5.** neo- **6.** a-/an-/de- **7.** hemi-/semi- **8.** dys- **9.** hyper- **10.** epi- **11.** poly-/multi- **12.** brady- **13.** auto- **14.** trans- **15.** bi-

D. **1.** cardiomalacia **2.** gastrostomy **3.** rhinoplasty **4.** hypertrophy **5.** pathology **6.** neuroma **7.** gastroenterology **8.** otitis **9.** chemotherapy **10.** carcinogen

E. **1.** life **2.** cancer **3.** heart **4.** chemical **5.** to cut **6.** skin **7.** small intestine **8.** stomach **9.** female **10.** blood **11.** immunity **12.** voice box **13.** disease **14.** kidney **15.** nerve **16.** eye **17.** ear **18.** lung **19.** nose

Chapter 2 Answers

Practice As You Go

A. **1.** cells, tissues, organs, systems, body **2.** cell membrane, cytoplasm, nucleus **3.** epithelial **4.** cardiac, skeletal, smooth **5.** connective **6.** neurons

B. **1.** integumentary, d **2.** cardiovascular, i **3.** digestive, g **4.** female reproductive, b **5.** musculoskeletal (skeletal), a **6.** respiratory, j **7.** urinary, c **8.** male reproductive, f **9.** nervous, h **10.** musculoskeletal (muscular), e

C. **1.** c **2.** a **3.** b

D. **1.** cephalic **2.** pubic **3.** crural **4.** gluteal **5.** cervical **6.** brachial **7.** dorsum **8.** thoracic

E. **1.** anatomical **2.** right lower **3.** cranial, spinal **4.** nine **5.** right inguinal **6.** pleural, pericardial

Practice Exercises

A. **1.** epi-; above **2.** peri-; around or about **3.** hypo-; under or below **4.** retro-; behind or backward

B. **1.** n **2.** f **3.** k **4.** d **5.** a **6.** e **7.** m **8.** i **9.** b **10.** j **11.** h **12.** l **13.** c **14.** g

C. **1.** MS **2.** lat **3.** RUQ **4.** CV **5.** GI **6.** AP **7.** OB **8.** LLQ

D. **1.** dorsal **2.** thoracic **3.** superior **4.** caudal **5.** visceral **6.** lateral **7.** distal **8.** neural **9.** pulmonology **10.** muscular **11.** ventral **12.** anterior **13.** cephalic **14.** medial

E. **1.** internal organ **2.** back **3.** abdomen **4.** chest **5.** middle **6.** belly **7.** front **8.** tissues **9.** epithelium **10.** skull **11.** cell **12.** near to **13.** head

F. **1.** a **2.** c **3.** f **4.** e **5.** a **6.** d **7.** b **8.** e **9.** c **10.** b

G. **1.** otorhinolaryngology **2.** cardiology **3.** gynecology **4.** orthopedics **5.** ophthalmology **6.** urology **7.** dermatology **8.** gastroenterology

Labeling Exercises

A. **1.** cephalic **2.** cervical **3.** thoracic **4.** brachial **5.** abdominal **6.** pelvic **7.** pubic **8.** crural **9.** trunk **10.** vertebral **11.** dorsum **12.** gluteal

B. **1.** frontal or coronal plane **2.** sagittal or median plane **3.** transverse or horizontal plane

Chapter 3 Answers

Practice As You Go

A. **1.** epidermis, dermis **2.** hypodermis or subcutaneous layer **3.** basal cell **4.** adipose **5.** dermis **6.** keratin **7.** melanin **8.** corium **9.** nail bed **10.** sebaceous, sweat

B. **1.** ungual **2.** dermal, cutaneous **3.** epidermal **4.** hypodermic, subcutaneous **5.** intradermal

C. **1.** e **2.** f **3.** i **4.** j **5.** a **6.** c **7.** l **8.** g **9.** k **10.** h **11.** d **12.** b

D. **1.** h **2.** i **3.** j **4.** e **5.** c **6.** a **7.** f **8.** g **9.** b **10.** d

E. **1.** FS **2.** I & D **3.** ID **4.** Subq, Subc **5.** UV **6.** BX, bx **7.** C&S **8.** BCC **9.** decub **10.** Derm, derm

Real-World Applications

Medical Record Analysis

1. basal cell carcinoma—Cancerous tumor of the basal cell layer of the epidermis. A frequent type of skin cancer that rarely metastasizes or spreads. These cancers can arise on sun-exposed skin.
2. lesions—A general term for a wound, injury, or abnormality.
3. biopsies—A piece of tissue is removed by syringe and needle, knife, punch, or brush to examine under a microscope. Used to aid in diagnosis.
4. excised—To surgically cut out.
5. pruritus—Severe itching.
6. anterior—Pertaining to the front side of the body.
7. erythema—Redness or flushing of the skin.
8. depigmentation—Loss of normal skin color or pigment.
9. epidermis—The superficial layer of the skin.
10. dermis—The middle layer of the skin.
11. dermatoplasty—Skin grafting; transplantation of skin.

Chart Note Transcription

1. ulcer **2.** dermatologist **3.** pruritus **4.** erythema **5.** pustules **6.** dermis **7.** necrosis **8.** culture and sensitivity **9.** cellulitis **10.** debridement

Case Study

1. Systemic lupus erythematosus; another example is rheumatoid arthritis.
2. Erythema—skin redness; photosensitivity—intolerance to strong light; alopecia—baldness; stiffness in joints.
3. Exfoliative cytology and fungal scrapings—in both tests cells are scraped away from the skin and examined under a microscope in order to make a diagnosis; in order to make sure the rash was not caused by something else like a fungal infection.
4. Internist—anti-inflammatory—to reduce pain, swelling, and stiffness in joints; dermatologist—corticosteroid cream to anti-inflammatory to reduce the red rash.
5. Completing examinations and various diagnostic tests in order to collect information necessary for a diagnosis.

Practice Exercises

A. **1.** cold **2.** skin **3.** profuse sweating **4.** pus **5.** to burn **6.** nail **7.** fat **8.** sweat **9.** wrinkles **10.** oil **11.** hair **12.** death **13.** skin condition **14.** other, different from usual **15.** foreign

B. **1.** redness involving superficial layer of skin **2.** burn damage through epidermis and into dermis causing vesicles **3.** burn damage to full thickness of epidermis and dermis

C. **1.** flat, discolored area **2.** small, solid raised spot less than 0.5 cm **3.** fluid-filled sac **4.** cracklike lesion **5.** raised spot containing pus **6.** small, round swollen area **7.** fluid-filled blister **8.** open sore **9.** firm, solid mass larger than 0.5 cm **10.** torn or jagged wound

D. **1.** dermatitis **2.** dermatosis **3.** dermatome **4.** dermatologist **5.** dermatoplasty **6.** dermatology **7.** melanoma **8.** melanocyte **9.** ichthyoderma **10.** leukoderma **11.** erythroderma **12.** onychomalacia **13.** paronychia **14.** onychophagia **15.** onychectomy

E. **1.** culture and sensitivity **2.** basal cell carcinoma **3.** dermatology **4.** skin graft **5.** decubitus ulcer **6.** malignant melanoma

F. **1.** xeroderma **2.** petechiae **3.** tinea **4.** scabies **5.** paronychia **6.** Kaposi's sarcoma **7.** impetigo **8.** keloid **9.** exfoliative cytology **10.** frozen section

G. **1.** antifungal, e **2.** antipruritic, c **3.** antiparasitic, a **4.** corticosteroid cream, b **5.** anesthetic, f **6.** antibiotic, d

Labeling Exercise

A. **1.** epidermis **2.** dermis **3.** subcutaneous layer **4.** sweat gland **5.** sweat duct **6.** hair shaft **7.** sebaceous gland **8.** arrector pili muscle **9.** sensory receptors

B. **1.** epidermis **2.** dermis **3.** subcutaneous layer **4.** sebaceous gland **5.** arrector pili muscle **6.** hair shaft **7.** hair follicle **8.** hair root **9.** papilla

C. **1.** free edge **2.** lateral nail groove **3.** lunula **4.** nail bed **5.** nail body **6.** cuticle **7.** nail root

Chapter 4 Answers

Practice As You Go

A. **1.** axial, appendicular **2.** frame, protect vital organs, work with muscles for movement, store minerals, red blood cell production **3.** short **4.** periosteum **5.** cancellous **6.** synovial **7.** foramen **8.** diaphysis

B. **1.** femoral **2.** sternal **3.** clavicular **4.** coccygeal **5.** maxillary **6.** tibial **7.** patellar **8.** phalangeal **9.** humeral **10.** pubic

C. **1.** c **2.** h **3.** f **4.** g **5.** d **6.** e **7.** a **8.** b

D. **1.** TKR **2.** HNP **3.** UE **4.** L5 **5.** AK **6.** fx/FX **7.** NSAID

E. **1.** smooth **2.** myoneural **3.** skeletal, smooth, cardiac

F. **1.** e **2.** d **3.** b **4.** c **5.** a **6.** h **7.** g **8.** f

G. **1.** IM **2.** DTR **3.** MD **4.** EMG **5.** CTS

Real-World Applications

Medical Record Analysis

1. osteoarthritis—Joint inflammation resulting in degeneration of the bones and joints, especially those bearing weight. Results in bone rubbing against bone.
2. bilateral—Pertaining to both sides.
3. TKA—Surgical reconstruction of a knee joint by implanting a prosthetic knee joint. Also called *total knee replacement (TKR).*
4. orthopedic surgeon—Physician that specializes in the diagnosis and treatment of conditions of the musculoskeletal system using surgical means.
5. CT scan—Computed tomography scan; imaging technique that produces cross-sectional view of the body.
6. physical therapy—Treats disorders using physical means and methods; includes joint motion and muscle strength.
7. ROM—Range of movement of a joint, from maximum flexion through maximum extension; it is measured as degrees of a circle.
8. gait training—Learning how to walk.
9. occupational therapy—Assists patients to regain, develop, and improve skills that are important for independent functioning.
10. ADLs—Activities of daily living.

Chart Note Transcription

1. Colles' fracture (fx) **2.** cast **3.** fracture **4.** orthopedist **5.** osteoporosis **6.** computerized axial tomography (CT or CAT scan) **7.** flexion **8.** extension **9.** comminuted fracture (fx) **10.** femur **11.** total hip arthroplasty (THA)

Case Study

1. Rheumatoid arthritis.
2. Cartilage damage and crippling deformities.
3. Osteoarthritis.
4. Bone scan—Radioactive dye is used to visualize the body; erythrocyte sedimentation rate—A blood test that can determine if a person has an inflammatory disease.
5. Anti-inflammatory medication to reduce inflammation and provide some pain relief; physical therapy—Treatment using warm water and exercises to maintain the flexibility of the joints.
6. Acute—Brief disease, also used to mean sudden and severe disease; chronic—Disease of a long duration.

Practice Exercises

A. **1.** osteocyte **2.** osteoblast **3.** osteoporosis **4.** osteopathy **5.** osteotomy **6.** osteotome **7.** osteomyelitis **8.** osteomalacia **9.** osteochondroma **10.** myopathy **11.** myoplasty **12.** myorrhaphy **13.** electromyogram **14.** myasthenia **15.** tenodynia **16.** tenorrhaphy **17.** arthrodesis **18.** arthroplasty **19.** arthrotomy **20.** arthritis **21.** arthrocentesis **22.** arthralgia **23.** chondrectomy **24.** chondroma **25.** chondromalacia

B. **1.** -desis **2.** -asthenia **3.** -listhesis **4.** -clasia **5.** -kinesia **6.** -porosis

C. **1.** cervical, 7 **2.** thoracic, 12 **3.** lumbar, 5 **4.** sacrum, 1 (5 fused) **5.** coccyx, 1 (3–5 fused)

D. **1.** S = -scopy; visual examination of the inside of a joint **2.** P = inter-, S = -al; pertaining to between vertebrae **3.** S = -malacia; abnormal softening of cartilage **4.** S = -ectomy; surgical removal of a disk **5.** P = intra- S = -al; pertaining to within the skull **6.** -osis = abnormal condition; abnormal condition of the vertebrae

E. **1.** lamina **2.** stiff joint **3.** cartilage **4.** vertebrae **5.** muscle **6.** straight **7.** hump **8.** tendon **9.** bone marrow **10.** joint

F. **1.** osteoporosis **2.** rickets **3.** lateral epicondylitis **4.** herniated nucleus pulposus **5.** osteogenic sarcoma **6.** scoliosis **7.** pseudotrophic muscular dystrophy **8.** systemic lupus erythematosus **9.** spondylolisthesis **10.** carpal tunnel syndrome

G. **1.** patella **2.** tarsus **3.** clavicle **4.** femur **5.** phalanges **6.** carpus **7.** tibia **8.** scapula **9.** phalanges

H. **1.** degenerative joint disease **2.** electromyogram **3.** first cervical vertebra **4.** sixth thoracic vertebra **5.** intramuscular **6.** deep tendon reflexes **7.** juvenile rheumatoid arthritis **8.** left lower extremity **9.** orthopedics **10.** carpal tunnel syndrome

I. **1.** surgical repair of cartilage **2.** slow movement **3.** porous bone **4.** abnormal increase in lumbar spine curve (swayback) **5.** lack of development/nourishment **6.** bone marrow tumor **7.** artificial substitute for a body part **8.** cutting into skull **9.** puncture of a joint to withdraw fluid **10.** bursa inflammation

J. **1.** nonsteroidal anti-inflammatory drugs, b **2.** corticosteroids, e **3.** skeletal muscle relaxants, a **4.** bone reabsorption inhibitors, c **5.** calcium supplements, d

Labeling Exercise

A. **1.** skull **2.** cervical vertebrae **3.** sternum **4.** ribs **5.** thoracic vertebrae **6.** lumbar vertebrae **7.** ilium **8.** pubis **9.** ischium **10.** femur **11.** patella **12.** tibia **13.** fibula **14.** tarsus **15.** metatarsus **16.** phalanges **17.** maxilla **18.** mandible **19.** scapula **20.** humerus **21.** ulna **22.** radius **23.** sacrum **24.** coccyx **25.** carpus **26.** metacarpus **27.** phalanges

B. **1.** proximal epiphysis **2.** diaphysis **3.** distal epiphysis **4.** articular cartilage **5.** epiphyseal line **6.** spongy or cancellous bone **7.** compact or cortical bone **8.** medullary cavity

C. **1.** periosteum **2.** synovial membrane **3.** articular cartilage **4.** joint cavity **5.** joint capsule

Chapter 5 Answers

Practice As You Go

A. **1.** cardiology **2.** endocardium, myocardium, epicardium **3.** sinoatrial node **4.** away from **5.** tricuspid, pulmonary, mitral (bicuspid), aortic **6.** atria, ventricles **7.** pulmonary **8.** apex **9.** septum **10.** systole, diastole

B. **1.** cardiac or coronary **2.** interventricular **3.** arterial **4.** venule **5.** myocardial **6.** atrial

C. **1.** f **2.** h **3.** d **4.** g **5.** b **6.** i **7.** a **8.** c **9.** e **10.** j

D. **1.** c **2.** g **3.** j **4.** a **5.** d **6.** b **7.** i **8.** e **9.** f **10.** h

E. **1.** MVP **2.** VSD **3.** PTCA **4.** Vfib **5.** DVT **6.** LDH **7.** CoA **8.** tPA **9.** CV **10.** ECC

Real-World Applications

Medical Record Analysis

1. hypertension—Blood pressure above the normal range.
2. tachycardia—The condition of having a fast heart rate, typically more than 100 beats/minute while at rest.
3. congestive heart failure (CAD)—Pathological condition of the heart in which there is a reduced outflow of blood from the left side of the heart because the left ventricle myocardium has become too weak to efficiently pump blood. Results in weakness, breathlessness, and edema.
4. mitral valve prolapse—Condition in which the cusps or flaps of the heart valve are too loose and fail to shut tightly, allowing blood to flow backward through the valve when the heart chamber contracts. Most commonly occurs in the mitral valve, but may affect any of the heart valves.
5. palpitations—Pounding, racing heartbeats.
6. electrocardiography (EKG)—Process of recording the electrical activity of the heart. Useful in the diagnosis of abnormal cardiac rhythm and heart muscle (myocardium) damage.
7. cardiac enzymes—Blood test to determine the level of enzymes specific to heart muscles in the blood. An increase in the enzymes may indicate heart muscle damage such as a myocardial infarction. These enzymes include creatine phosphokinase (CPK), lactate dehydrogenase (LDH), and glutamic oxaloacetic transaminase (GOT).
8. echocardiography—Noninvasive diagnostic method using ultrasound to visualize internal cardiac structures. Cardiac valve activity can be evaluated using this method.
9. stress test—Method for evaluating cardiovascular fitness. The patient is placed on a treadmill or a bicycle and then subjected to steadily increasing levels of work. An EKG and oxygen levels are taken while the patient exercises. The test is stopped if abnormalities occur on the EKG. Also called an *exercise test* or a *treadmill test*.
10. angiocardiography—X-rays taken after the injection of an opaque material into a blood vessel. Can be performed on the aorta as an aortic angiogram, on the heart as an angiocardiogram, and on the brain as a cerebral angiogram.
11. coronary artery disease (CAD)—Insufficient blood supply to the heart muscle due to an obstruction of one or more coronary arteries. May be caused by atherosclerosis and may cause angina pectoris and myocardial infarction.
12. myocardial infarction—Condition caused by the partial or complete occlusion or closing of one or more of the coronary arteries. Symptoms include a squeezing pain or heavy pressure in the middle of the chest (angina pectoris). A delay in treatment could result in death. Also referred to as a *heart attack*.
13. mitral valve replacement—Removal of a diseased heart valve and replacement with an artificial valve.

Chart Note Transcription

1. angina pectoris **2.** bradycardia **3.** hypertension **4.** myocardial infarction (MI) **5.** electrocardiogram (EKG, ECG) **6.** cardiac enzymes **7.** coronary artery disease (CAD) **8.** cardiac catheterization **9.** stress test (treadmill test) **10.** percutaneous transluminal coronary angioplasty (PTCA) **11.** coronary artery bypass graft (CABG)

Case Study

1. Heart attack; condition caused by the partial or complete occlusion or closing of one or more of the coronary arteries. Symptoms include a squeezing pain or heavy pressure in the middle of

the chest (angina pectoris). A delay in treatment could result in death.

2. The main complaint, the one the patient is most aware of or most anxious about.
3. Angina pectoris—Condition in which there is severe pain with a sensation of constriction around the heart; caused by a deficiency of oxygen to the heart muscle.
4. Nausea—Feeling of need to vomit; dyspnea—Difficulty breathing; diaphoresis—Profuse sweating.
5. Cardiac enzymes; angiocardiography; cardiac scan; electrocardiography; stress testing; cardiac catheterization; Holter monitor.
6. Smokes; overweight; family history; sedentary lifestyle. He can stop smoking, lose weight, and become more active.

Practice Exercises

A. **1.** cardiac **2.** cardiomyopathy **3.** cardiomegaly **4.** tachycardia **5.** bradycardia **6.** electrocardiogram **7.** angiostenosis **8.** angiitis **9.** angiospasm **10.** arterial **11.** arteriosclerosis **12.** arteriole **13.** endocarditis **14.** epicarditis **15.** myocarditis

B. **1.** heart **2.** valve **3.** chest **4.** artery **5.** vein **6.** vessel **7.** ventricle **8.** clot **9.** atrium **10.** fatty substance

C. **1.** venous **2.** cardiology **3.** venogram **4.** electrocardiography **5.** hypertension **6.** hypotension **7.** valvoplasty **8.** interventricular **9.** atherectomy **10.** arteriostenosis

D. **1.** -tension **2.** -stenosis **3.** -manometer **4.** -ule, -ole **5.** -sclerosis

E. **1.** blood pressure **2.** congestive heart failure **3.** myocardial infarction **4.** coronary care unit **5.** premature ventricular contraction **6.** cardiopulmonary resuscitation **7.** coronary artery disease **8.** chest pain **9.** electrocardiogram **10.** first heart sound

F. **1.** thin flexible tube **2.** an area of dead tissue **3.** a blood clot **4.** pounding heartbeat **5.** backflow **6.** weakened and ballooning arterial wall **7.** complete stoppage of heart activity **8.** serious cardiac arrhythmia **9.** heart attack **10.** varicose veins in anal region

G. **1.** murmur **2.** defibrillation **3.** hypertension **4.** pacemaker **5.** varicose veins **6.** angina pectoris **7.** CCU **8.** MI **9.** angiography **10.** echocardiogram **11.** Holter monitor **12.** CHF

H. **1.** antiarrhythmic, e **2.** antilipidemic, g **3.** cardiotonic, f **4.** diuretic, h **5.** anticoagulant, b **6.** thrombolytic, a **7.** vasodilator, d **8.** calcium channel blocker, c

Labeling Exercise

A. **1.** pulmonary arteries **2.** vena cavae **3.** right atrium **4.** right ventricle **5.** systemic veins **6.** capillary bed lungs **7.** pulmonary veins **8.** aorta **9.** left atrium **10.** left ventricle **11.** systemic arteries **12.** systemic capillary beds

B. **1.** superior vena cava **2.** aorta **3.** pulmonary trunk **4.** pulmonary valve **5.** right atrium **6.** tricuspid valve **7.** right ventricle **8.** inferior vena cava **9.** pulmonary artery **10.** pulmonary vein **11.** left atrium **12.** aortic valve **13.** mitral or bicuspid valve **14.** left ventricle **15.** endocardium **16.** myocardium **17.** pericardium

Chapter 6 Answers

Practice As You Go

A. **1.** hematology **2.** phagocytosis **3.** erythrocytes (red blood cells), leukocytes (white blood cells), platelets (thrombocytes) **4.** plasma **5.** hemostasis

B. **1.** hematic or sanguinous **2.** leukocytic **3.** thrombocytic **4.** fibrinous **5.** erythrocytic

C. **1.** d **2.** e **3.** c **4.** b **5.** a

D. **1.** c **2.** e **3.** a **4.** b **5.** d

E. **1.** ALL **2.** BMT **3.** eosins, eos **4.** HCT, Hct, crit **5.** PA **6.** CBC **7.** diff **8.** WBC

F. **1.** spleen, tonsils, thymus **2.** thoracic duct, right lymphatic duct **3.** axillary, cervical, mediastinal, inguinal **4.** active acquired **5.** antibody-mediated

G. **1.** splenic **2.** lymphatic **3.** tonsillar **4.** thymic **5.** lymphangial

H. **1.** c **2.** a **3.** d **4.** e **5.** b

I. **1.** e **2.** c **3.** d **4.** a **5.** b

J. **1.** AIDS **2.** ARC **3.** HIV **4.** mono **5.** KS **6.** Ig **7.** SCIDS **8.** PCP

Real-World Applications

Medical Record Analysis

1. splenomegaly—An enlarged spleen.
2. non-Hodgkin's lymphoma—Cancer of the lymphatic tissues other than Hodgkin's lymphoma.
3. spleen—An organ located in the upper left quadrant of the abdomen. Consists of lymphatic tissue that is highly infiltrated with blood vessels. It filters out and destroys old red blood cells.
4. splenectomy—The surgical removal of the spleen.
5. Monospot—A blood test for infectious mononucleosis.
6. enzyme-linked immunosorbent assay (ELISA)—A blood test for an antibody to the AIDS virus. A positive test means that the person has been exposed to the virus. There may be a false-positive reading, and then the Western blot test would be used to verify the results.

7. Magnetic resonance imaging (MRI)—Medical imaging that uses radio-frequency radiation as its source of energy. It does not require the injection of contrast medium or exposure to ionizing radiation. The technique is useful for visualizing large blood vessels, the heart, the brain, and soft tissues.
8. tumor—Abnormal growth of tissue that may be benign or malignant.
9. biopsy—A piece of tissue is removed by syringe and needle, knife, punch, or brush to examine under a microscope. Used to aid in diagnosis.
10. oncologist—A physician who specializes in the treatment of cancer.
11. metastases—The spreading of a cancerous tumor from its original site to different locations of the body.

Chart Note Transcription

1. hematologist **2.** ELISA **3.** prothrombin time **4.** complete blood count (CBC) **5.** erythropenia **6.** thrombopenia **7.** leukocytosis **8.** bone marrow aspiration **9.** leukemia **10.** homologous transfusion

Case Study

1. Acute lymphocytic leukemia.
2. High fever; thrombopenia—Too few platelets; epistaxis—Nosebleed; gingival bleeding—Gums bleeding; petechiae—Pinpoint bruises; ecchymoses—Large black and blue bruises.
3. Bone marrow aspiration—Sample of bone marrow is removed by aspiration with a needle and examined for diseases.
4. A diagnosis based on the results of the physician's direct examination rather than based on other tests like X-rays and labwork.
5. Chemotherapy—Treating disease by using chemicals that have a toxic effect upon the body, especially cancerous tissue.
6. Remission—A period during which the symptoms of a disease or disorder leave. Can be temporary.

Practice Exercises

A. **1.** splenomegaly **2.** splenectomy **3.** splenotomy **4.** lymphocytes **5.** lymphoma **6.** lymphadenopathy **7.** lymphadenoma **8.** lymphadenitis **9.** immunologist **10.** immunoglobulin **11.** immunology **12.** hematic **13.** hematoma **14.** hematopoiesis **15.** hemolytic **16.** hemoglobin **17.** leukopenia **18.** erythropenia **19.** pancytopenia **20.** leukocytosis **21.** erythrocytosis **22.** thrombocytosis **23.** erythrocyte **24.** leukocyte **25.** lymphocyte

B. **1.** basophil **2.** complete blood count **3.** hemoglobin **4.** prothrombin time **5.** graft versus host disease **6.** red blood count/red blood cell **7.** packed cell volume **8.** erythrocyte sedimentation rate **9.** differential **10.** lymphocyte

C. **1.** lymphaden/o **2.** thromb/o **3.** sanguin/o, hem/o, hemat/o **4.** tonsill/o **5.** tox/o **6.** phag/o **7.** lymphangi/o **8.** path/o **9.** splen/o **10.** lymph/o

D. **1.** polycythemia vera **2.** mononucleosis **3.** anaphylactic shock **4.** HIV **5.** Kaposi's sarcoma **6.** AIDS **7.** Hodgkin's disease **8.** Pneumocystis **9.** aplastic **10.** pernicious

E. **1.** reverse transcriptase inhibitor, e **2.** anticoagulant, a **3.** antihemorrhagic, d **4.** antihistamine, h **5.** immunosuppressant, f **6.** thrombolytic, b **7.** hematinic, g **8.** corticosteroid, c **9.** antiplatelet agent, i

F. **1.** d **2.** f **3.** b **4.** g **5.** a **6.** e **7.** c

G. **1.** treatment with an antibody injection **2.** blood test for HIV in addition to ELISA **3.** infections seen in immunocompromised patients **4.** intense itching **5.** tissue's response to injury **6.** blood transfusion from another person **7.** caused by vitamin B_{12} deficiency **8.** cancer of blood forming bone marrow **9.** rapid flow of blood, bleeding **10.** blood poisoning

Labeling Exercise

A. **1.** plasma **2.** red blood cells or erythrocytes **3.** platelets or thrombocytes **4.** white blood cells or leukocytes

B. **1.** cervical nodes **2.** mediastinal nodes **3.** axillary nodes **4.** inguinal nodes

C. **1.** thymus gland **2.** lymph node **3.** tonsil **4.** spleen **5.** lymphatic vessels

Chapter 7 Answers

Practice As You Go

A. **1.** nasal cavity, pharynx, larynx, trachea, bronchial tubes, lungs **2.** pharynx **3.** epiglottis **4.** diaphragm **5.** 3; 2 **6.** alveoli **7.** pleura **8.** bronchioles, alveoli

B. **1.** laryngeal **2.** pulmonary **3.** paranasal **4.** alveolar **5.** nasal **6.** diaphragmatic

C. **1.** e **2.** i **3.** h **4.** a **5.** j **6.** d **7.** b **8.** g **9.** f **10.** c

D. **1.** f **2.** c **3.** e **4.** a **5.** d **6.** b

E. **1.** URI **2.** PFT **3.** O_2 **4.** CO_2 **5.** COPD **6.** Bronch **7.** TB **8.** IRDS

Real-World Applications

Medical Record Analysis

1. asthma—Disease caused by various conditions, such as allergens, and resulting in constriction of the bronchial airways, dyspnea, coughing,

and wheezing. Can cause violent spasms of the bronchi (bronchospasms) but is generally not a life-threatening condition. Medication can be very effective.

2. dyspnea—Term describing difficult or labored breathing.
3. cyanosis—Refers to the bluish tint of skin that is receiving an insufficient amount of oxygen or circulation.
4. expiration—To breath out; exhale.
5. phlegm—Thick mucus secreted by the membranes that line the respiratory tract. When phlegm is coughed through the mouth, it is called *sputum*. Phlegm is examined for color, odor, and consistency.
6. auscultation—To listen to body sounds, usually using a stethoscope.
7. rhonchi—Somewhat musical sound during expiration, often found in asthma or infection. Caused by spasms of the bronchial tubes. Also called *wheezing*.
8. arterial blood gases (ABGs)—Testing for the gases present in the blood. Generally used to assist in determining the levels of oxygen (O_2) and carbon dioxide (CO_2) in the blood.
9. hypoxemia—The condition of having an insufficient amount of oxygen in the bloodstream.
10. spirometry—Procedure to measure lung capacity using a *spirometer*.
11. Proventil—Medication that relaxes muscle spasms in bronchial tubes. Used to treat asthma.
12. bronchospasms—An involuntary muscle spasm of the smooth muscle in the wall of the bronchus.

Chart Note Transcription

1. dyspnea **2.** tachypnea **3.** arterial blood gases (ABGs) **4.** hypoxemia **5.** auscultation **6.** crackles **7.** purulent **8.** sputum **9.** CXR **10.** pneumonia **11.** endotracheal intubation

Case Study

1. Pneumonia.
2. Dyspnea—Difficulty breathing; dizziness; orthopnea—comfortable breathing only while sitting up; elevated temperature, cough.
3. Auscultation (listening to the body sounds) revealed crackles (abnormal sound); chest X-ray revealed fluid in the upper lobe of the right lung.
4. A method of determining a patient's general health and heart and lung function by measuring pulse (100 BPM and rapid), respiratory rate (24 breaths/min and labored), temperature (102°F), and blood pressure (180/110).
5. IV antibiotics—medicine to kill bacteria given into a vein; intermittent positive pressure breathing—method of assisting patients in breathing by using a machine that produces an increased pressure.
6. The IV antibiotics were changed to oral antibiotics—she started taking pills.

Practice Exercises

A. **1.** exchange of O_2 and CO_2 **2.** ventilation **3.** exchange of O_2 and CO_2 in the lungs **4.** exchange of O_2 and CO_2 at cellular level

B. **1.** dilation **2.** carbon dioxide **3.** voice **4.** chest **5.** breathing **6.** spitting **7.** smell

C. **1.** rhinitis **2.** rhinorrhea **3.** rhinoplasty **4.** laryngitis **5.** laryngospasm **6.** laryngoscopy **7.** laryngeal **8.** laryngectomy **9.** laryngoplasty **10.** laryngoplegia **11.** bronchial **12.** bronchitis **13.** bronchoscopy **14.** bronchogenic **15.** bronchospasm **16.** thoracotomy **17.** thoracalgia **18.** thoracic **19.** tracheotomy **20.** tracheostenosis **21.** endotracheal **22.** dyspnea **23.** tachypnea **24.** orthopnea **25.** apnea

D. **1.** trachea or windpipe **2.** larynx **3.** bronchus **4.** breathing **5.** lung or air **6.** nose **7.** dust **8.** pleura **9.** epiglottis **10.** alveolus or air sac **11.** lung **12.** oxygen **13.** sinus **14.** lobe **15.** nose

E. **1.** inhalation or inspiration **2.** hemoptysis **3.** pulmonary emboli **4.** sinusitis **5.** pharyngitis **6.** pneumothorax **7.** pertussis **8.** pleurotomy **9.** pleurodynia **10.** nasopharyngitis

F. **1.** chest X-ray **2.** tidal volume **3.** temperature, pulse, respirations **4.** arterial blood gases **5.** dyspnea on exertion **6.** right upper lobe **7.** sudden infant death syndrome **8.** total lung capacity **9.** adult respiratory distress syndrome **10.** metered-dose inhaler **11.** clear to auscultation **12.** severe acute respiratory syndrome

G. **1.** volume of air in the lungs after a maximal inhalation or inspiration **2.** amount of air entering lungs in a single inspiration or leaving air in single expiration of quiet breathing **3.** air remaining in the lungs after a forced expiration

H. **1.** cardiopulmonary resuscitation **2.** thoracentesis **3.** respirator **4.** supplemental oxygen **5.** patent **6.** ventilation-perfusion scan **7.** sputum cytology **8.** hyperventilation **9.** rhonchi **10.** anthracosis

I. **1.** decongestant, f **2.** antitussive, a **3.** antibiotic, c **4.** expectorant, g **5.** mucolytic, h **6.** bronchodilator, d **7.** antihistamine, e **8.** corticosteroid, b

Labeling Exercise

A. **1.** pharynx and larynx **2.** trachea **3.** nasal cavity **4.** bronchial tubes **5.** lungs

B. **1.** nares **2.** paranasal sinuses **3.** nasal cavity **4.** hard palate **5.** soft palate **6.** palatine tonsil **7.** epiglottis **8.** vocal cords **9.** esophagus **10.** trachea

C. **1.** trachea **2.** right upper lobe **3.** right middle lobe **4.** right lower lobe **5.** apex of lung **6.** left upper lobe **7.** left lower lobe **8.** diaphragm

Chapter 8 Answers

Practice As You Go

A. **1.** gastrointestinal **2.** gut, alimentary canal, mouth, anus **3.** salivary glands, liver, gallbladder, pancreas **4.** digesting food, absorbing nutrients, eliminating waste **5.** cutting, grinding **6.** peristalsis **7.** hydrochloric acid, chyme **8.** duodenum, jejunum, ileum **9.** sigmoid **10.** bile, eumulsification, gallbladder

B. **1.** duodenal **2.** nasogastric **3.** hepatic **4.** pancreatic **5.** cholecystic or cystic **6.** sublingual **7.** esophageal **8.** sigmoidal

C. **1.** i **2.** f **3.** c **4.** a **5.** j **6.** l **7.** e **8.** b **9.** k **10.** d **11.** g **12.** o **13.** h **14.** n **15.** m

D. **1.** f **2.** g **3.** e **4.** h **5.** b **6.** a **7.** d **8.** c

E. **1.** NG **2.** GI **3.** HBV **4.** FOBT **5.** IBD **6.** HSV-1 **7.** AST **8.** pc **9.** PUD **10.** GERD

Real-World Applications

Medical Record Analysis

1. epigastric—Pertaining to the area above the stomach.
2. anemia—A large group of conditions characterized by a reduction in the number of red blood cells or the amount of hemoglobin in the blood; results in less oxygen reaching the tissues.
3. melena—Passage of dark tarry stools. Color is the result of digestive enzymes working on blood in the gastrointestinal tract.
4. dyspepsia—An "upset stomach."
5. antacids—Medication to neutralize stomach acid.
6. complete blood count (CBC)—A combination of blood tests including red blood cell count, white blood cell count, hemoglobin, hematocrit, white blood cell differential, and platelet count.
7. fecal occult blood—Laboratory test on the feces to determine if microscopic amounts of blood are present. Also called *hemoccult* or *stool guaiac*.
8. *Helicobacter pylori*—A bacteria that may damage the lining of the stomach setting up the conditions for peptic ulcer disease to develop.
9. gastroscopy—Procedure in which a flexible *gastroscope* is passed through the mouth and down the esophagus in order to visualize inside the stomach. Used to diagnose peptic ulcers and gastric carcinoma.
10. ulcer—An open sore or lesion in the skin or mucous membrane.
11. peptic ulcer disease—Ulcer occurring in the lower portion of the esophagus, stomach, and/or duodenum; thought to be caused by the acid of gastric juices. Initial damage to the protective lining of the stomach may be caused by a *Helicobacter pylori* (*H. pylori*) bacterial infection. If the ulcer extends all the way through the wall of the stomach, it is called a *perforated ulcer*, which requires immediate surgery to repair.
12. gastrectomy—Surgical removal of the stomach.

Chart Note Transcription

1. gastroenterologist **2.** constipation **3.** cholelithiasis **4.** cholecystectomy **5.** gastroesophageal reflux disease **6.** ascites **7.** lower gastrointestinal series **8.** polyposis **9.** colonoscopy **10.** sigmoid colon **11.** colectomy **12.** colostomy

Case Study

1. Severe RUQ pain—Severe pain is located in the upper right corner of the abdomen; nausea—Feeling the urge to vomit; emesis—Vomiting; scleral jaundice—The whites of the eye have a yellowish cast to them.
2. Gallbladder, right kidney, majority of the liver, a small portion of the pancreas, portion of colon and small intestine.
3. Gallstones blocking the common bile duct so bile can't drain into the small intestine.
4. Abdominal ultrasound—The use of high-frequency sound waves to produce an image of an organ, such as the uterus and ovaries or a fetus; percutaneous transhepatic cholangiography (PTC)—Procedure in which contrast medium is injected directly into the liver to visualize the bile ducts; used to detect obstructions such as gallstones in the common bile duct.
5. Cholelithiasis is the condition of having gallstones present in the gallbladder, they may not be causing any symptoms; cholecystitis is the inflammation of the gallbladder that occurs when gallstones block the flow of bile out of the gallbladder.
6. Laparoscopic cholecystectomy—The gallbladder was removed through a very small abdominal incision with the assistance of a laparoscope.

Practice Exercises

A. **1.** gastritis **2.** gastroenterology **3.** gastrectomy **4.** gastroscopy **5.** gastralgia **6.** gastromegaly **7.** gastrotomy **8.** esophagitis **9.** esophagoscopy **10.** esophagoplasty **11.** esophageal **12.** esophagectasis **13.** proctopexy **14.** proctoptosis **15.** proctitis **16.** proctologist **17.** cholecystectomy **18.** cholecystolithiasis **19.** cholecystolithotripsy

20. cholecystitis 21. laparoscope 22. laparotomy 23. laparoscopy 24. hepatoma 25. hepatomegaly 26. hepatic 27. hepatitis 28. pancreatitis 29. pancreatic 30. colostomy 31. colitis

B. 1. esophagus 2. liver 3. ileum 4. anus and rectum 5. tongue 6. lip 7. jejunum 8. sigmoid colon 9. rectum 10. gum 11. gallbladder 12. duodenum 13. anus 14. small intestine 15. tooth

C. 1. postprandial 2. cholelithiasis 3. anorexia 4. dysphagia 5. hematemesis 6. bradypepsia

D. 1. bowel movement 2. upper gastrointestinal series 3. barium enema 4. bowel sounds 5. nausea and vomiting 6. ova and parasites 7. by mouth 8. common bile duct 9. nothing by mouth 10. postprandial

E. 1. visual exam of the colon 2. tooth X-ray 3. bright red blood in the stools 4. blood test to determine amount of waste product in the bloodstream 5. weight loss and wasting from a chronic illness 6. use NG tube to wash out stomach 7. surgical repair of hernia 8. pulling teeth 9. surgical crushing of common bile duct stone 10. surgically create a connection between two organs

F. 1. liver biopsy 2. colostomy 3. barium swallow 4. lower GI series 5. colectomy 6. fecal occult blood test 7. choledocholithotripsy 8. total parenteral nutrition 9. gastric stapling 10. intravenous cholecystography 11. colonoscopy 12. ileostomy

G. 1. d 2. g 3. h 4. e 5. f 6. b 7. c 8. a

H. 1. antidiarrheal, f 2. proton pump inhibitor, h 3. antiemetic, d 4. H_2-receptor antagonist, a 5. anorexiant, b 6. laxative, c 7. antacid, e 8. antiviral, g

Labeling Exercise

A. 1. salivary glands 2. esophagus 3. pancreas 4. small intestine 5. oral cavity 6. stomach 7. liver and gallbladder 8. colon

B. 1. esophagus 2. cardiac or lower esophageal sphincter 3. pyloric sphincter 4. duodenum 5. antrum 6. fundus of stomach 7. rugae 8. body of stomach

C. 1. cystic duct 2. common bile duct 3. gallbladder 4. duodenum 5. liver 6. hepatic duct 7. pancreas 8. pancreatic duct

Chapter 9 Answers

Practice As You Go

A. 1. nephrons 2. filtration, reabsorption, secretion 3. electrolytes 4. retroperitoneal 5. glomerulus 6. calyx 7. two, one 8. micturition, voiding

B. 1. ureteral 2. renal 3. glomerular 4. urinary 5. urethral

C. 1. c 2. g 3. h 4. i 5. f 6. e 7. d 8. b 9. a 10. j

D. 1. f 2. e 3. h 4. a 5. g 6. c 7. d 8. b

E. 1. kidneys, ureters, bladder 2. catheter/catheterization 3. cystoscopy 4. genitourinary 5. extracorporeal shockwave lithotripsy 6. urinary tract infection 7. urine culture 8. retrograde pyelogram 9. acute renal failure 10. blood urea nitrogen 11. chronic renal failure 12. water

Real-World Applications

Medical Record Analysis

1. hematuria—The presence of blood in the urine.
2. pyelonephritis—Inflammation of the renal pelvis and the kidney. One of the most common types of kidney disease. It may be the result of a lower urinary tract infection that moved up to the kidney by way of the ureters. There may be large quantities of white blood cells and bacteria in the urine. Blood (hematuria) may even be present in the urine in this condition. Can occur with any untreated or persistent case of cystitis.
3. chronic cystitis—Urinary bladder inflammation.
4. dysuria—Difficult or painful urination.
5. clean catch urinalysis—Laboratory test that consists of the physical, chemical, and microscopic examination of urine.
6. pyuria—The presence of pus in the urine.
7. culture and sensitivity—Laboratory test of urine for bacterial infection. Attempt to grow bacteria on a culture medium in order to identify it and determine which antibiotics it is sensitive to.
8. pathogen—Anything, such as bacteria, viruses, fungi, or toxins, that may cause disease.
9. antibiotic—Medication used to treat bacterial infections of the urinary tract.
10. cystoscopy—Visual examination of the urinary bladder using an instrument called a *cystoscope*.
11. bladder neck obstruction—Blockage of the bladder outlet. Often caused by an enlarged prostate gland in males.
12. congenital—Present from birth.
13. catheterized—Insertion of a tube through the urethra and into the urinary bladder for the purpose of withdrawing urine or inserting dye.

Chart Note Transcription

1. urologist 2. hematuria 3. cystitis 4. clean-catch specimen 5. urinalysis (U/A, UA) 6. pyuria 7. retrograde pyelogram 8. ureter 9. ureterolith 10. extracorporeal shockwave lithotripsy (ESWL) 11. calculi

Case Study

1. Cystitis—Inflammation of the urinary bladder; pyelonephritis—Inflammation of the renal pelvis and the kidney. One of the most common types

of kidney disease. It may be the result of a lower urinary tract infection that moved up to the kidney by way of the ureters. There may be large quantities of white blood cells and bacteria in the urine. Blood (hematuria) may even be present in the urine in this condition. Can occur with any untreated or persistent case of cystitis.

2. Fever; chills; fatigue; urgency—Feeling the need to urinate immediately; frequency—Urge to urinate more often than normal; dysuria—Difficult or painful urination; hematuria—Blood in the urine; cloudy urine with a fishy smell—Urine was not clear and smelled bad.
3. Clean catch specimen—Urine sample obtained after cleaning off the urinary opening and catching or collecting a urine sample in midstream (halfway through the urination process) to minimize contamination from the genitalia; U/A (urinalysis)—A physical, chemical, and microscopic examination of the urine; urine C&S (culture & sensitivity)—Test for the presence and identification of bacteria in the urine; KUB (kidney, ureters, and bladder)—An X-ray of the urinary organs.
4. Pyuria—Pus in the urine; bacteriuria—Bacteria in the urine; acidic pH—Indicates a urinary tract infection; culture and sensitivity—Revealed a common type of bacteria; KUB—Pyelonephritis.
5. Antibiotic—To kill the bacteria; push fluids—To flush out the bladder.
6. Clear yellow to deep gold color, aromatic odor, specific gravity between 1.010–1.030, pH between 5.0–8.0, very little protein, no glucose, ketones, or blood.

Practice Exercises

A. **1.** nephropexy **2.** nephrogram **3.** nephrolithiasis **4.** nephrectomy **5.** nephritis **6.** nephropathy **7.** nephrosclerosis **8.** cystitis **9.** cystorrhagia **10.** cystoplasty **11.** cystoscope **12.** cystalgia **13.** pyeloplasty **14.** pyelitis **15.** pyelogram **16.** ureterolith **17.** ureterectasis **18.** ureterostenosis **19.** urethritis **20.** urethroscope

B. **1.** urine **2.** meatus **3.** urinary bladder **4.** kidney **5.** renal pelvis **6.** sugar **7.** night **8.** scanty **9.** ureter **10.** glomerulus

C. **1.** antispasmodic, b **2.** antibiotic, c **3.** diuretic, a

D. **1.** urination, voiding **2.** increases urine production **3.** pain associated with kidney stone **4.** inserting a tube through urethra into the bladder **5.** inflammation of renal pelvis **6.** inflammation of glomeruli in the kidney **7.** cutting into an organ to remove stone **8.** bedwetting **9.** enlargement of urethral opening **10.** damage to glomerulus secondary to diabetes mellitus **11.** lab test of chemical composition of urine **12.** decrease in force of urine stream

E. **1.** anuria **2.** hematuria **3.** calculus/nephrolith **4.** lithotripsy **5.** urethritis **6.** pyuria **7.** bacteriuria **8.** dysuria **9.** ketonuria **10.** proteinuria **11.** polyuria

F. **1.** K^+ **2.** Na^+ **3.** UA **4.** BUN **5.** SG, sp.gr. **6.** IVP **7.** BNO **8.** I & O **9.** ATN **10.** ESRD

G. **1.** drooping **2.** condition of the urine **3.** stone **4.** surgical crushing **5.** condition of stones

H. **1.** renal transplant **2.** nephropexy **3.** urinary tract infection **4.** pyelolithectomy **5.** renal biopsy **6.** ureterectomy **7.** cystostomy **8.** cystoscopy **9.** IVP

Labeling Exercise

A. **1.** kidney **2.** urinary bladder **3.** ureter **4.** male urethra **5.** female urethra

B. **1.** cortex **2.** medulla **3.** calyx **4.** renal pelvis **5.** renal papilla **6.** renal pyramid **7.** ureter

C. **1.** efferent arteriole **2.** glomerular (Bowman's) capsule **3.** glomerulus **4.** afferent arteriole **5.** proximal convoluted tubule **6.** descending nephron loop **7.** distal convoluted tubule **8.** collecting tubule **9.** ascending nephron loop **10.** peritubular capillaries

Chapter 10 Answers

Practice As You Go

A. **1.** uterine tubes **2.** gestation **3.** dilation, expulsion, placental **4.** menopause **5.** ovum **6.** endometrium **7.** uterus

B. **1.** embryonic **2.** fetal **3.** uterine **4.** ovarian **5.** mammary **6.** vaginal

C. **1.** b **2.** h **3.** g **4.** c **5.** a **6.** i **7.** j **8.** d **9.** e **10.** f

D. **1.** e **2.** g **3.** d **4.** a **5.** h **6.** c **7.** b **8.** f

E. **1.** GI, grav I **2.** AI **3.** UC **4.** FTND **5.** IUD **6.** D & C **7.** HRT **8.** gyn/GYN **9.** AB **10.** OCPs

F. **1.** urinary, reproductive **2.** testes, epididymis, penis **3.** foreskin **4.** testes **5.** bulbourethral glands **6.** testosterone **7.** perineum

G. **1.** testicular **2.** spermatic **3.** vesicular **4.** penile **5.** prostatic

H. **1.** b **2.** e **3.** a **4.** c **5.** f **6.** d

I. **1.** c **2.** a **3.** d **4.** b **5.** e

J. **1.** ED **2.** GC **3.** DRE **4.** TURP **5.** STI

Real-World Applications

Medical Chart Analysis

1. gestation—The length of time of pregnancy, normally about 40 weeks.
2. amniocentesis—Puncturing of the amniotic sac using a needle and syringe for the purpose of withdrawing amniotic fluid for testing. Can assist in determining fetal maturity, development, and genetic disorders.

3. fetus—The unborn infant from approximately week 9 until birth.
4. obstetrician—Branch of medicine specializing in the diagnosis and treatment of women during pregnancy and childbirth, and immediately after childbirth. Physician is called an *obstetrician*.
5. multigravida—A woman who has been pregnant two or more times.
6. nullipara—A woman who has not given birth to a live infant.
7. miscarriage—Unplanned loss of a pregnancy due to the death of the embryo or fetus before the time it is viable, also referred to as a *spontaneous abortion*.
8. pelvic ultrasound—Use of high-frequency sound waves to produce an image or photograph of an organ, such as the uterus, ovaries, or fetus.
9. placenta previa—A placenta that is implanted in the lower portion of the uterus and, in turn, blocks the birth canal.
10. abruptio placentae—Emergency condition in which the placenta tears away from the uterine wall prior to delivery of the infant. Requires immediate delivery of the baby.
11. placenta—The organ that connects the fetus to the mother's uterus, supplies fetus with oxygen and nutrients.
12. C-section—Surgical delivery of a baby through an incision into the abdominal and uterine walls.

Chart Note Transcription

1. ejaculation **2.** cryptorchidism **3.** orchidopexy **4.** vasectomy **5.** ejaculation **6.** digital rectal exam (DRE) **7.** prostate cancer **8.** prostate-specific antigen (PSA) **9.** benign prostatic hyperplasia (BPH) **10.** transurethral resection (TUR)

Case Study

1. Genital herpes.
2. Fever—She has a temperature; malaise—A feeling of general discomfort; dysuria—Painful urination; vaginal leukorrhea—A white discharge or flow from the vagina.
3. Vesicles—Small fluid-filled blisters; ulcers–Craterlike erosions of the skin; erythema–redness; edema–Swelling.
4. An abnormality located on the body in some area outside of the genital region.
5. To feel with your hands.
6. There is a risk of passing the virus to the baby as it passes through the birth canal.

Practice Exercises

A. **1.** suprapubic prostatectomy **2.** transurethral resection **3.** genitourinary **4.** benign prostatic hyperplasia **5.** prostate-specific antigen **6.** cervix **7.** last menstrual period **8.** fetal heart rate **9.** pelvic inflammatory disease **10.** gynecology **11.** cesarean section **12.** newborn **13.** premenstrual syndrome **14.** toxic shock syndrome **15.** low birth weight

B. **1.** the formation of mature sperm **2.** accumulation of fluid within the testes **3.** surgical removal of the prostate gland by inserting a device through the urethra and removing prostate tissue **4.** inability to father children due to a problem with spermatogenesis **5.** surgical removal of the testes **6.** surgical removal of part or all of the vas deferens **7.** removal of the testicles in the male or the ovaries in the female **8.** the normal length of time of pregnancy, about 37 weeks **9.** first bowel movement of newborn **10.** a woman who has never been pregnant **11.** difficult labor and childbirth **12.** discharge from the uterus other than the menstrual flow **13.** a benign fibrous growth **14.** benign cysts forming in the breast **15.** placenta implants in lower uterus and blocks birth canal

C. **1.** colposcopy **2.** colposcope **3.** cervicectomy **4.** cervicitis **5.** hysteropexy **6.** hysterectomy **7.** hysterorrhexis **8.** oophoritis **9.** oophorectomy **10.** mammogram **11.** mammoplasty **12.** amniotomy **13.** amniorrhea **14.** prostatectomy **15.** prostatitis **16.** orchiectomy **17.** orchioplasty **18.** orchiotomy **19.** aspermia **20.** oligospermia **21.** spermatogenesis **22.** spermatolysis

D. **1.** uterus **2.** uterus **3.** female **4.** vulva **5.** ovary **6.** ovary **7.** uterine tube **8.** menstruation or menses **9.** vagina **10.** breast **11.** sperm **12.** testes **13.** male **14.** penis **15.** prostate

E. **1.** labor, childbirth **2.** pregnancy **3.** beginning **4.** pregnancy **5.** childbirth **6.** to bear (offspring) **7.** uterine tube **8.** sperm condition

F. **1.** conization **2.** stillbirth **3.** puberty **4.** premenstrual syndrome **5.** laparoscopy **6.** fibroid tumor **7.** D & C **8.** eclampsia **9.** endometriosis **10.** cesarean section

G. **1.** e **2.** i **3.** h **4.** c **5.** a **6.** d **7.** g **8.** b **9.** f

H. **1.** androgen therapy, f **2.** oxytocin, a **3.** antiprostatic agent, b **4.** birth control pills, g **5.** spermatocide, d **6.** erectile dysfunction agent, h **7.** hormone replacement therapy, i **8.** abortifacient, e **9.** fertility drug, c

Labeling Exercise

A. **1.** uterine tube **2.** ovary **3.** fundus of uterus **4.** corpus (body) of uterus **5.** cervix **6.** vagina **7.** clitoris **8.** labium majora **9.** labium minora

B. **1.** seminal vesicle **2.** vas deferens **3.** prostate gland **4.** bulbourethral gland **5.** urethra **6.** epididymis **7.** glans penis **8.** testis

C. **1.** areola **2.** nipple **3.** lactiferous gland **4.** lactiferous duct **5.** fat

Chapter 11 Answers

Practice As You Go

A. **1.** endocrinology **2.** pituitary **3.** gonads **4.** corticosteroids **5.** testosterone **6.** estrogen, progesterone **7.** antidiuretic hormone (ADH) **8.** thymus gland

B. **1.** thymic **2.** pancreatic **3.** thyroidal **4.** ovarian **5.** testicular

C. **1.** b **2.** a **3.** e **4.** h **5.** j **6.** i **7.** f **8.** g **9.** c **10.** d

D. **1.** e **2.** d **3.** a **4.** f **5.** c **6.** b **7.** h **8.** g

E. **1.** NIDDM **2.** IDDM **3.** ACTH **4.** PTH **5.** T_3 **6.** TSH **7.** FBS **8.** PRL

Real-World Applications

Medical Record Analysis

1. hyperglycemia—The condition of having a high level of sugar in the blood; associated with diabetes mellitus.
2. ketoacidosis—Acidosis due to an excess of acidic ketone bodies (waste products). A serious condition requiring immediate treatment that can result in death for the diabetic patient if not reversed. Also called *diabetic acidosis.*
3. glycosuria—Having a high level of sugar excreted in the urine.
4. type 1 diabetes mellitus—Also called *insulin-dependent diabetes mellitus.* It develops early in life when the pancreas stops insulin production. Patient must take daily insulin injections.
5. polyuria—The condition of producing an excessive amount of urine.
6. polydipsia—Excessive feeling of thirst.
7. fasting blood sugar—Blood test to measure the amount of sugar circulating throughout the body after a 12-hour fast.
8. insulin—Medication administered to replace insulin for type 1 diabetics or to treat severe type 2 diabetics.
9. glucose tolerance test—Test to determine the blood sugar level. A measured dose of glucose is given to a patient either orally or intravenously. Blood samples are then drawn at certain intervals to determine the ability of the patient to use glucose. Used for diabetic patients to determine their insulin response to glucose.
10. glucometer—A device designed for a diabetic to use at home to measure the level of glucose in the bloodstream.

Chart Note Transcription

1. endocrinologist **2.** obesity **3.** hirsutism **4.** radio immunoassay (RIA) **5.** cortisol **6.** adenoma **7.** adrenal cortex **8.** Cushing's syndrome **9.** adenoma **10.** adrenal cortex **11.** adrenalectomy

Case Study

1. Diabetes mellitus.
2. Diaphoresis—Profuse sweating; rapid respirations—Breathing fast; rapid pulse—Fast heart rate; disorientation—Confused about his surroundings.
3. Blood serum test—Lab test to measure the levels of different substances in the blood, used to determine the function of endocrine glands.
4. Hyperglycemia—Blood level of glucose is too high; ketoacidosis—an excessive amount of acidic ketone bodies in the body.
5. Type 1, insulin-dependent, or juvenile diabetes mellitus because he has had it since childhood and he is taking insulin shots.
6. Type 2, non-insulin-dependent diabetes mellitus typically develops later in life. The pancreas produces normal to high levels of insulin, but the cells fail to respond to it. Patients may take oral hypoglycemic agents to improve insulin function, or may eventually have to take insulin.

Practice Exercises

A. **1.** thyroidectomy **2.** thyroidal **3.** hyperthyroidism **4.** pancreatic **5.** pancreatitis **6.** pancreatectomy **7.** pancreatotomy **8.** adrenal **9.** adrenomegaly **10.** adrenopathy **11.** thymoma **12.** thymectomy **13.** thymic **14.** thymitis

B. **1.** sodium **2.** female **3.** pineal gland **4.** pituitary gland **5.** potassium **6.** calcium **7.** parathyroid glands **8.** extremities **9.** sugar **10.** sex glands

C. **1.** protein-bound iodine **2.** potassium **3.** thyroxine **4.** glucose tolerance test **5.** diabetes mellitus **6.** basal metabolic rate **7.** sodium **8.** antidiuretic hormone

D. **1.** glycosuria **2.** vasopressin **3.** polyuria **4.** hypercalcemia **5.** polydipsia **6.** gonadotropin **7.** postprandial

E. **1.** hormone obtained from cortex of adrenal gland **2.** having excessive hair **3.** a nerve condition characterized with spasms of extremities; can occur from imbalance of pH and calcium or disorder of parathyroid gland **4.** disorder of the retina occurring with diabetes mellitus **5.** increase in blood sugar level **6.** decrease in blood sugar level **7.** another term for epinephrine; produced by inner portion of adrenal gland **8.** hormone produced by pancreas; essential for metabolism of blood sugar **9.** toxic condition due to hyperactivity of thyroid gland **10.** a condition resulting when the endocrine gland secretes more hormone than is needed by the body

F. **1.** insulinoma **2.** ketoacidosis **3.** panhypopituitarinism **4.** pheochromocytoma **5.** Hashimoto's thyroiditis **6.** gynecomastia

G. **1.** corticosteroids, e **2.** human growth hormone therapy, a **3.** oral hypoglycemic agent, d **4.** antithyroid agent, c **5.** insulin, f **6.** vasopressin, b

Labeling Exercise

A. **1.** pineal gland **2.** thyroid and parathyroid glands **3.** adrenal glands **4.** pancreas **5.** pituitary gland **6.** thymus gland **7.** ovary **8.** testis

B. **1.** pituitary gland **2.** bone and soft tissue **3.** GH **4.** testes **5.** FSH, LH **6.** ovary **7.** FSH, LH **8.** thyroid gland **9.** TSH **10.** adrenal cortex **11.** ACTH **12.** breast **13.** PRL

C. **1.** liver **2.** stomach **3.** pancreas **4.** beta cell **5.** alpha cell **6.** islets of Langerhans

Chapter 12 Answers

Practice As You Go

A. **1.** brain, spinal cord, nerves **2.** peripheral nervous system, central nervous system **3.** efferent or motor; afferent or sensory **4.** cerebrum **5.** cerebellum **6.** eyesight **7.** hearing, smell **8.** parasympathetic, sympathetic

B. **1.** cerebrospinal **2.** meningeal **3.** subdural **4.** encephalic **5.** neural **6.** intracranial

C. **1.** b **2.** f **3.** g **4.** h **5.** i **6.** j **7.** e **8.** c **9.** d **10.** a

D. **1.** e **2.** c **3.** g **4.** b **5.** a **6.** d **7.** d **8.** f

E. **1.** CSF **2.** CVD **3.** EEG **4.** ICP **5.** PET **6.** CVA **7.** ANS

Real World Applications

Medical Chart Analysis

1. paraplegia—Paralysis of the lower portion of the body and both legs.
2. comminuted fracture—Fracture in which the bone is shattered, splintered, or crushed into many small pieces or fragments.
3. epidural hematoma—Mass of blood in the space outside the dura mater of the brain and spinal cord.
4. spinal cord injury—Damage to the spinal cord as a result of trauma. Spinal cord may be bruised or completely severed.
5. unconscious—State of being unaware of surroundings, with the inability to respond to stimuli.
6. anesthesia—The lack of feeling or sensation.
7. paralysis—Temporary or permanent loss of function or voluntary movement.
8. computed tomography scan (CT scan)—An imaging technique that is able to produce a cross-sectional view of the body.
9. laminectomy—Removal of a portion of a vertebra, called the *lamina*, in order to relieve pressure on the spinal nerve.
10. spinal fusion—Surgical immobilization of adjacent vertebrae. This may be done for several reasons, including correction for a herniated disk.
11. physical therapy (PT)—Treats disorders using physical means and methods; includes joint motion and muscle strength.
12. occupational therapy (OT)—Assists patients to regain, develop, and improve skills that are important for independent functioning.

Chart Note Transcription

1. neurologist **2.** dysphasia **3.** hemiplegia **4.** convulsions **5.** electroencephalography (EEG) **6.** lumbar puncture (LP) **7.** brain scan **8.** cerebral cortex **9.** astrocytoma **10.** craniotomy **11.** cryosurgery

Case Study

1. Cerebrovascular accident (CVA or stroke).
2. aphasia—Inability to speak; hemiparesis—Weakness on one side of the body; syncope—Fainting; delirium—Abnormal mental state with confusion, disorientation, and agitation.
3. hypertension—High blood pressure; atherosclerosis—Hardening of arteries due to buildup of yellow fatty substances; diabetes mellitus—Inability to make or use insulin properly to control blood sugar levels.
4. brain scan—An image of the brain after injection of radioactive isotopes into the circulation; revealed an infarct in the right cerebral hemisphere.
5. infarct—An area of tissue within an organ that undergoes necrosis (death) following the loss of its blood supply.
6. hemorrhage—Ruptured blood vessel; thrombus—Stationary clot; embolus—Floating clot; compression—Pinching off a blood vessel.

Practice Exercises

A. **1.** h **2.** k **3.** d **4.** g **5.** a **6.** b **7.** f **8.** j **9.** e **10.** l **11.** i **12.** c

B. **1.** neuritis **2.** neurologist **3.** neuralgia **4.** polyneuritis **5.** neurectomy **6.** neuroplasty **7.** neuroma **8.** neurorrhaphy **9.** meningitis **10.** meningocele **11.** myelomeningocele **12.** encephalogram **13.** encephalopathy **14.** encephalitis **15.** encephalocele **16.** cerebrospinal **17.** cerebral

C. **1.** transient ischemic attack **2.** multiple sclerosis **3.** spinal cord injury **4.** central nervous system **5.** peripheral nervous system **6.** headache **7.** cerebral palsy **8.** lumbar puncture **9.** amyotrophic lateral sclerosis

D. **1.** injecting radiopaque dye into spinal canal to examine under X-ray the outlines made by the dye **2.** X-ray of the blood vessels of the brain after the injection of radiopaque dye **3.** reflex test on bottom of foot to detect lesion and abnormalities of nervous system **4.** test that measures how fast an impulse travels along a nerve to pinpoint an area of nerve damage **5.** laboratory examination of fluid taken from the brain and spinal cord **6.** positron emission tomography to measure cerebral blood flow, blood volume, oxygen, and glucose uptake **7.** recording the ultrasonic echoes of the brain **8.** needle puncture into the spinal cavity to withdraw fluid

E. **1.** paralysis **2.** muscular coordination **3.** pertaining to development **4.** weakness **5.** speech

F. **1.** meninges **2.** brain **3.** cerebellum **4.** spinal cord **5.** head **6.** thalamus **7.** nerve **8.** nerve root **9.** cerebrum **10.** pons

G. **1.** tumor of astrocyte cells **2.** seizure **3.** without sensation **4.** weakness of one-half of body **5.** physician that treats nervous system with surgery **6.** without sense of pain **7.** localized seizure of one limb **8.** paralysis of all four limbs **9.** accumulation of blood in the subdural space **10.** within the meninges

H. **1.** d **2.** e **3.** f **4.** g **5.** b **6.** a **7.** c **8.** j **9.** h **10.** i

I. **1.** delirium **2.** amyotrophic lateral sclerosis **3.** Bell's palsy **4.** cerebral aneurysm **5.** Parkinson's disease **6.** cerebrospinal fluid shunt **7.** transient ischemic attack **8.** subdural hematoma **9.** cerebral palsy **10.** nerve conduction velocity

J. **1.** anesthetic, e **2.** dopaminergic drugs, a **3.** hypnotic, d **4.** analgesic, g **5.** sedative, b **6.** narcotic analgesic, c **7.** anticonvulsant, f

Labeling Exercise

A. **1.** brain **2.** spinal nerves **3.** spinal cord

B. **1.** dendrites **2.** nerve cell body **3.** unmyelinated region **4.** myelinated axon **5.** nucleus **6.** axon **7.** terminal end fibers

C. **1.** cerebrum **2.** diencephalon **3.** thalamus **4.** hypothalamus **5.** brain stem **6.** midbrain **7.** cerebellum **8.** pons **9.** medulla oblongata

Chapter 13 Answers

Practice As You Go

A. **1.** ophthalmology **2.** cilia **3.** lacrimal **4.** cornea **5.** retina **6.** iris

B. **1.** pupillary **2.** optic or optical **3.** retinal **4.** lacrimal **5.** intraocular **6.** extraocular

C. **1.** h **2.** g **3.** a **4.** d **5.** b **6.** i **7.** c **8.** f **9.** e **10.** j

D. **1.** d **2.** a **3.** f **4.** e **5.** b **6.** c

E. **1.** PE tube **2.** EM **3.** XT **4.** OS **5.** EOM **6.** VA

F. **1.** malleus, incus, stapes **2.** otology **3.** tympanic membrane **4.** cerumen **5.** eustachian or auditory **6.** vestibulocochlear nerve

G. **1.** cochlear **2.** otic, aural, or auricular **3.** vestibular **4.** acoustic or auditory **5.** monoaural

H. **1.** e **2.** h **3.** a **4.** g **5.** j **6.** c **7.** i **8.** b **9.** d **10.** f

I. **1.** c **2.** b **3.** d **4.** a **5.** g **6.** h **7.** e **8.** f

J. **1.** OE **2.** EENT **3.** BC **4.** AU **5.** OM

Real-World Applications

Medical Record Analysis

1. photophobia—Although the term translates into *fear of light*, it actually means a strong sensitivity to bright light.
2. hyperopia—With this condition a person can see things in the distance but has trouble reading material at close range. Also known as *farsightedness.* This condition is corrected with converging or biconvex lenses.
3. visual acuity test—Measurement of the sharpness of a patient's vision. Usually, a Snellen chart is used for this test in which the patient identifies letters from a distance of 20 feet.
4. intraocular—Pertaining to inside the eye.
5. ophthalmoscopy—Examination of the interior of the eyes using an instrument called an *ophthalmoscope*. The physician dilates the pupil in order to see the cornea, lens, and retina. Used to identify abnormalities in the blood vessels of the eye and some systemic diseases.
6. mydriatic drops—Any substance that causes the pupil to dilate by paralyzing the iris and/or ciliary body muscles. Particularly useful during eye examinations and eye surgery.
7. cataract—Damage to the lens causing it to become opaque or cloudy, resulting in diminished vision. Treatment is usually surgical removal of the cataract or replacement of the lens.
8. retinopathy—A general term for disease affecting the retina.
9. macular degeneration—Deterioration of the macular area of the retina of the eye. May be treated with laser surgery to destroy the blood vessels beneath the macula.
10. phacoemulsification—Use of high-frequency sound waves to emulsify (liquefy) a lens with a cataract, which is then aspirated (removed by suction) with a needle.
11. prosthetic lens implant—The use of an artificial lens to replace the lens removed during cataract surgery.

Chart Note Transcription

1. otorhinolaryngologist (ENT) **2.** otitis media (OM) **3.** AU, binaural **4.** otoscopy **5.** tympanic membrane **6.** cerumen **7.** tympanometry **8.** audiometric test **9.** conductive hearing loss **10.** myringotomy

Case Study

1. Conductive hearing loss results from disease or malformation of the outer or middle ear; all sound is weaker because it is not conducted correctly to the inner ear.
2. Sensorineural hearing loss as a result of damage or malformation of the inner ear or the cochlear nerve.
3. Otoscopy examination of the auditory canal and middle ear; tympanometry measurement of the movement of the tympanic membrane; audiometry test for hearing ability; Rinne and Weber tuning-fork tests assess both the nerve and bone conduction of sound.
4. Hearing aids or amplification devices amplify sound and will work best for conductive hearing loss; cochlear implant is a device that converts sound signals into magnetic impulses to stimulate the auditory nerve and is used to treat profound sensorineural hearing loss.
5. Protect his ears better during playing music by wearing earplugs.

Practice Exercises

A. **1.** artificial tears, h **2.** antiglaucoma medication, c **3.** antibiotic otic solution, i **4.** mydriatic, a **5.** antiemetic, g **6.** antibiotic ophthalmic solution, j **7.** anti-inflammatory otic solution, b **8.** miotic, f **9.** wax emulsifier, e **10.** anesthetic ophthalmic solution, d

B. **1.** blepharitis **2.** blepharoplasty **3.** blepharoptosis **4.** retinopathy **5.** retinopexy **6.** ophthalmology **7.** ophthalmic **8.** ophthalmoscopy **9.** iridoplegia **10.** iridectomy **11.** otoplasty **12.** otopyorrhea **13.** otalgia **14.** otitis **15.** tympanorrhexis **16.** tympanotomy **17.** tympanitis **18.** audiogram **19.** audiometer **20.** audiology

C. **1.** -tropia **2.** -opia **3.** -itis **4.** -logy **5.** -otomy **6.** -plasty **7.** -pexy **8.** -algia **9.** -otia **10.** -cusis

D. **1.** tear or tear duct **2.** choroid **3.** water **4.** light **5.** cornea **6.** glassy **7.** double **8.** gray **9.** old age **10.** dull or dim **11.** ear **12.** stapes **13.** hearing **14.** eustachian or auditory tube **15.** eardrum or tympanic membrane

E. **1.** conductive—problem with outer or middle ear, muffles sound; sensorineural—damage of inner ear or nerve **2.** cornea, pupil, lens, retina **3.** mucous membrane that covers and protects front of eyeball **4.** incus, malleus, stapes, vibrate to amplify and conduct sound waves from outer ear to inner ear

F. **1.** otology **2.** both eyes **3.** rapid eye movement **4.** hertz **5.** senile macular degeneration **6.** pupils equal, round, react to light and accommodation **7.** intraocular pressure **8.** decibel **9.** right eye **10.** visual field

G. **1.** tonometry **2.** emmetropia **3.** conjunctivitis **4.** myopia **5.** cataract **6.** hordeolum **7.** strabismus **8.** hyperopia **9.** presbycusis **10.** otorhinolaryngologist **11.** inner ear **12.** Ménière's disease **13.** acoustic neuroma

H. **1.** dull/dim vision **2.** double vision **3.** enlarge or widen pupil **4.** constrict pupil **5.** diminished vision of old age **6.** ringing in the ears **7.** middle ear bone **8.** measure movement in eardrum **9.** auditory tube **10.** inner ear **11.** results of hearing test **12.** middle ear infection

Labeling Exercise

A. **1.** iris **2.** lens **3.** conjunctiva **4.** pupil **5.** cornea **6.** suspensory ligaments **7.** ciliary body **8.** fovea centralis **9.** optic nerve **10.** retina **11.** choroid **12.** sclera

B. **1.** pinna **2.** external auditory meatus **3.** auditory canal **4.** tympanic membrane **5.** malleus **6.** incus **7.** semicircular canals **8.** vestibular nerve **9.** cochlear nerve **10.** cochlea **11.** round window **12.** stapes **13.** Eustachian tube

Chapter 14 Answers

Real-World Applications

Chart Note Transcription

1. oncologist **2.** exploratory surgery **3.** biopsies **4.** malignant **5.** neoplasm **6.** Grade II **7.** encapsulated **8.** metastases **9.** nephrocarcinoma **10.** protocol **11.** chemotherapy

Case Study

1. Bronchogenic carcinoma—lung cancer that begins in the bronchial tubes.
2. Dyspnea—difficulty breathing; cough producing thick sputum—coughing up thick mucus material; hemoptysis—coughing up blood.
3. Computed tomography scan (CT scan)—An imaging technique that is able to produce a cross-sectional view of the body. X-ray pictures are taken at multiple angles through the body. A computer then uses all these images to construct a composite cross-section, scan revealed a mass in the right lung.
4. Sputum culture and sensitivity—testing sputum by placing it on a culture medium and observing any bacterial growth. The specimen is then tested to determine antibiotic effectiveness, there was no bacterial growth; sputum cytology examining sputum for malignant cells, cells were found

that confirmed the presence of bronchogenic carcinoma.

5. Lobectomy—removal of a lobe of the lung.
6. The tumor has spread to other areas of the body.

Practice Exercises

A. **1.** *Physician's Desk Reference* (PDR) **2.** pharmacist **3.** generic or nonproprietary **4.** brand or proprietary **5.** the chemical formula **6.** Drug Enforcement Agency

B. **1.** sublingual **2.** rectal **3.** topical **4.** intradermal **5.** intramuscular **6.** intravenous **7.** oral

C. **1.** unusual or abnormal response to a drug **2.** administration of a drug through a needle and syringe under the skin, or into a muscle, vein, or body cavity **3.** harmless substance to satisfy patient's desire for medication **4.** extent to which a substance is poisonous **5.** response to drug other than the expected response **6.** prepackaged and prelabeled method of medication distribution **7.** emotional dependence on a drug **8.** substance that neutralizes poisons **9.** condition under which a particular drug should not be used **10.** prevention of disease

D. **1.** grain **2.** two times a day **3.** three times a day **4.** as desired **5.** as needed **6.** before **7.** over the counter **8.** drop **9.** label as follows/directions **10.** immediately **11.** milligram **12.** aqueous **13.** night **14.** nothing by mouth **15.** at bedtime **16.** intravenous **17.** telephone order **18.** drops **19.** after meals **20.** discontinue

E. **1.** Pravachol, 20 milligrams each, take one every day at bedtime, supply with 30, refill three times with no substitutions **2.** Lanoxin, 0.125 milligram each, take three now and then 2 every morning, supply with 100 and may refill as needed **3.** Synthroid, 0.075 milligram each, take 1 every day, supply with 100 and may refill four times **4.** Norvasc, 5 milligrams each, take 1 every morning, supply with 60 and may refill

F. **1.** i **2.** k **3.** h **4.** j **5.** e **6.** f **7.** b **8.** a **9.** d **10.** c **11.** g

G. **1.** minor tranquilizers **2.** humanistic psychotherapy **3.** lithium **4.** antipsychotic drugs **5.** psychoanalysis **6.** antidepressant drugs

H. **1.** general anesthesia **2.** local anesthesia **3.** topical anesthesia **4.** regional anesthesia

I. **1.** h **2.** c **3.** b **4.** g **5.** f **6.** a **7.** d **8.** e **9.** i

J. **1.** range of motion **2.** occupational therapy **3.** activities of daily living **4.** lower extremity **5.** electromyogram **6.** transcutaneous electrical nerve stimulation **7.** physical therapy **8.** passive range of motion **9.** electrical stimulation **10.** ultrasound

K. **1.** massage **2.** debridement **3.** hydrotherapy **4.** postural drainage with clapping **5.** active exercises **6.** phonophoresis **7.** cryotherapy **8.** traction

L. **1.** h **2.** e **3.** j **4.** g **5.** a **6.** i **7.** c **8.** f **9.** b **10.** d

M. **1.** magnetic resonance imaging **2.** barium **3.** anteroposterior **4.** computerized tomography **5.** right lateral **6.** posteroanterior **7.** left lateral **8.** positron emission tomography **9.** upper gastrointestinal series **10.** kidneys, ureters, bladder

N. **1.** h **2.** d **3.** g **4.** j **5.** f **6.** b **7.** i **8.** a **9.** e **10.** c

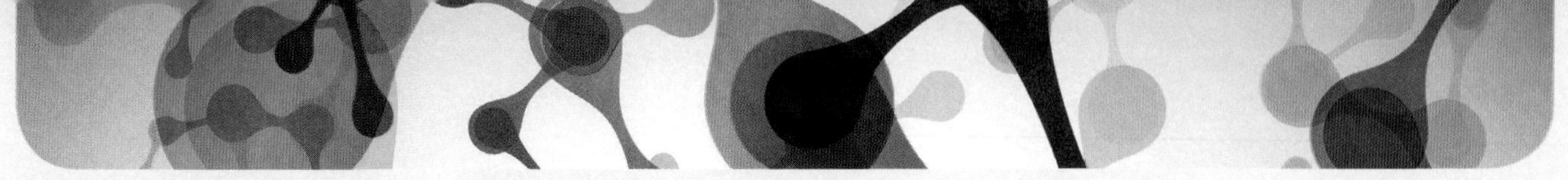

Glossary/Index

Note: Headings in **bold** indicate definitions. Page numbers with *t* indicate tables; those with *f* indicate figures.

Additive, sum of action of two (or more) drugs given; in this case, total strength of medications is equal to sum of strength of each individual drug, 506
Adduction, directional term meaning to move toward median or middle line of body, 11, 118*t*, 118*f*
Adenocarcinoma, malignant adenoma in a glandular organ, 404
Adenoidectomy, surgical removal of adenoids, 208
Adenoiditis, inflammation of adenoids, 204
Adenoids, another term for pharyngeal tonsils; tonsils are a collection of lymphatic tissue found in nasopharynx to combat microorganisms entering body through nose or mouth, 199, 206
Adhesion, scar tissue forming in fascia surrounding a muscle making it difficult to stretch muscle, 121
Adipose, type of connective tissue; also called *fat*; stores energy and provides protective padding for underlying structures, 25
Adjective suffixes, 9
Adrenal, pertaining to adrenal glands, 398
Adrenal cortex, outer layer of adrenal glands; secretes several families of hormones: mineralocorticoids, glucocorticoids, and steroid sex hormones, 388*t*, 390
Adrenal feminization, development of female secondary sexual characteristics (such as breasts) in a male; often as a result of increased estrogen secretion by adrenal cortex, 400
Adrenal glands, pair of glands in endocrine system located just above each kidney; composed of two sections, cortex and medulla, that function independently of each other; cortex secretes steroids, such as aldosterone, cortisol, androgens, estrogens, and progestins; medulla secretes epinephrine and norepinephrine; regulated by adrenocorticotropic hormone, which is secreted by pituitary gland, 31, 387, 390, 390*f*, 400
Adrenal medulla, inner portion of adrenal gland; secretes epinephrine and norepinephrine, 388*t*, 390
Adrenal virilism, development of male secondary sexual characteristics (such as deeper voice and facial hair) in a female; often as a result of increased androgen secretion by adrenal cortex, 400
Adrenalectomy, surgical removal of one or both adrenal glands, 406
Adrenaline, hormone produced by adrenal medulla; also known as epinephrine; some of its actions include increasing heart rate and force of contraction, bronchodilation, and relaxation of intestinal muscles, 390
Adrenalitis, inflammation of adrenal gland, 400
Adrenocorticotropic hormone (ACTH), hormone secreted by anterior pituitary; regulates function of adrenal gland cortex, 389*t*, 393
Adrenomegaly, enlarged adrenal gland, 398
Adrenopathy, adrenal gland disease, 399
Adult respiratory distress syndrome (ARDS), acute respiratory failure in adults characterized by tachypnea, dyspnea, cyanosis, tachycardia, and hypoxemia, 239
Adverse reaction. *See* Side effect
Aerosol, drugs inhaled directly into nose and mouth, 505*t*
Aerosol therapy, medication suspended in mist intended to be inhaled; delivered by a *nebulizer*, which delivers mist for period of time while patient breathes, or a *metered-dose inhaler* (MDI), which delivers a single puff of mist, 246
Afferent, moving toward, 307
Afferent arteriole, arteriole that carries blood into glomerulus, 307, 308*f*, 310*f*
Afferent neurons, neurons that carry impulses to brain and spinal cord from skin and sense organs; also called *sensory neurons*, 426
Agglutinate, clumping together to form small clusters; platelets agglutinate to start clotting process, 184
Agranulocytes, nongranular leukocyte; one of two types of leukocytes found in plasma that are classified as either monocytes or lymphocytes, 183, 183*t*
AIDS-related complex (ARC), early stage of AIDS; there is a positive test for virus but only mild symptoms of weight loss, fatigue, skin rash, and anorexia, 206
Alanine transaminase (ALT), enzyme normally present in blood; levels are increased in persons with liver disease, 285
Albinism, genetic condition in which person is not able to produce melanin; an albino has white hair and skin and pupils of eyes are red, 62
Albumin, protein normally found circulating in bloodstream; it is abnormal for albumin to be in urine, 183, 311
Aldosterone, hormone produced by adrenal cortex; regulates levels of sodium and potassium in body and as a side effect volume of water lost in urine, 390
Alimentary canal, also known as gastrointestinal system or digestive system; covers area between mouth and anus and includes 30 feet of intestinal tubing; has a wide range of functions; serves to store and digest food, absorb nutrients, and eliminate waste; major organs include mouth, pharynx, esophagus, stomach, small intestine, colon, rectum, and anus, 264
Allergen, antigen capable of causing a hypersensitivity or allergy in body, 204
Allergist, physician who specializes in testing for and treating allergies, 203
Allergy, hypersensitivity to a substance in environment or medication, 204
Allograft, skin graft from one person to another; donor is usually a cadaver, 69
Alopecia, absence or loss of hair, especially of head, 67
Alveolar, pertaining to alveoli, 233
Alveoli, tiny air sacs at end of each bronchiole; surrounded by capillary network; gas exchange takes place as oxygen and carbon dioxide diffuse across alveolar and capillary walls, 227, 228*f*
Alzheimer's disease (AD), chronic, organic mental disorder consisting of dementia, which is more prevalent in adults after 65 years of age; involves progressive disorientation, apathy, speech and gait disturbances, and loss of memory, 432, 511

Angiospasm, involuntary muscle contraction of a vessel, 154
Angiostenosis, narrowing of a vessel, 154
Anhidrosis, abnormal condition of no sweat, 57
Ankylosing spondylitis, inflammatory spinal condition that resembles rheumatoid arthritis; results in gradual stiffening and fusion of vertebrae; more common in men than in women, 103
Anorchism, absence of one or both testes; may be congenital or result of accident or surgery, 368
Anorexia, loss of appetite that can accompany other conditions such as gastrointestinal (GI) upset, 277
Anorexia nervosa, type of eating disorder characterized by distorted body image, a pathological fear of becoming fat, and severe weight loss due to excessive dieting, 277, 511, 511*f*
Anorexiant, substance that treats obesity by suppressing appetite, 290
Anosmia, loss of sense of smell, 235
Anoxia, lack of oxygen, 235
Antacid, substance that neutralizes acid in stomach, 290
Antagonistic pairs, pair of muscles arranged around a joint that produce opposite actions, 117, 118–19*t*
Anteflexion, while uterus is normally in this position, exaggeration of forward bend of uterus is abnormal; forward bend is near neck of uterus; position of cervix, or opening of uterus, remains normal, 340
Antepartum, before birth, 348
Anterior, directional term meaning more toward the front or belly side of body, 39*f*, 39*t*
Anterior lobe, anterior portion of pituitary gland; secretes adrenocorticotropic hormone, follicle-stimulating hormone, growth hormone, luteinizing hormone, melanocyte-stimulating hormone, prolactin, and thyroid-stimulating hormone, 393
Anterior pituitary gland, 393–94*f*
Anterior tibial artery, 148*f*
Anterior tibial vein, 150*f*
Anteroposterior view (AP), positioning patient so that X-rays pass through body from anterior side to posterior side, 517
Anthracosis, type of pneumoconiosis that develops from collection of coal dust in lung; also called *black lung* or *miner's lung*, 240
Anti-inflammatory otic solution, reduces inflammation, itching, and edema associated with otitis externa, 488
Antiarrhythmic, controls cardiac arrhythmias by altering nerve impulses within heart, 166
Antibiotic, substance that destroys or prohibits growth of microorganisms; used to treat bacterial infections; not found effective in treating viral infections; to be effective, it must be taken regularly for specified period, 71, 249, 324
Antibiotic ophthalmic solution, eyedrops for treatment of bacterial eye infections, 473
Antibiotic otic solution, eardrops to treat otitis externa, 488
Antibody, protein material produced in body as a response to invasion of foreign substance, 200
Antibody-mediated immunity, production of antibodies by B cells in response to an antigen; also called *humoral immunity*, 200
Anticoagulant, substance that prevents or delays clotting or coagulation of blood, 166, 192
Anticonvulsant, prevents or relieves convulsions; drugs such as phenobarbital reduce excessive stimulation in brain to control seizures and other symptoms of epilepsy, 411
Antidepressant drugs, medications classified as stimulants that alter patient's mood by affecting levels of neurotransmitters in brain, 514
Antidiarrheal, prevents or relieves diarrhea, 290
Antidiuretic hormone (ADH), hormone secreted by posterior pituitary; promotes water reabsorption by kidney tubules, 389*t*, 393
Antidote, substance that will neutralize poisons or their side effects, 506
Antiemetic, substance that treats nausea, vomiting, and motion sickness, 291, 488
Antifungal, substance that kills fungi, 71
Antigen, substance capable of inducing formation of antibody; antibody then interacts with antigen in antigen–antibody reaction, 200
Antigen–antibody complex, combination of antigen with its specific antibody; increases susceptibility to phagocytosis and immunity, 201
Antiglaucoma medications, group of drugs that reduce intraocular pressure by lowering amount of aqueous humor in eyeball; may achieve this by either reducing production of aqueous humor or increasing its outflow, 473
Antihemorrhagic, substance that prevents or stops hemorrhaging, 192
Antihistamine, substance that acts to control allergic symptoms by counteracting histamine, which exists naturally in body, and is released in allergic reactions, 209, 249
Antilipidemic, substance that reduces amount of cholesterol and lipids in bloodstream; treats hyperlipidemia, 166
Antiparasitic, substance that kills mites or lice, 71
Antiplatelet agent, substance that interferes with action of platelets; prolongs bleeding time; used to prevent heart attacks and strokes, 166, 192
Antiprostatic agent, medication to treat early cases of benign prostatic hyperplasia; may prevent surgery for mild cases, 373
Antipruritic, substance that reduces severe itching, 71
Antipsychotic drugs, major tranquilizer drugs that have transformed treatment of patients with psychoses and schizophrenia by reducing patient agitation and panic and shortening schizophrenic episodes, 514
Antiseptic, substance used to kill bacteria in skin cuts and wounds or at a surgical site, 71
Antisocial personality disorder, personality disorder in which patient engages in behaviors that are illegal or outside of social norms, 512
Antispasmodic, medication to prevent or reduce bladder muscle spasms, 324

Asphyxia, lack of oxygen that can lead to unconsciousness and death if not corrected immediately; some common causes are drowning, foreign body in respiratory tract, poisoning, and electric shock, 235

Asphyxiation. *See* Asphyxia

Aspiration, for respiratory system, refers to inhaling food, liquid, or a foreign object into airways; term also refers to withdrawing fluid from body cavity using suction, 235

Aspirator, surgical instrument used to suction fluids, 530*t*

Asthma, disease caused by various conditions, such as allergens, and resulting in constriction of bronchial airways and labored respirations; can cause violent spasms of the bronchi (bronchospasms) but is generally not a life-threatening condition; medication can be very effective, 239

Astigmatism (Astigm), condition in which light rays are focused unevenly on eye, which causes distorted image due to abnormal curvature of cornea, 464

Astrocytoma, tumor of brain or spinal cord composed of astrocytes, 432

Ataxia, having lack of muscle coordination as a result of disorder or disease, 431

Atelectasis, condition in which lung tissue collapses, preventing respiratory exchange of oxygen and carbon dioxide; can be caused by a variety of conditions, including pressure upon lung from tumor or other object, 240

Atherectomy, surgical removal of fatty substance from an artery", 164

Atheroma, a deposit of fatty substance in an artery wall, 155, 159

Atherosclerosis, most common form of arteriosclerosis; caused by formation of yellowish plaques of cholesterol buildup on inner walls of arteries, 159

Atherosclerotic plaque, 155, 155*f*

Atonia, lack of tone, 121

Atria, two upper chambers of heart; left atrium receives blood returning from lungs, and right atrium receives blood returning from body, 143

Atrial, pertaining to atrium, 152

Atrial septal defect (ASD), a congenital septal defect between the atria, 156

Atrioventricular, pertaining to the atrium and ventricle, 152

Atrioventricular bundle, located in interventricular septum; receives electrical impulse from atrioventricular node and distributes it through ventricular walls, causing them to contract simultaneously, 145, 146*f*

Atrioventricular node, this area at junction of right atrium and ventricle receives stimulus from sinoatrial node and sends impulse to ventricles through bundle of His, 145, 146*f*

Atrioventricular valve (AV, A-V), heart valves located between atrium and ventricle; includes tricuspid valve in right side of heart and bicuspid or mitral valve in left side of heart, 144

Atrophy, lack or loss of normal development, 121

Attention-deficit/hyperactivity disorder (ADHD), type of mental disorder diagnosed in childhood characterized by poor attention and inability to control behavior; child may or may not be hyperactive, 511

Audiogram, chart that shows faintest sounds patient can hear during audiometry testing, 484

Audiologist, provides comprehensive array of services related to prevention, diagnosis, and treatment of hearing impairment and its associated communication disorders, 482

Audiology, study of hearing, 477, 482

Audiometer, instrument to measure hearing, 484

Audiometry, process of measuring hearing, 484, 484*f*

Auditory, pertaining to hearing, 481

Auditory canal, canal that leads from external opening of ear to eardrum, 477, 477*f*

Auditory tube, another name for eustachian tube connecting middle ear and nasopharynx, 226, 478

Aura, sensations, such as seeing colors or smelling unusual odor, that occur just prior to an epileptic seizure or a migraine headache, 431

Aural, pertaining to ear, 481

Auricle, also called pinna; external ear; functions to capture sound waves as they go past outer ear, 476, 477

Auricular, pertaining to ear, 481

Auscultation, listening to sounds within body by using stethoscope, 161

Autism spectrum disorder, range of conditions in which child exhibits deficits in social interaction, communication skills, and restricted patterns of behavior, 511

Autograft, skin graft from person's own body, 69, 69*f*

Autoimmune disease, disease resulting from the body's immune system attacking its own cells as if they were pathogens; examples include systemic lupus erythematosus, rheumatoid arthritis, and multiple sclerosis, 204

Autologous transfusion, procedure for collecting and storing patient's own blood several weeks prior to actual need; can then be used to replace blood lost during surgical procedure, 192

Autonomic nervous system (ANS), portion of nervous system consisting of nerves to internal organs that function involuntarily; regulates functions of glands (especially salivary, gastric, and sweat glands), adrenal medulla, heart, and smooth muscle tissue; system is divided into two parts: sympathetic and parasympathetic, 145, 426–27

Axial skeleton, axial skeleton includes bones in head, spine, chest, and trunk, 86, 87–90, 88*f*

Axillary, pertaining to armpit, 197*t*, 198*f*, 203

Axillary nodes, 197*t*

Axon, single projection of a neuron that conducts impulse away from nerve cell body, 420, 421*f*

Azotemia, accumulation of nitrogenous waste in bloodstream; occurs when kidney fails to filter these wastes from blood, 314

B

B cells, common name for B lymphocytes, responds to foreign antigens by producing protective antibodies, 200
B lymphocytes, humoral immunity cells, which respond to foreign antigens by producing protective antibodies; simply referred to as *B cells*, 200
Babinski's reflex, reflex test to determine lesions and abnormalities in nervous system; Babinski reflex is present if great toe extends instead of flexes when lateral sole of foot is stroked; normal response to this stimulation would be flexion, or upward movement, of toe, 439
Bacteria, primitive, single-celled microorganisms that are present everywhere; some are capable of causing disease in humans, 199
Bacteriuria, bacteria in urine, 314
Balanic, pertaining to glans penis, 366
Balanitis, inflammation of skin covering glans penis, 368
Balanoplasty, surgical repair of glans penis, 371
Balanorrhea, discharge from glans penis, 367
Balloon angioplasty. *See* Percutaneous transluminal coronary angioplasty
Bariatric surgery, group of surgical procedures such as stomach stapling and restrictive banding to reduce size of stomach; treatment for morbid (extreme) obesity, 288
Barium (Ba), soft metallic element from earth used as radiopaque X-ray dye, 517
Barium enema (BE). *See* Lower gastrointestinal series
Barium swallow. *See* Upper gastrointestinal series
Barrier contraception, prevention of pregnancy using a device to prevent sperm from meeting ovum; includes condoms, diaphragms, and cervical caps, 356
Bartholin's glands, glands located on either side of vaginal opening that secrete mucus for vaginal lubrication, 341
Basal cell carcinoma (BCC), tumor of basal cell layer of epidermis; frequent type of skin cancer that rarely metastasizes or spreads; these cancers can arise on sun-exposed skin, 62, 62*f*
Basal layer, deepest layer of epidermis; this living layer constantly multiplies and divides to supply cells to replace cells that are sloughed off skin surface, 52
Base, directional term meaning bottom or lower part, 40*t*, 228
Basilic vein, 150*f*
Basophil (Basos), granulocyte white blood cell that releases histamine and heparin in damaged tissues, 181, 183*f*, 183*t*
Basophilic, pertaining to basophils, 186
Bell jar apparatus, 230*f*
Bell's palsy, one-sided facial paralysis due to inflammation of facial nerve, 436
Benign, not cancerous; benign tumor is generally not progressive or recurring, 535
Benign prostatic hyperplasia (BPH), enlargement of prostate gland commonly seen in males over age 50, 368
Beta-blocker drugs, medication that treats hypertension and angina pectoris by lowering heart rate, 166
Biceps, arm muscle named for number of attachment points; *bi-* means "two" and biceps have two heads attached to bone, 116
Bicuspid valve, valve between left atrium and ventricle; prevents blood from flowing backward into atrium; has two cusps or flaps; also called *mitral valve*, 144, 145*f*
Bicuspids, premolar permanent teeth having two cusps or projections that assist in grinding food; humans have eight bicuspids, 265*f*, 266, 267*f*
Bilateral, pertaining to two sides, 5
Bile, substance produced by liver and stored in gallbladder; added to chyme in duodenum and functions to emulsify fats so they can be digested and absorbed, 271
Bile duct, 272*f*, 284*f*
Bilirubin, waste product produced from destruction of worn-out red blood cells; disposed of by liver, 183
Binaural, referring to both ears, 481
Biopsy (Bx, bx), piece of tissue is removed by syringe and needle, knife, punch, or brush to examine under a microscope; used to aid in diagnosis, 69, 538
Bipolar disorder (BPD), mental disorder in which patient has alternating periods of depression and mania, 512
Bite-wing X-ray, X-ray taken with part of film holder held between teeth, and film held parallel to teeth, 285
Black lung. *See* Anthracosis
Bladder cancer, cancerous tumor that arises from cells lining bladder; major symptom is hematuria, 308*f*
Bladder neck obstruction (BNO), blockage of bladder outlet into urethra, 318
Blepharectomy, surgical removal of eyelid, 471
Blepharitis, inflammatory condition of eyelash follicles and glands of eyelids that results in swelling, redness, and crusts of dried mucus on lids; can be result of allergy or infection, 467
Blepharoplasty, surgical repair of eyelid, 471
Blepharoptosis, drooping eyelid, 463
Blood, major component of hematic system; consists of watery plasma, red blood cells, and white blood cells, 179–93
  abbreviations, 193
  ABO system, 184
  adjective forms of anatomical terms, 186
  anatomy and physiology, 182–85
  diagnostic procedures, 190–91
  erythrocytes, 182–83, 183*f*
  leukocytes, 183, 183*f*, 183*t*
  pathology, 187–90
  pharmacology, 192
  plasma, 182
  platelets, 184, 184*f*
  Rh factor, 185
  terminology, 185–90
  therapeutic procedures, 192
  typing, 184–85

impulses to be conducted between brain and spinal cord; also contains centers that control respiration, heart rate, and blood pressure; in addition, 12 pairs of cranial nerves begin in brain stem, 422, 422*f*

Brain tumor, intracranial mass, either benign or malignant; benign tumor of brain can be fatal since it will grow and cause pressure on normal brain tissue, 432, 432*f*

Brand name, name a pharmaceutical company chooses as trademark or market name for its drug; also called *proprietary* or *trade name*, 501

Breast cancer, malignant tumor of breast; usually forms in milk-producing gland tissue or lining of milk ducts, 352, 352*f*

Breasts, milk-producing glands to provide nutrition for newborn; also called *mammary glands*, 337, 338, 342, 342*f*, 352, 352*f*

Breech presentation, placement of fetus in which buttocks or feet are presented first for delivery rather than head, 344, 345*f*

Bridge, dental appliance attached to adjacent teeth for support to replace missing teeth, 287

Broad spectrum, ability of drug to be effective against a wide range of microorganisms, 506

Bronchial, pertaining to the bronchi, 233

Bronchial tree, 227, 227*f*

Bronchial tube, organ of respiratory system that carries air into each lung, 223, 224, 227, 227–28*f*

Bronchiectasis, results from dilation of bronchus or bronchi that can result from infection; this abnormal stretching can be irreversible and result in destruction of bronchial walls; major symptom is large amount of purulent (pus-filled) sputum; rales (bubbling chest sound) and hemoptysis may be present, 235, 239

Bronchiolar, pertaining to a bronchiole, 233

Bronchioles, narrowest air tubes in lungs; each bronchiole terminates in tiny air sacs called alveoli, 227, 227–28*f*

Bronchitis, acute or chronic inflammation of lower respiratory tract that often occurs after other childhood infections such as measles, 239

Bronchodilator, medication that dilates or opens bronchi (airways in lungs) to improve breathing, 249

Bronchogenic carcinoma, malignant lung tumor that originates in bronchi; usually associated with history of cigarette smoking, 239, 239*f*

Bronchogram, X-ray record of lungs and bronchial tubes, 244

Bronchography, process of taking X-ray of lung after radiopaque substance has been placed into trachea or bronchial tube, 244

Bronchoplasty, surgical repair of a bronchial defect, 246

Bronchoscope, instrument to view inside a bronchus, 244

Bronchoscopy (Bronch), using bronchoscope to visualize bronchi; instrument can also be used to obtain tissue for biopsy and to remove foreign objects, 244, 245*f*

Bronchospasm, involuntary muscle spasm in bronchi, 235

Bronchus, distal end of trachea splits into left and right main bronchi as it enters each lung; each main bronchus is subdivided into smaller branches; smallest bronchi are bronchioles; each bronchiole ends in tiny air sacs called alveoli, 226*f*, 227, 227*f*

Buccal, (1) pertaining to cheeks; (2) drugs that are placed under lip or between cheek and gum, 274, 506*t*

Buccolabial, pertaining to cheeks and lips, 274

Buffers, chemicals that neutralize acid, particularly stomach acid, 272

Bulbourethral gland, also called *Cowper's gland*; these two small male reproductive system glands are located on either side of urethra just distal to prostate; secretion from these glands neutralizes acidity in urethra and vagina, 362 363, 363*f*, 365

Bulimia, eating disorder characterized by recurrent binge eating and then purging of food with laxatives and vomiting, 512

Bundle branch block (BBB), occurs when electrical impulse is blocked from travelling down bundle of His or bundle branches; results in ventricles beating at a different rate than atria; also called a *heart block*, 155

Bundle branches, part of conduction system of heart; electrical signal travels down interventricular septum, 145, 146*f*

Bundle of His. *See* Atrioventricular bundle

Bunion, inflammation of bursa of the great toe, 105

Bunionectomy, removal of bursa at joint of great toe, 108

Burn, full-thickness burn exists when all layers are burned, called *third-degree burn*; partial-thickness burn exists when first layer of skin, epidermis, is burned, and second layer of skin, dermis, is damaged, called *second-degree burn*; *first-degree burn* damages only epidermis, 62, 63*f*

Bursa, saclike connective tissue structure found in some joints; protects moving parts from friction; some common bursa locations are elbow, knee, and shoulder joints, 94

Bursectomy, surgical removal of a bursa, 108

Bursitis, inflammation of bursa between bony prominences and muscles or tendons; common in shoulder and knee, 94, 99

C

Cachexia, loss of weight and generalized wasting that occurs during a chronic disease, 277

Calcitonin (CT), hormone secreted by thyroid gland; stimulates deposition of calcium into bone, 389*t*, 396

Calcium (Ca^+), inorganic substance found in plasma; is important for bones, muscles, and nerves, 182, 392

Calcium channel blocker drugs, medication that treats hypertension, angina pectoris, and congestive heart failure by causing heart to beat less forcefully and less often, 166

Calcium supplements, maintaining high blood levels of calcium in association with vitamin D helps maintain bone density and treats osteomalacia, osteoporosis, and rickets, 110

Calculus, stone formed within organ by accumulation of mineral salts; found in kidney, renal pelvis, ureters, bladder, or urethra; plural is *calculi*, 314, 314*f*

Callus, mass of bone tissue that forms at fracture site during its healing, 99
Calyx, duct that connects renal papilla to renal pelvis; urine flows from collecting tubule through calyx and into renal pelvis, 306, 307*f*
Cancellous bone, bony tissue found inside a bone; contains cavities that hold red bone marrow; also called *spongy bone*, 85, 86*f*
Cancerous tumors, malignant growths in the body, 199
Candidiasis, yeastlike infection of skin and mucous membranes that can result in white plaques on tongue and vagina, 351
Canines, also called *cuspid teeth* or *eyeteeth*; permanent teeth located between incisors and bicuspids that assist in biting and cutting food; humans have four canine teeth, 266, 267*f*
Canker sores. *See* Aphthous ulcers
Capillaries, smallest blood or lymphatic vessels; blood capillaries are very thin to allow gas, nutrient, and waste exchange between blood and tissues; lymph capillaries collect lymph fluid from tissues and carry it to larger lymph vessels, 139, 140, 147*f*, 149
Capillary bed, network of capillaries found in a given tissue or organ, 149
Carbon dioxide (CO_2), waste product of cellular energy production; removed from cells by blood and eliminated from body by lungs, 141, 224
Carbuncle, inflammation and infection of skin and hair follicle that may result from several untreated boils; most commonly found on neck, upper back, or head, 67
Carcinogen, substance or chemical agent that produces or increases risk of developing cancer; for example, cigarette smoke and insecticides are considered to be carcinogens, 536
Carcinoma, new growth or malignant tumor that occurs in epithelial tissue; can spread to other organs through blood or direct extension from organ, 535
Carcinoma in situ (CIS), malignant tumor that has not extended beyond original site, 536
Cardiac, pertaining to the heart, 152
Cardiac arrest, when heart stops beating and circulation ceases, 156
Cardiac catheterization (CC), passage of thin tube (catheter) through arm vein and blood vessel leading into heart; used to detect abnormalities, to collect cardiac blood samples, and to determine pressure within cardiac area, 162
Cardiac enzymes, complex protein molecules found only in heart muscle; taken by blood sample to determine amount of heart disease or damage, 161
Cardiac muscle, involuntary muscle found in heart, 25, 26*f*, 114, 114*f*, 115, 115*f*, 141
Cardiac scan, patient is given radioactive thallium intravenously and then scanning equipment is used to visualize heart; especially useful in determining myocardial damage, 162
Cardiac sphincter, also called *lower esophageal sphincter*; prevents food and gastric juices from backing up into esophagus, 269
Cardiologist, physician specializing in treating diseases and conditions of cardiovascular system, 153
Cardiology, branch of medicine specializing in conditions of cardiovascular system, 153
Cardiomegaly, abnormally enlarged heart, 156
Cardiomyopathy, general term for disease of myocardium that may be caused by alcohol abuse, parasites, viral infection, and congestive heart failure, 156
Cardiopulmonary resuscitation (CPR), emergency treatment provided by trained persons and given to patients when their respirations and heart stop; provides oxygen to brain, heart, and other vital organs until medical treatment can restore normal heart and pulmonary function, 163, 248
Cardiotonic, substance that strengthens the heart muscle, 166
Cardiovascular, pertaining to the heart and blood vessels, 28*t*
Cardiovascular system (CV), system that transports blood to all areas of body; organs include heart and blood vessels (arteries, veins, and capillaries); also called *circulatory system*, 137–68
  abbreviations, 167–68
  adjective forms of anatomical terms, 152–53
  anatomy and physiology, 140–50
  diagnostic procedures, 161–63
  pathology, 153–60
  pharmacology, 166
  terminology, 151–60
  therapeutic procedures, 163–66
Cardioversion. *See* Defibrillation
Carotid artery, 148*f*
Cardiovascular technician, healthcare professional trained to perform a variety of diagnostic and therapeutic procedures including electrocardiography, echocardiography, and exercise stress tests, 154
Carotid endarterectomy, surgical procedure for removing obstruction within carotid artery, major artery in neck that carries oxygenated blood to brain; developed to prevent strokes but found to be useful only in severe stenosis with TIA, 440
Carpal, pertaining to the wrist, 92, 92*t*, 96
Carpal tunnel release, surgical cutting of ligament in wrist to relieve nerve pressure caused by carpal tunnel syndrome, which can be caused by repetitive motion such as typing, 124
Carpal tunnel syndrome (CTS), painful disorder of wrist and hand, induced by compression of median nerve as it passes under ligaments on palm side of wrist; symptoms include weakness, pain, burning, tingling, and aching in forearm, wrist, and hand, 123
Carpals, wrist bones in upper extremity, 96
Carpus, collective name for the eight wrist bones in each upper extremity, 91*f*, 92, 92*f*, 92*t*
Cartilage, strong, flexible connective tissue found in several locations in body, such as covering ends of bones in synovial joint, nasal septum, external ear, eustachian tube, larynx, trachea, bronchi, and intervertebral disks, 25, 84, 477*f*

Cartilaginous joints, joint that allows slight movement but holds bones firmly in place by solid piece of cartilage; example is pubic symphysis; fetal skeleton is composed of cartilaginous tissue, 94, 94*f*

Cast, application of solid material to immobilize extremity or portion of body as a result of fracture, dislocation, or severe injury; most often made of plaster of Paris or fiberglass, 109

Castration, surgical removal of testicles in male or ovaries in female, 371

Cataract, diminished vision resulting from lens of eye becoming opaque or cloudy; treatment is usually surgical removal of cataract, 465, 465*f*

Catheter (cath), flexible tube inserted into body for purpose of moving fluids into or out of body; used in cardiovascular system to place dye into blood vessels so they may be visualized on X-rays; used in urinary system to drain urine from bladder, 162, 321

Catheterization, insertion of a tube through urethra and into urinary bladder for purpose of withdrawing urine or inserting dye, 321

Caudal, directional term meaning toward feet or tail, or below, 39*f*, 39*t*

Cauterization, destruction of tissue by using caustic chemicals, electric currents, or by heating or freezing, 70, 352

Cecal, pertaining to the cecum, 274

Cecum, first portion of colon; a blind pouch off beginning of large intestine; appendix originates at end, 269*f*, 270*f*

Cell, basic unit of all living things; composes all tissues and organs in body; performs survival functions such as reproduction, respiration, metabolism, and excretion; some also able to carry on specialized functions, such as contraction by muscle cells and electrical impulse transmission by nerve cells, 24

Cell membrane, outermost boundary of the cell, 24

Cell-mediated immunity, immunity resulting from activation of sensitized T lymphocytes; immune response causes antigens to be destroyed by direct action of cells; also called *cellular immunity*, 200

Cellular immunity, also called *cell-mediated immunity*; process results in production of T cells and natural killer (NK) cells that directly attach to foreign cells; immune response fights invasion by viruses, bacteria, fungi, and cancer, 200

Cellulitis, inflammation of cellular or connective tissues, 64

Cementum, anchors root of a tooth into socket of jaw, 266, 267*f*

Central canal, canal that extends down length of spinal cord; contains cerebrospinal fluid, 425

Central fissure, 423*f*

Central nervous system (CNS), portion of nervous system consisting of brain and spinal cord; receives impulses from all over body, processes information, and then responds with action; consists of both gray and white matter, 420, 421–25
- brain, 422–24, 422*f*, 423*f*
- meninges, 425, 425*f*
- spinal cord, 424–25, 424*f*

Cephalalgia, a headache, 431

Cephalic, directional term meaning toward the head, or above, 39*f*, 39*t*

Cephalic region, head region of the body, 34*t*, 35*f*

Cephalic vein, 150*f*

Cerebellar, pertaining to cerebellum, 429

Cerebellitis, inflammation of cerebellum, 433

Cerebellum, second largest portion of brain, located beneath posterior portion of cerebrum; part of brain that aids in coordinating voluntary body movements and maintaining balance and equilibrium; attached to brain stem by pons; refined muscular movement is initiated in cerebrum, 422, 422*f*, 423*f*

Cerebral, pertaining to the cerebrum, 429

Cerebral aneurysm, localized abnormal dilatation of blood vessel, usually artery; result of congenital defect or weakness in wall of vessel; ruptured aneurysm is a common cause for hemorrhagic CVA, 433, 433*f*

Cerebral angiography, X-ray of blood vessels of brain after injection of radiopaque dye, 439

Cerebral contusion, bruising of brain from blow or impact; symptoms last longer than 24 hours and include unconsciousness, dizziness, vomiting, unequal pupil size, and shock, 433

Cerebral cortex, outer layer of cerebrum; composed of folds of gray matter called gyri, which are separated by sulci, 422–23

Cerebral hemispheres, division of cerebrum into right and left halves, 423

Cerebral palsy (CP), brain damage resulting from a defect, trauma, infection, or lack of oxygen before, during, or shortly after birth, 433

Cerebrospinal, pertaining to cerebrum and spine, 429

Cerebrospinal fluid (CSF), watery, clear fluid found in ventricles of brain; provides protection from shock or sudden motion to brain, 424

Cerebrospinal fluid analysis, laboratory examination of clear, watery, colorless fluid from within brain and spinal cord; can detect infections and abnormal presence of blood, 439

Cerebrospinal fluid shunts, surgical procedure in which bypass is created to drain cerebrospinal fluid; used to treat hydrocephalus by draining excess cerebrospinal fluid from brain and diverting it to abdominal cavity, 440

Cerebrovascular accident (CVA), also called a *stroke*; development of infarct due to loss in blood supply to area of brain; blood flow can be interrupted by ruptured blood vessel (hemorrhage), floating clot (embolus), stationary clot (thrombosis), or compression; extent of damage depends on size and location of infarct and often includes speech problems and muscle paralysis, 433, 433*f*

Cerebrum, largest section of brain; located in upper portion, and possesses thoughts, judgment, memory, association skills, and ability to discriminate between items; outer layer is cerebral cortex, which is composed of folds of gray matter; elevated portions, or *convolutions*, are called gyri and are separated by fissures or sulci; has both a left

Clamp, surgical instrument used to grasp tissue and control bleeding, 530*t*
Clavicle, also called *collar bone*; bone of pectoral girdle, 92, 92*f*, 92*t*
Clavicular, pertaining to clavicle or collar bone, 96
Clean catch specimen (CC), urine sample obtained after cleaning off urinary opening and catching or collecting a sample in midstream (halfway through urination process) to minimize contamination from genitalia, 319
Cleft lip, congenital anomaly in which upper lip fails to come together; often seen along with cleft palate; corrected with surgery, 279
Cleft palate, congenital anomaly in which roof of mouth has split or fissure; corrected with surgery, 279
Clinical psychologist, diagnoses and treats mental disorders; specializes in using individual and group counseling to treat patients with mental and emotional disorders, 510
Clitoris, small organ containing erectile tissue covered by labia minora; contains sensitive tissue aroused during sexual stimulation and is similar to penis in male, 338*f*, 341, 341*f*
Closed fracture, simple fracture with no open skin wound, 100, 100*f*
Clubbing, abnormal widening and thickening of ends of fingers and toes associated with chronic oxygen deficiency; seen in patients with chronic respiratory conditions or circulatory problems, 235
Coagulate, convert liquid to gel or solid, as in blood coagulation, 187
Coarctation of the aorta (CoA)**,** severe congenital narrowing of aorta, 159
Coccygeal, pertaining to coccyx or tailbone, 96
Coccyx, tailbone, three to five very small vertebrae attached to sacrum; often become fused, 88*f*, 89, 90*f*, 90*t*
Cochlea, portion of labyrinth associated with hearing; rolled in shape of snail shell; lined by organs of Corti, 478
Cochlear, pertaining to cochlea, 481
Cochlear implant, mechanical device surgically placed under skin behind outer ear (pinna); converts sound signals into magnetic impulses to stimulate auditory nerve; can be beneficial for those with profound sensorineural hearing loss, 486, 486*f*
Cochlear nerve, branch of vestibulocochlear nerve that carries hearing information to brain, 477, 477*f*
Coitus, sexual intercourse, 364
Cold sores. *See* Herpes labialis
Colectomy, surgical removal of colon, 288
Collagen fibers, fibers made up of insoluble fibrous protein present in connective tissue that forms flexible mat to protect skin and other parts of body, 52
Collecting tubule, portion of renal tubule, 307, 308*f*, 310*f*
Colles' fracture, specific type of wrist fracture, 100, 100*f*
Colon, also called *large intestine*; functions to reabsorb most of fluid in digested food; material that remains after water reabsorption is feces; sections include cecum, ascending colon, transverse colon, descending colon, and sigmoid colon, 264, 270
Colonic, pertaining to colon, 275
Colonoscope, instrument to view inside colon, 286
Colonoscopy, flexible fiberscope passed through anus, rectum, and colon used to examine upper portion of colon; polyps and small growths can be removed during procedure, 286
Color vision tests, use of polychromic (multicolored) charts to determine ability of patient to recognize color, 469
Colorectal, pertaining to colon and rectum, 275
Colorectal carcinoma, cancerous tumor originating in the colon or rectum, 281
Colostomy, surgical creation of opening in some portion of colon through abdominal wall to outside surface; fecal material (stool) drains into bag worn on abdomen, 289, 289*f*
Colostrum, thin fluid first secreted by breast after delivery; does not contain much protein, but is rich in antibodies, 348
Colposcope, instrument to view inside vagina, 355
Colposcopy, visual examination of cervix and vagina using colposcope, 355
Coma, profound unconsciousness resulting from illness or injury, 431
Combining form, word root plus combining vowel; always written with a "/" between word root and combining vowel; for example, *cardi* is word root and *o* is combining vowel, 3–4
Combining vowel, vowel inserted between word parts that makes it possible to pronounce long medical terms; usually the vowel *o*, 2, 3–4
Comedo, medical term for blackhead; an accumulation of sebum in sebaceous gland that has become blackened, 57
Comminuted fracture, fracture in which bone is shattered, splintered, or crushed into many pieces or fragments; fracture is completely through bone, 100
Common bile duct (CBD), duct that carries bile from gallbladder to duodenum, 272, 272*f*
Common iliac artery, 148*f*
Common iliac vein, 150*f*
Compact bone, hard exterior surface bone; also called *cortical bone*, 85, 86*f*, 94*f*
Complemental air. *See* Inspiratory reserve volume
Complete blood count (CBC), a combination of blood tests; includes red blood cell count, white blood cell count, hemoglobin, hematocrit, white blood cell differential, and platelet count, 190
Compound fracture, fracture in which the bone has broken through the skin, 100
Compression fracture, fracture involving loss of height of vertebral body, 101
Computed tomography scan (CT scan)**,** imaging technique able to produce cross-sectional view of body; X-ray pictures are taken at multiple angles through body and computer constructs composite cross-section from images, 518
Conception, fertilization of ovum by a sperm, 340
Concussion, injury to brain resulting from blow or impact; symptoms may include headache, blurred vision, nausea or vomiting, dizziness, and balance problems, 434

Conductive hearing loss, loss of hearing as a result of blocking of sound transmission in middle ear and outer ear, 479
Condyle, refers to rounded portion at end of a bone, 86, 87*f*
Cones, sensory receptors of retina that are active in bright light and see in color, 457
Confidentiality, 16
Congenital anomalies, birth defects, 343
Congenital hypothyroidism, congenital condition due to lack of thyroid secretion that may result in arrested physical and mental development; formerly called *cretinism*, 403
Congenital septal defect (CSD), defect, present at birth, in wall separating two chambers of heart; results in a mixture of oxygenated and deoxygenated blood being carried to surrounding tissues; there can be atrial septal defect (ASD) and ventricular septal defect (VSD), 156
Congestive heart failure (CHF), pathological condition of heart in which there is reduced outflow of blood from left side of heart; results in weakness, breathlessness, and edema, 156
Conization, surgical removal of core of cervical tissue; also refers to partial removal of cervix, 357
Conjunctiva, protective mucous membrane lining on underside of each eyelid and across anterior surface of each eyeball, 456, 456*f*, 459, 467
Conjunctival, pertaining to conjunctiva, 462
Conjunctivitis, also referred to as *pinkeye* or inflammation of conjunctiva, 467
Conjunctivoplasty, surgical repair of conjunctiva, 471
Connective tissue, supporting and protecting tissue in body structures; examples are fat or adipose tissue, cartilage, and bone, 25, 26*f*
Conscious, condition of being awake and aware of surroundings, 431
Constipation, experiencing difficulty in defecation or infrequent defecation, 277
Consultation reports, document in patient's medical record; reports given by specialists who physician has requested to evaluate patient, 14
Contracture, abnormal shortening of muscle, making it difficult to stretch muscle, 122
Contraindication, condition in which particular drug should not be used, 506
Contrast studies, radiopaque substance is injected or swallowed; X-rays are then taken that outline body structure containing radiopaque substance, 519, 519*f*
Controlled substances, drugs that have potential for being addictive (habit forming) or can be abused, 502, 502*t*
Contusion, injury caused by blow to body; causes swelling, pain, and bruising; skin is not broken, 57
Conversion disorder, disorder in which patient unconsciously substitutes physical signs or symptoms for anxiety; most common physical signs or symptoms are blindness, heart palpitations, and paralysis, 513
Convulsion, severe involuntary muscle contractions and relaxations; caused by a variety of things, such as epilepsy, fever, and toxic conditions, 431
Corium, living layer of skin located between epidermis and subcutaneous layer; also referred to as *dermis*, contains hair follicles, sweat glands, sebaceous glands, blood vessels, lymph vessels, sensory receptors, nerve fibers, and muscle fibers, 52
Cornea, portion of sclera that is clear and transparent and allows light to enter interior of eye; also plays role in bending light rays, 455, 456, 456*f*
Corneal, pertaining to cornea, 462
Corneal abrasion, scraping injury to cornea; if not allowed to heal, may develop into ulcer, 465
Coronal plane, vertical plane that divides body into front (anterior or ventral) and back (posterior or dorsal) sections; also called *frontal plane*, 33, 33*f*
Coronal section, sectional view of body produced by cut along frontal plane; also called *frontal section*, 33
Coronary, pertaining to heart, 147, 152
Coronary arteries, group of three arteries that branch off aorta and carry blood to myocardium, 147, 147*f*
Coronary artery bypass graft (CABG), open-heart surgery in which blood vessel is grafted to route blood around point of constriction in diseased coronary artery, 164
Coronary artery disease (CAD), insufficient blood supply to heart muscle due to obstruction of one or more coronary arteries; may be caused by atherosclerosis and may cause angina pectoris and myocardial infarction, 156, 156*f*
Corpus, body or central portion of uterus, 338*f*, 340
Corpus albicans, 339*f*
Corpus luteum, 339*f*
Cortex, outer layer of organ; within endocrine system, refers to outer layer of adrenal glands; within urinary system, refers to outer layer of kidney, 306, 307*f*, 390, 390*f*
Cortical, pertaining to cortex, 85
Cortical bone, hard exterior surface bone; also called *compact bone*, 85, 86*f*
Corticosteroid cream, powerful anti-inflammatory cream, 71
Corticosteroids, general term for group of hormones secreted by adrenal cortex; include mineralocorticoid hormones, glucocorticoid hormones, and steroid sex hormones; used as medication for its strong anti-inflammatory properties, 110, 209, 249, 390, 407
Cortisol, glucocorticoid hormone secreted by adrenal cortex; regulates carbohydrate metabolism, 390
Costal, pertaining to ribs, 96
Cowper's glands, also called *bulbourethral glands*; these two small male reproductive system glands are located on either side of urethra just distal to prostate; secretion from these glands neutralizes acidity in urethra and vagina, 365
Crackles, abnormal crackling or bubbling sound made during aspiration usually indicates presence of fluid or mucus in small airways; also called *rales*, 235
Cranial, pertaining to skull, 97, 429
Cranial bones, 89*t*
Cranial cavity, dorsal body cavity; within skull and contains brain, 36, 36*f*, 37*t*
Cranial nerves, nerves that arise from brain, 420, 426*t*

Craniotomy, incision into skull, 108
Cranium, skull; bones that form protective covering over brain, 87, 88*f*
Creatine phosphokinase (CPK), muscle enzyme found in skeletal muscle and cardiac muscle; blood levels become elevated in disorders such as heart attack, muscular dystrophy, and other skeletal muscle pathologies, 123
Creatinine, waste product of muscle metabolism, 182
Creatinine clearance, test of kidney function; creatinine is waste product cleared from bloodstream by kidneys; for test, urine is collected for 24 hours and amount of creatinine in urine is compared to amount of creatinine that remains in bloodstream, 319
Crepitation, noise produced by bones or cartilage rubbing together, 99
Crick in the neck, 123
Cricoid cartilage, 225*f*
Crohn's disease, form of chronic inflammatory bowel disease affecting ileum and/or colon; also called *regional ileitis*, 281
Cross infection, occurs when person, either patient or healthcare worker, acquires pathogen from another patient or healthcare worker, 201
Cross-eyed. *See* Esotropia
Cross-section, internal view of body produced by slice perpendicular to long axis of structure, 23
Croup, acute viral respiratory infection common in infants and young children and characterized by hoarse cough, 238
Crown, portion of tooth covered by enamel; also artificial covering for tooth created to replace original enamel, 266, 267*f*, 287
Crowning, when head of baby is visible through vaginal opening; a sign that birth is imminent, 344
Crural, pertaining to leg, 35*f*
Crural region, lower extremity region of body, 34*t*
Cryoextraction, procedure in which cataract is lifted from lens with extremely cold probe, 471
Cryoretinopexy, surgical fixation of retina by using extreme cold, 471
Cryosurgery, exposing tissues to extreme cold in order to destroy them; used in treating malignant tumors and to control pain and bleeding, 70, 532
Cryotherapy, using cold for therapeutic purposes, 525
Cryptorchidism, failure of testes to descend into scrotal sac before birth; usually the testes will descend before birth; surgical procedure called orchidopexy may be required to bring testes down into scrotum permanently; failure of testes to descend could result in sterility in male, 368
Culdoscopy, examination of female pelvic cavity by introducing endoscope through wall of vagina, 355
Culture and sensitivity (C&S), laboratory test in which colony of pathogens that have been removed from infected area are grown to identify pathogen and then determine its sensitivity to a variety of antibiotics, 69
Cumulative action, action that occurs in body when drug is allowed to accumulate or stay in body, 506
Curettage, removal of superficial skin lesions with curette (surgical instrument shaped like spoon) or scraper, 70
Curette, surgical instrument used to scrape and remove tissue, 530*t*
Cushing's syndrome, set of symptoms that result from hypersecretion of adrenal cortex; may be result of tumor of adrenal glands; symptoms include weakness, edema, excess hair growth, skin discoloration, and osteoporosis, 400, 400*f*
Cuspids, permanent teeth located between incisors and bicuspids that assist in biting and cutting food; humans have four cuspids; also called *canine teeth* or *eyeteeth*, 265*f*, 266, 267*f*
Cusps, leaflets or flaps of heart valve, 144
Cutaneous, pertaining to skin, 56
Cutaneous membrane, another term for skin, 50
Cuticle, thin skinlike layer overlapping base of nail, 53, 53*f*
Cyanosis, slightly bluish color of skin due to deficiency of oxygen and excess of carbon dioxide in blood; caused by a variety of disorders, ranging from chronic lung disease to congenital and chronic heart problems, 53, 236, 236*f*
Cycloplegia, paralysis of ciliary body, 463
Cyst, fluid-filled sac under skin, 57, 57*f*
Cystalgia, bladder pain, 315
Cystectomy, surgical removal of bladder, 323
Cystic, (1) pertaining to urinary bladder; (2) pertaining to gallbladder, 275, 313
Cystic duct, duct leading from gallbladder to common bile duct; carries bile, 271, 272*f*
Cystic fibrosis (CF), hereditary condition causing exocrine glands to malfunction; patient produces very thick mucus that causes severe congestion within lungs and digestive system; through more advanced treatment, many children are now living into adulthood with this disease, 240
Cystitis, inflammation of bladder, 309, 318
Cystocele, protrusion (or herniation) of urinary bladder into wall of vagina; may cause urinary frequency and urgency, 318, 351
Cystogram, record of bladder, 320
Cystography, process of instilling contrast material or dye into bladder by catheter to visualize urinary bladder on X-ray, 320
Cystolith, bladder stone, 315
Cystopexy, surgical fixation of bladder, 323
Cystoplasty, surgical repair of bladder, 323
Cystorrhagia, profuse bleeding from bladder, 315
Cystoscope, instrument used to visually examine bladder, 321
Cystoscopy (cysto), visual examination of urinary bladder using instrument called cystoscope, 321
Cystostomy, creation of opening through abdominal wall and into bladder, 323
Cystotomy, incision into bladder, 323
Cytologic testing, examination of cells to determine structure and origin; example includes Pap smears, 538
Cytology, study of cells, 24
Cytoplasm, watery internal environment of a cell, 24
Cytotoxic, pertaining to poisoning cells, 201

D

Dacryoadenitis, inflammation of lacrimal gland, 467
Dacryocystitis, inflammation of tear sac, 467
Day surgery, type of outpatient surgery in which patient is discharged on same day as being admitted; also called *ambulatory surgery*, 532
Deafness, inability to hear or having some degree of hearing impairment, 482
Debridement, removal of foreign material and dead or damaged tissue from wound, 70, 525
Decibel (dB), measures intensity or loudness of sound; zero decibels is quietest sound measured and 120 dB is loudest sound commonly measured, 485
Deciduous teeth, 20 teeth that begin to erupt around six months of age; eventually pushed out by permanent teeth, 266
Decongestant, substance that reduces nasal congestion and swelling, 249
Decubitus ulcer (decub), bedsore or pressure sore formed from pressure over bony prominences on body; caused by lack of blood flow, 64
Deep, directional term meaning away from surface of body, 40*t*
Deep tendon reflex (DTR), muscle contraction in response to stretch caused by striking muscle tendon with reflex hammer; test used to determine if muscles are responding properly, 124
Deep vein thrombosis, formation of blood clots in a vein deep in the body, usually in the legs, 159
Defecation, evacuation of feces from rectum, 270
Defibrillation, procedure that converts serious irregular heartbeats, such as fibrillation, by giving electric shocks to heart, 163, 163*f*
Delirium, state of mental confusion with lack of orientation to time and place, 431
Delivery, emergence of baby from birth canal, 344
Delusional disorder, false belief held with conviction even in face of strong evidence to contrary, 512
Dementia, progressive impairment of intellectual function that interferes with performing activities of daily living; patients have little awareness of their condition; found in disorders such as Alzheimer's, 431, 511
Dendrite, branched process off a neuron that receives impulses and carries them to cell body, 420, 421*f*
Dental, pertaining to teeth, 275
Dental caries, gradual decay and disintegration of teeth caused by bacteria that can result in inflamed tissue and abscessed teeth; commonly called a *tooth cavity*, 279
Dentalgia, tooth pain, 277
Dentin, main bulk of tooth; covered by enamel, 266, 267*f*
Dentist, practitioner of dentistry, 277
Dentistry, branch of healthcare involved with prevention, diagnosis, and treatment of conditions involving teeth, jaw, and mouth; practitioner is *dentist* or *oral surgeon*, 277
Denture, partial or complete set of artificial teeth that are set in plastic materials; substitute for natural teeth and related structures, 288
Deoxygenated, blood in veins that is low in oxygen content, 140
Depigmentation, loss of normal skin color or pigment, 57
Depression, downward movement, as in dropping shoulders, 119*t*
Depressive disorders, a classification of psychiatric disorders in the DSM-5 characterized by instability in mood; includes major depressive disorder and mania, 512
Dermabrasion, abrasion or rubbing using wire brushes or sandpaper, 70
Dermal, pertaining to skin, 56
Dermatitis, inflammation of skin, 64
Dermatologist, physician specialized in diagnosis and treatment of diseases of integumentary system, 57
Dermatology (Derm, derm), branch of medicine specializing in conditions of integumentary system, 57
Dermatome, instrument for cutting skin or thin transplants of skin, 69
Dermatoplasty, surgical repair of skin, 69
Dermatosis, abnormal condition of skin, 64
Dermis, living layer of skin located between epidermis and subcutaneous layer; also referred to as *corium* or *true skin*; contains hair follicles, sweat glands, sebaceous glands, blood vessels, lymph vessels, sensory receptors, nerve fibers, and muscle fibers, 50, 51*f*, 52
Descending aorta, 145*f*
Descending colon, section of colon that descends left side of abdomen, 269*f*, 270, 270*f*
Descending tracts, nerve tracts carrying motor signals down spinal cord to muscles, 425
Diabetes insipidus (DI), disorder caused by inadequate secretion of hormone by posterior lobe of pituitary gland; there may be polyuria and polydipsia, 393, 402
Diabetes mellitus (DM), serious disease in which pancreas fails to produce insulin or insulin does not work properly; consequently, patient has very high blood sugar; kidney will attempt to lower high blood sugar level by excreting excess sugar in urine, 401
Diabetic acidosis. *See* Ketoacidosis
Diabetic nephropathy, accumulation of damage to glomerulus capillaries due to chronic high blood sugars of diabetes mellitus, 317
Diabetic retinopathy, secondary complication of diabetes affecting blood vessels of retina, resulting in visual changes and even blindness, 401
Diagnostic and Statistical Manual of Mental Disorders, Fifth Edition (DSM-5), 510
Diagnostic imaging (DI), 516–21
  abbreviations, 521
  procedures, 518–21
  vocabulary, 517–18
Diagnostic reports, found in patient's medical record; consists of results of all diagnostic tests performed on patient, principally from lab and medical imaging (e.g., X-ray and ultrasound), 14
Diaphoresis, excessive or profuse sweating, 57
Diaphragm, major muscle of inspiration; separates thoracic from abdominal cavity, 36, 36*f*, 141*f*, 229, 229*f*

E

Electrolyte, chemical compound that separates into charged particles, or ionizes, in solution; sodium (Na+, chloride (Cl^-), and potassium (K^+) are examples of electrolytes, 309

Electromyogram (EMG), record of muscle electricity, 124, 525

Electromyography, recording of electrical patterns of muscle in order to diagnose diseases, 124, 525

Elephantiasis, inflammation, obstruction, and destruction of lymph vessels that results in enlarged tissues due to edema, 205

Elevation, muscle action that raises body part, as in shrugging the shoulders, 119*t*

Elimination disorders, a classification of psychiatric disorders in the DSM-5 involving inappropriate voiding of urine or feces; includes enuresis and encopresis, 514

Embolectomy, surgical removal of embolus or clot from a blood vessel, 164

Embolus, obstruction of blood vessel by blood clot that moves from another area, 154, 154*f*

Embryo, term to describe developing infant from fertilization until end of eighth week, 343, 343*f*

Embryonic, pertaining to embryo, 347

Emesis, vomiting, usually with some force, 278

Emmetropia (EM)**,** state of normal vision, 463

Emphysema, pulmonary condition that can occur as result of long-term heavy smoking; air pollution also worsens this disease; patient may not be able to breathe except in sitting or standing position, 240

Empyema, pus within pleural space, usually result of infection, 242

Emulsification, to make fats and lipids more soluble in water, 271

Enamel, hardest substance in body; covers outer surface of teeth, 266, 267*f*

Encapsulated, growth enclosed in sheath of tissue that prevents tumor cells from invading surrounding tissue, 536

Encephalic, pertaining to brain, 429

Encephalitis, inflammation of brain due to disease factors such as rabies, influenza, measles, or smallpox, 434

Encopresis, elimination disorder characterized by voiding feces in inappropriate places after toilet training, 514

Endarterectomy, removal of inside layer of an artery, 165

Endings
- plural, 12
- singular, 12

Endocarditis, inflammation of inner lining layer of heart; may be due to microorganisms or to abnormal immunological response, 157

Endocardium, inner layer of heart, which is very smooth and lines chambers of heart, 142, 142*f*

Endocervicitis, inflammation of inner aspect of cervix, 350

Endocrine glands, glandular system that secretes hormones directly into bloodstream rather than into duct; endocrine glands are frequently referred to as ductless glands; endocrine system includes thyroid gland, adrenal glands, parathyroid glands, pituitary gland, pancreas (islets of Langerhans), testes, ovaries, and thymus gland, 388, 388–89t

Endocrine system, body system consisting of glands that secrete hormones directly into bloodstream; endocrine glands include adrenal glands, parathyroid glands, pancreas, pituitary gland, testes, ovaries, thymus gland, and thyroid gland, 385–407
- abbreviations, 407
- adjective forms of anatomical terms, 398
- adrenal glands, 390, 390*f*
- anatomy and physiology, 388–96
- diagnostic procedures, 404–05
- ovaries, 390, 391*f*
- pancreas, 391–92, 391*f*
- parathyroid glands, 392, 392*f*
- pathology, 398–404
- pharmacology, 407
- pineal gland, 392, 392*f*
- pituitary gland, 392–93, 393*f*, 394*f*
- terminology, 397–98
- testes, 394, 394*f*
- therapeutic procedures, 405–06
- thymus gland, 395, 395*f*
- thyroid gland, 395–96, 396f

Endocrinologist, physician who specializes in treatment of endocrine glands, 398

Endocrinology, branch of medicine specializing in conditions of endocrine system, 398

Endocrinopathy, disease of endocrine system, 399

Endometrial, pertaining to the endometrium, 347

Endometrial biopsy (EMB), taking sample of tissue from lining of uterus to test for abnormalities, 356

Endometrial cancer, cancer of endometrial lining of uterus, 350

Endometriosis, abnormal condition of endometrium tissue appearing throughout pelvis or on abdominal wall; this tissue is usually found within uterus, 351

Endometritis, inflammation of endometrial lining of uterus, 350

Endometrium, inner lining of uterus; contains rich blood supply and reacts to hormonal changes every month, which results in menstruation; during pregnancy, lining of uterus does not leave body but remains to nourish unborn child, 340, 340*f*

Endoscopic retrograde cholangiopancreatography (ERCP), using endoscope to X-ray bile and pancreatic ducts, 287

Endoscopic surgery, use of lighted instrument to examine interior of cavity, 533

Endothelium, 147*f*

Endotracheal intubation, placing tube through mouth to create airway, 246, 246*f*

Enteric, pertaining to small intestine, 275

Enteritis, inflammation of only small intestine, 281

Enucleated, loss of cell's nucleus, 182

Enucleation, surgical removal of an eyeball, 471

Enuresis, elimination disorder characterized by the involuntary discharge of urine after age by which bladder control should have been established; usually occurs by age 5; also called *bed-wetting* at night, 315, 514

Enzyme-linked immunosorbent assay (ELISA), blood test for antibody to AIDS virus; positive test means that person has been exposed to virus; in case of false-positive reading, Western blot test would be used to verify results, 207
Eosinophil (eosins, eos), granulocyte white blood cells that destroy parasites and increase during allergic reactions, 181, 183*f*, 183*t*
Eosinophilic, pertaining to eosinophils, 186
Epicardium, outer layer of heart; forms part of pericardium, 142
Epicondyle, projection located above or on condyle, 86, 87*f*
Epidermal, pertaining to above the skin, 56
Epidermis, superficial layer of skin; is composed of squamous epithelium cells; these are flat scalelike cells that are arranged in layers, called stratified squamous epithelium; many layers of epidermis create a barrier to infection; epidermis does not have a blood supply, so is dependent on deeper layers of skin for nourishment; however, deepest epidermis layer is called basal layer; these cells are alive and constantly dividing; older cells are pushed out toward surface by new cells forming beneath; during this process, they shrink and die, becoming filled with a protein called keratin; keratin-filled cells are sloughed off as dead cells, 50–52, 51*f*
Epididymal, pertaining to epididymis, 366
Epididymectomy, surgical removal of epididymis, 371
Epididymis, coiled tubule that lies on top of testes within scrotum; stores sperm as they are produced and turns into vas deferens, 362, 363, 364, 368, 394*f*
Epididymitis, inflammation of epididymis causing pain and swelling in inguinal area, 368
Epidural hematoma, mass of blood in space outside dura mater of brain and spinal cord, 437
Epidural space, 425*f*
Epigastric, pertaining to above stomach; anatomical division of abdomen, middle section of upper row, 37*t*
Epigastric region, 37*t*
Epiglottic, pertaining to epiglottis, 233
Epiglottis, flap of cartilage that covers larynx when swallowing; prevents food and drink from entering larynx and trachea, 225*f*, 226, 266*f*, 268
Epilepsy, recurrent disorder of brain in which convulsive seizures and loss of consciousness occur, 434
Epinephrine, hormone produced by adrenal medulla; also known as *adrenaline*; actions include increased heart rate and force of contraction, bronchodilation, and relaxation of intestinal muscles, 388*t*, 390
Epiphyseal line, 86*f*
Epiphysis, wide ends of a long bone, 85, 86*f*
Episiorrhaphy, suture vulva, 357
Episiotomy, surgical incision of perineum to facilitate delivery process; can prevent irregular tearing of tissue during birth, 357
Epispadias, congenital opening of urethra on dorsal surface of penis, 369
Epistaxis, nosebleed, 225, 236
Epithelial, pertaining to epithelium, 25
Epithelial tissue, tissue found throughout body as skin, outer covering of organs, and inner lining for tubular or hollow structures, 25, 26*f*
Epithelium, epithelial tissue composed of close-packed cells that form covering for and lining of body structures, 25
Equilibrium, sense of balance, 477
Erectile dysfunction (ED), inability to copulate due to inability to maintain erection; also called *impotence*, 369, 514
Erectile dysfunction agents, medications that temporarily produce erection in patients with erectile dysfunction, 373
Erectile tissue, tissue with numerous blood vessels and nerve endings; becomes filled with blood and enlarges in size in response to sexual stimulation, 341, 364
Ergonomics, study of human work including how requirements for performing work and work environment affect musculoskeletal and nervous system, 524
Erythema, redness or flushing of skin, 58
Erythroblastosis fetalis. *See* Hemolytic disease of the newborn
Erythrocyte, also called *red blood cells (RBCs)*; cells that contain hemoglobin, an iron-containing pigment that binds oxygen in order to transport it to cells of body, 182–83, 183*f*, 188–89
Erythrocyte sedimentation rate (ESR, sed rate), blood test to determine rate at which mature red blood cells settle out of blood after addition of anticoagulant; indicator of presence of inflammatory disease, 190
Erythrocytic, pertaining to red blood cells, 186
Erythrocytosis, too many red cells, 188
Erythroderma, red skin, 58
Erythropenia, too few red cells, 188
Eschar, thick layer of dead tissue and tissue fluid that develops over deep burn area, 58
Esophageal, pertaining to esophagus, 275
Esophageal varices, enlarged and swollen varicose veins in lower end of esophagus; they can rupture and result in serious hemorrhage, 279
Esophagogastroduodenoscopy (EGD), use of flexible fiber-optic scope to visually examine esophagus, stomach, and beginning of duodenum, 287
Esophagus, tube that carries food from pharynx to stomach, 225*f*, 263, 264, 266*f*, 268, 268*f*, 279
Esotropia, inward turning of eye; example of a form of strabismus (muscle weakness of eye), 467
Estrogen, one of hormones produced by ovaries; works with progesterone to control menstrual cycle and is responsible for producing secondary sexual characteristics, 339, 389*t*, 390
Ethmoid bone, cranial bone, 87, 89*t*
Eupnea, normal breathing, 236
Eustachian tube, tube or canal that connects middle ear with nasopharynx and allows for balance of pressure between outer and middle ear; infection can travel via mucous membranes of eustachian tube, resulting in middle ear infections, 477*f*, 478

F

Follicle-stimulating hormone (FSH), hormone secreted by anterior pituitary gland; stimulates growth of eggs in females and sperm in males, 339, 389*t*, 393

Foramen, passage or opening through bone for nerves and blood vessels, 86

Forceps, surgical instrument used to grasp tissues, 530*t*

Formed elements, solid, cellular portion of blood; consists of erythrocytes, leukocytes, and platelets, 182

Fossa, shallow cavity or depression within or on surface of a bone, 86

Fovea capitis, 87*f*

Fovea centralis, area of retina that has sharpest vision, 456f, 457

Fowler position, surgical position in which patient is sitting with back positioned at 45° angle, 531*f*, 532*t*

Fracture (FX, Fx), injury to bone that causes it to break; named to describe type of damage to bone, 100–102

Fraternal twins, twins that develop from two different ova fertilized by two different sperm; although twins, these siblings do not have identical DNA, 348

Free edge, exposed edge of a nail that is trimmed when nails become too long, 53, 53*f*

Frequency, greater than normal occurrence in urge to urinate, without increase in total daily volume of urine; frequency is indication of inflammation of bladder or urethra, 315

Frontal bone, forehead bone of skull, 87, 89*f*, 89*t*

Frontal lobe, one of four cerebral hemisphere lobes; controls motor functions, 423, 423*f*

Frontal plane, vertical plane that divides body into front (anterior or ventral) and back (posterior or dorsal) sections; also called *coronal plane*, 33, 33*f*

Frontal section, sectional view of body produced by cut along frontal plane; also called *coronal section*, 33

Frozen section (FS), thin piece of tissue is cut from frozen specimen for rapid examination under a microscope, 69

Full-term pregnancy, 343*f*

Functional bowel syndrome. *See* Irritable bowel syndrome

Functional residual capacity (FRC), air that remains in lungs after normal exhalation has taken place, 229*t*

Fundus, domed upper portion of organ such as stomach or uterus, 268, 268*f*, 338*f*, 340, 340*f*, 343*f*

Fungal scrapings, scrapings, taken with curette or scraper, of tissue from lesions are placed on a growth medium and examined under a microscope to identify fungal growth, 69

Fungi, organisms found in Kingdom Fungi; some are capable of causing disease in humans, such as yeast infections or histoplasmosis, 199

Furuncle, staphylococcal skin abscess with redness, pain, and swelling; also called a *boil*, 67

G

Gait, manner of walking, 524

Gait training, assisting person to learn to walk again or how to use assistive device to walk, 525, 525*f*

Gallbladder (GB), small organ located just under liver; functions to store bile produced by liver; releases bile into duodenum through common bile duct, 263, 264, 271–72, 272*f*

Gambling disorder, addictive disorder in which patient is unable to control urge to gamble, 513

Gametes, reproductive sex cells—ova and sperm, 390

Gamma globulin, protein component of blood containing antibodies that help to resist infection, 182

Ganglion, knotlike mass of nerve tissue located outside brain and spinal cord, 426

Ganglion cyst, cyst that forms on tendon sheath, usually on hand, wrist, or ankle, 123

Gangrene, necrosis of skin usually due to deficient blood supply, 64

Gastralgia, stomach pain, 278

Gastrectomy, surgical removal of stomach, 289

Gastric, pertaining to stomach, 275

Gastric carcinoma, cancerous tumor of stomach, 279

Gastric stapling, procedure that closes off large section of stomach with rows of staples; results in a much smaller stomach to assist very obese patients to lose weight, 289

Gastritis, inflammation of stomach that can result in pain, tenderness, nausea, and vomiting, 279

Gastroenteritis, inflammation of stomach and small intestine, 279

Gastroenterologist, physician specialized in treating diseases and conditions of gastrointestinal tract, 277

Gastroenterology, branch of medicine specializing in conditions of gastrointestinal system, 277

Gastroesophageal reflux disease (GERD), acid from stomach backs up into esophagus, causing inflammation and pain, 279

Gastrointestinal system (GI), digests food and absorbs nutrients; organs include mouth, pharynx, esophagus, stomach, small and large intestines, liver, gallbladder, and anus; also called *digestive system*, 264, 275

Gastrointestinal tract, continuous tube that extends from mouth to anus; also called *gut* or *alimentary canal*, 264

Gastroscope, instrument to view inside stomach, 287

Gastroscopy, flexible gastroscope is passed through mouth and down esophagus in order to visualize inside stomach; used to diagnose peptic ulcers and gastric carcinoma, 287

Gastrostomy, surgical creation of gastric fistula or opening through abdominal wall; opening is used to place food into stomach when esophagus is not entirely open (esophageal stricture), 289

Gavage, using nasogastric tube to place liquid nourishment directly into stomach, 288

Gender dysphoria, person identifies as gender contrary to the gender of his or her birth, 513

General anesthesia (GA)**,** produces a loss of consciousness including absence of pain sensation; administered to patient by either intravenous or inhalation method; patient's vital signs must be carefully monitored when in use, 530*t*

General anxiety disorder, feeling dread in absence of clearly identifiable stress trigger, 510

Grade, tumor can be graded from grade I through grade IV; based on microscopic appearance of tumor cells; grade I tumor is well differentiated and is easier to treat than more advanced grades, 536, 536*t*

Graft versus host disease (GVHD), serious complication of bone marrow transplant; immune cells from donor bone marrow (graft) attack recipient's (host's) tissues, 206

Grand mal seizure. *See* Tonic-clonic seizure

Granulocytes, granular polymorphonuclear leukocytes; three types: neutrophil, eosinophil, and basophil, 183, 183*t*

Graves' disease, condition resulting in overactivity of thyroid gland and can result in crisis situation; also called *hyperthyroidism*, 403

Gray matter, tissue within central nervous system; consists of unsheathed or uncovered nerve cell bodies and dendrites, 421

Great saphenous vein, 150*f*

Greenstick fracture, fracture in which there is incomplete break; one side of bone is broken and other side is bent; commonly found in children due to their softer and more pliable bone structure, 101

Gross motor skills, use of large muscle groups that coordinate body movements such as walking, running, jumping, and balance, 524

Growth hormone (GH), hormone secreted by anterior pituitary that stimulates growth of body, 389*t*, 393

Guillain-Barré syndrome, disease of nervous system in which nerves lose their myelin covering; may be caused by autoimmune reaction; characterized by loss of sensation and/or muscle control in arms and legs; symptoms then move toward trunk and may even result in paralysis of diaphragm, 436

Gums, tissue around teeth; also called *gingival*, 265

Gut, name for continuous muscular tube that stretches between mouth and anus; also called *alimentary canal*, 264

Gynecologist, physician specialized in treating conditions and diseases of female reproductive system, 349

Gynecology (GYN, gyn), branch of medicine specializing in conditions of female reproductive system, 349

Gynecomastia, development of breast tissue in males; may be symptom of adrenal feminization, 399

Gyri, convoluted, elevated portions of cerebral cortex; separated by fissures or sulci; singular is *gyrus*, 423

H

H_2-receptor antagonist, blocks production of stomach acids, 291

Habituation, development of emotional dependence on drug due to repeated use, 507

Hair, structure in integumentary system, 52, 53*f*, 67

Hair follicle, cavities in dermis that contain hair root; hair grows longer from root, 52, 53*f*

Hair root, deeper cells that divide to grow hair longer, 52, 53*f*

Hair shaft, older keratinized cells that form most of length of a hair, 52, 53*f*

Hallucination, perception of something that is not there; may be visual, auditory, gustatory, or tactile, 512

Hammer. *See* Malleus

Hard palate, 265*f*–66*f*

Hashimoto's thyroiditis, chronic form of thyroiditis, 403

Head, large ball-shaped end of a bone; may be separated from shaft of bone by area called neck, 86, 87*f*

Health Insurance Portability and Accountability Act (HIPAA), 16

Health Maintenance Organization (HMO), organization that contracts with group of physicians and other healthcare workers to provide care exclusively for its members, 15

Healthcare settings, 15

Hearing, one of special senses; sound waves detected by ear, 477, 479, 479*f*, 482

Hearing aid, apparatus or mechanical device used by persons with impaired hearing to amplify sound; same as amplification device, 486

Hearing impairment, 479

Heart, organ of cardiovascular system that contracts to pump blood through blood vessels, 139, 140, 141–46, 155–58, 196*f*, 229*f*, 395*f*
- chambers, 143–44
- conduction system of, 145, 146*f*
- layers, 142, 142*f*
- valves, 143*f*, 144

Heart attack. *See* Myocardial infarction

Heart transplantation, replacement of diseased or malfunctioning heart with donor's heart, 165

Heart valve prolapse, cusps or flaps of heart valve are too loose and fail to shut tightly, allowing blood to flow backward through valve when heart chamber contracts; most commonly occurs in mitral valve, but may affect any of heart valves, 157

Heart valve stenosis, cusps or flaps of heart valve are too stiff; therefore, they are unable to open fully, making it difficult for blood to flow through, or to shut tightly, allowing blood to flow backward; condition may affect any of heart valves, 157

Heartburn. *See* Pyrosis

Heimlich maneuver, technique for removing foreign body or food from trachea or pharynx when it is choking a person; maneuver consists of applying pressure just under diaphragm to pop obstruction out, 248

***Helicobacter pylori* (*H. pylori*),** bacteria responsible for causing some cases of peptic ulcer disease, 280

Hematemesis, to vomit blood from gastrointestinal tract, 278

Hematic, pertaining to blood, 186

Hematic system, consists of plasma and blood cells—erythrocytes, leukocytes, and platelets; responsible for transporting oxygen, protecting against pathogens, and controlling bleeding, 28*t*

Hematinic, substance that increases number of erythrocytes or amount of hemoglobin in blood, 192

Hematochezia, passing bright red blood in stool, 278

also called *hyaline membrane disease (HMD)* and *respiratory distress syndrome of the newborn*, 241

Infarct, area of tissue within organ that undergoes necrosis (death) following loss of blood supply, 154

Inferior, directional term meaning toward feet or tail, or below, 39*f*, 39*t*

Inferior vena cava, branch of vena cava that drains blood from abdomen and lower body, 142*f*, 144, 145*f*, 150*f*, 390*f*

Infertility, inability to produce children; generally defined as no pregnancy after properly timed intercourse for one year, 353

Inflammation, tissue response to injury from pathogens or physical agents; characterized by redness, pain, swelling, and feeling hot to touch, 204, 204*f*

Inflammatory bowel disease (IBD). *See* Ulcerative colitis

Influenza, viral infection of respiratory system characterized by chills, fever, body aches, and fatigue; commonly called the *flu*, 241

Informed consent, medical record document, voluntarily signed by patient or responsible party, that clearly describes purpose, methods, procedures, benefits, and risks of diagnostic or treatment procedure, 14

Inguinal, pertaining to groin area; there is a collection of lymph nodes in this region that drain each leg, 197*t*, 198*f*, 203

Inguinal hernia, hernia or protrusion of intestine into inguinal region of body, 282, 282*f*

Inguinal nodes, 198*f*

Inhalation, (1) to breathe air into lungs; also called *inspiration*; (2) to introduce drugs into body by inhaling them, 224, 505*f*, 505*t*, 530*t*

Innate immunity, 200

Inner ear, innermost section of ear; contains cochlea, semicircular canals, saccule, and utricle, 476, 477, 478, 479*f*, 483

Inner ear infection. *See* Labyrinthitis

Innominate bone, also called *os coxae* or *hipbone*; pelvis portion of lower extremity; consists of ilium, ischium, and pubis and unites with sacrum and coccyx to form pelvis, 92

Insertion, attachment of skeletal muscle to more movable bone in joint, 117, 117*f*

Insomnia disorder, sleeping disorder characterized by marked inability to fall asleep, 513

Inspiration. *See* Inhalation

Inspiratory capacity (IC), volume of air inhaled after normal exhale, 229*t*

Inspiratory reserve volume (IRV), air that can be forcibly inhaled after normal respiration has taken place; also called *complemental air*, 229*t*

Insulin, hormone secreted by pancreas; regulates level of sugar in bloodstream; the more insulin present in blood, the lower blood sugar will be, 389*t*, 391, 391*f*, 407

Insulin-dependent diabetes mellitus (IDDM), also called *type 1 diabetes mellitus*; develops early in life when pancreas stops insulin production; people with IDDM must take daily insulin injections, 401

Insulinoma, tumor of islets of Langerhans cells of pancreas that secretes excessive amount of insulin, 401

Integument, another term for skin, 50

Integumentary system, skin and its appendages including sweat glands, oil glands, hair, and nails; sense organs that allow humans to respond to changes in temperature, pain, touch, and pressure are located in skin; largest organ in body, 47–80, 49*f*
- abbreviations, 72
- accessory organs, 52–54
- adjective forms of anatomical terms, 56
- anatomy and physiology of, 50–54
- diagnostic procedures, 69
- pathology, 57–68
- pharmacology, 71
- skin, 50–52
- terminology, 55–56
- therapeutic procedures, 69–70

Intellectual development disorder, disorder characterized by below average intellectual functions, 511

Interatrial, pertaining to between atria, 153

Interatrial septum, wall or septum that divides left and right atria, 143

Intercostal muscles, muscles between ribs; when contracted, they raise ribs, which helps to enlarge thoracic cavity, 299

Intercostal nerve, 427*f*

Intermittent claudication, attacks of severe pain and lameness caused by ischemia of muscles, typically calf muscles; brought on by walking even very short distances, 122

Intermittent positive pressure breathing (IPPB), method for assisting patients to breathe using mask connected to a machine that produces increased pressure, 246

Internal genitalia, 338–41

Internal iliac artery, 148*f*

Internal iliac vein, 150*f*

Internal medicine, branch of medicine involving diagnosis and treatment of diseases and conditions of internal organs such as respiratory system; physician is *internist*, 234

Internal respiration, process of oxygen and carbon dioxide exchange at cellular level when oxygen leaves bloodstream and is delivered to tissues, 224

Internal sphincter, ring of involuntary muscle that keeps urine within bladder, 308

Internist, physician specialized in treating diseases and conditions of internal organs such as respiratory system, 234

Internodal pathway, 146*f*

Interstitial cystitis, disease of unknown cause in which there is inflammation and irritation of bladder; most commonly seen in middle-aged women, 318

Interventricular, pertaining to between ventricles, 153

Interventricular septum, wall or septum that divides left and right ventricles, 145*f*, 146*f*

Intervertebral, pertaining to between vertebrae, 97

J

K

L

Left upper quadrant (LUQ), clinical division of abdomen; contains left lobe of liver, spleen, stomach, portion of pancreas, and portion of small and large intestines, 38*t*

Left ventricle, 140*f*, 142*f*, 145*f*

Legally blind, describes person who has severely impaired vision; usually defined as having visual acuity of 20/200, 466

Legionnaires' disease, severe, often fatal bacterial infection characterized by pneumonia and liver and kidney damage; named after people who came down with it at American Legion convention in 1976, 241

Lens, transparent structure behind pupil and iris; functions to bend light rays so they land on retina, 455, 456*f*, 457

Lesion, general term for wound, injury, or abnormality, 58

Leukemia, cancer of WBC-forming bone marrow; results in large number of abnormal WBCs circulating in blood, 189

Leukocytes, also called *white blood cells (WBCs)*; group of several different types of cells that provide protection against invasion of bacteria and other foreign material; able to leave bloodstream and search out foreign invaders (bacteria, viruses, and toxins), where they perform phagocytosis, 182, 183, 183*f*, 183*t*, 189, 198*f*

Leukocytic, pertaining to white blood cells, 186

Leukocytosis, too many white blood cells, 189

Leukoderma, disappearance of pigment from skin in patches, causing milk-white appearance; also called *vitiligo*, 58

Leukopenia, too few white (cells), 189

Leukorrhea, whitish or yellowish vaginal discharge, 349

Ligaments, very strong bands of connective tissue that bind bones together at a joint, 84, 94

Ligation and stripping, surgical treatment for varicose veins; damaged vein is tied off (ligation) and removed (stripping), 165

Lingual tonsils, tonsils located on very posterior section of tongue as it joins with pharynx, 166*f*

Lipocytes, medical term for cells that contain fat molecules, 52

Lipoma, fatty tumor that generally does not metastasize, 58

Liposuction, removal of fat beneath skin by means of suction, 70

Lips, anterior opening of oral cavity, 265, 265f, 266*f*

Lithium, special category of drug used successfully to calm patients who suffer from bipolar disorder, 514

Lithotomy, surgical incision to remove kidney stones, 323

Lithotomy position, lying face up with hips and knees bent at 90° angles, 531*f*, 532*t*

Lithotripsy, destroying or crushing kidney stones in bladder or urethra with device called lithotriptor, 323

Liver, large organ located in right upper quadrant of abdomen; serves many functions in body; digestive system role includes producing bile, processing absorbed nutrients, and detoxifying harmful substances, 263, 264, 271, 272*f*

Liver transplant, transplant of a liver from a donor, 290

Lobe, ear, 477*f*

Lobectomy, surgical removal of a lobe from an organ, such as a lung; often treatment of choice for lung cancer; may also be removal of one lobe of thyroid gland, 247, 406

Lobes, subdivisions of organ such as lungs or brain, 228, 229*f*

Local anesthesia, substance that produces a loss of sensation in one localized part of body; patient remains conscious when using this type of anesthetic; administered either topically or via subcutaneous route, 530*t*

Long bone, type of bone longer than it is wide; examples include femur, humerus, and phalanges, 85, 85*f*, 86*f*

Long-term care facility, facility that provides long-term care for patients who need extra time to recover from illness or accident before they return home or for persons who can no longer care for themselves; also called a *nursing home*, 15

Longitudinal section, internal view of body produced by lengthwise slice along long axis of structure, 33

Loop of Henle, portion of renal tubule, 307

Lordosis, abnormal increase in forward curvature of lumbar spine; also known as *swayback*, 104, 104*f*

Lower esophageal sphincter, also called *cardiac sphincter*; prevents food and gastric juices from backing up into esophagus, 269

Lower extremity (LE), the leg, 90, 91*f*, 93*t*, 524

Lower gastrointestinal series (lower GI series), X-ray image of colon and rectum is taken after administration of barium by enema; also called *barium enema*, 286, 286*f*

Lumbar, pertaining to five low back vertebrae, 97

Lumbar puncture (LP), puncture with needle into lumbar area (usually fourth intervertebral space) to withdraw fluid for examination and for injection of anesthesia; also called *spinal puncture* or *spinal tap*, 440, 440*f*

Lumbar vertebrae, five vertebrae in low back region, 89, 90*f*, 90*t*

Lumbosacral plexus, 427*f*

Lumen, space, cavity, or channel within tube or tubular organ or structure in body, 146, 147*f*

Lumpectomy, surgical removal of only a breast tumor and tissue immediately surrounding it, 358

Lung metastases, 537*f*

Lung volumes/capacities, 228, 229*f*

Lungs, major organs of respiration; consist of air passageways, bronchi and bronchioles, and air sacs, or alveoli; gas exchange takes place within alveoli, 141*f*, 223, 224, 228, 229*f*, 239–42, 395*f*

Lunula, lighter-colored, half-moon region at base of a nail, 53, 53*f*

Luteinizing hormone (LH), secreted by anterior pituitary; regulates function of male and female gonads and plays a role in releasing ova in females, 339, 389*t*, 393

Lymph, clear, transparent, colorless fluid found in lymphatic vessels, 196

Lymph glands, another name for *lymph nodes*; small organs composed of lymphatic tissue located along route of lymphatic vessels; remove impurities from

lymph and manufacture lymphocytes and antibodies, 197
Lymph nodes, small organs in lymphatic system that filter bacteria and other foreign organisms from body fluids, 195, 196, 197, 197*t*, 198*f*
Lymphadenectomy, removal of a lymph node; this is usually done to test for malignancy, 208
Lymphadenitis, inflammation of lymph glands; referred to as swollen glands, 205
Lymphadenopathy, disease of lymph nodes, 205
Lymphangial, pertaining to lymph vessels, 203
Lymphangiogram, X-ray taken of lymph vessels after injection of dye; lymph flow through chest is traced, 207
Lymphangiography, process of taking X-ray of lymph vessels after injection of dye, 207
Lymphangioma, lymph vessel tumor, 205
Lymphatic, pertaining to lymph, 203
Lymphatic and immune system, 194–209
abbreviations, 209
adjective forms of anatomical terms, 203
anatomy and physiology, 196–201
diagnostic procedures, 207–08
immunity, 199–201
lymph nodes, 197, 197*t*, 198*f*
pathology, 203–06
pharmacology, 209
spleen, 199
terminology, 202–08
therapeutic procedures, 208
thymus gland, 199
tonsils, 199
Lymphatic capillaries, smallest lymph vessels; collect excessive tissue fluid, 196
Lymphatic ducts, two largest vessels in lymphatic system, right lymphatic duct and thoracic duct, 197, 198*f*
Lymphatic system, helps body fight infection; organs include spleen, lymph vessels, and lymph nodes, 29*t*, 195
Lymphatic vessels, extensive network of vessels throughout entire body; conduct lymph from tissue toward thoracic cavity, 195, 196–197, 196f, 197*f*, 198*f*
Lymphedema, edema appearing in extremities due to obstruction of lymph flow through lymphatic vessels, 204
Lymphocyte (lymphs), agranulocyte white blood cell that provides protection through immune response, 181, 183*f*, 183*t*
Lymphocytic, pertaining to lymphocytes, 186
Lymphoma, tumor of lymphatic tissue, 205

M

Macrophage, phagocytic cells found in large quantities in lymph nodes; engulf foreign particles, 199
Macrotia, abnormally large ears, 482
Macula lutea, area of retina onto which straight-ahead images are projected, 457
Macular, pertaining to macula lutea, 462
Macular degeneration, deterioration of macular area of retina of eye; may be treated with laser surgery to destroy blood vessels beneath macula, 466
Macule, flat, discolored area flush with skin surface; example would be freckle or birthmark, 58, 58*f*
Magnetic resonance imaging (MRI)**,** medical imaging that uses radio-frequency radiation as its source of energy; does not require injection of contrast medium or exposure to ionizing radiation; useful for visualizing large blood vessels, heart, brain, and soft tissues, 519, 519*f*
Major depressive disorder, mood disorder characterized by marked loss of interest in usually enjoyable activities, disturbances in sleep and eating patterns, fatigue, suicidal thoughts, and feelings of hopelessness, helplessness, and worthlessness, 512
Male reproductive system, responsible for producing sperm for reproduction; organs include penis, testes, epididymis, vas deferens, seminal vesicles, prostate gland, and bulbourethral glands, 361–73, 363*f*
abbreviations, 373
adjective forms of anatomical terms, 366–67
anatomy and physiology, 363–65
bulbourethral glands, 365
diagnostic procedures, 371
epididymis, 364
external organs of, 363–64
internal organs of, 365
pathology, 367–70
penis, 364
pharmacology, 373
prostate gland, 365
seminal vesicles, 365
terminology, 366–70
testes, 363–64
therapeutic procedures, 371–72
vas deferens, 365
Male urethra, 305, 309*f*
Malignant, cancerous tumor; generally progressive and recurring, 535
Malignant melanoma (MM), cancerous, darkly pigmented tumor or mole on skin, 65, 65*f*
Malleus, one of three ossicles of middle ear; also called *hammer*, 477*f*, 478, 478*f*
Mammary, pertaining to breast, 347
Mammary glands, breasts; milk-producing glands to provide nutrition for newborn, 342
Mammogram, X-ray record of breast, 354
Mammography, process of X-raying breast, 354
Mammoplasty, surgical repair of breast, 358
Mandible, lower jawbone, 87, 89*f*, 89*t*, 225*f*
Mandibular, pertaining to mandible or lower jaw, 97
Mania, depressive disorder characterized by extreme elation and euphoria; patient displays rapid speech, flight of ideas, decreased sleep, distractibility, grandiosity, and poor judgment, 512
Massage, kneading or applying pressure by hands to a part of patient's body to promote muscle relaxation and reduce tension, 526
Mastalgia, breast pain, 349
Mastectomy, surgical removal of breast, 358

N

Neonatologist, specialist in treatment of newborn, 349
Neonatology, study of newborn, 349
Neoplasm, abnormal growth of tissue that may be benign or malignant; also called a *tumor*, 537
Nephrectomy, surgical removal of a kidney, 323
Nephritis, inflammation of kidney, 317
Nephrogram, X-ray of kidney, 320
Nephrolith, kidney stone, 315
Nephrolithiasis, presence of calculi in kidney, 317
Nephrolithotomy, incision into kidney to remove a stone, 323
Nephrologist, specialist in treatment of kidney disorders, 314
Nephrology, branch of medicine specializing in conditions of urinary system, 314
Nephroma, kidney tumor, 317
Nephromalacia, softening of kidney, 315
Nephromegaly, enlarged kidney, 315
Nephron, functional or working unit of kidney that filters blood and produces urine; more than 1 million in adult kidney; each consists of renal corpuscle and renal tubules, 306, 307, 308*f*
Nephropathy, kidney disease, 317
Nephropexy, surgical fixation of kidney, 323
Nephroptosis, drooping kidney, 317
Nephrosclerosis, hardening of kidney, 315
Nephrosis. *See* Nephrotic syndrome
Nephrostomy, creating new opening across body wall into kidney, 323
Nephrotic syndrome (NS), damage to glomerulus resulting in protein appearing in urine, proteinuria, and corresponding decrease in protein in bloodstream, 317
Nephrotomy, incision into kidney, 323
Nerve block, also referred to as *regional anesthesia*; anesthetic interrupts patient's pain sensation in particular region of body; anesthetic injected near nerve that will be blocked from sensation; patient usually remains conscious, 440, 530*t*
Nerve cell body, portion of nerve cell that includes nucleus, 420, 421*f*
Nerve cells. *See* Neuron
Nerve conduction velocity, test to determine if nerves have been damaged by recording rate at which electrical impulse travels along nerve; if nerve is damaged, velocity will be decreased, 440, 526
Nerve root, point where spinal or cranial nerve is attached to CNS, 426
Nerves, structures in nervous system that conduct electrical impulses from brain and spinal cord to muscles and other organs, 25, 31*t*, 419, 420, 436–37
Nervous system, coordinates all conscious and subconscious activities of body; organs include brain, spinal cord, and nerves, 417–42
  abbreviations, 442
  adjective forms of anatomical terms, 429–30
  anatomy and physiology, 420–27
  central, 421–25
  diagnostic procedures, 439–40
  nervous tissue, 420, 421*f*
  pathology, 430–38
  peripheral, 426–27
  pharmacology, 441–42
  terminology, 428–30
  therapeutic procedures, 440–41
Nervous tissue, conducts electrical impulses to and from brain and rest of body, 25, 26*f*, 420, 421*f*
Neural, pertaining to nerves, 429
Neuralgia, nerve pain, 431
Neurectomy, surgical removal of a nerve, 440
Neurocognitive disorders, a classification of psychiatric disorders in the DSM-5 characterized by deterioration of mental functions due to temporary brain or permanent brain dysfunction; includes dementia and Alzheimer's disease, 511
Neurodevelopmental disorders, a classification of psychiatric disorders in the DSM-5 associated with impairment in the growth or development of the CNS; includes intellectual development disorder, attention-deficit/hyperactivity disorder, and autism spectrum disorder, 511
Neurogenic bladder, loss of nervous control that leads to retention; may be caused by spinal cord injury or multiple sclerosis, 318
Neuroglial, pertaining to glial cells, 429
Neuroglial cells, nervous tissue cells that perform support functions for neurons, 420
Neurologist, physician who specializes in disorders of nervous system, 430
Neurology, branch of medicine specializing in conditions of nervous system, 430
Neuroma, nerve tumor, 437
Neuron, name for individual nerve cell; neurons group together to form nerves and other nervous tissue, 420, 421*f*
Neuropathy, disease of nerves, 437
Neuroplasty, surgical repair of nerves, 440
Neurorrhaphy, suture a nerve, 441
Neurosurgery, branch of medicine specializing in surgery on nervous system, 430
Neurotransmitter, chemical messenger that carries electrical impulse across gap between two neurons, 420
Neutrophil, granulocyte white blood cells that are important for phagocytosis; also most numerous of leukocytes, 181, 183*f*, 183*t*
Neutrophilic, pertaining to neutrophils, 186
Nevus, pigmented (colored) congenital skin blemish, birthmark, or mole; usually benign but may become cancerous, 59
Night blindness. *See* Nyctalopia
Nipple, point at which milk is released from breast, 342, 342*f*
Nitrogenous wastes, waste products that contain nitrogen; products, such as ammonia and urea, are produced during protein metabolism, 311
Nocturia, excessive urination during night; may or may not be abnormal, 315
Nocturnal enuresis. *See* Enuresis
Nodule, solid, raised group of cells, 59, 59*f*
Non-Hodgkin's lymphoma (NHL), cancer of lymphatic tissues other than Hodgkin's lymphoma, 205, 205*f*

O

Ophthalmology (Ophth), branch of medicine specializing in condition of eye, 456, 463
Ophthalmoplegia, paralysis of eye, 464
Ophthalmorrhagia, bleeding from the eye, 464
Ophthalmoscope, instrument to view inside eye, 469, 470*f*
Ophthalmoscopy, examination of interior of eyes using instrument called ophthalmoscope; physician dilates pupil in order to see cornea, lens, and retina; identifies abnormalities in blood vessels of eye and some systemic diseases, 469
Opiates. *See* Narcotic analgesic
Opportunistic infections, infectious diseases associated with patients who have compromised immune systems and lowered resistance to infections and parasites, 206
Opposition, moves thumb away from palm; ability to move thumb into contact with other fingers, 119*t*
Optic, pertaining to eye, 462
Optic disk, area of retina associated with optic nerve; also called *blind spot*, 457
Optic nerve, second cranial nerve that carries impulses from retinas to brain, 426*t*, 456, 456*f*
Optical, pertaining to eye or vision, 462
Optician, grinds and fits prescription lenses and contacts as prescribed by physician or optometrist, 463
Optometer, instrument to measure vision, 470
Optometrist (OD), doctor of optometry; provides care for eyes including examining eyes for diseases, assessing visual acuity, prescribing corrective lenses and eye treatments, and educating patients, 463
Optometry, process of measuring vision, 463
Oral, (1) pertaining to mouth; (2) administration of medication through mouth, 275, 504*t*
Oral cavity, the mouth, 263, 264–66, 265f–266*f*
Oral contraceptive pills (OCPs), birth control medication that uses low doses of female hormones to prevent conception by blocking ovulation, 359
Oral hypoglycemic agents, medication taken by mouth that causes decrease in blood sugar; not used for insulin-dependent patients; no proof that medication will prevent long-term complications of diabetes mellitus, 407
Oral surgeon, practitioner of oral surgery, 277
Oral surgery, branch of dentistry that uses surgical means to treat dental conditions; specialist is *oral surgeon*, 277
Orbit, 89*f*
Orchidectomy, surgical removal of one or both testes, 371
Orchidopexy, surgical fixation to move undescended testes into scrotum and attaching to prevent retraction, 368, 371
Orchiectomy, surgical removal of one or both testes, 371
Orchioplasty, surgical repair of testes, 371
Orchiotomy, to cut into testes, 371
Orchitis, inflammation of a testis, 368
Organs, group of different types of tissue coming together to perform special functions; for example, heart contains muscular fibers, nerve tissue, and blood vessels, 27, 27–31*t*
Organs of Corti, sensory receptor hair cells lining cochlea; these cells change sound vibrations to electrical impulses and send impulses to brain via vestibulocochlear nerve, 478
Origin, attachment of skeletal muscle to less movable bone in joint, 116, 117*f*
Oropharynx, middle section of pharynx that receives food and drink from mouth, 225*f*, 226, 268
Orthodontic, pertaining to straight teeth, 266
Orthodontics, dental specialty concerned with straightening teeth, 277
Orthodontist, dental specialist in straightening teeth, 277
Orthopedic surgeon, 99
Orthopedic surgery, branch of medicine specializing in surgical treatments of musculoskeletal system, 28*t*, 99
Orthopedics (Ortho), branch of medicine specializing in diagnosis and treatment of conditions of musculoskeletal system, 28*t*, 99
Orthopedist, 99
Orthopnea, term to describe patient who needs to sit up straight in order to breathe comfortably, 237
Orthostatic hypotension, sudden drop in blood pressure person experiences when standing up suddenly, 154
Orthotics, use of equipment, such as splints and braces, to support paralyzed muscle, promote specific motion, or correct musculoskeletal deformities, 99, 108, 524
Os coxae, also called *innominate bone* or *hipbone*; pelvis portion of lower extremity; consists of ilium, ischium, and pubis and unites with sacrum and coccyx to form pelvis, 92, 93*t*
Osseous tissue, bony tissue; one of hardest materials in body, 84
Ossicles, three small bones in middle ear; bones are incus, malleus, and stapes; ossicles amplify and conduct sound waves to inner ear, 478
Ossification, process of bone formation, 84
Ostealgia, bone pain, 99
Osteoarthritis (OA), noninflammatory type of arthritis resulting in degeneration of bones and joints, especially those bearing weight, 3, 105
Osteoblast, immature bone cell, 84
Osteochondroma, tumor composed of both cartilage and bony substance, 102
Osteoclasia, intentional breaking of bone in order to correct deformity, 108
Osteocyte, mature bone cell, 84
Osteogenic sarcoma, most common type of bone cancer; usually begins in osteocytes found at ends of long bones, 102
Osteomalacia, softening of bones caused by deficiency of calcium; thought to be caused by insufficient sunlight and vitamin D in children, 102
Osteomyelitis, inflammation of bone and bone marrow due to infection; can be difficult to treat, 99
Osteopathy, form of medicine that places great emphasis on musculoskeletal system and body system as a whole; manipulation is also used as part of treatment, 102
Osteoporosis, decrease in bone mass that results in thinning and weakening of bone with resulting fractures; bone becomes more porous, especially in spine and pelvis, 103

P

Pansinusitis, inflammation of all sinuses, 237
Pap (Papanicolaou) **smear,** test for early detection of cancer of cervix named after developer of test, George Papanicolaou, a Greek physician; a scraping of cells is removed from cervix for examination under a microscope, 354
Papilla, 53*f*
Papilledema, swelling of optic disk, often a result of increased intraocular pressure; also called *choked disk*, 464
Papule, small, solid, circular raised spot on surface of skin, often a result of inflammation in oil gland, 59, 59*f*
Paracentesis, insertion of needle into abdominal cavity to withdraw fluid; tests to diagnose disease may be conducted on fluid, 287
Paralysis, temporary or permanent loss of function or voluntary movement, 432
Paranasal, pertaining to the sinuses beside the nose, 233
Paranasal sinuses, air-filled cavities within facial bones that open into nasal cavity; act as echo chamber during sound production, 225, 225*f*
Paranoid personality disorder, personality disorder characterized by exaggerated feelings of persecution, 512
Paraphilic disorders, a classification of psychiatric disorders in the DSM-5 involving aberrant sexual activity; includes pedophilic disorder, sexual masochism disorder, and voyeuristic disorder, 513
Paraplegia, paralysis of lower portion of body and both legs, 432
Parasympathetic branch, branch of autonomic nervous system; serves as counterbalance for sympathetic nerves; causes heart rate to slow down, lowers blood pressure, constricts eye pupils, and increases digestion, 427
Parathyroid glands, four small glands located on back surface of thyroid gland; regulate amount of calcium in blood by secreting parathyroid hormone, 387, 389*t*, 392, 392*f*, 401
Parathyroid hormone (PTH), secreted by parathyroid glands; the more hormone, the higher the calcium level in blood and the lower the level stored in bone; low hormone level will cause tetany, 389*t*, 392
Parenteral, route for introducing medication into body through needle with syringe inserted either under the skin or into a muscle, vein, or body cavity, 505*f*, 505*t*
Parathyroidal, pertaining to parathyroid glands, 398
Parathyroidectomy, surgical removal of one or more of parathyroid glands; performed to halt progress of hyperparathyroidism, 406
Parenteral administration of drugs, 505*t*
Paresthesia, abnormal sensation such as burning or tingling, 432
Parietal bone, cranial bone, 87, 89*f*, 89*t*
Parietal layer, outer pleural layer around lungs; lines inside of chest cavity, 36
Parietal lobe, one of four cerebral hemisphere lobes; receives and interprets nerve impulses from sensory receptors, 423, 423*f*
Parietal pericardium, outer layer of pericardium surrounding heart, 142
Parietal peritoneum, outer layer of serous membrane sac lining abdominopelvic cavity, 36
Parietal pleura, outer layer of serous membrane sac lining thoracic cavity, 228
Parkinson's disease, chronic disorder of nervous system with fine tremors, muscular weakness, rigidity, and shuffling gait, 434
Paronychia, infection around nail, 68, 68*f*
Parotid duct, 271*f*
Parotid glands, pair of salivary glands located in front of ears, 271, 271*f*
Passive acquired immunity, results when person receives protective substances produced by another human or animal; may take form of maternal antibodies crossing placenta to baby or antitoxin injection, 200
Passive range of motion (PROM), therapist putting patient's joints through full range of motion without assistance from patient, 526
Patella, also called *kneecap*; lower extremity bone, 92, 93*f*, 93*t*
Patellar, pertaining to patella or kneecap, 97
Patent, open or unblocked, such as patent airway, 237
Patent ductus arteriosus (PDA), congenital heart anomaly in which opening between pulmonary artery and aorta fails to close at birth; condition requires surgery, 160
Pathogenic, pertaining to microscopic organisms, such as bacteria, capable of causing disease, 200
Pathogens, disease-bearing organisms, 50, 183
Pathologic fracture, caused by diseased or weakened bone, 101
Pathologist, physician who specializes in evaluating specimens removed from living or dead patients, 203, 536
Pathologist's report, medical record report given by pathologist who studies tissue removed from patient (e.g., bone marrow, blood, or tissue biopsy), 14
Pathology, branch of medicine specializing in studying how disease affects body, 203
Pectoral girdle, consists of clavicle and scapula; functions to attach upper extremity to axial skeleton, 90, 91*f*, 92*t*
Pediculosis, infestation with lice, 66
Pedophilic disorder, paraphilic disorder characterized by having sexual interest in children, 513
Pelvic, pertaining to pelvis, 34
Pelvic cavity, inferior portion of abdominopelvic cavity, 36, 36*f*, 37*t*, 351
Pelvic examination, physical examination of vagina and adjacent organs performed by physician placing fingers of one hand into vagina; visual examination is performed using speculum, 356
Pelvic girdle, consists of ilium, ischium, and pubis; functions to attach lower extremity to axial skeleton, 90, 91*f*, 93*t*
Pelvic inflammatory disease (PID), any inflammation of female reproductive organs, generally bacterial in nature, 351
Pelvic region, lowest anterior region of trunk, 34*t*, 35*f*

Placenta previa, occurs when placenta is in lower portion of uterus and thus blocks birth canal, 353, 353*f*

Placental stage, third stage of labor, which takes place after delivery of infant; uterus resumes strong contractions and placenta detaches from uterine wall and is delivered through vagina, 344, 344*f*

Plantar flexion, bending sole of foot; pointing toes downward, 118*f*, 118*t*

Plaque, yellow, fatty deposit of lipids in artery, 155, 159

Plasma, liquid portion of blood containing 90% water; remaining 10% consists of plasma proteins (serum albumin, serum globulin, fibrinogen, and prothrombin), inorganic substances (calcium, potassium, and sodium), organic components (glucose, amino acids, cholesterol), and waste products (urea, uric acid, ammonia, and creatinine), 181, 182

Plasma proteins, found in plasma; includes serum albumin, serum globulin, fibrinogen, and prothrombin, 182

Plasmapheresis, method of removing plasma from body without depleting formed elements; whole blood is removed and cells and plasma are separated; cells are returned to patient along with donor plasma transfusion, 192

Plastic surgery, surgical specialty involved in repair, reconstruction, or improvement of body structures such as skin that are damaged, missing, or misshapen; physician is *plastic surgeon*, 57

Platelet count, blood test to determine number of platelets in given volume of blood, 191

Platelets, cells responsible for coagulation of blood; also called *thrombocytes* and contain no hemoglobin, 181, 182, 184, 184*f*, 190

Pleura, protective double layer of serous membrane around lungs; parietal membrane is outer layer and visceral layer is inner membrane; secretes thin, watery fluid to reduce friction associated with lung movement, 36, 228

Pleural, pertaining to pleura, 233

Pleural cavity, cavity formed by serous membrane sac surrounding lungs, 36, 36*f*, 37*t*, 228, 242–43

Pleural effusion, abnormal presence of fluid or gas in pleural cavity; physicians can detect presence of fluid by tapping chest (percussion) or listening with stethoscope (auscultation), 242

Pleural rub, grating sound made when two surfaces, such as pleural surfaces, rub together during respiration; caused when one of surfaces becomes thicker as a result of inflammation or other disease conditions; rub can be felt through fingertips when placed on chest wall or heard through stethoscope, 237

Pleurectomy, surgical removal of pleura, 247

Pleurisy, inflammation of pleura, 242

Pleuritis. *See* Pleurisy

Pleurocentesis, puncture of pleura to withdraw fluid from thoracic cavity in order to diagnose disease, 247

Pleurodynia, pleural pain, 237

Plural endings, 12

Pneumoconiosis, condition resulting from inhaling environmental particles that become toxic, such as coal dust (anthracosis) or asbestos (asbestosis), 241

Pneumocystis pneumonia (PCP), pneumonia caused by fungus *Pneumocystis jiroveci*; opportunistic infection often seen in those with weakened immune systems, such as AIDS patients, 206

Pneumonia, inflammatory condition of lung, which can be caused by bacterial and viral infections, diseases, and chemicals, 241

Pneumonectomy, surgical removal of an entire lung, 247

Pneumothorax, collection of air or gas in pleural cavity, which can result in collapse of lung, 243, 243*f*

Podiatrist, 99

Podiatry, healthcare profession specializing in diagnosis and treatment of disorders of feet and lower legs; healthcare professional is *podiatrist*, 99

Poliomyelitis, acute viral disease that causes inflammation of gray matter of spinal cord, resulting in paralysis in some cases; has been brought under almost total control through vaccinations, 435

Polyarteritis, inflammation of many arteries, 160

Polycystic kidneys, formation of multiple cysts within kidney tissue; results in destruction of normal kidney tissue and uremia, 317, 317*f*

Polycythemia vera, production of too many red blood cells in bone marrow, 189

Polydipsia, condition of having excessive amount of thirst, such as in diabetes, 400

Polymyositis, disease involving muscle inflammation and weakness from unknown cause, 123

Polyneuritis, inflammation of many nerves, 437

Polyp, small tumor with pedicle or stem attachment; commonly found in vascular organs such as nose, uterus, and rectum, 283, 283*f*

Polyphagia, to eat excessively, 278

Polyposis, small tumors that contain pedicle or footlike attachment in mucous membranes of large intestine (colon), 283, 283*f*

Polysomnography, monitoring a patient while sleeping to identify sleep apnea; also called *sleep apnea study*, 245

Polyuria, condition of having excessive urine production; can be a symptom of disease conditions such as diabetes, 316, 400

Pons, portion of brain stem that forms bridge between cerebellum and cerebrum, 422*f*, 423–24, 423*f*

Pontine, pertaining to pons, 429

Popliteal artery, 148*f*

Popliteal vein, 150*f*

Positron emission tomography (PET), use of positive radionuclides to reconstruct brain sections; measurements can be taken of oxygen and glucose uptake, cerebral blood flow, and blood volume, 439, 520, 520*f*

Posterior, directional term meaning near or on back or spinal cord side of body, 39*f*, 39*t*

Posterior lobe, posterior portion of pituitary gland; secretes antidiuretic hormone and oxytocin, 393

Posterior pituitary gland, 393*f*

Prosthesis, artificial device used as substitute for body part either congenitally missing or absent as result of accident or disease; for instance, artificial leg or hip prosthesis, 108

Prosthetic hip joint, 109*f*

Prosthetic lens implant, use of artificial lens to replace lens removed during cataract surgery, 472

Prosthetics, artificial devices, such as limbs and joints, that replace missing body part, 99, 524

Prosthetist, 99

Protease inhibitor drugs, medications that inhibit protease, enzyme viruses need to reproduce, 209

Protein-bound iodine test (PBI), blood test to measure concentration of thyroxine (T_4) circulating in bloodstream; iodine becomes bound to protein in blood and can be measured; useful in establishing thyroid function, 405

Proteinuria, protein in urine, 316

Prothrombin, protein element within blood that interacts with calcium salts to form thrombin, 184

Prothrombin time (pro-time), measurement of time it takes for sample of blood to coagulate, 191

Protocol (prot), actual plan of care, including medications, surgeries, and treatments for care of patient; often, entire healthcare team—including physician, oncologist, radiologist, nurse, and patient—will assist in designing treatment plan, 535

Proton pump inhibitor, blocks stomach's ability to secrete acid; used to treat peptic ulcers and gastroesophageal reflux disease, 291

Protozoans, single-celled organisms that can infect body, 199

Proximal, directional term meaning located closest to point of attachment to body, 39*f*, 39*t*

Proximal convoluted tubule, portion of renal tubule, 307, 308*f*, 310*f*

Pruritus, severe itching, 60

Pseudocyesis, false pregnancy, 353

Pseudohypertrophic muscular dystrophy, one type of inherited muscular dystrophy in which muscle tissue is gradually replaced by fatty tissue, giving the appearance of a strong and healthy muscle, 123

Psoriasis, chronic inflammatory condition consisting of crusty papules forming patches with circular borders, 66, 66*f*

Psychiatric nurse, nurse with additional training in care of patients with mental, emotional, and behavioral disorders, 510

Psychiatric social work, social worker with additional training in care of patients with mental, emotional, or behavioral disorders, 510

Psychiatrist, physician with specialized training in diagnosing and treating mental disorders; prescribes medication and conducts counseling, 510

Psychiatry, branch of medicine that deals with the diagnosis, treatment, and prevention of mental disorders, 510

Psychoanalysis, method of obtaining a detailed account of past and present emotional and mental experiences from patient to determine source of problem and eliminate effects, 515

Psychology, study of human behavior and thought process; behavioral science is primarily concerned with understanding how human beings interact with their physical environment and with each other, 510

Psychopharmacology, study of effects of drugs on mind and particularly use of drugs in treating mental disorders; main classes of drugs for treatment of mental disorders are antipsychotic drugs, antidepressant drugs, minor tranquilizers, and lithium, 514

Psychotherapy, method of treating mental disorders by mental rather than chemical or physical means; includes psychoanalysis, humanistic therapies, and family and group therapy, 515

Pterygium, hypertrophied conjunctival tissue in inner corner of eye, 467

Puberty, series of events leading up to a child becoming capable of reproduction, 341

Pubic, pertaining to pubis; one of pelvic bones, 97

Pubic region, genital region of body, 34*t*

Pubis, one of three bones that form os coxae or innominate bone, 92, 93*f*, 93*t*

Pulmonary, pertaining to lung, 233

Pulmonary angiography, injecting dye into blood vessel for purpose of taking X-ray of arteries and veins of lungs, 244

Pulmonary artery, large artery that carries deoxygenated blood from right ventricle to lung, 144, 145*f*

Pulmonary capillaries, network of capillaries in lungs that tightly encase each alveolus; site of gas exchange, 227

Pulmonary circulation, transports deoxygenated blood from right side of heart to lungs where oxygen and carbon dioxide are exchanged; then carries oxygenated blood back to left side of heart, 140, 140*f*

Pulmonary edema, condition in which lung tissue retains excessive amount of fluid; results in labored breathing, 241

Pulmonary embolism, blood clot or air bubble in pulmonary artery or one of its branches, 241

Pulmonary fibrosis, formation of fibrous scar tissue in lungs, which leads to decreased ability to expand lungs; may be caused by infections, pneumoconiosis, autoimmune diseases, and toxin exposure, 241

Pulmonary function test (PFT), group of diagnostic tests that give information regarding air flow in and out of the lungs, lung volumes, and gas exchange between the lungs and bloodstream, 245

Pulmonary semilunar valve, 143*f*, 144

Pulmonary trunk, 141*f*, 142*f*

Pulmonary valve, semilunar valve between right ventricle and pulmonary artery in heart; prevents blood from flowing backward into ventricle, 142*f*, 143*f*, 144

Pulmonary vein, large vein that returns oxygenated blood from lungs to left atrium, 144, 145*f*

Pulmonologist, physician specialized in treating diseases and disorders of respiratory system, 234

Pulmonology, branch of medicine specializing in conditions of respiratory system, 234

Pulp cavity, hollow interior of tooth; contains soft tissue made up of blood vessels, nerves, and lymph vessels, 266, 267*f*

Pulse (P), expansion and contraction produced by blood as it moves through artery; can be taken at several pulse points throughout body where artery is close to surface, 149

Pupil, hole in center of iris; size is changed by iris dilating or constricting, 455, 456*f*, 457

Pupillary, pertaining to pupil, 462

Purified protein derivative (PPD). *See* Tuberculin skin test

Purkinje fibers, part of conduction system of heart; found in ventricular myocardium, 145, 146*f*

Purpura, hemorrhages into skin and mucous membranes, 60, 60*f*

Purulent, containing pus or an infection that is producing pus, 60

Pustule, raised spot on skin containing pus, 60, 60*f*

Pyelitic, pertaining to renal pelvis, 313

Pyelitis, inflammation of renal pelvis, 318

Pyelogram, X-ray record of the renal pelvis, 320

Pyelonephritis, inflammation of renal pelvis and kidney; one of most common types of kidney disease; may be result of lower urinary tract infection that moved up to kidney by way of ureters; may be large quantities of white blood cells and bacteria in urine, and blood (hematuria) may even be present in urine in this condition; can occur with any untreated or persistent case of cystitis, 318

Pyeloplasty, surgical repair of renal pelvis, 323

Pyloric, pertaining to pylorus, 276

Pyloric sphincter, located at distal end of stomach; controls passage of food into duodenum, 268*f*, 269, 272*f*

Pyoderma, pus-producing skin infection, 60

Pyosalpinx, condition of having pus in fallopian tubes, 350

Pyothorax, condition of having pus in chest cavity, 237, 242

Pyromania, impulse control disorder in which patient is unable to control impulse to start fires, 512

Pyrosis, pain and burning sensation usually caused by stomach acid splashing up into the esophagus; commonly called *heartburn*, 278

Pyuria, presence of pus in urine, 316

Q

Quadriplegia, paralysis of all four extremities; same as tetraplegia, 432

R

Radial, pertaining to radius; lower arm bone, 97

Radial artery, 148*f*

Radial keratotomy, spokelike incisions around cornea that result in it becoming flatter; surgical treatment for myopia, 472

Radial nerve, 427*f*

Radial vein, 150*f*

Radiation therapy, use of X-rays to treat disease, especially cancer, 538

Radical mastectomy, surgical removal of breast tissue plus chest muscles and axillary lymph nodes, 358

Radical surgery, extensive surgery to remove as much tissue associated with tumor as possible, 538

Radiculitis, nerve root inflammation, 437

Radiculopathy, disease of nerve root, 437

Radioactive implant, embedding radioactive source directly into tissue to provide highly localized radiation dosage to damage nearby cancerous cells; also called *brachytherapy*, 538

Radiography, making of X-ray pictures, 107, 517

Radioimmunoassay (RIA), test used to measure levels of hormones in plasma of blood, 405

Radioisotope, radioactive form of element, 517

Radiologist, physician who practices diagnosis and treatment by use of radiant energy; responsible for interpreting X-ray films, 517

Radiology, branch of medicine that uses radioactive substances such as X-rays, isotopes, and radiation to prevent, diagnose, and treat diseases, 520

Radiolucent, structures that allow X-rays to pass through and expose photographic plate, making it appear as black area on X-ray, are termed *radiolucent*, 517

Radiopaque, structures impenetrable to X-rays, appearing as light area on radiograph (X-ray), 517

Radius, one of forearm bones in upper extremity, 92, 92*f*, 92*t*

Range of motion (ROM), range of movement of a joint, from maximum flexion through maximum extension; measured as degrees of a circle, 525

Raynaud's phenomenon, periodic ischemic attacks affecting extremities of body, especially fingers, toes, ears, and nose; affected extremities become cyanotic and very painful; attacks are brought on by arterial constriction due to extreme cold or emotional stress, 160

Reabsorption, second phase of urine production; substances needed by body are reabsorbed as filtrate passes through kidney tubules, 310, 310*f*

Recklinghausen disease, excessive production of parathyroid hormone, which results in degeneration of bones, 401

Rectal, (1) pertaining to rectum; (2) substances introduced directly into rectal cavity in form of suppositories or solution; drugs may have to be administered by this route if patient is unable to take them by mouth due to nausea, vomiting, and surgery, 276, 506*t*

Rectocele, protrusion or herniation of rectum into vagina, 351

Rectum, area at end of digestive tube for storage of feces that leads to anus, 264, 270, 270*f*, 338*f*, 341*f*, 343*f*, 363*f*

Rectus abdominis, muscle named for its location and direction of its fibers: rectus means "straight" and abdominis means "abdominal," 116

Rectus muscles, rectus means "straight"; four of eye muscles are rectus muscles, 458

Red blood cell count (RBC), blood test to determine number of erythrocytes in volume of blood; decrease in red blood cells may indicate anemia; increase may indicate polycythemia, 191

Semen, contains sperm and fluids secreted by male reproductive system glands; leaves body through urethra, 363

Semen analysis, procedure used when performing fertility workup to determine if male is able to produce sperm; semen is collected by patient after abstaining from sexual intercourse for a period of three to five days; sperm in semen are analyzed for number, swimming strength, and shape; also used to determine if vasectomy has been successful; after a period of six weeks, no sperm should be present in sample from patient, 371

Semicircular canals, portion of labyrinth associated with balance and equilibrium, 477*f,* 478

Semiconscious, state of being aware of surroundings and responding to stimuli only part of time, 432

Semilunar valve, heart valves located between ventricles and great arteries leaving heart; pulmonary valve is located between the right ventricle and the pulmonary artery aortic valve is located between left ventricle and aorta, 144

Seminal vesicles, two male reproductive system glands located at base of bladder; secrete fluid that nourishes sperm into vas deferens; fluid plus sperm constitutes much of semen, 362, 363, 363*f,* 365

Seminiferous tubules, network of coiled tubes that make up bulk of testes; sperm development takes place in walls of tubules and mature sperm are released into tubule in order to leave testes, 364, 394*f*

Sensorineural hearing loss, type of hearing loss in which sound is conducted normally through external and middle ear but there is a defect in inner ear or with cochlear nerve, resulting in inability to hear; hearing aid may help, 479

Sensory neurons, nerves that carry sensory information from sensory receptors to brain; also called *afferent neurons*, 426

Sensory receptors, nerve fibers located directly under skin surface; detect temperature, pain, touch, and pressure; messages for these sensations are conveyed to brain and spinal cord from nerve endings in skin, 420

Sepsis. *See* Septicemia

Septal, pertaining to nasal septum, 233

Septicemia, having bacteria in bloodstream; commonly referred to as *sepsis* or *blood poisoning*, 188

Sequential multiple analyzer computer (SMAC), machine for doing multiple blood chemistry tests automatically, 191

Serous fluid, watery secretion of serous membranes, 228

Serum, clear, sticky fluid that remains after blood has clotted, 182

Serum bilirubin, blood test to determine amount of waste product bilirubin in bloodstream; elevated levels indicate liver disease, 285

Serum lipoprotein level, laboratory test to measure amount of cholesterol and triglycerides in blood, 161

Severe acute respiratory syndrome (SARS), acute viral respiratory infection that begins like the flu but quickly progresses to severe dyspnea; high fatality rate in persons over age 65; first appeared in China in 2003, 242

Severe combined immunodeficiency syndrome (SCIDS), disease seen in children born with nonfunctioning immune system; often forced to live in sealed sterile rooms, 206

Sex hormones, secreted by gonads and adrenal cortex; estrogen and progesterone in females; testosterone in males, 338, 363

Sexual dysfunctions, a classification of psychiatric disorders in the DSM-5 characterized by having difficulty during any stage of normal sexual activity that negatively impacts quality of life; includes erectile dysfunction and premature ejaculation, 514

Sexual masochism disorder, paraphilic disorder characterized by receiving sexual gratification from being hurt or abused, 513

Sexually transmitted disease (STD), disease usually acquired as a result of sexual intercourse; formerly referred to as *venereal disease*, 370

Shield, protective device used to protect against radiation, 518

Shingles, eruption of painful blisters along a nerve path; thought to be caused by a *Herpes zoster* virus infection of the nerve root, 437, 437*f*

Short bone, type of bone that is roughly cube shaped; carpals are short bones, 85, 85*f*

Shortness of breath (SOB), term used to indicate that patient is having some difficulty breathing; cause can range from mild SOB after exercise to SOB associated with heart disease, 238

Sialadenitis, inflammation of salivary gland, 279

Sickle cell anemia, severe, chronic, incurable disorder that results in anemia and causes joint pain, chronic weakness, and infections; actual blood cell is crescent shaped, 189, 189*f*

Side effect, response to drug other than effect desired, 507

Sigmoid colon, final section of colon; follows S-shaped path and terminates in rectum, 269*f,* 270, 270*f*

Sigmoidal, pertaining to sigmoid colon, 276

Sigmoidoscope, instrument to view inside sigmoid colon, 287

Sigmoidoscopy, using flexible sigmoidoscope to visually examine sigmoid colon; commonly done to diagnose cancer and polyps, 287

Silicosis, form of respiratory disease resulting from inhalation of silica (quartz) dust; considered an occupational disease, 242

Simple fracture. *See* Closed fracture

Simple mastectomy, surgical removal of breast tissue, 358

Singular endings, 12

Sinoatrial node (SA), also called *pacemaker of heart*; area of right atria that initiates electrical pulse that causes heart to contract, 145, 146*f*

Sinus, hollow cavity within bone, 86

Skeletal, pertaining to skeleton, 125

Skeletal muscle, voluntary muscle attached to bones by tendon, 25, 114, 114*f,* 115, 115*f*

Skeletal muscle relaxant, produces relaxation of skeletal muscle, 125

Skeletal muscle tissue, 25

Thoracic vertebrae (T1, T2, etc.), 12 vertebrae in chest region, 89, 90*f*, 90*t*
Thoracostomy, insertion of tube into chest for purpose of draining off fluid or air, 247
Thoracotomy, incision into chest, 247
Thrombin, clotting enzyme that converts fibrinogen to fibrin, 184
Thrombocytes, also called *platelets*; play critical part in blood-clotting process by agglutinating into small clusters and releasing thrombokinase, 184
Thrombocytic, pertaining to platelets, 186
Thrombocytosis, too many clotting cells (platelets), 190
Thrombolytic, able to dissolve existing blood clots, 166, 192
Thrombolytic therapy, drugs, such as streptokinase or tissue plasminogen activator, are injected into blood vessel to dissolve clots and restore blood flow, 164
Thrombopenia, too few clotting cells, 190
Thrombophlebitis, inflammation of vein that results in formation of blood clots within vein, 160
Thromboplastin, substance released by platelets; reacts with prothrombin to form thrombin, 184
Thrombus, blood clot, 155, 155*f*
Thymectomy, removal of thymus gland, 208, 406
Thymic, pertaining to thymus gland, 203, 398
Thymitis, inflammation of thymus gland, 403
Thymoma, malignant tumor of thymus gland, 205, 403
Thymosin, hormone secreted by thymus gland; causes lymphocytes to change into T lymphocytes, 199, 389*t*, 395
Thymus gland, endocrine gland located in upper mediastinum that assists body with immune function and development of antibodies; as part of immune response it secretes hormone, thymosin, that changes lymphocytes to T cells, 195, 196, 199, 199*f*, 387, 389*t*, 395, 395*f*, 403
Thyroid cartilage, piece of cartilage associated with larynx; commonly called *Adam's apple* and is larger in males, 225*f*, 226
Thyroid echography, ultrasound examination of thyroid that can assist in distinguishing thyroid nodule from cyst, 405
Thyroid function test (TFT), blood tests used to measure levels of T_3, T_4, and TSH in bloodstream to assist in determining thyroid function, 405
Thyroid gland, endocrine gland located on either side of trachea; shape resembles butterfly with large left and right lobe connected by narrow isthmus; produces hormones thyroxine (T_4), triiodothyronine (T_3), and calcitonin (CT), 387, 389*t*, 395–96, 396*f*, 403–04
Thyroid replacement hormone, given to replace thyroid in patients with hypothyroidism or who have had thyroidectomy, 407
Thyroid scan, test in which radioactive element is administered that localizes in thyroid gland; gland can then be visualized with scanning device to detect pathology such as tumors, 405
Thyroid-stimulating hormone (TSH), hormone secreted by anterior pituitary; regulates function of thyroid gland, 389*t*, 393
Thyroidal, pertaining to thyroid gland, 398
Thyroidectomy, removal of entire thyroid or portion (partial thyroidectomy) to treat variety of conditions, including nodes, cancer, and hyperthyroidism, 406
Thyromegaly, enlarged thyroid, 400
Thyrotoxicosis, condition that results from excessive secretion of thyroid gland hormones; symptoms include rapid heart action, tremors, enlarged thyroid gland, exophthalmos, and weight loss, 404
Thyroxine (T_4), hormone produced by thyroid gland; also known as T_4 and requires iodine for production; regulates level of cell metabolism; the greater the level of hormone in the bloodstream, the higher the cell metabolism, 389*t*, 395
Tibia, also called *shin bone*; lower extremity bone, 92, 93*f*, 93*t*
Tibial, pertaining to tibia or shin bone, 98
Tidal volume (TV), amount of air that enters lungs in single inhalation or leaves lungs in single exhalation of quiet breathing, 229*t*
Tinea, fungal skin disease resulting in itching, scaling lesions, 67
Tinea capitis, fungal infection of scalp; commonly called *ringworm*, 67
Tinea pedis, fungal infection of foot; commonly called *athlete's foot*, 67
Tinnitus, ringing in ears, 482
Tissues, formed when cells of same type are grouped to perform one activity; for example, nerve cells combine to form nerve fibers; there are four types: nervous, muscle, epithelial, and connective
connective, 25, 26*f*
epithelial, 25, 26*f*
muscle, 25, 26*f*
nervous, 25, 26*f*, 420, 421*f*
Tolerance, development of capacity for withstanding large amount of substance, such as foods, drugs, or poison, without any adverse effect; decreased sensitivity to further doses will develop, 507
Tongue, muscular organ in floor of mouth; works to move food around inside mouth and is also necessary for speech, 225*f*, 265, 265*f*–266*f*, 271*f*
Tonic-clonic seizure, type of severe epileptic seizure characterized by loss of consciousness and convulsions; seizure alternates between strong continuous muscle spasms (tonic) and rhythmic muscle contraction and relaxation (clonic); also called *grand mal seizure*, 432
Tonometry, measurement of intraocular pressure of eye using tonometer to check for condition of glaucoma; generally part of normal eye exam for adults, 470
Tonsillar, pertaining to tonsils, 203
Tonsillectomy, surgical removal of tonsils, 208
Tonsillitis, inflammation of tonsils, 205
Tonsils, collections of lymphatic tissue located in pharynx to combat microorganisms entering body through nose or mouth; include pharyngeal tonsils, palatine tonsils, and lingual tonsils, 195, 196, 199, 199*f*
Tooth cavity. *See* Dental caries

Topical, applied directly to skin or mucous membranes; distributed in ointment, cream, or lotion form; used to treat skin infections and eruptions, 506*t*, 530*t*

Topical anesthesia, applied using either liquid or gel placed directly onto specific area; patient remains conscious; used on skin, cornea, and mucous membranes in dental work, 529, 530*t*

Torticollis, severe neck spasms pulling head to one side; commonly called *wryneck* or *crick in the neck*, 123

Total abdominal hysterectomy–bilateral salpingo-oophorectomy (TAH-BSO), removal of entire uterus, cervix, both ovaries, and both fallopian tubes, 358

Total calcium, blood test to measure total amount of calcium to assist in detecting parathyroid and bone disorders, 405

Total hip arthroplasty (THA), surgical reconstruction of hip by implanting prosthetic or artificial hip joint; also called *total hip replacement*, 109, 109*f*

Total hip replacement (THR). *See* Total hip arthroplasty

Total knee arthroplasty (TKA), surgical reconstruction of knee joint by implanting prosthetic knee joint; also called *total knee replacement*, 109

Total knee replacement (TKR). *See* Total knee arthroplasty

Total lung capacity (TLC), volume of air in lungs after maximal inhalation, 229*t*

Total parenteral nutrition (TPN), providing 100% of patient's nutrition intravenously; used when patient is unable to eat, 288

Toxemia. *See* Preeclampsia

Toxic shock syndrome (TSS), rare and sometimes fatal staphylococcus infection that generally occurs in menstruating women, 351

Toxicity, extent or degree to which substance is poisonous, 507

Toxins, substances poisonous to body; many are filtered out of blood by kidney, 199

Tracheal, pertaining to trachea, 233

Trachea, also called *windpipe*; conducts air from larynx down to main bronchi in chest, 223, 225*f*, 226–27, 226*f*, 227*f*, 229, 266*f*, 395*f*

Tracheostenosis, narrowing and stenosis of lumen or opening into trachea, 238

Tracheostomy, surgical procedure used to make opening in trachea to create airway; tracheostomy tube can be inserted to keep opening patent, 247

Tracheotomy, surgical incision into trachea to provide airway, 247, 248*f*

Tract, bundle of fibers located within central nervous system, 421

Traction, process of pulling or drawing, usually with mechanical device; used in treating orthopedic (bone and joint) problems and injuries, 110, 526

Tractotomy, incision into spinal cord tract, 441

Trademark, pharmaceutical company's brand name for drug, 501

Transcutaneous electrical nerve stimulation (TENS), application of mild electrical stimulation to skin via electrodes placed over painful area, causing interference with transmission of painful stimuli; can be used in pain management to interfere with normal pain mechanism, 526

Transdermal, route of drug administration; medication coats underside of patch applied to skin; medication is then absorbed across skin, 506*t*

Transfusion reaction. *See* Hemolytic reaction

Transient ischemic attack (TIA), temporary interference with blood supply to brain, causing neurological symptoms such as dizziness, numbness, and hemiparesis; may lead eventually to full-blown stroke (CVA), 435

Transurethral resection of the prostate (TUR, TURP), surgical removal of prostate gland by inserting device through urethra and removing prostate tissue, 372

Transverse colon, section of colon that crosses upper abdomen from right side of body to left, 269*f*, 270, 270*f*

Transverse fracture, complete fracture straight across bone at right angles to long axis of bone, 102, 102*f*

Transverse plane, horizontal plane that divides body into upper (superior) and lower (inferior) sections; also called *horizontal plane*, 33, 33*f*

Transverse section, sectional view of body produced by cut along transverse plane, 33

Trauma- and Stressor-related disorders, a classification of psychiatric disorders in the DSM-5 involving exposure to actual or implied death, injury, or violence; includes posttraumatic stress disorder, 513

Traumatic brain injury (TBI), brain damage resulting from impact (such as a car accident), blast waves (such as from an explosion), or a penetrating projectile (such as caused by a bullet); symptoms may be mild, moderate, or severe and may include loss of consciousness, headache, vomiting, loss of motor coordination, and dizziness, 435

Treadmill test. *See* Stress testing

Tremor, involuntary quivering movement of part of body, 432

Trendelenburg position, surgical position in which patient is lying face up and on incline with head lower than legs, 531*f*, 532*t*

Trephine, surgical saw used to remove disk-shaped piece of tissue, 530*t*

Trichomoniasis, genitourinary infection usually without symptoms (asymptomatic) in both males and females; disease in women can produce itching and/or burning and foul-smelling discharge, and can result in vaginitis, 370

Trichomycosis, abnormal condition of hair fungus, 67

Tricuspid valve, between right atrium and ventricle of heart; prevents blood from flowing backward into atrium; has three cusps or flaps, 142*f*, 143*f*, 144, 145*f*

Trigeminal nerve, 426*t*

Triiodothyronine (T_3), hormone produced by thyroid gland known as T_3 that requires iodine for its production; regulates level of cell metabolism; the greater the level of hormone in bloodstream, the higher the cell metabolism, 389*t*, 395

Trochanter, large blunt process that provides attachment for tendons and muscles, 86, 87*f*

Trochlear nerve, 426*t*

Trunk, torso region of body, 34*t*, 35*f*

Tubal ligation, surgical tying-off of fallopian tubes to prevent conception from taking place; results in sterilization of female, 358
Tubal pregnancy. *See* Salpingocyesis
Tubercle, small, rounded process that provides attachment for tendons and muscles, 86
Tuberculin skin tests (TB test), applying chemical agent (Tine or Mantoux tests) under surface of skin to determine if patient has been exposed to tuberculosis, 245
Tuberculosis (TB), infectious disease caused by tubercle bacillus, *Mycobacterium tuberculosis"*; most commonly affects respiratory system and causes inflammation and calcification of system; incidence is on the increase and is seen in many patients with weakened immune systems, 242
Tuberosity, large, rounded process that provides attachment to tendons and muscles, 86
Tumor, abnormal growth of tissue that may be benign or malignant; also called *neoplasm*, 535
Two-hour postprandial glucose tolerance test, assists in evaluating glucose metabolism; patient eats high-carbohydrate diet and fasts overnight before test; blood sample is then taken two hours after meal, 405
Tympanectomy, surgical removal of eardrum, 487
Tympanic, pertaining to eardrum, 481
Tympanic membrane, also called *eardrum*; as sound moves along auditory canal, it strikes tympanic membrane causing it to vibrate; this conducts sound wave into middle ear, 477, 478, 478*f*
Tympanitis, eardrum inflammation, 483
Tympanogram, graphic record that illustrates results of tympanometry, 485
Tympanometer, instrument to measure eardrum's movement, 485
Tympanometry, measurement of movement of tympanic membrane; can indicate presence of pressure in middle ear, 485
Tympanoplasty, another term for surgical reconstruction of eardrum; also called *myringoplasty*, 487
Tympanorrhexis, ruptured eardrum, 482
Tympanotomy, incision into eardrum, 487
Type A blood, one of ABO blood types; person with type A markers on his or her RBCs; type A blood will make anti-B antibodies, 184
Type AB blood, one of ABO blood types; person with both type A and type B markers on his or her RBCs; since it has both markers, it will not make antibodies against either A or B blood, 184
Type B blood, one of ABO blood types; person with type B markers on his or her RBCs; type B blood will make anti-A antibodies, 184
Type O blood, one of ABO blood types; person with no markers on his or her RBCs; type O blood will not react with anti-A or anti-B antibodies; therefore, is considered universal donor, 184
Type and cross-match, lab test performed before person receives blood transfusion; double-checks blood type of both donor's and recipient's blood, 192

U

Ulcer, open sore or lesion in skin or mucous membrane, 61, 61*f*
Ulcerative colitis, ulceration of unknown origin of mucous membranes of colon; also known as *inflammatory bowel disease* (IBD), 283
Ulna, one of forearm bones in upper extremity, 92, 92*f*, 92*t*
Ulnar, pertaining to ulna, one of lower arm bones, 98
Ulnar artery, 148*f*
Ulnar nerve, 427*f*
Ulnar vein, 150*f*
Ultrasound (US), use of high-frequency sound waves to create heat in soft tissues under skin; particularly useful for treating injuries to muscles, tendons, and ligaments, as well as muscle spasms; in radiology, ultrasound waves can be used to outline shapes of tissues, organs, and fetus, 521, 521*f*, 527, 527*f*
Ultraviolet (UV), 72
Umbilical, anatomical division of abdomen; middle section of middle row, 37*t*
Umbilical cord, extends from baby's umbilicus (navel) to placenta; contains blood vessels that carry oxygen and nutrients from mother to baby and carbon dioxide and wastes from baby to mother, 343–44, 343*f*
Unconscious, condition or state of being unaware of surroundings with inability to respond to stimuli, 432
Ungual, pertaining to nails, 56
Unit dose, drug dosage system that provides prepackaged, prelabeled, individual medications ready for immediate use by the patient, 507
Universal donor, type O blood is considered universal donor; with no markers on RBC surface, will not trigger reaction with anti-A or anti-B antibodies, 184
Universal recipient, person with type AB blood has no antibodies against other blood types and therefore, in emergency, can receive any type of blood, 184
Upper extremity (UE), the arm, 90, 91*f*, 92*t*, 525
Upper gastrointestinal (UGI) **series,** administering barium contrast material orally and then taking X-ray to visualize esophagus, stomach, and duodenum, 286
Uptake, absorption of radioactive material and medicines into organ or tissue, 518
Urea, waste product of protein metabolism; diffuses through tissues in lymph and is returned to circulatory system for transport to kidneys, 182
Uremia, excess of urea and other nitrogenous waste in blood, 306, 316
Ureteral, pertaining to ureter, 313
Ureterectasis, dilation of ureter, 316
Ureterolith, a calculus in ureter, 316
Ureterostenosis, narrowing of ureter, 316
Ureters, organs in urinary system that transport urine from kidney to bladder, 305, 306, 307, 307*f*, 308, 308*f*
Urethra, tube that leads from urinary bladder to outside of body; in male it is also used by reproductive system to release semen, 305, 306, 308, 309, 309*f*, 338*f*, 363*f*
Urethral, pertaining to urethra, 313
Urethralgia, urethral pain, 316

V

Vasal, pertaining to vas deferens, 367
Vascular, pertaining to vessels, 153
Vasectomy, removal of segment or all of vas deferens to prevent sperm from leaving male body; used for contraception purposes, 372, 372*f*
Vasoconstrictor, contracts smooth muscle in walls of blood vessels; raises blood pressure, 166
Vasodilator, produces relaxation of blood vessels to lower blood pressure, 166
Vasopressin, substance given to control diabetes insipidus and promote reabsorption of water in kidney tubules, 407
Vasovasostomy, creation of new opening between two sections of vas deferens; used to reverse vasectomy, 372
Vegetation, 157
Veins, blood vessels of cardiovascular system that carry blood toward heart, 139, 140, 147*f,* 149, 150*f*, 196*f*
Vena cava, 140*f*
Venereal disease (VD). *See* Sexually transmitted disease
Venipuncture. *See* Phlebotomy
Venous, pertaining to vein, 153
Ventilation, movement of air in and out of lungs, 224
Ventilation-perfusion scan, nuclear medicine diagnostic test especially useful in identifying pulmonary emboli; radioactive air is inhaled for ventilation portion to determine if air is filling entire lung; radioactive intravenous injection shows whether blood is flowing to all parts of lung, 244
Ventilator, machine that provides artificial ventilation for patient unable to breathe on his or her own; also called *respirator*, 246
Ventral, directional term meaning more toward the front or belly side of body, 39*f,* 39*t*
Ventral cavities, 37*t*
Ventricles, two lower chambers of heart that receive blood from atria and pump it back out of heart; left ventricle pumps blood to body, and right ventricle pumps blood to lungs; also fluid-filled spaces within cerebrum; contain cerebrospinal fluid (watery, clear) that provides protection from shock or sudden motion to brain, 142*f,* 145*f*, 424
Ventricular, pertaining to ventricle, 153, 430
Ventricular septal defect (VSD), a congenital septal defect between the ventricles, 156
Venules, smallest veins; receive deoxygenated blood leaving capillaries, 149, 153
Vermiform appendix, small outgrowth at end of cecum; function or purpose is unknown, 270
Verruca, warts; benign neoplasm (tumor) caused by virus; has rough surface that is removed by chemicals and/or laser therapy, 67
Vertebrae, 88*f*
Vertebral, pertaining to vertebrae, 98, 430
Vertebral canal, bony canal through vertebrae that contains spinal cord, 424, 424*f*
Vertebral column, part of axial skeleton; a column of 26 vertebrae that forms backbone and protects spinal cord; divided into five sections: cervical, thoracic, and lumbar vertebrae, sacrum, and coccyx; also called *spinal column*, 89, 424
Vertebral region, spinal column region of body, 34*t*
Vertigo, sensation of spinning or whirling around; incorrectly used to mean dizziness, 482
Vesicle, small, fluid-filled raised spot on skin, 61, 61*f*
Vesicular, pertaining to seminal vesicle, 367
Vestibular, pertaining to vestibule, 481
Vestibular nerve, branch of vestibulocochlear nerve responsible for sending equilibrium information to brain, 477, 477*f*
Vestibulocochlear nerve, eighth cranial nerve; responsible for hearing and balance, 426*t*, 477
Viruses, group of infectious particles that cause disease, 199
Viscera, name for internal organs of body, such as lungs, stomach, and liver, 36
Visceral, pertaining to viscera or internal organs, 41
Visceral layer, inner pleural layer; adheres to surface of lung, 36
Visceral muscle, muscle found in walls of internal organs such as stomach, 115, 115*f*
Visceral pericardium, inner layer of pericardium surrounding heart, 142
Visceral peritoneum, inner layer of serous membrane sac encasing abdominopelvic viscera, 36
Visceral pleura, inner layer of serous membrane sac encasing thoracic viscera, 228
Vision, 459, 460*f,* 468
Visual acuity (VA) **test,** measurement of sharpness of patient's vision; a Snellen chart is usually used for this test and patient identifies letters from distance of 20 feet, 470
Vital capacity (VC), total volume of air that can be exhaled after maximum inhalation; amount will be equal to sum of tidal volume, inspiratory reserve volume, and expiratory reserve volume, 229*t*
Vital signs (VS), respiration, pulse, temperature, skin color, blood pressure, and reaction of pupils; signs of condition of body functions, 230
Vitamin D therapy, maintaining high blood levels of calcium in association with vitamin D helps maintain bone density and treats osteomalacia, osteoporosis, and rickets, 110
Vitiligo, disappearance of pigment from skin in patches, causing a milk-white appearance; also called *leukoderma*, 67
Vitreous body, 456*f*
Vitreous humor, transparent jellylike substance inside eyeball, 457
Vocal cords, structures within larynx that vibrate to produce sound and speech, 225*f,* 226
Voiding, another term for urination, 308
Voiding cystourethrography (VCUG), X-ray taken to visualize urethra while patient is voiding after contrast dye has been placed in bladder, 320
Voluntary muscles, those that person can consciously choose to contract; skeletal muscles of arm and leg are examples, 114
Volvulus, condition in which bowel twists upon itself and causes painful obstruction that requires immediate surgery, 283, 283*f*
Vomer bone, facial bone, 89, 89*f,* 89*t*

W

X

Y

Z